POCKET COMPANION TO

Textbook of SMALL ANIMAL SURGERY

Douglas Slatter, B.V.Sc., M.S., Ph.D., F.R.C.V.S.

Diplomate, American College of Veterinary Surgeons
Diplomate, European College of Veterinary Surgeons
Diplomate, American College of Veterinary Ophthalmologists

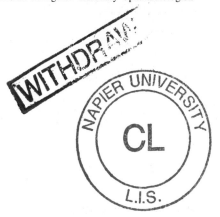
W.B. SAUNDERS COMPANY
A Division of Harcourt Brace & Company
Philadelphia   London   Toronto   Montreal   Sydney   Tokyo

W.B. SAUNDERS COMPANY
A Division of
Harcourt Brace & Company

The Curtis Center
Independence Square West
Philadelphia, Pennsylvania 19106

Library of Congress
Cataloging-in-Publication Data

Slatter, Douglas H.

Pocket companion to Textbook of small animal
surgery / Douglas Slatter.—1st ed.

p.   cm.

Includes index.

ISBN 0–7216–5544–0

1. Dogs—Surgery.   2. Cats—Surgery.   3. Veterinary surgery.   I. Textbook of small animal
   surgery.   II. Title.

SF991.S58   1995

636.089′7—dc20   94–13110

Pocket Companion to
Textbook of Small Animal Surgery   ISBN 0–7216–5544–0

Copyright © 1995 by W.B. Saunders Company

Printed in the United States of America.

Last digit is the print number: 9   8   7   6   5   4   3   2   1

COMPILING EDITORS

David Holmberg, D.V.M., M.V.Sc.
Diplomate, American College of Veterinary Surgeons
Guelph
Ontario

Giselle Hosgood, B.V.Sc., M.S.
Diplomate, American College of Veterinary Surgeons
Baton Rouge
Louisiana

A. Wendell Nelson, D.V.M., M.S., Ph.D.
Diplomate, American College of Veterinary Surgeons
Fort Collins
Colorado

Ghery Pettit, B.S., D.V.M.
Diplomate, American College of Veterinary Surgeons
Pullman
Washington

Douglas Slatter, B.V.Sc., M.S., Ph.D., F.R.C.V.S.
Diplomate, American College of Veterinary Surgeons
Diplomate, European College of Veterinary Surgeons
Diplomate, American College of Veterinary Ophthalmologists
Incline Village
Nevada

Phil Vasseur, D.V.M.
Diplomate, American College of Veterinary Surgeons
Davis
California

NOTICE

PREFACE

The purpose of this handbook is to provide an accessible, portable reference for students, residents, and practitioners for use outside the operating room. With the increase in information available, a concise source is necessary when use of the *Textbook of Small Animal Surgery* is impractical. A summary table of drugs commonly used in surgery, and referred to in the main text, is included.

Subjects abstracted are keyed to the same discussion and chapters in the main text, where much greater detail will be found. Detailed descriptions of surgical procedures have been omitted. ***Before any surgical procedure is performed, the full description should be referred to in the main text.*** In all situations, the reader is referred to the Textbook for a full discussion. The Pocket Companion is also designed as a summary and introduction to, and refresher for, the material in the Textbook.

I am most grateful to the compiling editors for their assistance in reducing the original volumes to the current handbook size. Comments by readers for improvement of the handbook will be gratefully received.

DOUGLAS SLATTER

Address for reader comments:

Veterinary Editor
W.B. Saunders Company
The Curtis Center
Independence Square West
Philadelphia, Pennsylvania 19106

CONTENTS

Surgical Biology (pages 1–113)

CHAPTER 1

Shock: Pathophysiology and Management of Hypovolemia and Sepsis

(pages 1–11)

Shock is defined as a state in which the amount of oxygen delivered to the tissues is inadequate to maintain normal cellular respiration.

TYPES OF SHOCK (pp. 1–2)

Hypovolemic shock is most commonly recognized in the form of hemorrhagic shock, or loss of blood volume. The loss of blood may be due to trauma, hemorrhagic diatheses, surgery, or organ damage due to disease, or it may be experimental. Additionally, hypovolemic shock may be due to fluid loss, without any loss of blood, as may occur with extreme dehydration.

Loss of intravascular fluid results in a decrease in venous pressure. As a result, there is a decrease in venous return of blood to the heart and, consequently, a decrease in cardiac output.

Cardiogenic shock is a failure of the pump, with a primary decrease in cardiac output. Ventricular tachycardia, cardiac arrest, and myocardial suppression due to drugs are potential causes of cardiogenic shock.

Obstructive shock (restrictive shock) refers to states of shock in which the primary cause of the reduced cardiac output is an obstruction or restriction to the flow of blood. The classic example of obstructive shock in veterinary medicine is gastric dilatation volvulus. Distension of the stomach results in compression of the portal vein and caudal vena cava, with reduction of venous return and cardiac output.

Distributive shock (neurogenic, vasculogenic) refers to a state in which the volume of intravascular fluid remains the same but the vascular space is increased. Examples include fainting, anaphylactic shock, endotoxic shock, and septic shock.

HEMORRHAGIC SHOCK (pp. 2–5)

Clinical Findings

The decrease in cardiac output results in a secondary decrease in arterial blood pressure. A high priority of the body is to maintain arterial blood pressure. It does this in the shock state by means of the baroreflex mechanisms, release of catecholamines, and increase in total systemic vascular resistance. This results in pale mucous membranes and increased capillary refill time, an increase in the toe web temperature differential, and cold extremities.

1

The pulse rate should increase in shock. Pulse rate changes are inconsistent in the dog. The pulse character is consistently weak and thready.

Laboratory Findings

With hemorrhage and the loss of red blood cells, there is a decrease in the packed cell volume (PCV). PCV does not immediately decrease with hemorrhage. It decreases owing to shifts of fluid from the extravascular to intravascular spaces shortly after hemorrhage but does not totally equilibrate to its new level until normal vascular volume has been re-established.

Blood Gases

Measurement of arterial and central venous blood gases provides useful information in shock states. An arterial sample is not always easy to obtain. A venous sample is satisfactory for determining nonrespiratory status and base deficit.

An oxygen pressure of 40 mm Hg is adequate to maintain cellular oxygenation. When the venous P_{O_2} is low, for example 20 mm Hg, there is inadequate oxygen to maintain normal cellular oxygenation.

Fluid Therapy

The large volume of fluids required for successful resuscitation of hypovolemic shock cannot be overemphasized. A starting volume of 90 ml/kg (one blood volume) is given rapidly and intravenously.

Extracellular replacement fluids consist of those fluids that have a sodium concentration approximately equal to that of serum. These include lactated Ringer's solution and normal saline.

Small-volume (4 ml/kg) resuscitation with hypertonic saline resulted in improved hemodynamic parameters compared with an equivalent volume of normal saline. It is likely that hypertonic saline is effective in hemorrhagic shock by drawing water from the intracellular space into the extravascular space.

Much research remains to be conducted, including controlled trials that critically evaluate the effect of hypertonic saline on organ function and survival in shock. We recommend that hypovolemic shock be treated with the appropriate volumes of isotonic extracellular replacement fluid, as described earlier.

Whole blood is indicated in hemorrhagic shock when the hemoglobin levels drop to the point that the oxygen-carrying capacity of the blood is seriously impaired. If hemorrhage is controlled and the patient is clinically stable with no risk of further deterioration or surgery, transfusion of blood is not necessary, even at a low PCV of 15 per cent. If the patient is unstable with further risk of hemorrhage, whole blood is considered at a PCV of 20 to 25 per cent.

Other Therapies

Bicarbonate

The patient in hypovolemic shock invariably has metabolic acidosis. This acidosis usually reverses itself with adequate fluid resuscitation and restoration of blood flow to the tissues. Bicarbonate therapy is frequently unnecessary in shock. It is recommended that HCO_3^- be given if the pH <7.2 and not if the pH >7.2.

The bicarbonate deficit is the normal bicarbonate concentration (21 mEq/L) minus the measured bicarbonate concentration.

$$\text{Amount of HCO}_3{}^- = \text{BD} \times 0.3 \times \text{BW*}$$

The 0.3 fraction from this equation represents distribution of the bicarbonate to the entire extracellular space, with some spillover into the intracellular space. This distribution of bicarbonate requires at least 30 minutes.

Steroids

Steroids block the arachidonic acid cascade at the level of phospholipase, which is one step higher than the cyclooxygenase inhibitors, and prevent the accumulation of the prostaglandins and thromboxanes. Steroids have been reported to improve microvascular integrity and stabilize lysosomal and cell membranes. Steroids cause vasodilation and should not be administered without appropriate and concurrent fluid therapy.

Antibiotics

The shock state is associated with cellular hypoxia and depressed immune function and gastrointestinal tract function, which results in bacteremia and endotoxemia. Antibiotics are indicated to prevent or ameliorate the possibility of a secondary toxemia, bacteremia, or soft-tissue infection.

Monitoring the Patient in Shock

Monitoring of the patient in shock is directed primarily toward determination of adequate flow of blood to tissues. The clinician should frequently assess mental status and mucous membrane color and capillary refill time. Adequate resuscitation is associated with the return of strong pulses with a good pulse pressure.

Urine output is an excellent means to assess organ perfusion. With hypovolemic shock and decreased blood pressure and kidney blood flow, urine production ceases. Restoration of adequate pressures and flow is associated with return of urine production. It is strongly emphasized that the anuria is almost certainly due to the fluid deficit, and fluids should be aggressively administered in almost all cases. The exceptions are left heart failure, pre-existing pulmonary hemorrhage, and true primary renal failure.

SEPTIC SHOCK (pp. 5–7)

In septic shock, there are components of hypovolemic and distributive shock, with cardiogenic shock occurring late in the shock syndrome. Additionally, septic shock is unique in that there is also *inability of the cells to effectively use existing metabolic substrate.*

Septic shock occurs when circulatory shock is superimposed on sepsis. Endotoxic shock is the occurrence of circulatory shock due to endotoxin, the lipopolysaccharide portion of the cell membrane of gram-negative bacteria. Major injury depresses immunity and predisposes the animal to sepsis. Chemotherapy, immunosuppressive treatments, improved care and survival of older patients, invasive devices (catheters), and antibiotic-resistant organisms all have contributed to an increased incidence of septic shock. Causes of septic shock in the dog include bacteremia, burns, trauma, shock, peritonitis, mastitis,

---

*BD = base deficit as calculated earlier; BW = body weight in kilograms; and 0.3 = volume of distribution of $HCO_3{}^-$.

prostatic and other abscesses, metritis, intestinal ischemia, enteritis, liver disease, and gastric dilatation volvulus.

Metabolism

There is increased energy expenditure in sepsis. This is due to increased energy expenditure by the heart, increased oxygen consumption by the wound, increased oxygen for conversion of lactate to glucose in the liver, and the effect of the increased body temperature. At the same time there is a need for increased energy, an insulin resistance of the tissues also exists, with glucose intolerance and decreased use of glucose. The inability of muscle cells to oxidize glucose effectively results in a block in the Krebs cycle, with accumulation of pyruvate and lactate.

Clinical and Laboratory Findings

The clinical and laboratory findings associated with sepsis and septic shock include an increased or decreased body temperature, mental confusion, hypotension, hyperventilation, edema, increased or decreased white blood cell count, falling platelet count with or without evidence of disseminated intravascular coagulation, positive blood culture, a source of infection, altered vascular resistance, oliguria, hypoxemia, and acidosis.

Treatment

The principal and most important aspects of treatment of the septic patient include drainage of the septic focus, appropriate antibiotic treatment, and aggressive fluid therapy.

Drainage may entail lancing an abscess or maintaining open abdominal drainage for peritonitis. Wounds and drainage should be cultured for aerobic and anaerobic bacteria, and the patient should be started on appropriate antimicrobial therapy with a bactericidal antibiotic. Antibiotics are continued until the temperature and white blood cell count have returned to normal.

Fluid is given that restores hemodynamic and clinical parameters to normal (color, capillary refill time, pulse). Urine output is monitored by a urinary catheter and maintained at >1 ml/kg/hr. Monitoring of central venous pressures via a jugular catheter is appropriate.

Pulmonary damage and pulmonary hypertension also occur in septic shock; the etiology is not known. The patient is monitored for signs of pulmonary edema (increased respiratory rate, moist rales, decreased arterial PO_2, radiography), and if pulmonary edema occurs, less aggressive fluid therapy is indicated. Positive end-expiratory pressure respiration has been recommended if respiratory distress is suspected and PO_2 decreases.

Three clinical prospective trials concluded that steroids were not efficacious in septic shock.

MEDIATORS OF SHOCK AND MULTIPLE ORGAN FAILURE (pp. 7–9)

Multiple Organ Failure

Multiple organ failure is most frequently due to sepsis, shock, and trauma, although it may occur in the absence of infection. The organs that fail in multiple organ failure are primarily the lung, liver, heart, and kidney, although all organ systems, including the nervous, gastrointestinal, metabolic, and immune systems, may fail.

Oxygen Radicals

Oxygen radicals, produced by macrophages and polymorphonuclear leukocytes, destroy microorganisms They are implicated in many disease states, including multiple organ failure. Oxygen radicals induce lipid peroxidation, thus resulting in the formation of the prostaglandins. At this time, clinical research protocols have not been completed that demonstrate efficacy of therapy against oxygen radicals.

Cytokines

The cytokines include tumor necrosis factor, interleukins-1 and -6, and interferon gamma. Tumor necrosis factor is a macrophage-derived polypeptide that is a potential mediator of tissue injury. High levels of tumor necrosis factor have been observed in states not accompanied by shock.

Prostanoids

The prostanoids are potent vasoactive substances and important mediators in disease, including inflammation, burns, hypertension, peptic ulcers, diarrhea, platelet function, and shock. The prostanoids are synthesized from arachidonic acid released from the cell membrane by the action of phospholipase.

Disseminated Intravascular Coagulation

Disseminated intravascular coagulation refers to a syndrome secondary to another disease state and in which there is activation of the clotting cascade and fibrinolytic system. The etiology of disseminated intravascular coagulation is not precisely known. Endotoxin directly activates the Hageman factor, which initiates the intrinsic clotting cascade and the kinin system.

Disseminated intravascular coagulation is frequently recognized when the animal is in the terminal stages of the syndrome and bleeding is occurring. Therapy at that stage is usually unrewarding. Specific treatment of disseminated intravascular coagulation includes removal of the underlying cause and administration of fluids, heparin, and antithrombin III.

Adenosine Triphosphate–MgCl$_2$

Treatment with ATP-MgCl$_2$ improves survival from hemorrhagic shock and hepatic ischemia.

Narcotic Antagonists

Their use in the management of shock cannot be recommended.

Platelet-Activating Factor

Its role in shock and organ failure has not been defined.

CHAPTER 2

Fluid, Electrolyte, and Acid-Base Therapy in the Surgical Patient (pages 11–28)

FLUID THERAPY (pp. 11–17)

General Principles

Body Water

Body water is divided into extracellular and intracellular spaces. The extracellular space may be subdivided into intravascular and interstitial spaces. The intracellular compartment contributes 30 to 40 per cent of total body water, with the extracellular compartment contributing 20 to 30 per cent. The intravascular compartment contributes approximately 5 per cent of total body water, and the interstitial compartment contributes approximately 15 per cent of total body water.

Intercompartmental water balance is maintained by an equilibrium between pressure gradients. Factors that affect hydrostatic pressure (blood pressure) or oncotic pressure (plasma protein) disturb the normal distribution of water between tissue compartments.

Intercompartmental water balance is also affected by tissue integrity. Vascular injury produces increased tissue permeability. Following injury, the difference in intercompartmental oncotic pressure is lost owing to increased endothelial permeability. Thus, "pooling" of water in the interstitial space results, with the formation of edema.

Reduction in salt concentration in the extracellular space causes redistribution of free water to the intracellular compartment. As water shifts between compartments, the intracellular osmotic pressure falls until a new equilibrium is established.

The degree of dehydration can be estimated by clinical evaluation (Table 2–1).

Electrolytes

Electrolyte evaluation should be routinely performed in animals that demonstrate fluid imbalance.

Sodium. Sodium is the largest cation in the body, with approximately 45 mEq (1 gm) distributed per kilogram body weight. Changes in sodium balance mainly affect the extracellular fluid space.

Hyponatremia (sodium levels less than 132 mEq/l) signifies a primary water or sodium imbalance in the plasma compartment. In many cases, hyponatremia is associated with primary diseases of the gastrointestinal or renal system. Other factors contributing to hyponatremia may include antidiuretic hormone (ADH) release secondary to pain, anesthetic drugs, metabolic response to injury, hemorrhage, shock, or sepsis. Endocrine lesions related to adrenal and thyroid function may also impair sodium conservation. Pre-existing diseases characterized by edema, cardiac failure, and hepatic disease also cause hyponatremia.

Clinical signs of hyponatremia may include generalized weakness, mental depression, inappetence, and hypotension. Therapy is directed at re-establishing a normal sodium and water ratio in the vascular compartment. This is accomplished by correction of the underlying

TABLE 2-1. CLINICAL SIGNS OF DEHYDRATION

Per Cent Dehydration	Mucous Membrane Dryness	Skin Turgor	Slowed Capillary Refill Time	Sunken Eyes	Tachycardia	Poor Pulse Quality
5–8%	+	+	0	0	0	0
9–12%	+ +	+ +	+	+	+	+
13–15%	+ + +	+ + +	+ + +	+ + +	+ + +	+ +

0 = normal; + = slight increase; + + = moderate increase; + + + = large increase.

disease and administration of saline-containing solutions. Saline is not recommended in pre-existing acidosis.

Hypernatremia occurs when the sodium level exceeds 155 mEq/l. Hypernatremia is usually a result of water loss. Pure water loss may result from water deprivation, loss through sweat or pulmonary tissue, or diabetes insipidus. Hypotonic loss may result from gastrointestinal lesions, sweat, salivary secretions, osmotic diuresis from glucose, urea, or mannitol, and serosal cavity loss during surgery or peritoneal dialysis. Salt gain may result from endogenous or exogenous corticosteroids, epinephrine, vasopressin, adrenocorticotropic hormone (ACTH) liberation, or inappropriate administration of saline-rich fluids.

Hypernatremia is often treated by administration of water.

Potassium. Potassium is considered the ''osmotic skeleton'' of the intracellular space, with 98 per cent of total body potassium located within cells.

Hyperkalemia is defined as serum values greater than 5.5 mEq/l. Hyperkalemia may result from acid-base disturbance, insulin deficiency, hypoaldosteronism, pharmacological agents, massive cell necrosis, and renal tubular lesions. The primary danger associated with hyperkalemia is development of life-threatening cardiac arrhythmias and myocardial depression.

Therapy for hyperkalemia is directed at correction of the underlying lesion. Correction of acidosis by administration of sodium bicarbonate is useful in correction of excessive potassium levels. Administration of glucose solutions with supplemental insulin has been successful.

Hypokalemia may be defined as serum potassium levels less than 3.5 mEq/L. Hypokalemia may be associated with disturbances in acid-base balance, gastrointestinal or renal disease, pharmacological agents, administration of low-potassium fluids or diet, and overzealous administration of sodium-containing fluids or drugs.

Clinical signs of hypokalemia include muscle weakness and paralysis, intestinal ileus, and alteration in electrocardiographic complexes.

Therapy is directed at replacing potassium salts. If oral methods are available, administration of supplemental potassium chloride is appropriate at a rate of 1 mEq KCl/kg/day. If parenteral routes are necessary, administration of supplemental potassium chloride in glucose or maintenance fluids is preferred. Inclusion of 20 to 40 mEq/l of potassium chloride per liter of fluid is safe if normal renal function is present.

Calcium. Serum calcium is divided into ionized and protein-bound (nonionized) fractions. Ionized calcium is physiologically important because of its effect on the cardiovascular system and coagulation.

Hypercalcemia is defined as serum levels greater than 12.5 mg/dl. Hypercalcemia can occur secondary to a variety of diseases, including neoplasia, renal disease, hypoadrenocorticism, or primary hyperparathyroidism. Hypercalcemia affects the renal, gastrointestinal, cardiovascular, and central nervous systems.

Therapy for hypercalcemia depends on the presence of clinical signs. If significant clinical signs are present, therapy including calcium-free fluid administration and diuretics is initiated. Acute reduction of serum calcium levels by administration of supplemental phosphate, sodium bicarbonate, glucocorticoids, and calcitonin administration or intravenous sodium ethylenediaminetetra-acetic acid (EDTA) may be necessary.

Hypocalcemia is defined as serum levels less than 9.0 mg/dl. Hypocalcemia may be associated with hypoalbuminemia, renal failure, soft-tissue injury, calcium-free fluid administration, acidosis, and blood transfusion (citrate chelation). Therapy is administration of calcium chloride or calcium gluconate. The recommended administration is 0.25 to 1.0 mEq/kg for the initial dose.

Magnesium. Magnesium plays an essential role in energy transfer related to adenosine triphosphate (ATP) use, neuromuscular function, thermoregulation, and protein synthesis. Primary hypermagnesemia, characterized by serum levels greater than 3.2 mg/dl, is rare in domestic species. Hypomagnesemia occurs when plasma levels are less than 1 mg/dl. Clinical appearance is similar to that of hypocalcemia. Therapy is directed at magnesium replacement through diet or parenteral means.

Chloride. Chloride is the predominant extracellular anion. Renal regulation of electroneutrality usually causes interaction of chloride with bicarbonate ions to maintain anion equilibrium.

Hyperchloremia occurs when serum levels exceed 110 mEq/L. Hyperchloremia is most commonly seen with overadministration of chloride-rich fluids by oral or parenteral route. Clinical signs associated with hyperchloremia include gastrointestinal irritation, anorexia, weight loss, lethargy, and persistent hyperventilation. Therapy consists of removing the source of chloride ions, administration of sodium bicarbonate by oral or parenteral route, and infusion of buffers.

Hypochloremia is noted when plasma values are less than 94 mEq/l. Gastrointestinal lesions, elevated bicarbonate levels, and hypokalemia may cause hypochloremia. Clinical signs of hypochloremia are interrelated with disturbances in acid-base balance. Metabolic alkalosis is noted with clinical signs associated with this disturbance. Therapy is chloride-rich fluids such as sodium or potassium chloride.

Bicarbonate. Normal values and disturbances in bicarbonate balance are discussed under acid-base regulation.

Phosphorus. The majority of phosphorus is stored in bone, with lesser quantities in the interstitial space.

Hypophosphatemia is present when serum levels fall below 2.5 mg/dl. Hypophosphatemia may be a result of dietary insufficiency, malabsorption, renal disease, diabetes mellitus, hyperparathyroidism, translocation associated with tissue trauma, acid-base disturbance, insulin, or hypoalbuminemia, or it may be of an undefined nature. Most clinical signs are related to reduced neuromuscular function exhibited by weakness, coma, tremors, paresis, and seizures. Treatment includes dietary supplementation and parenteral administration of potassium phosphate at a rate of 0.5 mg/kg/hr for 6 hours.

Fluid Plan Formulation

Fluid Volume

Fluid requirements can be divided into replacement and maintenance therapy. Replacement therapy is aimed at correcting pre-existing or continuing losses. The magnitude of loss is based on the parameters listed earlier, as well as on additional information concerning anticipated continuation of fluid loss. Maintenance therapy is judged on the basis of known obligatory water metabolism and routes of loss that are common to all surgical patients.

Replacement therapy is calculated and added to maintenance requirements for the surgical and postoperative periods. For dogs, we use a maintenance protocol of 20 ml/kg for the first hour, followed by 10 ml/kg for each additional hour. In cats, we initiate and maintain perioperative fluid therapy at 10 ml/kg/hr.

Postoperative fluid administration is readjusted to continue maintenance requirements based on body weight and additional volume for contemporary losses that may continue during the postoperative period. The calculated administration rate is continued until oral ingestion of water can be re-established.

Electrolyte Balance and Fluid Composition

If minimal blood loss is anticipated during the surgical procedure, use of a hypotonic maintenance solution appears acceptable in mature animals. With the exception of the upper gastrointestinal tract, most losses encountered during anesthesia and surgery are hypotonic in composition with predominant water loss. Contemporary water and electrolyte losses from hemorrhage are replaced with isotonic balanced electrolyte solutions such as lactated Ringer's solution. In young animals, sodium conservation mechanisms are immature. Most authors recommend isotonic balanced electrolyte solutions in these animals because the composition of loss more closely approximates an isotonic composition.

Additional Therapeutic Considerations

A priority rank assigned to fluid therapy goals is (1) replacement volume of fluid, (2) osmolality: sodium concentration, (3) potassium concentration, (4) pH: bicarbonate concentration, (5) chloride concentration, (6) water-soluble vitamins, (7) energy supplied as carbohydrates or lipids, (8) amino acids for tissue repair, and (9) trace elements.

Monitoring Response to Fluid Therapy

Water balance may be evaluated by monitoring urine production and estimating fluid loss from the wound. Replacement fluid volume approximates urine loss. Serial determinations of packed cell volume and total solids provide information of trends in fluid balance when interpreted along with urine production.

Products Available for Fluid Therapy (pp. 17–18)

COLLOID THERAPY (pp. 17–20)

Colloids are substances that do not diffuse across cell membranes owing to their molecular size or structure. Their role in maintenance of water balance is due to osmotic effect in the vascular compartment.

Under normal conditions, albumin plays a vital role in maintenance of intercompartmental fluid balance by acting as the major source of colloidal oncotic pressure in the vascular compartment. In hypoalbuminemic surgical patients, colloid administration maintains intravascular water balance during surgery. In addition, colloids are beneficial in resuscitation from hypovolemia and shock

Available Colloids

Plasma Protein. Plasma protein is produced by separation of erythrocytes from stored blood. Plasma is a mixture of albumin, globulins, platelets, and clotting factors. The main component for colloid replacement is albumin.

Plasma protein has several advantages over synthetic substances. It is inexpensive, has a long half-life (4 to 15 days), and provides vascular compartment stabilization in chronic disease states. Its disadvantages include direct protein allergy, anticolloid antibodies, complement activation, and histamine release.

Dextrans. Two forms of dextrans are commercially available: low molecular weight (mean molecular weight 40,000) and high molecular weight (mean molecular weight 60,000 to 75,000). Low molecular weight has a 2-hour half-life, and high molecular weight has a 6-hour half-life.

Anaphylactoid reactions have been associated with administration of dextrans. Hemostasis may be affected through reduced platelet adhesiveness, reduced factor VIII activity, and increased clot lysability.

Starch. Hydroxyethyl (hetastarch) is commercially available as a 6 per cent solution and is effective in resuscitation of hypovolemia. Hetastarch has a volume-expanding effect that lasts 24 to 36 hours. It has been shown to elicit immune reactions *in vivo*.

Hetastarch is metabolized by a complex series of pathways. Hydrolysis and renal filtration as well as phagocytosis play a role in excretion.

Indications for Use

Colloids are not a substitute for crystalloid solutions to restore water balance in dehydrated animals but are useful in volume re-expansion associated with acute hypovolemia. Colloids are also beneficial with crystalloid solutions to prevent translocation of free water from vascular to interstitial compartments.

ACID-BASE BALANCE (pp. 20–28)

Buffer Systems

Maintenance of cellular function requires an exacting environment. One of the most important factors in this environment is hydrogen ion regulation. Under normal conditions, buffer systems are responsible for the regulation of pH within narrow limits. The buffers include bicarbonate, hemoglobin, plasma protein, and phosphates.

Bicarbonate

The bicarbonate system is the predominant and most quickly responding buffer. Buffered acids may be subsequently excreted by the pulmonary or renal route. The bicarbonate system can be represented as follows:

$$CO_2 + H_2O \rightleftarrows H_2CO_3 \rightleftarrows H^+ + HCO_3^-$$

An interrelationship between metabolic acid (H^+ ion) and carbon dioxide allows for chemical transformation of a metabolic product (fixed acid) into a volatile product (carbon dioxide). In addition, CO_2 (volatile acid) can be transformed to a fixed product for systemic transport to the kidney or lung. Thus, CO_2 can be transformed into bicarbonate at the cellular level for transportation to sites of elimination.

Hemoglobin

When acids are buffered, approximately 60 per cent of the buffering capacity is in the hemoglobin buffer system, with 30 per cent in the bicarbonate system. The remaining 10 per cent is provided by organic phosphate buffers, which are intracellular. Hemoglobin is integral in buffering carbonic acid.

Protein

Plasma proteins provide a broad spectrum of buffers. Their function is similar to that in the hemoglobin system.

Phosphate

The phosphate buffer system is similar to the bicarbonate system and is capable of buffering strong and weak alkalis. Its main importance is acid-base balance in renal tubules and in intracellular fluids owing to the increased phosphate concentration.

Distribution of Buffers

Extracellular fluid has bicarbonate, protein, and phosphate systems. Intracellular fluid (including erythrocytes) has hemoglobin, phosphate, and protein buffering systems.

Pulmonary Regulation of Acid-Base Balance

Arterial CO_2 tension is the direct and immediate reflection of alveolar ventilation in relation to metabolic rate. Ineffective alveolar ventilation creates retention of CO_2 and effectively induces retention of H^+ (acidosis). Increased alveolar ventilation enhances removal of CO_2 and effectively reduces H^+ concentration (alkalosis).

Renal Regulation of Acid-Base Balance

Changes in bicarbonate ion concentration and buffer base reflect renal regulation and excretion of fixed (noncarbonic) acids.

Bicarbonate Reabsorption. Bicarbonate undergoes dynamic regulation in the kidney. Reabsorption takes place through hydrogen ion secretion and selective recirculation of bicarbonate. As hydrogen ion is excreted, disturbance in electroneutrality occurs, which is balanced by reabsorption of sodium ion from the tubular lumen.

Ammonium Ion. Bicarbonate conservation may also occur in distal renal tubules, where intraluminal volumes are diminished and the previous interaction is exhausted. To further conserve bicarbonate, ammonia (NH_3) formed from amino acid deamination diffuses into the tubular cells and combines with hydrogen ion to form ammonium (NH_4^+). By this process, ammonia acts as a urine buffer. Once NH_4^+ is formed, it penetrates cell membrane poorly and remains in the tubular lumen. Thus, a unidirectional flow is established.

Measurement of Metabolic Acid-Base Balance

Base Excess. Base excess specifies the number of milliequivalents of acid or base required to titrate 1 liter of blood to pH 7.40 and 37°C with constant P_{CO_2} of 40 mm Hg. Base excess may be determined by actual titration or can be derived from nomogram calculations following measurement of pH, P_{CO_2}, and hematocrit values. Base excess is expressed in milliequivalents per liter above or below the normal buffer-base range.

Carbon Dioxide Content (Total CO_2). CO_2 content represents the total amount of CO_2 that can be recovered from a plasma sample collected under anaerobic conditions. It is equal to bicarbonate plus carbonic acid concentrations. Measurement of carbon dioxide content is an estimate of the *metabolic* component of acid-base balance. Normal values for total carbon dioxide approximate those for bicarbonate.

Anion Gap. The anion gap accounts for the difference between measured cations and anions. The anion gap is calculated from the following equation:

$$\text{Anion gap (mEq/l)} = (Na^+ + K^+) - (Cl^- + HCO_3^-)$$

An **elevated anion gap** represents **metabolic acidosis;** a **reduced value** represents **metabolic alkalosis.**

Abnormalities of Acid-Base Balance

Simple Acid-Base Disturbances

Respiratory Acidosis. If an increase in CO_2 levels occurs, increased ventilation occurs to increase elimination. Inadequate elimination occurs with pulmonary disease. Predictable changes have been demonstrated regarding changes in CO_2 and pH during this period. HCO_3^- increases 1 mEq/l for each 10 mm Hg P_{CO_2} elevation. A similar relationship between pH and P_{CO_2} occurs; 0.01 pH unit change accompanies each 1 mm Hg change in P_{CO_2}.

If CO_2 retention persists, plasma bicarbonate concentration increases beyond the initial mass action response. The elevation is a result of renal conservation and synthesis of bicarbonate. This compensation normalizes overall balance.

Respiratory Alkalosis. Arterial P_{CO_2} (hypocapnia) falls whenever pulmonary CO_2 excretion (increased alveolar ventilation) exceeds CO_2 production.

A fall in bicarbonate values occurs within minutes and is unassociated with any significant renal bicarbonate loss. Bicarbonate decreases 2 mEq/l for every 10 mm Hg decrease in P_{CO_2}.

Hypocapnia lasting for more than 6 hours results in increased renal bicarbonate excretion. Bicarbonate values are reduced 5 mEq/l for every 10 mm Hg reduction in P_{CO_2} level.

Metabolic Acidosis. Metabolic acidosis is characterized by reduced plasma bicarbonate values due to secretory loss (diarrhea, renal disease) or consumption of bicarbonate to buffer nonvolatile acids (ketoacidosis, lactic acidosis).

With normal renal function, bicarbonate loss is usually associated with the gastrointestinal tract. Diabetes mellitus, exercise, shock, cyanide intoxication, and lactic acidosis produce abnormal quantities of acid. The kidney attempts to secrete excess acid to compensate for bicarbonate loss but may be unsuccessful if the loss is large and occurs rapidly. Dehydration may further contribute to acidosis.

Metabolic Alkalosis. Metabolic alkalosis is a common acid-base disorder, characterized by primary elevation of plasma bicarbonate concentration with a reduction in plasma chloride concentration. Contributory factors to the development of metabolic alkalosis include administration of exogenous base substances, gastrointestinal loss or sequestration of nonvolatile acid, and increased loss of urinary hydrogen ion. Regardless of underlying disturbance, most compensatory mechanisms are mediated by the kidney. Renal integrity, electrolyte values, and therapeutic course are evaluated to prevent further metabolic disturbance.

Mixed Acid-Base Disturbances

The previous discussion defined the four primary alterations in acid-base disturbance and indicated the expected response. *Overcompensation* of the primary disorder is rare, and deviation from the guidelines may suggest coexistence of more than one primary disturbance.

Therapy of Acid-Base Disturbances

Acute lesions are treated quickly, and chronic lesions slowly. Rapid intervention and correction of a chronic lesion may upset compensatory mechanisms that have occurred.

Respiratory-Related Disturbance

If hypoxemia is confirmed by blood gas analysis, oxygen therapy is used. The only direct effects of supplemental oxygenation are improved alveolar oxygen tensions, decreased work of breathing, and decreased myocardial work to maintain oxygenation.

Refractory hypoxemia usually exists with cardiovascular shunts, pulmonary vascular fistulas (i.e., neoplastic metastasis), alveolar atelectasia, surfactant-related diseases, and acute pulmonary injury (respiratory distress syndrome, shock lung).

Respiratory Acidosis (Ventilatory Failure). Animals that retain carbon dioxide (hypercapnia), with or without diminished oxygenation, have respiratory acidosis or ventilatory failure. They are unable to provide muscular work to exchange an adequate volume of air for elimination of carbon dioxide. Support of ventilation is provided until the underlying factor can be reversed.

Respiratory Alkalosis. Respiratory alkalosis without hypoxemia is usually secondary to central nervous system–mediated events, including pain and excitement. If hypoxemia is present, primary cardiopulmonary lesions such as alveolar disease, myocardial lesions, pulmonary edema, postoperative compromise, pregnancy, and musculoskeletal disease affecting ventilation are considered. Lesions affecting oxygen-carrying capacity such as anemia or carbon monoxide poisoning may also cause respiratory alkalosis.

Metabolic-Related Disturbance

Metabolic Acidosis. The main therapeutic consideration in metabolic acidosis involves treating the underlying cause of the acid-base disturbance. Primary therapy of acidosis is palliative and bridges the time interval until the primary disease can be treated. The bicarbonate deficit is usually derived from the formula:

$$0.3 \times \text{body weight (kg)} \times \text{base deficit} = \text{bicarbonate replacement}$$

Base deficit is derived from the base excess value or by subtracting actual bicarbonate from desired bicarbonate values. The factor of 0.3 is a value for interstitial fluid volume.

Metabolic Alkalosis. Metabolic alkalosis may be pure or mixed. It is compensated for by ventilatory depression. This compensatory mechanism is limited owing to activation of oxygen receptors from decreased Pao_2.

Therapy of metabolic alkalosis involves correction of underlying disturbances. Administration of normal saline (0.9% NaCl) corrects volume depletion associated with alkalosis and also replaces chloride ions.

Collection of Blood Gas Samples

Accuracy of data provided by blood gas analysis or titration techniques depends on adherence to appropriate collection techniques. Arterial sites are preferred. Central venous sampling provides data with respect to acid-base status; however, no conclusions regarding respiratory function can be inferred.

Prior to collection, an anticoagulant is introduced into the syringe-needle unit. Heparin is preferred because other anticoagulants (EDTA, CPD, ACD, sodium fluoride, and concentrated heparin) may induce *in vitro* changes in acid-base status.

Sample collection is anaerobically performed so that room air cannot influence results. Slow aspiration of the sample is preferred to minimize trapped air. Collected samples with more than minor gas bubbles are discarded. After the needle is withdrawn, rotation of the syringe barrel with the needle pointed up enhances dispersion of heparin and allows air to collect at the liquid surface, facilitating gas expulsion. Blood is introduced to the needle tip, and a rubber or cork stopper is placed over the tip to maintain an anaerobic environment.

After collection, immediate analysis is preferred to provide accurate measurements. Delay in evaluation (greater than 15 minutes) permits continued oxygen consumption by leukocytes and reticulocytes as well as glycolysis in erythrocytes. If a delay longer than 15 minutes between collection and analysis is expected, the sample is placed in an ice bath.

CHAPTER 3

Hemostasis: Physiology, Diagnosis, and Treatment of Bleeding Disorders in Surgical Patients (pages 29–52)

PHYSIOLOGY OF HEMOSTASIS (pp. 29–30)

Primary System

Hemostasis depends on an interaction among vessel walls, platelets, and the soluble coagulation factors (procoagulants). Not only does the normal vessel wall fail to support coagulation but it actually functions in an inhibitory capacity.

When a vessel is injured, it undergoes local reflex vasoconstriction. Vasoconstriction decreases blood flow at the site of the injury, allowing activated platelets and soluble coagulation factors to accumulate locally and function in clot formation. When vessels are injured and endothelium is denuded, subendothelial collagen is exposed. The exposed collagen activates platelets and soluble coagulation factors. A fibrin network is laid down on the primary platelet plug, cross-linked by factor XIII, to form a secondary, or stable, plug.

Secondary System

The soluble coagulation factors are synthesized by the liver and circulate primarily as zymogens or procoagulants, with half-lives varying from a few hours to a few days. Other compounds or electrolytes are occasionally referred to as factors. Calcium is sometimes referred to as factor IV and tissue thromboplastin as factor III.

Hemostasis Control Mechanisms

Maintaining control of activated soluble coagulation factors is essential in localizing clot formation to the site of vascular damage. Two important inhibitors of activated soluble coagulation factors are alpha$_2$-macroglobulin and antithrombin III (AT III). Antithrombin III, occasionally referred to as the heparin cofactor, is considered the most important natural inhibitor. It inhibits all activated serine proteinase factors (factors XII, XI, IX, VII, X, and II) by binding at the active site of the factor and forming a stable complex.

Fibrinolysis

Plasminogen is the inactive plasma zymogen that, when activated to plasmin, breaks down fibrin and fibrinogen to aid in dissolution of deposited fibrin strands and clots.

During fibrin clot formation, plasminogen is entrapped from the plasma, and surrounding vascular endothelial cells release plasminogen activator into the clot. Both plasminogen and plasminogen activator are absorbed onto the fibrin meshwork of the clot, localizing plasminogen's activation to plasmin, and thus minimizing release of plasmin into the general circulation.

DIAGNOSTIC APPROACH TO BLEEDING DISORDERS
(pp. 30–34)

Initial Diagnostic Approach to Bleeding Disorders
Signalment

Breed is an important consideration when considering potential inherited bleeding disorders. Although purebreds are most commonly affected by inherited disorders such as coagulation factor VIII (FVIII:C) deficiency (hemophilia A), mixed-breed dogs may also be affected. Age may indicate certain bleeding disorders but is not reliable.

History

Episodes of historical weakness, lameness, or illness are recorded. Also, one should inquire about prior bleeding episodes including severity, age of occurrence, number of episodes, and association with disease or drug therapy. Previous drug therapy should be addressed because many drugs suppress megakaryocytopoiesis, inhibit platelet function, increase platelet destruction, and decrease absorption or synthesis of vitamin K. Dates of vaccination are determined, because transient mild to moderate thrombocytopenia associated with platelet or endothelial dysfunction (between days 1 and 10 after modified live virus vaccination) or both occurs as does mild spontaneous clinical bleeding associated with severe thrombocytopenia and concurrent underlying disease.

Physical Examination

Physical examination should be complete, including an ocular fundic examination. Primary system abnormalities (platelet and vascular disorders) more typically are manifested as superficial bleeding into the skin or mucous membranes or from body orifices. Blood loss from primary system abnormalities is generally not as severe as blood loss associated with the secondary system (coagulation system). With a pure secondary system disorder, petechiation does not occur. Hematomas, hemarthrosis, and bleeding into body cavities are typical.

Laboratory Evaluation

Initial laboratory evaluation in the patient with a suspected bleeding disorder should include not only tests to differentiate between primary and secondary system abnormalities but also tests to assess the overall condition of the patient. A complete blood count is performed. Urinalysis and serum biochemistries are useful in detecting underlying or concurrent disease and in evaluation of the patient's overall health.

Primary System Disorders. Platelet numbers can be estimated from a well-made blood smear, or an actual platelet count can be performed. Various function tests, such as bleeding time and clot retraction tests, can be performed in the clinic.

Thrombocytopenia is recognized by either platelet estimation or platelet count and may be due to decreased platelet production, platelet sequestration, or increased platelet destruction or use.

Bone marrow evaluation with special emphasis on megakaryocyte number, stage, and morphology can be useful for differentiating general mechanisms of thrombocytopenia. Thrombocytopenia due to increased platelet use or destruction results in normal to increased marrow megakaryocyte numbers; thrombocytopenia due to platelet sequestration results in normal marrow megakaryocyte numbers; and thrombocytopenia due to decreased platelet production results in decreased marrow megakaryocyte numbers.

Bleeding time is used to assess the primary system. Prolonged bleeding time is caused by quantitative or qualitative platelet disorders and vascular disease. The buccal mucosal bleeding time (BMBT) using a spring-loaded disposable device is a sensitive test of primary system function abnormalities. With this procedure, normal dogs had bleeding times of 2.62 ± 0.49 minutes. Dogs with severe thrombocytopenia or thrombopathy (secondary to von Willebrand's disease or uremia) were easily identified before surgery by prolongation of the BMBT, and they exhibited deficient hemostasis during surgical procedures.

Secondary System Disorders. In animals with a secondary system bleeding disorder or that have potential for prolonged bleeding with surgery (e.g., animals with severe hepatic disease), assessment of the secondary system is indicated. The most readily available and least costly test is the activated clotting time (ACT).

The more common *in vitro* tests used to evaluate the soluble coagulation factors are the APTT and the one-stage prothrombin time (OSPT).

Fibrin degradation products (FDPs) are elevated when fibrin or fibrinogen is broken down at an accelerated rate. When excessive fibrinolysis occurs, as with disseminated intravascular coagulation (DIC) or primary fibrinolysis, FDP concentration increases to more than 10 μg/ml (frequently >40 μg/ml).

Assessment of the Patient with a Bleeding Disorder

The initial diagnostic step usually is measurement of platelet numbers. Next, OSPT, APTT, and FDP results are determined. In patients not exhibiting evidence of bleeding but suspected of having an increased bleeding potential with surgical challenge because of a qualitative primary system disorder, measurement of bleeding time using the BMBT technique is a clinically useful first step to determine whether a qualitative primary system defect exists.

DIAGNOSIS AND TREATMENT OF BLEEDING DISORDERS (pp. 34–45)

Vascular Disorders Associated with Abnormalities of Hemostasis

Degenerative diseases of collagen (e.g., hyperadrenocorticism, diabetes mellitus, dysproteinemia) may also lead to increased bruising, especially in the patient that is challenged surgically.

Vasculitis may be primary or secondary (associated with collagen vascular disease (infectious vasculitis) or idiopathic.

In patients with primary vasculitis, systemic signs of illness such as fever, listlessness, and anorexia may be present. These signs may be present in the patient with secondary and idiopathic vasculitis as well. Diagnosis of vasculitis is based on the history and clinical appearance initially. To confirm a diagnosis of vasculitis, biopsies of affected tissues, usually of the skin, are collected for histology.

All unnecessary drug therapy is stopped. In primary or idiopathic vasculitis, immunosuppressive doses of prednisone (1 to 2 mg/kg/day) with or without concurrent administration of antibiotics are recommended. Other immunosuppressive drugs, such as cyclophosphamide, are reserved for cases that do not respond.

Thrombocytopenic Disorders

Decreased Production of Platelets

Immune-Mediated Disorders. Diagnostically, an antimegakaryocyte antibody test, using direct immunofluorescence, can be performed on bone marrow cells to confirm the disease. Prognosis of immune-mediated suppression of megakaryocytes is guarded because treatment is difficult and response to therapy is slow.

Infectious Disorders. Diseases that suppress thrombopoiesis include parvovirus, feline leukemia virus, canine distemper virus, and chronic canine ehrlichiosis.

Neoplastic Disorders. Neoplastic diseases leading to decreased production of platelets include the myeloproliferative and infiltrative extramedullary neoplastic diseases (myelophthisis), in which thrombocytopoiesis is disturbed owing to environmental changes, and tumors secreting estrogens.

Toxicity Disorders. Chemotherapeutic drugs, used to treat a variety of neoplastic and immune-mediated diseases, have been associated most commonly with bone marrow suppression, inclusive of megakaryocytes. Chloramphenicol has minimal toxic effects in domestic animals. Nonsteroidal anti-inflammatory drugs, such as phenylbutazone, have been associated with severe granulocytopenia in the dog, with milder suppression of erythrocytes and megakaryocytes. Administration of estrogens, for a variety of conditions, is a well-established cause of aplastic anemia, particularly megakaryocytic aplasia, in dogs.

Sequestration of Platelets

With sequestration, the body mass of platelets is unchanged; therefore, megakaryopoiesis is not changed. Circulating platelets may be markedly decreased, resulting in increased bleeding time, especially with surgical challenge.

Etiology of Sequestration. Splenomegaly creating sequestration thrombocytopenia (hypersplenism) may be associated with a variety of inflammatory diseases, neoplastic and non-neoplastic infiltrative diseases, congestion, and hyperplasia splenomegaly. The liver, when enlarged or diseased, also serves as a site of platelet sequestration.

Diagnosis and Management. Patients with splenic or hepatic disease should have, as part of the diagnostic evaluation, a platelet count performed prior to surgical intervention. Treatment for platelet sequestration involves management of the primary disease.

Increased Destruction of Platelets

Usually, with accelerated platelet destruction, platelet numbers are low, an increased percentage of megaplatelets is seen, and megakaryocytic activity is high.

Immune-Mediated Thrombocytopenia. Primary immune-mediated thrombocytopenia (IMTP) occurs when antiplatelet antibody is produced and attaches to circulating platelets, and the antibody-platelet complex is removed by the mononuclear phagocytic system (primarily in the spleen). Physical findings in dogs with IMTP relate only to the thrombocytopenia (evidence of primary system bleeding), and mild splenomegaly is seen occasionally. The platelet count is usually less than 20,000 to 30,000/µl at the time of diagnosis. Hematological changes vary, with the most common findings being regenerative anemia with leukocytosis.

Treatment of IMTP includes supportive care in the form of an atraumatic environment, immunosuppressive therapy (initially oral prednisone at 2.2 to 4.4 mg/kg/day, divided bid for 7 to 10 days, depending on patient response), and blood or blood component therapy if needed. Splenectomy is reserved for patients that do not adequately respond to conventional medical therapy.

Excessive Platelet Use and Consumption

Etiology of Use and Consumption. Thrombocytopenia associated with disseminated intravascular coagulation is due to consumption of platelets because of excessive formation of thrombin and intravascular fibrin thrombi. Diseases in which vascular damage is present (e.g., immune-mediated vasculitis, heartworm disease) may result in thrombosis. Severe hemorrhage should not be overlooked as a cause of use and loss thrombocytopenia.

Diagnosis and Management. Thrombocytopenia due to use or consumption is always secondary to an underlying disease; however, with thrombotic thrombocytopenic purpura the underlying stimulus is not known. Specific therapy should be used when possible. Supportive therapy such as blood or blood component replacement may be necessary.

Thrombocytopathic Disorders

Inherited Thrombocytopathic Disorders

Hereditary defects may involve platelet adhesion or platelet release or may be miscellaneous in nature.

von Willebrand's Disease. This disorder of defective platelet adhesion is due to deficient endothelial cell and megakaryocyte production of a glycoprotein (von Willebrand's factor [vWf]). Genetic transmission in humans and dogs is autosomal and may be either recessive or dominant. In the more common autosomal incompletely dominant form (with variable penetrance), both heterozygotes and homozygotes have an increased tendency to bleed.

In many patients with von Willebrand's disease, bleeding tendencies are not evident on physical examination unless the patient is suffering from concurrent disease, suffers emotional stress, is receiving drugs that alter platelet numbers or function, or is challenged with trauma or surgery. Normal physiological events, such as estrus and whelping, may alter a bitch's hemostatic response, resulting in severe hemorrhage from the reproductive tract. Association of increased bleeding tendencies in Doberman pinschers with concurrent hypothyroidism has been made. Buccal mucosal bleeding time is prolonged in patients with von Willebrand's disease and should be tested in suspect animals and in the surgical patient with a strong breed tendency to carry the trait (e.g., Doberman pinscher). Diagnosis is confirmed by measurement of vWf.

Treatment of von Willebrand's disease in the symptomatic patient involves supportive therapy in the form of an atraumatic environment and blood or blood component therapy (e.g., fresh plasma, fresh frozen plasma, or cryoprecipitate). It is reported that daily supplementation of L-thyroxine at the standard dose (0.1 mg/10 lbs bid PO) increases plasma concentration of vWf:Ag, increases platelet adhesiveness, and corrects bleeding times in both normal dogs and dogs with von Willebrand's disease or other thrombopathies. Desmopressin acetate (DDAVP), 1 μg/kg IV or SQ, increased the higher molecular weight forms of vWf along with increasing vWf activity (as measured by botrocetin cofactor) in normal dogs and in 11 of 12 Doberman pinschers affected with von Willebrand's disease. Buccal mucosal bleeding time and surgical complications due to hemorrhage were reduced in 11 of 12 treated dogs for up to 3 hours.

Acquired Thrombocytopathic Disorders (p. 40)

Thrombopathies may occur naturally or they may occur secondary to treatment. Drug-induced thrombopathia must always be considered in the differential diagnosis of a patient with a recent history of primary system bleeding.

Coagulopathies

Inherited Coagulopathies

Inherited disorders of the secondary system (coagulopathies) occur most commonly in purebred dogs that are inbred or linebred. Coagulopathies have been reported in cats, mixed-breed dogs, and other species. The defect in coagulation is usually a result of deficient production of a factor (quantitative), although production of an abnormal factor may occur. This quantitative or qualitative disorder results in the inability of the secondary system to stabilize the primary platelet plug.

Clinical Findings. Potential for hemorrhage depends on which factor is deficient, the degree of deficiency, and whether hemostatic challenge has occurred. Delayed blood oozing from an unstabilized platelet plug may result in hematoma formation, hemarthrosis, hemorrhage into body cavities, or continual external blood loss.

Laboratory findings in the patient with inherited coagulopathy that has not experienced a bleeding episode are unremarkable. Diagnostic testing by buccal mucosal bleeding time is normal because the primary plug is produced but rebleeding occurs. Presurgical screening tests (OSPT, APTT) of the secondary system are prolonged in dogs and cats with less than 30 per cent of factor present.

Treatment. An atraumatic, exercise-restricted environment, followed by intravenous fluid support, if necessary, is indicated. Specific therapy is replacement of the coagulation factors, which are absent, with fresh whole blood or plasma, fresh frozen plasma, or cryoprecipitate.

Acquired Coagulopathies

Disseminated Intravascular Coagulation. DIC is characterized by a simultaneous disturbance of the coagulation and fibrinolytic systems. The pathophysiology involves an inciting cause, because DIC is not a disease entity in itself but requires initiation. Any disorder that induces vascular damage or favors vascular stasis, involves bacterial endotoxins, or allows release of tissue thromboplastin has the potential to initiate microthrombus formation. When microthrombi develop, homeostatic mechanisms work to locally restrict thrombus development.

Initially, fibrinolysis is beneficial for resolving the microthrombi and limiting clot formation. In the patient with DIC, excessive triggering of these homeostatic mechanisms occurs. Coagulation proteins are activated in excess, fibrinogen is converted to fibrin, platelets are activated, and accelerated fibrinolysis occurs. Consumption of clotting factors, fibrinolytic enzymes, and platelets occurs if production of these elements is hindered, if removal of these activated elements by the mononuclear phagocytic system occurs, if AT III concentrations are subnormal, or if shock or acidosis (respiratory or metabolic, which inhibits activation of heparin and AT III) is present.

Diagnostic evaluation of the surgical patient with a disease process known to initiate DIC, or a patient that is exhibiting evidence of abnormal hemostasis, should include hematological, biochemical, and coagulation screening tests. Thrombocytopenia is expected in most canine patients with DIC. Other sensitive indicators of naturally occurring DIC in dogs include alterations in red blood cell morphology (fragmentation), prolonged OSPT and APTT, and decreased concentration of AT III. Less sensitive indicators include increased concentrations of FDPs and decreased concentrations of fibrinogen.

Treatment of DIC begins with correction of the initiating condition or disease, if possible. Therapy for DIC initially is directed toward rehydration, maintenance of normovolemia, and prevention of ischemia by means of intravenous fluid administration.

In patients with severe hemorrhage, the next treatment chosen is administration of fresh whole blood or plasma. The rationale is replacement of clotting factors, AT III, and platelets.

Antiplatelet therapy (aspirin) is contraindicated with thrombocytopenia. The use of heparin, a potentiator of AT III, in the management of naturally occurring DIC remains controversial because of its mechanism of action, side effects, and management dilemma. Because AT III is often decreased or depleted in DIC and heparin requires AT III for activity, administration of heparin alone is questionable. Pretreatment or concurrent administration of fresh whole blood or fresh plasma to supply depleted clotting factors and AT III is recommended when heparin therapy is used. Heparin therapy should be continued intravenously (5 to 10 IU/kg/hr) or subcutaneously (50 to 100 IU/kg tid to qid). Heparin dosage is tailored to prolong the APTT 1.5 to 2.0 times normal. Once heparin therapy is begun, it is continued until DIC has resolved, because abrupt cessation of therapy may predispose the patient to thromboembolism due to drug-induced depression of AT III.

Liver Disease. With hepatic insufficiency, synthesis of coagulation proteins is depressed. In addition, the half-life of proteins that are produced may be shortened because of consumption.

Platelet disorders (thrombocytopenia and thrombocytopathia) may also exist. Last, DIC and primary fibrinolysis have been known to occur secondary to hepatic disease.

Diagnostic evaluation of the patient with liver disease, both before and after surgery, should include assessment of a coagulation profile (OSPT, APTT). However, the coagulation profile may be normal, because these tests are only prolonged in patients with less than 30 per cent of normal factor levels. Additional readily available tests that should be performed include a platelet count, FDPs and fibrinogen concentrations, and BMBT.

Treatment of the patient with liver disease requiring surgery should begin with carefully selected intravenous fluid therapy to maintain tissue perfusion. Administration of fresh whole blood or plasma is indicated prior to surgery to replace red blood cells, platelets, and coagulation factors. Presurgical treatment with vitamin K_1 may help restore hepatic protein synthesis within 24 hours (p. 44).

Vitamin K Deficiency and Antagonism. Vitamin K is required for the production of functional forms of the prothrombin group (FII, FVII, FIX, and FX) and the production of protein C (inhibitor of FV and FVIII). Vitamin K deficiency is rare in companion animals today because of the quality of commercial diets.

Hypercoagulable Disorders (Thrombosis and Thromboembolic Disease)

Pathophysiology. In small animals, most thrombotic conditions are due to vascular endothelial injuries caused by infectious agents. AT III deficiency, usually due to renal loss, is a well-described cause of thromboembolism. Saddle thrombus formation in cats with cardiomyopathy, presumably caused by altered arterial blood flow and endocardial damage, is a recognized clinical entity.

Clinical Findings. Physical examination findings in animals with hypercoagulable disorders vary depending on localization of the thrombus, function of the affected organ or tissues, and whether sufficient perfusion is maintained.

Diagnostic Evaluation. Evaluation techniques to confirm the clinical suspicion of thrombotic or thromboembolic disease (e.g., contrast angiography, ultrasonography, and nuclear medicine imaging) may not be readily available except at large institutions. In some patients, shortening of coagulation times (APTT, OSPT) is apparent. AT III concentration may help to reveal hypercoagulable states in that levels below 50 per cent in humans are associated with markedly increased risk.

Treatment and Prognosis. Prophylactic therapy such as antiplatelet drugs in patients with cardiomyopathy should be considered. Thrombolytic therapy must be considered in patients with documented thrombosis or thromboembolism.

BLOOD AND BLOOD COMPONENT REPLACEMENT THERAPY (pp. 45–50)
Objectives

Replacement of red blood cell mass by means of fresh whole blood or packed cells is performed in the anemic patient when the packed cell volume and hemoglobin fall to a level that fails to deliver sufficient oxygen to tissues. Replacement of platelet numbers in thrombocytopenic or thrombocytopathic patients with fresh whole blood, fresh plasma, or platelet-rich plasma is performed in patients with primary system bleeding due to platelet disorders. Replacement of clotting factors in patients with coagulopathies and those with von Willebrand's disease with fresh whole blood, fresh or fresh frozen plasma, or cryoprecipitate is performed in actively bleeding patients or those with a potential to bleed.

Blood Groups and Blood Compatibility
Dogs

Grouping is based on specific dog erythrocyte antigens (DEA), and eight blood groups have been identified. Administration of blood or red blood cells to a patient that lacks that particular red blood cell (RBC) antigen results in production of isoantibodies. The combination of DEA antibodies and complement results in a transfusion reaction in the form of hemolysis or hemagglutination.

Reasons to type blood donors and crossmatch the recipient are (1) to avoid sensitization of the recipient to future incompatible transfusions; (2) to avoid the occurrence of an immediate transfusion reaction in a previously sensitized recipient; (3) to avoid formation of isoantibodies 7 to 10 days after administration of the first incompatible blood, resulting in delayed destruction and decreased RBC survival; and (4) to avoid sensitization of a brood bitch, which could cause subsequent hemolytic disease in newborns after ingestion of colostral isoantibodies. A blood donor 27 kg or larger can donate 500 ml of blood every 3 weeks for at least 2 years without any adverse effects.

Cats

Three feline blood groups have been identified in an AB system (A, B, and AB). In the United States, 99.6 per cent of cats surveyed were type A, which correlated well with findings in England In contrast, 73.3 per cent of cats in Australia were found to be type A, 26.3 per cent type B, and 0.4 per cent type AB. A high incidence of type B was found among Abyssinian, Birman, British shorthair, Devon Rex, Himalayan, Persian, and Somali breeds. A blood donor, 5 to 7 kg in body weight, can supply 40 ml of blood every 3 weeks.

Collection and Storage of Whole Blood and Blood Products

Blood Collection

If chemical restraint is necessary, thiamylal sodium is preferred for the dog. Ketamine hydrochloride or thiamylal sodium can be used in the cat. For repeated donations, the femoral artery or the jugular vein can be used. The collection site should be surgically prepared. Following collection, pressure is applied to the site for 5 to 10 minutes to avoid the formation of a hematoma. Mixing of blood and anticoagulant is performed by gentle rotation throughout the collection process.

Anticoagulants. Citrate products work by binding ionized calcium, thus blocking several steps in the cascade. Results of a recent study evaluating citrate phosphate dextrose adenine-1 (CPDA-1) as a storage medium for packed canine erythrocytes revealed that posttransfusion viability of RBCs stored up to 20 days, but not longer, complied with the Food and Drug Administration standard. Heparin can be used as an anticoagulant because of its ability to potentiate the action of AT III.

Equipment. CPDA-1 is supplied in plastic bags and bottles with the appropriate amount of anticoagulant added to produce a ratio of 1 part anticoagulant to 9 parts blood when the receptacle is filled with donor blood. When needed, volumes of blood (less than 50 ml) can be drawn into syringes for small dog or cat recipients, using the 9:1 ratio of blood to anticoagulant.

Whole Blood Storage

At 4° to 6°C, platelets become nonfunctional 12 to 72 hours after collection; coagulation factors are nonfunctional after 24 hours. The metabolic changes that occur in stored blood are reversed by the recipient 12 to 24 hours after transfusion, making stored blood acceptable for the surgical patient with anticipated blood loss The acutely anemic patient needs fresh blood.

Blood Components—Preparation and Storage

Administration of blood components permits specific replacement therapy. By dividing whole blood into components, more efficient use of available blood is possible. At the same time, blood component therapy may reduce the risk of transfusion reactions.

Routes of Administration

Intravenous Administration. Intravenous administration is performed via a cephalic or jugular catheter. Solutions containing calcium, such as lactated Ringer's solution, should not be administered through this intravenous line, because the calcium in the fluids could exceed the citrate-binding ability of the anticoagulant.

Intramedullary Administration. Neonatal puppies or kittens, or small hypovolemic patients can be transfused in this manner when access to a peripheral vein is not possible. A 20-gauge needle can be inserted through the greater tubercle into the humerus or through the trochanteric fossa into the femur.

Intraperitoneal Administration. This technique should be reserved for the neonate and the very obese patient. RBC absorption is 50 per cent after 24 hours.

Volume

An estimated dose of whole blood to be administered to a dog or cat is 20 ml/kg of body weight. A more specific guideline based on increasing the PCV to a desired level is displayed in Table 3–1.

Rates of Administration

Initially, the rate of intravenous administration should be slow (<0.25 ml/kg/min) to allow for detection of incompatibility reactions. After 10 to 30 minutes, the rate may be increased if problems are not detected. In the patient suffering from hypovolemia due to massive hemorrhage, a rapid rate of intravenous replacement, up to 22 ml/kg/hr, along with administration of a balanced electrolyte fluid to combat shock, is recommended.

Transfusion of the Patient with Anemia

The chronically anemic presurgical patient is better adapted to existing with a decreased number of RBCs. Transfusions of whole fresh blood or RBCs should not be considered until the PCV reaches 20 per cent or less. Cats tolerate very low PCVs; transfusion may not be needed until the PCV reaches 10 per cent unless the patient requires anesthesia and surgery.

Transfusion of the Patient with Thrombocytopenia or Thrombocytopathia

In the thrombocytopenic or thrombocytopathic patient with a PCV greater than 20 per cent, transfusion of blood components should be

TABLE 3–1. CALCULATION FOR VOLUME OF BLOOD TO BE TRANSFUSED

$$\begin{matrix} \text{ml of blood}_D \\ \text{in} \\ \text{anticoagulant} \end{matrix} = \begin{matrix} \text{wt in kg}_R \times 90 \text{ (dog)} \\ \\ \times 70 \text{ (cat)} \end{matrix} \times \frac{\text{PCV desired} - \text{PCV}_R}{\text{PCV}_D \text{ in anticoagulant}}$$

D = Donor; R = recipient; PCV = packed cell volume.
Modified from Turnwald GH, Pichler ME: Blood transfusion in dogs and cats. Part II. Administration, adverse effects, and component therapy. *Comp Cont Educ Pract Vet* 7:115, 1985. Used with permission.

considered. Fresh plasma or platelet-rich plasma should be administered at a dose of 6 to 10 ml/kg of body weight sid to tid until bleeding stops. Pretreatment with antihistamines is advocated when transfusing plasma to decrease the occurrence of urticaria and help maintain plasma in the circulation.

Transfusion of the Patient with Coagulopathy (p. 49)
Transfusion Reactions

Transfusion reactions may be immunologically or nonimmunologically mediated. Examples of immunologically mediated reactions include urticaria, hemolytic reactions, fever, and isoerythrolysis neonatorum. Nonimmunologically mediated reactions include fever, circulatory overload, citrate intoxication, and coagulation. Pretreatment with antihistamines is beneficial in stopping development of urticaria.

SURGICAL HEMOSTASIS (pp. 50–51)
Local Management of Hemostasis

Intraoperative hemorrhage in animals without clotting disorders is usually caused by ineffective local hemostasis. Local hemostasis may be achieved by closure of a defect in a blood vessel wall or by interruption of blood flow to the affected area. Methods used to control local hemorrhage include application of pressure, instruments, and ligatures; thermal cauterization; and hemostatic agents to aid coagulation.

CHAPTER 4
Wound Healing and Specific Tissue Regeneration (pages 53–63)

STAGES OF WOUND REPAIR (pp. 53–57)
The Inflammatory Stage

Regardless of the nature of the injury, the response is the same. The immediate response to injury is vasoconstriction of the small vessels in the area of the wound. Vascular occlusion occurs at the point of trauma, tending to control hemorrhage. This response lasts 5 to 10 minutes and is followed by active vasodilation involving all elements of the local vasculature.

Fluid leaking from venules provides fibrinogen and other clotting elements to form fibrin clots, which quickly plug the damaged lymphatics, preventing drainage from the injured area. Thus, the inflammatory reaction is localized to an area immediately surrounding the injury.

Within 30 to 60 minutes, the entire endothelium of local venules may be covered with adherent leukocytes, which begin to move through the gaps in the vessel walls and eventually concentrate at the site of injury. Initially, the predominant cell is the polymorphonuclear leukocyte (PMN), whose primary role is destruction of bacteria. PMNs are short-lived compared with monocytes; therefore, monocytes predominate in older wounds.

Monocytes are essential for wound healing. Circulating monocytes originate from precursor cells found in the bone marrow. On entering the wound, they become macrophages, which phagocytize necrotic tissue and debris. Persistence of mononuclear cells at the site of injury indicates the presence of foreign material that granulocytes have been unable to remove.

Macrophages precede the onset of fibroplasia during wound healing and might even regulate the process. There is ample evidence that macrophages release a chemotactic substance that attracts mesenchymal cells and influences their differentiation into fibroblasts.

The Repair Stage

Fibroblastic Phase

Shortly after injury, undifferentiated mesenchymal cells begin to change into migratory fibroblasts. As soon as necrotic tissue, blood clots, and other debris are removed by granulocytes and macrophages, fibroblasts move into the injured area.

Fibroblasts move by forming a cytoplasmic extension called a *ruffled membrane*, which extends from the cell and adheres to a solid substrate (e.g., a fiber or capillary). The cell then moves in the direction of the ruffled membrane. When the ruffled membranes of two like cells meet, the cells adhere to each other and movement ceases. This process is called *contact inhibition*.

Fibroblasts do not contain fibrinolytic enzymes but, when migrating into a wound, are closely followed by new capillaries. New capillaries are formed by endothelial budding and are a prominent feature of new granulation tissue. The endothelial cells of these new capillaries contain a plasminogen activator. Thus, as new capillaries grow into a wound immediately behind the fibroblasts, fibrinolysis occurs and the fibrin network is broken down and removed.

After the fibroblasts have entered the wound, they secrete protein-polysaccharides and various glycoproteins that make up the ground substance. Mucopolysaccharides of the ground substance surround the fibroblast and influence the aggregation and orientation of collagen. Collagen is synthesized by the fibroblasts beginning on about the fourth or fifth day. As young collagen fibrils bond together, collagen fibers are formed and the collagen becomes less soluble. The collagen bundles are small but gradually enlarge to form dense collagen that binds the edges of the wound.

The fibroblastic phase of wound healing lasts 2 to 4 weeks.

Epithelialization Phase

The initial response of cells immediately adjacent to a wound is mobilization. These cells must detach from their substrate and prepare for migration.

After mobilization, epithelial cells enlarge and begin to migrate down and across the wound. The main regenerative activity occurs in the marginal basal cell layer. Migrating epidermal cells move by rolling or sliding over one another. Isolated cells move randomly if the substrate on which they are placed is not oriented. Epithelial cells migrating across a wound usually move across the rest of the basal lamina or along fibrin deposits. This phenomenon is called *contact guidance*. As with fibroblasts, the migrating epithelial cells stop moving when they come in contact with a like cell (contact inhibition).

If the full thickness of dermis has not been removed, as with split-thickness skin grafts, mobilization and migration of epithelial cells from skin appendages (primarily hair follicles) also occur. An open wound is almost always initially covered by a blood clot and then by granulation tissue. The migrating epithelium moves under the clot (not through it) and over or into the granulation tissue. The epithelial cells secrete a proteolytic enzyme that dissolves the base of the clot and permits unhindered cell migration. The undermining of the clot, and later the scab, by migrating epithelium is seen as separation of the scab as epithelialization progresses.

In large open wounds, all stages of epithelial repair occur simultaneously. Epithelial migration is rapid initially, but as the migrating cells move farther from the wound's edge, the epithelium becomes a monolayer and progresses more slowly.

Contraction Phase

Contraction involves the movement of existing tissue at the wound edge, not the formation of new skin.

There are five theories of contraction of open wounds: (1) the push theory, in which the wound edges are pushed inward by extension of surrounding skin; (2) the growth and push theory, in which the wound edges grow; (3) the sphincter theory, in which contractile material at the wound margin acts as a constricting sphincter; (4) the picture frame theory, in which active cells within the wound margin migrate inward, pulling the edges of the defect; and (5) the pull theory, in which material within the defect exerts tension. The first three theories are unlikely to be correct.

During contraction, the skin surrounding the wound is stretched, thinned, and under tension; however, this state does not persist. New collagen is gradually laid down in the dermis, and new epithelial cells are formed. This process continues until the full thickness of the stretched skin is restored. This process is called *intussusceptive growth*.

Wound contraction is an extremely valuable process in the healing of open wounds, but it is not without some disadvantages. Contraction of wounds near joints may result in the formation of a tight band of scar tissue limiting flexion or extension of the joint. Also, contraction of wounds near body openings, such as the anus, may cause stenosis.

Remodeling Phase

Early Wound Strength. A properly coapted wound has effective strength even during the first 24 hours. This strength is the result of the formation of a fibrin clot within the wound. Epithelialization across the wound also contributes to early wound strength, as does ingrowth of new capillaries into the wound's ground substance.

After the initial proliferative phase, wound strength increases significantly to reach an early maximum at 14 to 16 days. This increase in wound strength occurs during the period of rapid fibroplasia and parallels the increase in collagen content in the wound.

Late Wound Strength. Wounds continue to increase in strength even after the wound collagen content stabilizes. The increased strength results from intramolecular and intermolecular cross-linking of collagen fibers that render the collagen less accessible to tissue collagenases. A scar is never as strong as the tissue it replaces.

SYSTEMIC AND ENVIRONMENTAL FACTORS AFFECTING WOUNDS (pp. 57–60)

Secondary Wound Healing

Primary wounds that were allowed to heal undisturbed for short periods and were then dehisced and resutured immediately showed a significantly greater strength on the third day after resuturing than primary wounds after the same time. The immediate onset of fibroplasia in the resutured wounds, without the usual lag phase, seems to be responsible for this phenomenon. No time was necessary to activate and mobilize cells.

Hypoproteinemia

Although the rate of wound healing is not well correlated with plasma protein levels, if serum protein concentration is less than 2 g/100 ml, wound healing is inhibited. Decreased plasma protein levels decrease fibroplasia rather than prolong the lag phase.

Anemia and Blood Loss

A healing wound depends on the local microcirculation to furnish necessary oxygen and other nutrients; therefore, anything that interferes with the microcirculation inhibits wound healing. Hypovolemia is the major deterrent to wound healing in anemia, hemorrhage, and shock.

Oxygen

Oxygen is required for normal wound healing. Measurements of oxygen tension near the leading fibroblasts suggest that oxygen supply is at the lower limit for migration and too low for replication or protein synthesis. Therefore, the activities of fibroblasts depend on the rate at which new capillaries are formed. Anything that interferes with this process interferes with wound healing.

Uremia

Uremia decreases wound healing by altering enzyme systems, biochemical pathways, and cellular metabolism.

Anti-Inflammatory Drugs
Phenylbutazone, Aspirin, and Indomethacin

These commonly used anti-inflammatory agents have no effect on the course or quality of wound healing if they are administered in pharmacological doses.

Steroids

Cortisone and its derivatives decrease the rate of protein synthesis, stabilize lysosomal membranes, and inhibit the normal inflammatory reaction. High doses limit capillary budding, inhibit fibroblast proliferation, and decrease the rate of epithelialization. Generally, even with high doses of steroids, wound healing proceeds to completion, although at a slower rate.

Vitamins and Minerals
Vitamin A

Vitamin A stimulates fibroblasts and the accumulation of collagen; however, there is no evidence that administration of vitamin A alters the wound healing rate in animals not under the influence of steroids or vitamin E.

Vitamin E

Vitamin E, like cortisone, stabilizes membranes. High doses of vitamin E significantly retard wound healing and collagen production.

Vitamin C

Deficiency of vitamin C delays wound healing. Without vitamin C, collagen molecules remain incomplete and may not be secreted by fibroblasts. Dogs and cats are among the animals that do not require exogenous sources of vitamin C.

Cytotoxic Drugs and Radiation

Most cytotoxic drugs have their greatest effect on dividing cells. Systemic administration rarely produces high enough wound concentrations to influence cell division. However, chronic local application of these agents can prevent wound healing.

All radiant energy of short enough wavelength to change nuclear DNA and RNA is destructive. The effects of radiation on surrounding tissue are closure of precapillary shunts, vascular bed flooding, and a change in capillary permeability.

When considering adjunctive radiation therapy, a surgeon must weigh the beneficial effects of early radiation in treating a neoplasm against its detrimental effects on wound healing. If potential complications (e.g., wound dehiscence) of immediate postoperative radiation are unacceptable, radiation therapy should be delayed for 2 weeks to allow wound healing to begin.

Dehydration and Edema

Dehydration delays wound healing. Edema does not inhibit wound healing, but the factors that initiate edema do.

Infection

Infection delays healing. Bacteria produce collagenases that degrade collagen, and this effect, in combination with granulocyte and macrophage collagenases, may account for decreased wound strength.

Antiseptics

Antiseptics are lethal to fibroblasts and PMNs, cause capillary shutdown, inhibit epithelialization and granulation tissue formation, increase wound infection rates, and decrease wound strength. Only isotonic solutions should be directly applied to wounds.

TISSUE REGENERATION (pp. 60–62)

There is a relationship between the degree of tissue differentiation and its regenerative capacity. Generally, the more differentiated cells (e.g., neurons) do not regenerate, whereas less well differentiated cells (e.g., epithelial cells) are capable of dividing and replacing themselves.

Regeneration of Selected Tissues

Liver

The liver has the capacity to regenerate after 70 to 80 per cent of its volume is removed. Regeneration begins within 24 hours of partial hepatectomy and peaks in 3 days. The liver's weight usually returns to normal in about 6 weeks after 70 per cent hepatectomy.

Skeletal Muscle

Skeletal muscle is composed of many individual muscle fibers. Each muscle fiber is contained within a limiting membrane called the *sarcolemma*.

The degree of repair after injury can usually be directly related to the degree of sarcolemmal and endomysial derangement. Muscle regeneration does not occur to its fullest when even modest amounts of fibrous tissue are interposed between ends of growing fibers.

If significant muscle mass has been lost or if the ends of transected muscle cannot be accurately apposed, healing will occur by fibrous union between the transected muscle ends rather than by true regeneration.

Smooth Muscle

Smooth-muscle cells regenerate in cell cultures, and smooth-muscle cells and fibers have been found in healing wounds of blood vessels, the intestine, the urinary tract, and the uterus. The most likely explanation for the "new" smooth-muscle cells is that they are the result of hypertrophy, migration, and differentiation from connective tissue cells.

Epithelium and Endothelium

All body surfaces are covered with epithelium, including internal surfaces such as the genitourinary tract, gastrointestinal tract, and respiratory tract. The epithelial cells that line the heart, blood vessels, lymph vessels, and serous cavities of the body are referred to as *endothelium*. The process begins with mobilization of cells at the wound edge. The epithelial cells migrate down and across the wound, followed by increased mitosis of the basal cells. This process continues until migrating cells bridge the gap.

Peripheral Nerves

The entire process of nerve regeneration hinges on the survival of the nerve cell after injury. Shortly after birth, mitosis and division of nerve cells stop, and no new cells are formed during the rest of an individual's life.

Each nerve fiber is an extension of the cytoplasm and cell membrane of a neuron whose cell body may be as far away as a meter from the ending of the nerve fiber. The closer a lesion is to the cell body and the greater the distance between the cell body and the peripheral receptors, the greater the likelihood of diminishing functional results.

A surgeon can aid the processes of nerve regeneration by removing damaged tissue from the injury site, excising epineurium that could produce an obstructive scar, and properly coapting the nerve ends to reduce loss of regenerating fibers.

CHAPTER 5

Nutritional Support of Hospitalized Patients (pages 63–83)

Disease-induced anorexia results from interruption of the normal mechanisms that control food intake. Loss of appetite can be caused by a wide variety of medical problems, including fear, stress, organic disease, inflammation, trauma, and neoplasia. Patients with chronic diseases often lose their appetite and become nutrient depleted as the disease progresses. Animals with facial injuries or obstruction of the gastrointestinal tract may not eat because they are physically incapable of taking in, chewing, or swallowing food.

METABOLIC RESPONSE TO STARVATION (pp. 63–65)

The pathways shown in Figure 5–1, are coordinated to ensure maintenance of normal blood glucose concentrations, protein turnover, and

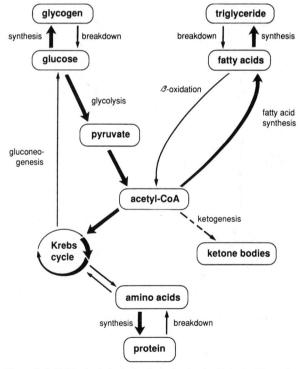

Figure 5–1. Nutrient substrate flux in fed animals. (Adapted from de Bruijne JJ: Ketone-body metabolism in fasting dogs. PhD dissertation, Utrecht, 1982.)

storage of excess ingested nutrients as triglyceride. Absence of food intake essentially reverses the pathways of anabolism, as shown in Figure 5–2. The metabolic response to starvation in dogs is somewhat different from that in food-deprived rats and humans.

The normal metabolic alterations of starvation do not occur in anorectic ill animals because of the superimposed disease stress. The initial metabolic events in these circumstances consist of mobilization of glycogen and lipid fuel stores: the ''fight or flight response.'' In hospitalized patients, no physical activity occurs to use the released energy substrates. The metabolic rate often declines initially. This phase of the response to injury has been called the *ebb phase*. The ebb period consists of massive sympathoadrenal discharge, and it typically lasts approximately 24 hours in human beings, depending on the severity of the injury and the treatment given.

If a patient survives the ebb phase, it proceeds into a more prolonged *flow phase*, characterized by increased metabolic rate and enhanced breakdown of lean body mass. The intensity and time course of this phase vary depending on the severity of the injury and have not been well defined for veterinary patients.

Protein (nitrogen) and amino acid metabolism are also affected by stress and trauma; an effective response requires movement of amino acids from peripheral tissues (primarily muscle) to the viscera. These

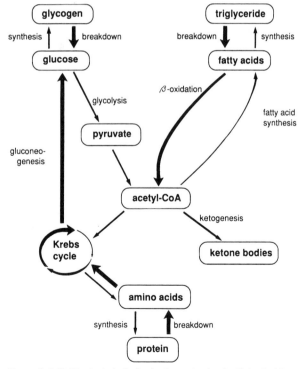

Figure 5–2. Nutrient substrate flux in starved animals. (Adapted from de Bruijne JJ: Ketone-body metabolism in fasting dogs. PhD dissertation. Utrecht, 1982.)

amino acids are used for gluconeogenesis, acute phase protein synthesis, wound healing, and immune function.

Although acute phase protein synthesis and plasma concentration are increasing, the plasma concentration of other proteins, including transferrin and albumin, is declining. The decrement in serum albumin concentration also results from an increase in the transcapillary escape rate. Hypoalbuminemia in severe injury and sepsis is often related to large, sustained increases in extracellular, extravascular water content and *not* to enhanced catabolism or depressed synthesis.

NUTRIENT REQUIREMENTS (pp. 65–68)

Water

Healthy animals can survive large losses of body fat and protein, yet the acute loss of 10 to 15 per cent of body water may be lethal. Water is necessary for temperature regulation and heat dispersal, transportation of nutrients and metabolic endproducts, and participation in chemical reactions. Dogs and cats require 50 to 100 ml of water per kilogram of body weight for daily maintenance, depending on environmental temperature, type of food, and level of activity. Dogs eating canned foods can obtain most of their total daily water intake from food, and cats eating canned food may not need to drink at all.

During anorexia, absence of the solute load of the diet causes water needs to decline significantly. Water requirements for ''maintenance'' of anorexic animals are only about 10 ml/kg of body weight per day.

Approximately 7 per cent of total water intake is excreted in the feces. The total daily volume of digestive secretions is greater than the plasma volume, but most of this fluid is reabsorbed along with the products of digestion. In the absence of diarrhea, fecal water loss from inappetent animals is minimal.

Approximately 70 per cent of daily water intake is excreted in urine. Because of the concentrating ability of the kidneys, decreased water intake is compensated for by reabsorption of nearly all filtered water and by excretion of small volumes of highly concentrated urine.

Insensible losses account for about 25 per cent of total water intake and production. In normal animals, the rate of loss is determined primarily by the environmental temperature and amount of exercise.

Energy

Caloric needs to maintain body substance depend on the rate of energy use. Basal energy requirements are those of an animal lying quietly in the postabsorptive state in a thermoneutral environment. Energy requirements of normal dogs have been estimated, but few actual determinations of energy expenditure of sick dogs are available. In the absence of direct measurements, estimates are made by accounting for requirements for basal metabolism, nutrient assimilation, body temperature maintenance, activity, and effects of disease.

Caloric needs of stressed, inappetent animals are for basal needs plus the effects of disease. Increased body temperature also increases energy expenditure in ill patients.

Energy needs may be estimated by assuming resting animals have basal energy needs, determined from Figure 5–3. This value is multiplied by the estimated degree of disease-related hypermetabolism: 1.25 times for mild, 1.5 times for moderate, and 2 times basal for severely hypermetabolic patients. Attempt to reach energy intake equal to the basal rate in 24 hours and to meet total estimated needs 48 hours after institution of nutritional therapy.

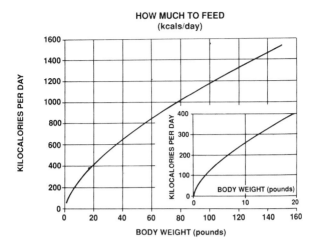

Figure 5-3. Approximate basal energy needs of dogs and cats. (Data from Abrams JT: The nutrition of the dog. *In* Rechcigl M (ed): *CRC Handbook.* CRC Press, Boca Raton, 1977, pp 1–27.)

Protein

Approximately half the body protein provides structural support: bones, tendons, and cartilage. The rest is present as muscle, plasma, and visceral protein. Proteins in metabolically active tissues are maintained in a dynamic steady state of constant synthesis and breakdown; the greater the importance of a protein in metabolic regulation, the more rapid its turnover.

Because reuse of amino acids released during protein degradation for new protein synthesis is inefficient, some are constantly lost. The more rapid the turnover rate, the more rapidly amino acids must be replaced. The diet normally provides amino acids and nitrogen to replace these daily losses, but in anorectic patients, the only source is body protein. After the first 2 or 3 days, muscle proteins are broken down. Normal animals lose approximately 1.2 to 1.6 g of protein per kilogram of body weight per day when adapted to starvation.

In disease, this adaptation does not occur, leading to large losses of nitrogen. Severely stressed patients may be unable to provide sufficient amino acids for high-priority protein synthesis, resulting in decreased wound healing, erythropoiesis, and immune function.

Minerals and Vitamins

Vitamin and mineral needs of hospitalized patients depend on the type and severity of disease. Oral diets for nutritional support contain necessary minerals, so supplementation is not necessary. Additions for intravenous solutions are discussed later.

PATIENT SELECTION (p. 68)

Identification of patients needing nutritional support is based on the history, physical examination, and laboratory evaluation. No single parameter is a dependable marker of malnutrition.

History

Important historical information includes types and amounts of all foods eaten; appetite and frequency of eating; recent weight changes; presence of vomiting, regurgitation, diarrhea, or constipation; and difficulty in chewing or swallowing food. Type and dosage of medication, including nutritional supplements, are determined.

Physical

Physical examination starts with determining the body condition. In underweight animals, one sees loss of subcutaneous fat, muscle wasting, easily pluckable hair, and thin, dry skin. Pressure sores and poor wound healing may be noted. Ill animals may have an "overcoat syndrome": disproportionate loss of lean versus fat body mass and may appear normal.

Laboratory

Serum albumin concentrations and total lymphocyte counts may provide information about nutritional status. The plasma half-life of albumin is 8.2 days in dogs. The serum albumin concentration is also affected by hydration status, vascular permeability, and the presence of gastrointestinal, liver, and kidney disease. The total lymphocyte count is a crude marker of immune status that may be depressed by protein depletion.

TREATMENT (pp. 69–81)

Fluids

The three goals of fluid therapy are rehydration and treatment of shock, electrolyte replacement, and normalization of acid-base status. Feeding begins only after these three goals are achieved (see Chapter 2).

Nutritional Support

There are two ways of providing nutrients: via the gastrointestinal tract or parenterally. The oral route should be used whenever possible.

A primary objective of nutrition support is to have an animal eating its own food in its own environment. The next best situation is for an animal to eat its own food in the hospital. Owners should be encouraged to provide and feed patients their normal food; animals are more likely to eat for owners than for strangers.

Food Intake Stimulation

Two commonly recommended pharmacological methods of stimulating eating are vitamin B injections and appetite-stimulating drugs. There is no evidence that administration of any of the individual B vitamins or combinations of them stimulates food intake in sick dogs or cats.

Psychogenic, fear-induced anorexia is common in dogs and cats in hospitalized situations because of the strange surroundings and personnel and the stress of disease and trauma. Administration of 0.2 mg/kg of body weight of diazepam intravenously stimulates food intake in these settings.

Other drugs, including glucocorticoids and the anabolic steroids, have been recommended to stimulate appetite. None of these drugs have been tested in controlled trials in veterinary patients; none are demonstrated to be of consistent value.

When an animal is in unfamiliar surroundings among strangers and is being subjected to unpleasant diagnostic procedures, fear-induced inhibition of food intake should be expected. Staying with an animal and encouraging it by petting and vocal reassurance may be sufficient to stimulate food intake. Warming the food to body temperature to enhance aroma or changing the type of food may be necessary. If dry foods have been offered, a canned, premium quality food may be more palatable. If an animal's nasal passages are occluded, clean them with warmed saline.

Force-Feeding (p. 70)

If all attempts to induce an animal to eat fail, force-feeding may be necessary.

Enteral Feeding

If a patient is too debilitated to tolerate repeated tube feedings, if feeding needs to continue for more than 2 to 3 days, or if the disease prevents periodic intubation, a nasogastric tube may be used. A nasogastric tube allows provision of fluid and nutritional support for extended periods of time.

Pharyngostomy

If the disease or injury prevents using the nasogastric route, or if a prolonged course of enteral feeding is anticipated, a feeding enterostomy may be created. Cervical pharyngostomy feeding tubes permit feeding of patients that have a functional gastrointestinal tract and no history of vomiting or regurgitation but that are unwilling or unable to eat. Pharyngostomy tubes are specifically indicated for patients requiring bypass of the oral cavity or oropharynx due to dysphagia, infection, inflammation, neoplasia, surgical procedures, or trauma.

Pharyngostomy tubes can be maintained for weeks with conscientious nursing care. A small amount of drainage may occur at the tube site. The surgical wound is cleaned and bandaged daily or every other day. Complications associated with pharyngostomy feeding tubes include hemorrhage, local infection and swelling, recurrent laryngeal nerve injury, epiglottic entrapment, laryngeal obstruction, respiratory stridor, coughing, vomiting, aspiration of food, esophageal erosion or esophagitis, gastroesophageal reflux, and premature displacement or occlusion of the tube.

Gastrostomy

When nutrient intake proximal to the stomach cannot occur in patients with normal gastrointestinal function, a gastrostomy feeding tube is an excellent method of temporary or permanent nutritional support. Gastrostomy feeding tubes are specifically indicated in patients that are comatose or that require bypass of the oral cavity, larynx, oral pharynx, and esophagus because of neurological or neuromuscular diseases, dysphagia, neoplasia, obstruction, inflammation, or stricture.

Gastrostomy feeding tubes are generally placed through a limited left paracostal laparotomy. Complications associated with the placement and maintenance of gastrostomy feeding tubes include leakage of food or fluid around the feeding tube, resulting in peritonitis, necrotizing fasciitis or subcutaneous abscess, vomiting, regurgitation, gastroesophageal reflux, aspiration pneumonia, and premature tube displacement. It is critical that the stomach not be overdistended to prevent vomiting or regurgitation, which would require feeding to be discontinued. Smaller and more frequent feedings may be required during the initial feeding of severely malnourished patients. Pharmacological stimulation of motility with drugs such as metoclopramide may stimulate gastric emptying.

Jejunostomy

When gastric atony, gastroduodenal obstruction, neoplasia, regurgitation, or vomiting prevents feeding via more proximal sites, a needle catheter jejunostomy may be placed. Patients requiring extensive surgical procedures of the stomach, duodenum, pancreas, or hepatobiliary system also can be provided with immediate postoperative nutritional support using this technique. Contraindications to jejunostomy feeding include adynamic ileus of the small intestine, persistent diarrhea, and intestinal obstruction distal to the feeding tube.

Complications associated with jejunostomy feeding tubes include diarrhea, excessive hemorrhage, infection, premature displacement of the feeding tube, and leakage of bowel contents or feeding solutions around the catheter into the peritoneal cavity or subcutaneously. Jejunostomy feeding tubes should also remain in place for at least 5 to 7 days to allow adhesion formation.

Diets

The choice of appropriate diet depends on disease-related nutrient modifications. Commercial products for enteral support fall into three groups—polymeric, defined formula, and concentrated sources of one nutrient: protein, fat, or carbohydrate.

Rate and Volume of Feeding

Anorectic patients may have decreased gastrointestinal functional capacity. The calculated goal for nutrients and fluids is approached over 48 hours to avoid vomiting, abdominal discomfort, and diarrhea. Slow rates of administration, particularly in patients that have been inappetent for prolonged periods, avoid diarrhea and cramping and maximize uptake of nutrients. Small volumes ($\leq$12-hour supply) of diet suspended in a fluid therapy buret or a gavage set minimize "overdosing" with excessive volumes of feeding solution.

Problems

Problems with enteral feeding are divided into mechanical, gastrointestinal, and metabolic. Mechanical problems are related to placement and maintenance of the tube. Nasogastric tubes must be flushed with water before feeding to confirm that the tube is still in position. Clogging is best prevented by prohibiting use of the tube for administration of nonliquid materials and properly flushing and capping it after use.

Most gastrointestinal problems caused by enteral feeding are due to too rapid administration of the solution or administration of solutions of high osmolality. When nutrient solutions enter the duodenum too rapidly, they cause vomiting, cramps, and diarrhea by overwhelming the normal neural and endocrine gastrointestinal control mechanisms. Hyperosmolar solutions cause rapid fluid and electrolyte influx into the gut lumen, leading to cramping and abdominal distension.

CHAPTER 6
Surgical Wound Infection and Use of Antibiotics (pages 84–95)

The proliferating use of antibiotics has not eliminated infection. Reducing infection to a minimum requires an understanding of the factors that determine whether an infection will occur in a wound.

DETERMINANTS OF WOUND INFECTION (p. 84)

All wounds are contaminated. A critical level of bacterial contamination is required before a wound infection results. The critical level of contamination for most bacteria is approximately 10^5 organisms per gram of tissue. Circumstances can significantly reduce the numbers of contaminating bacteria required to produce infection in a wound. Blood clots, ischemic tissue, pockets of fluid, and foreign materials all may inhibit normal body defenses and significantly decrease the numbers of contaminating microorganisms necessary.

Studies have shown little correlation between bacteria isolated from the operating room air, from surfaces in the operating room, from the wound at the conclusion of the surgery, and the bacteria eventually cultured from a postoperative wound infection. Considerable evidence supports the assumption that bacteria from a patient account for the majority of wound infections.

HOST DEFENSE MECHANISMS (pp. 84–85)

Normal host defense mechanisms are a complex combination of humoral factors present in wound fluid and phagocytic cells, predominately neutrophils, that migrate into the wound. Surgery is a severe injury that causes an immediate and sustained increase in capillary permeability in tissue at the wound site. Closure of the wound creates a compartment that rapidly fills with fluid. This wound fluid is a serosanguineous exudate derived from blood plasma as part of the acute inflammation caused by surgery. This fluid, along with the interstitial fluid in tissue at the perimeter of the wound, is the site of microorganism–host defense interaction and is the location of postoperative wound infection.

The single most important host defense against infection in the surgical wound is neutrophils. Within 10 hours after closure of an incision in a dog, the concentration of neutrophils in surgical wound fluid exceeds the concentrations of neutrophils in the blood. Neutrophils squeeze through blood vessel walls at the margins of a wound, migrate toward chemoattractants at the site of contamination, phagocytize bacteria with the help of complement and other opsonizing proteins, and kill bacteria by several intracellular mechanisms.

The second line of phagocytic response is macrophages, mobile cells with a long half-life. Macrophages, like neutrophils, require antibody and complement for effective phagocytosis. After phagocytosis and digestion by a macrophage, microbial antigens are presented to lymphocytes for specific antibody production.

INCIDENCE OF SURGICAL WOUND INFECTION (p. 85)

Wounds are classified on an estimate of contamination. Four categories are generally described (Table 6–1).

USE OF ANTIBIOTICS (pp. 85–89)

The use of antibiotics for treatment is perhaps less controversial than the use of prophylaxis.

Adverse Effects of Antibiotic Administration

The adverse reactions produced by antibiotics are of three types: toxic effects, hypersensitivity reactions, and biological alterations affecting the microbial system. No antibiotic now available is entirely free of side effects; these reactions may be induced in various degrees by their administration. The major toxic effects and hypersensitivity reactions of commonly used antibiotics are listed in Table 6–2.

In addition to causing adverse effects on individual patients, the injudicious use of antibiotics may contribute to the emergence of resistant bacterial strains. Drug-resistant bacteria that are selected by pressure of antibiotics are at a disadvantage, however slight, when the antibiotic is removed. Antibiotics should be used for the shortest time possible to minimize the risk of resistant mutant strains.

Mechanisms of Action

A working knowledge of the mechanisms of action of various antimicrobials becomes important when treating different types of wound

TABLE 6–1. WOUND CLASSIFICATION*

Clean	Nontraumatic
	No inflammation encountered
	No break in technique
	Respiratory, alimentary, genitourinary tracts not entered
Clean-contaminated	Gastrointestinal or respiratory tracts entered without significant spillage
	Oropharynx entered
	Vagina entered
	Genitourinary tract entered in absence of infected urine
	Biliary tract entered in absence of infected bile
	Minor break in technique
Contaminated	Major break in technique
	Gross spillage from gastrointestinal tract
	Traumatic wound, fresh
	Entrance of genitourinary tract or biliary tract in presence of infected urine or bile
Dirty	Acute bacterial inflammation encountered
	Transection of "clean" tissues for the purpose of surgical access to a collection of pus
	Traumatic wound with retained devitalized tissue, foreign bodies, fecal contamination, and/or delayed treatment

*Based on recommendations of the Committee on Control of Surgical Infections of the Committee on Pre- and Postoperative Care of the American College of Surgeons.

TABLE 6-2. ADVERSE EFFECTS OF COMMON ANTIMICROBIAL AGENTS

Drug	Adverse Effects
Bactericidal Drugs	
Penicillins	Hypersensitivity reactions: cutaneous eruptions, fever, angioedema, and anaphylaxis
	Mild GI problems: anorexia, vomiting
Cephalosporins	Hypersensitivity reactions, cross-reactivity with penicillins
	Minor GI problems: anorexia, vomiting
Aminoglycosides	Nephrotoxicity, potentially fatal (predisposing factors are dehydration and fever; synergistic toxicity seen with simultaneous administration of flunixin or furosemide)
	Ototoxicity, not well recognized in veterinary medicine; cats are more susceptible than dogs; exhibited as vestibular signs
Fluoroquinolones	Articular cartilage erosion in immature animals
	Mild GI problems: anorexia, vomiting
	CNS signs: confusion, dizziness
Metronidazole	Dose-dependent CNS signs: anorexia and vomiting progressing to ataxia and nystagmus
Trimethoprim/sulfonamides	Keratoconjunctivitis sicca
	Idiosyncratic reactions*: polyarthritis, fever, lymphadenopathy, cutaneous eruptions, hepatitis, focal retinitis, blood dyscrasias (anemia, leukopenia, thrombocytopenia), glomerulonephritis
Vancomycin	Ototoxicity, primarily the auditory nerve; deafness
	Hypersensitivity reactions: skin reactions, fever, anaphylaxis
	Thrombophlebitis at the injection site

Rifampin	Mild GI problems: anorexia, vomiting
	Cutaneous reactions, mild pruritus
	Turns body fluids red-orange (e.g., urine, tears, saliva, feces)
	Induces hepatic microsomal enzymes that may alter concurrent drug metabolism and/or progress to clinical hepatitis

Bacteriostatic Drugs

Tetracyclines	Mild GI problems, especially in cats
	Discoloration of erupting teeth
	Localization in newly formed bone
	Nephrotoxicity: ultrastructural changes in the renal proximal tubules, decreased concentrating ability
Chloramphenicol	GI problems: anorexia, vomiting
	Inhibition of drug-transforming enzymes
	Drug-related, reversible, bone marrow suppression with aplastic anemia and other dyscrasias possible
	Immune response alteration/inhibition
Macrolides	Dose-related GI problems
Erythromycin	Pain and swelling at the injection site
Tylosin	
Lincosamides	Minor GI problems, especially in cats
Lincomycin	Dose-dependent neuromuscular blockade leading to skeletal muscle paralysis
Clindamycin	

*Idiosyncratic reactions are unpredictable and can occur at appropriate dosages and dosing intervals. These reactions may depend on the type of sulfonamide used. Doberman pinschers seem to be predisposed to these reactions.

CNS, central nervous system; GI, gastrointestinal.

41

infection. Finally, combinations of bactericidal and bacteriostatic agents may antagonize each other.

ANTIMICROBIAL PROPHYLAXIS IN SURGERY (pp. 89–90)

Although antibiotics can be important in decreasing postoperative wound infection, the best way to reduce the incidence of surgical infection is to use excellent surgical technique. Antibiotics are not a substitute for asepsis, gentle handling of tissue, meticulous hemostasis, judicious use of suture materials, and accurate apposition of tissue without obstructing blood supply. In selected surgical procedures, prophylactic antibiotics in appropriate doses should be used.

The use of antibiotics to prevent infection is indicated in surgical procedures that have a high risk of infection (greater than 5 per cent) and in surgical procedures in which the consequences of infection seriously endanger a patient or the success of an operation.

Antibiotics selected for antimicrobial prophylaxis must be effective against the microorganism most likely to cause postoperative wound infection.

The importance of timing of the administration of antibiotics for surgical prophylaxis has been confirmed by experimental and clinical studies. Antibiotics should be present in the tissue at the surgical site during the time of bacterial contamination. The major antibiotic effect is over in approximately 1 hour, and systemic antibiotics have no effect on primary bacterial infection if the bacteria creating the lesion have been in the tissue longer than 3 hours before the antibiotic is given.

There is no reason to begin administration of an antibiotic before the operation or to continue the administration of the drug afterward. There is no evidence that continuing antibiotics after the immediate postoperative period decreases the incidence of wound infection.

PRINCIPLES OF ANTIMICROBIAL THERAPY (pp. 90–91)

Rational selection of an antibiotic to treat infection requires that two questions be answered:

1. What microorganism is most likely responsible for causing the infection?
2. To what antibiotic is this microorganism likely to be susceptible?

In dogs, osteomyelitis and surgical wound infections that do not involve the alimentary canal are most commonly caused by staphylococci. Intra-abdominal sepsis, traumatic wounds, and surgical wound infections involving or near the alimentary canal are often polymicrobial, with *Escherichia coli* being the prominent microorganism found. In cats, the bacteria most commonly responsible for soft-tissue infection, including traumatic wounds, are *Pasteurella* spp.

When selecting an antibiotic from several that may be effective against the probable pathogen(s), choose the antibiotic that is the least expensive, least toxic, and most convenient to administer. As a general rule, antibiotic treatment should be carried out for a minimum of 3 days and continued for 2 to 3 days after body temperature returns to normal and other signs of infection have subsided.

In many surgical infections, a cure is not achieved with antibiotic therapy alone. In such situations, the antibiotic administration is a valuable adjunct to surgical therapy. This situation pertains when large amounts of pus, exudate, necrotic or avascular infected tissue, or foreign bodies are present.

ANAEROBIC INFECTIONS (pp. 91–94)
Bacteriology

Anaerobic bacteria are now recognized as important causes of infection, often occurring with facultative aerobic bacteria. These mixed infections typically result from contamination with normal flora of the mouth, upper respiratory tract, lower gastrointestinal tract, and occasionally the skin.

Pathogenesis

In general, most anaerobic infections arise endogenously, usually as a result of contamination with indigenous flora. Clostridial wound infections, which usually occur secondary to wound contamination by clostridial spores or organisms present in the environment, are an important exception to this rule. The bacterial wound flora is distinctly different from normal flora, suggesting that those pathogenic anaerobes most often isolated from wounds possess factors that favor their growth and multiplication in tissues once they gain access.

Healthy tissues are resistant to anaerobic infection by virtue of both high redox potential and high oxygen tensions. Anaerobic infection may develop, however, when these defenses are impaired, especially by compromised blood supply and tissue death.

Clinical Syndromes

Clostridial wound infection, although uncommon, is an important sequel to wound contamination because if not treated appropriately, it may be rapidly fatal. The most important infection is clostridial myonecrosis, caused by *Clostridium perfringens*. Infection develops very rapidly, is characterized by excessive toxin production and massive muscle necrosis, and in some cases may not be associated with gas production; septic shock frequently develops as well.

Oropharyngeal infections are often mixed infections containing obligate anaerobes and facultative bacteria that have originated from oropharyngeal mucous membranes. Submandibular abscesses and necrotizing ulcerative gingivitis are typical examples.

Chronic pleuropulmonary infections (pyothorax, lung abscess, consolidating aspiration pneumonia) of dogs and cats are in many instances primarily anaerobic. These infections most likely originate as foreign bodies migrate caudally from the mouth or after bite wounds to the thorax; the result in either case is introduction of oral bacteria into the pleural space, which provides a favorable environment for anaerobic growth.

Other infections frequently associated with anaerobic bacteria in dogs and cats include peritoneal infections, chronic osteomyelitis, pyometra, chronic sinusitis, and brain abscess and subdural empyema.

Diagnosis

Anaerobic cultures are technically difficult, and culture results are often delayed. Therefore, a tentative diagnosis is usually made based on clinical features of the infection (Table 6–3) and the results of cytological examination of Gram-stained wound exudates. The presence of multiple types of bacteria, together with purulent inflammation, is strong presumptive evidence of anaerobic infection.

Treatment

Effective management of most anaerobic infections still relies primarily on drainage of pus and débridement of devitalized tissues. By so

TABLE 6–3. CLINICAL HINTS SUGGESTING
ANAEROBIC INFECTION

Foul-smelling exudate

Necrotic tissue; gangrene

Gas in wounds

Infections after bite wounds

Chronic osteomyelitis, especially after open fractures

Infections from penetrating foreign bodies

Infections associated with solid tumors

Bacteria seen on a Gram stain that fail to grow on routine culture

Endocarditis with negative routine blood cultures

Blackish discoloration of exudate; may fluoresce red under ultraviolet
    light if *Bacteroides melaninogenicus* is present

Sulfur granules in discharges (actinomycotic granules)

Infections nonresponsive to aminoglycosides, polymyxins,
    sulfonamides

Delayed-onset pneumonia after aspiration

Closed-space infections: pyothorax, pyometra, brain abscess, lung
    abscess, intra-abdominal abscess

Infections characterized by very high fever and white blood cell counts

Subacute onset of inflammation in a previously contaminated area (e.g.,
    after bowel surgery)

From Dow SW, et al: Anaerobic infections. *Comp Cont Educ Pract Vet* 9:828,
1987.

doing, tissue oxygenation is improved, environmental conditions favorable for anaerobic growth are eliminated, and blood flow to tissues is improved. Antimicrobial selection for treatment of anaerobic infections remains largely empirical.

Penicillins remain effective against most anaerobic pathogens, with the exception of *Bacteroides* and some strains of *Fusobacterium* and *Clostridium.*

Clindamycin is active against most anaerobes (including penicillin-resistant strains of *Bacteroides*), is well absorbed orally, and is widely distributed. Clindamycin penetrates well into tissues (including abscess cavities) and also reaches effective intracellular concentrations within leukocytes. Clinically, clindamycin is effective in oropharyngeal and pleuropulmonary infections of both dogs and cats and may be the drug of choice for pyothorax.

Metronidazole has the most consistent activity against *Bacteroides* and most other anaerobic pathogens, with the exception of *Actinomyces* and microaerophilic streptococci. Metronidazole is inactive against nearly all aerobic bacteria.

Chloramphenicol is active against nearly all strains of anaerobic bacteria, including *Bacteroides* and *Clostridium*, is well absorbed orally, and penetrates well into tissues.

Most cephalosporin antibiotics are ineffective against both *Bacteroides* and *Clostridium*. However, both cefoxitin and cefotetan (second-generation cephalosporins) are active against a broad range of anaerobic pathogens, as well as against aerobic gram-positive cocci and most gram-negative bacillary pathogens. These drugs are therefore useful as single-agent treatment of mixed infections, especially intra-abdominal infections.

CHAPTER 7

Organ Transplantation in Clinical Veterinary Practice
(pages 95–101)

Three overlapping "types" of organ rejection are recognized clinically. Hyperacute rejection is accelerated rejection associated with preformed circulatory antibody in the serum of the recipient that reacts with donor cells, particularly the endothelium of vessel walls. Polymorphonuclear leukocytes line the capillary walls, and most capillaries and arterioles are blocked by microthrombi, resulting in tissue necrosis. In hyperacute rejection, the recipient has been sensitized to the allograft antigens by previous blood transfusions, pregnancy, or transplantation.

Acute rejection occurs 7 to 21 days after transplantation or when effective immunosuppression is terminated. Pathological studies of the rejected organ reveal a predominant pattern of mononuclear leukocyte infiltration in the tissue.

Chronic rejection is characterized by gradual loss of organ function over months to years, often without any clear-cut clinical rejection. Kidneys undergoing chronic rejection show severe narrowing of numerous arteries and thickening of the glomerular capillary basement membrane. The lesions are formed by adherence of platelets and fibrin aggregates to the vessel walls. These deposits become covered by endothelium and incorporated in the intima, which often contains IgM and complement.

Without the use of immunosuppressive agents, matching the donor and recipient for similar or identical cell surface histocompatibility antigens prolongs allograft survival. Siblings may be matched (25 per cent), partially matched (50 per cent), or mismatched (25 per cent).

PROTOCOL FOR RENAL TRANSPLANTATION: CATS
(pp. 96–99)

Criteria for a Suitable Renal Recipient

Renal transplantation is one method of treatment for renal insufficiency. It cannot be regarded as an emergency treatment or last-ditch effort to save the life of a critically ill, malnourished patient. Surgical intervention has to take place before all medical means of therapy have been exhausted.

Body weight is an important indication of the status of a renal transplant candidate. If a cat has been in compensated renal failure and starts to lose body weight or is presented in renal failure with a history of chronic weight loss, transplantation is considered as an option before further weight loss occurs. Age, plasma creatinine levels, blood urea nitrogen values, and other clinical pathological assessments of renal function cannot identify patients suitable for transplantation. Candidates for renal transplantation should be free of bacterial urinary tract infection.

Feline candidates for renal transplantation should be free of feline leukemia virus infection and other complicating diseases. Cardiac enlargement determined by ultrasonographic examination, gallop rhythms, or electrocardiographic abnormalities all are indications to decline a candidate for transplantation.

The feline renal donor/recipient pair do not have to be related or tissue matched but must be blood crossmatched.

Criteria for the Renal Donor

The renal donor should be in excellent health and have no evidence of renal insufficiency based on clinical pathological testing; a complete blood count, serum chemistry panel, and urinalysis are performed. The feline donor should be free of feline leukemia virus infection and have blood compatible with the recipient. The renal donor has a normal life expectancy after unilateral nephrectomy.

Preoperative Preparation of a Recipient

Before surgery, a renal recipient is given balanced electrolyte solutions subcutaneously or intravenously at 1.5 to 2 times daily maintenance requirements. Whole blood transfusions are administered until a packed red blood cell volume of 30 per cent is achieved. Twenty-four to 48 hours before surgery, cyclosporine oral solution is administered. In cats, a level of 500 ng/ml is maintained for the first 30 postoperative days, reducing to 250 ng/ml by 3 months after transplantation. Prednisolone is also started the morning of surgery.

Surgery

Two teams perform renal transplantation. The two-team approach minimizes the warm ischemia time of the donor kidney, which is kept to less than 60 minutes.

Postoperative Care

The recipient receives balanced electrolyte solutions intravenously at a daily maintenance rate until eating and drinking resume. Cyclosporine is administered in amounts necessary to achieve whole blood levels of 500 ng/ml. Prednisolone is administered in tapering doses.

During the early postoperative period, needless venipuncture, blood sampling, and handling of patients is avoided. If the operation is a technical success, the urine specific gravity is increased and plasma creatinine level decreased by the third postoperative day.

Long-term Management

Management of a transplant recipient must be coordinated with the client, a local veterinarian(s), and the transplant center. Packed blood cell volume, total serum protein, plasma creatinine, and whole blood cyclosporine values are determined, and a urinalysis is performed.

PROTOCOL FOR RENAL TRANSPLANTATION: DOGS
(p. 99)

The primary difference in transplantation between dogs and cats is selection of a donor. Using cyclosporine and prednisolone to achieve immunosuppression, we use only mixed lymphocyte response matched, related donors.

CHAPTER 8
Trauma: Epidemiology and Mechanisms (pages 101–105)

TYPES (pp. 101–102)

Eight categories of trauma were defined and studied in dogs and cats at two institutional practices (Table 8–1).

INCIDENCE (p. 102)

The incidence of trauma among pet animals is unknown. In two studies, trauma was responsible for about 13 per cent of hospital accessions. However, these figures do not account for animals that were not brought in for attention because of the minor nature of the injury, early death, or neglect.

MECHANISMS OF TRAUMA (pp. 102–104)

All the energy delivered to an organism is absorbed and changed. The larger the volume of tissue involved, the greater the amount of energy that can be absorbed without damage because the stress per unit of volume of tissue is smaller. In addition to volume, the strength and physical characteristics of tissue involved play a part in wounding. Tissue strength is related to the amount of elastin, collagen, and water present. Whether or not the tissue is strong enough to absorb and dissipate the applied energy depends not only on the intermolecular

TABLE 8–1. TRAUMA AMONG URBAN AND SUBURBAN DOGS AND CATS*

	Urban		Suburban	
	Dogs	*Cats*	*Dogs*	*Cats*
Motor vehicle accidents	53.2	17.9	53.5	28.6
Unknown cause	12.2	36.5	17.0	25.7
Animal interactions	11.1	16.0	13.9	22.8
Sharp objects	11.2	3.2	5.3	11.4
Falls from height	6.3	13.5	3.8	2.8
Crush	2.6	10.9	0.8	2.8
Weapon	2.2	0	5.3	5.7
Burn	1.4	1.9	0	0

*Expressed as per cent of 970 urban dogs, 156 urban cats, 129 suburban dogs, and 35 suburban cats.

cohesion of its components but also on how the force is applied and on the stress condition of the tissue at the time it is applied. When a shear force is applied to a tendon in a relaxed state, the tendon can displace and absorb the force, whereas if the tendon is under tensile stress at the time of impact, the combination of tension and shear can result in failure.

Blunt Impact

Blunt impact is one of the most common ways that mechanical energy is delivered to pets (see Table 8–1). The transmission of energy at impact is by compression, stretching, shearing, or a combination. The rate at which force is applied is a factor in injury due to an important physical property of tissue—viscoelasticity. A tissue's resistance to changing shape on impact is a function of its viscosity, and the tendency for a tissue to resume its prestress configuration after impact is related to its elasticity. If a force (stress) is applied slowly, the tissues can displace at a rate low enough to dissipate the force over a large area without shock waves, and little or no injury results. If a force is applied rapidly and tissues cannot displace at a low rate and over a large area, the result is that shock or compression waves form and pass through the tissue. Local areas near the wave fronts move relative to one another and fail to maintain cohesion, resulting in injuries.

Bones, although stiffer than other tissues, are also viscoelastic and behave differently under slow or rapid loading. With slow loading to failure, fractures propagate as a single crack and generally have only two major fragments, but fractures due to very high velocity loading (rapid strain) have comminutions that are caused by the propagation of numerous fracture planes in a small area.

Penetrating or Lacerating Injuries

The mechanism of injury due to sharp objects can be reduced to two components, crush and stretch. Knives and sharp-edged objects create microscopic crush lesions along the path of the edge, and the rest of the blade stretches the tissues. The resulting injury is the consequence of disruption of tissues along a plane and division of the structure.

Gunshot

Because of the viscoelastic nature of tissues, when they are struck by a missile, a shock wave is propagated and moves ahead of and around the missile, stretching the tissues. The shock or compression wave created by the impact disrupts the tissues along the missile's leading edge. The missile crushes additional tissue as it expands, fragments, and tumbles along its path. If a tissue affected cannot stretch, it absorbs the energy by fragmenting. The severity of injury varies as a function of the weight of the missile and its velocity, because these govern the amount of energy delivered. Velocity is the critical factor, because the energy delivered by a missile only doubles if its weight is doubled but is increased four times if its velocity is doubled.

Bite Wounds

Bite wounds are a combination of crush and tear/avulsion, in which the tooth crushes a path into the tissue and stretches it as it penetrates. Once a tooth enters the tissues, its movement tears and avulses tissues. These wounds have great potential for infection.

CHAPTER 9

Biomaterials (pages 105–113)

BIOLOGICAL EVALUATION OF MATERIALS
(pp. 105–108)

Tissue responses to an implant material occur in two locations: a direct response of the tissue adjacent to the material, and a systemic effect in which breakdown products of the material may be present and affect tissues remote from the implant.

Both *in vitro* and *in vivo* testing of materials are performed to evaluate their suitability for implant applications. Biocompatibility evaluations categorize the kind and degree of response and are of two types: (1) toxicological effects and (2) blood compatibility. An ideal material would not denature plasma proteins, induce thrombus formation, damage blood elements, exhibit instability, produce adverse immune responses, stimulate cancer, produce toxic or teratological effects, have inadequate mechanical properties, diminish electrolytes, or be changed by sterilization.

METALS AND ALLOYS (pp. 108–109)
Stainless Steel

Alloys of steel with more than 12 per cent chromium exhibit corrosion resistance. The addition of nickel, molybdenum, and silicon to the alloy increases corrosion resistance.

Corrosion occurs (1) if the composition of elements in the metal is incorrect, (2) if incorrect metallurgical conditions of temperature and cooling rates are used during the formation of the implant, and (3) if an implant is improperly selected and handled.

Cobalt-Chromium Alloys

The cobalt-chromium alloys offer the best combination of high abrasion resistance, low-corrosion characteristics, high fatigue strength, and excellent biocompatibility for total hip replacements in man.

Titanium and Titanium Alloys

Titanium and its alloys offer outstanding corrosion resistance and good mechanical properties. The relatively low density of titanium and titanium alloy is useful when large volumes of the implant material are required.

POLYMERS (pp. 109–111)
Polyethylene

The chemical repeat unit of polyethylene is $-[CH_2CH_2-]_n$, where n is the number of repeating units (mers). Low-density polyethylene is used as a non–load-bearing implant material (ophthalmic reconstruction material, catheters, or tendon repair). High-density polyethylene is stronger and is especially useful in joint applications as the cup component of a total hip replacement.

Polymers like polyethylene are used extensively as implants or catheters and are hydrophobic rather than hydrophilic in association with minimal tissue response.

Polypropylene

The chemical repeat unit of polypropylene is $-[CH_2CH(CH_3)-]_n$. Polypropylene is harder than polyethylene. Polypropylene has good flexure characteristics and creep resistance and is commonly used for joints.

Nylon

There are thousands of types of nylons, including some of interest for routine as well as experimental implant applications. One disadvantage is its propensity to absorb liquid, which weakens it. Also, it exhibits a much greater tissue reactivity than polypropylene. It is relatively inexpensive and is satisfactory in many applications.

Polyvinylchloride

Polyvinylchloride tubing is widely used as cannulas and catheters. To have a flexible tube, commonly 50 per cent of the polyvinylchloride is a plasticizing agent such as di-2-ethylhexyl phthalate. Plasticizer additives are impure and can be a source of undesirable interaction with living systems and may cause local irritation or central nervous system depression.

Cyanoacrylates

When an initiator of a polymerization reaction is added to the monomer, polymerization occurs immediately. Water or blood can act as an initiator. The degradation products include formaldehyde and an alkyl cyanoacetate. Both of these substances are toxic.

Silicone Rubber

Silicone rubber is the most widely used implant material. It is commonly used in tubular form or as an encapsulant (potting) material for electronic components or device housings.

Dacron

Dacron is the most widely used artificial vascular prosthesis. Woven, knitted, or velour fabric implants are satisfactory in large diameters (>6 mm internal diameter); however, for small-diameter applications, Teflon or polyurethane may be preferred.

Teflon

Teflon (polytetrafluoroethylene) has been used as a vascular prosthetic material for about 30 years. As a replacement material for arteries, it is commonly in tubular or patch form.

Polyurethane (p. 110)

Polymethyl Methacrylate

Polymethyl methacrylate is commonly used as a bone cement or, in special applications, as an implant housing material. It is essentially the same material as Plexiglas or Lucite. To make it easy to use and place the material, it is supplied as a liquid and a powder that are combined in specific proportions before use. The liquid contains mostly the unpolymerized monomer (methyl methacrylate) and a small amount of hydroquinone (to extend shelf life). The reaction gives off heat capable of killing tissue in the immediate vicinity of the bone cement. To minimize formation of small pores or voids and consequent loss of strength in the polymerizing material, it is commonly placed under pressure.

Bioerodable Polymers (p. 111)

Collagen

Collagen can be purified from connective tissue and rendered nonantigenic. This material is being produced in new forms of interest in surgical applications. An artificial skin has been developed and tested in burn wound repair.

CERAMICS (pp. 111–112)

Calcium and phosphorus are major structural elements of skeletal tissue. These elements are present in bone as hydroxyapatite. Synthetic hydroxyapatite can be made with high purity and specific repeatable resorption characteristics. The commercial products that are available facilitate improvements in bone defect repair. Also, the calcium phosphates are being used in composites as coatings on metallic implants. This approach offers the potential for improvement over purely mechanical fixation.

Bioglass (p. 111)

Carbon

The principal forms of carbon are diamond, graphite, pyrolitic, carbon black, and activated carbon. Pyrolitic carbon is the variety most commonly used. It is stronger and tougher than glassy carbon. The high degree of cross-linking among carbon atoms for pyrolitic carbon results in a material of high strength with great abrasion resistance. Coupled with its excellent blood compatibility characteristics, is a useful implant material as a thin film coating on implant devices (e.g., struts on heart valves).

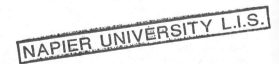

Surgical Methods (pages 114–259)

CHAPTER 10

Principles of Surgical Asepsis
(pages 114–123)

Wound infection remains an important factor, even under aseptic conditions, owing to increased use of surgical treatments when a patient has decreased resistance because of such factors as organ transplantation, old age, and neoplasia.

DEFINITION OF TERMS (p. 114)

The absence of pathogenic microbes in living tissue constitutes a state of *asepsis. Sterilization* is the process of killing all microorganisms with the use of either physical or chemical agents.

An *antiseptic* is a chemical agent that either kills pathogenic microorganisms or inhibits their growth as long as the agent and microbe remain in contact. The term *antiseptic* is reserved for agents applied to tissues. A *disinfectant* is a germicidal, chemical substance that kills microorganisms on inanimate objects, such as instruments and other equipment, that cannot be exposed to heat.

Antimicrobial drugs are used to alter the activity of microbial agents in a patient. A *bacteriostatic* antimicrobial agent inhibits bacterial growth; growth may resume on removal of the agent. *Bactericidal* agents kill bacteria.

HISTORICAL ASPECTS (pp. 114–115)
TYPES OF SURGICAL INFECTIONS (pp. 115–116)

Veterinary surgeons contend with infection in five major settings: (1) as a primary surgical disease, (2) as a complication of an operation not otherwise associated with infection, (3) as a complication of diagnostic or support procedures, (4) as an entity totally unrelated to the primary surgical disease, and (5) as a complication (short and long term) of prosthetic implants.

Infection as the Primary Surgical Disease

A significant portion of surgical treatment is directed at therapy of infections. These infections may be presented as abscesses, peritonitis, pleuritis, or other closed body cavity infections or as trauma that may include contamination with foreign material.

Patients are usually brought for treatment for the effects of the infection (anorexia, swelling, and pain). These infections are therapeutic problems requiring surgical drainage and antimicrobial therapy.

Postsurgical Wound Infection

During most surgical procedures, the skin and fascia are incised, altering the body's protective barrier against contamination. Supplementing the protection afforded by the skin and fascia, a group of tissues including the reticuloendothelial system and the leukocytes constantly combat infectious agents that do invade the body. These tissues aid a surgeon, provided the level of contamination is not overwhelming and the systems have not been compromised by previous disease, exposure to immunosuppressive drugs, or other immunodeficiencies.

Postoperative wound infection results from bacterial contamination during or after a surgical procedure and usually involves the subcutaneous tissues. Any factor that interferes with wound healing increases the possibility of wound infection.

Infectious Complications of Diagnostic and Support Procedures

It is not uncommon to perform lengthy and sophisticated procedures on very young, severely traumatized, or malnourished patients. A trio of support mechanisms accompanies these procedures: (1) continuous intravenous therapy, (2) endotracheal intubation, and (3) urinary catheter drainage. Each shares a common problem: if the therapy is continued long enough, infection develops, and if the device is left in place after superficial infection occurs, systemic infection follows.

Cautious technical insertion of these devices and careful nursing care are required to prevent infection.

Infections Unrelated to Primary Surgical Disease

Infection of Prosthetic Implants (p. 116)

PATHOGENESIS OF SURGICAL WOUND INFECTION (pp. 116–118)

There is no such thing as *sterile* surgery; all surgical wounds are contaminated with bacteria. Second, by breaking the integrity of the bacteria-resistant skin, the surgical incision provides an increased risk of infection. Numerous factors determine whether (microbial damage of tissue) will result: (1) those factors that reduce the host's resistance to bacterial infection, (2) the characteristics of the bacterial contaminants, and (3) the interaction between the host and the bacteria that results in a tissue-damaging infection.

Host Resistance to Infection

The pathophysiological conditions that increase the risk of infection are: extremes in age (very old or very young), poor physical condition, and malnutrition. Other conditions that may decrease resistance to bacterial infection include systemic disease such as diabetes, leukemia, hypogammaglobulinemia, suppression by corticosteroids or cytotoxic drugs, and metabolic or physiological alterations caused by anesthetics and hypothermia. Local conditions at the surgical site are some of the most important factors increasing susceptibility to infection. Necrotic tissue is a growth medium for bacteria and is often not accessible to a host's defense mechanisms. Phagocytosis and humoral immunity are significantly decreased when tissue integrity is interrupted during the operation. Hematomas and dead space are excellent locations for infection because bacteria can multiply in these areas, in which there is relatively little host response.

The most obvious mechanical factor reducing resistance to infection is a skin incision. The damage caused by clamps, ligatures, retractors, hemorrhage, and thrombosis alters the blood supply and decreases efficiency of host defenses.

Bacterial Contamination of the Surgical Wound

The most common source of bacteria that contaminate surgical wounds is an animal's endogenous microbial flora. Prevention of exposure to this flora and resulting infection is most important at the time of surgery.

Bacteria that infect surgical wounds use the opportunity offered by the weakened defense mechanisms of the host to become established and inflict tissue damage. They are often organisms of low virulence, unable to invade intact body surfaces, or do not survive well in the tissues and therefore must be present in large numbers. The most common bacteria involved *Staphylococcus intermedius* and *Streptococcus* spp.

Development of Infection

The development of a surgical wound infection then depends on the probability of sufficient bacteria falling on a small site where the host resistance has been decreased enough to allow sufficient bacterial growth to cause further tissue damage. Bacterial infections resulting in tissue damage generally require growth of the contaminating organisms to numbers of 10^6 *or greater per gram of tissue.*

PREVENTION OF SURGICAL INFECTION (pp. 118–120)

Proper Selection and Preparation of Surgical Patients

Some of the important historical considerations are acute or chronic corticosteroid therapy, long-term use of antimicrobials, or history and evidence of remote infection elsewhere in the patient's body.

Preoperative evaluation of patients should be comprehensive to assess the overall state of health, determine the risk of the impending surgical treatment, and guide the preoperative preparation. Most importantly, all the information gathered must be shared with the owner (including treatment options, risks, and costs) to enable both veterinarian and owner to form treatment plans.

Preparation of Surgical Personnel
(see Chapter 12)

Sterilization of Surgical Equipment and Materials (see Chapter 11)

Maintenance of the Operating Room (see Chapter 14)

Preparation of Patients (see Chapter 13)

Operative Technique (see Chapter 16)

All operations should be performed to minimize the disturbance of blood flow through the tissue involved; otherwise, healing is slowed and infection enhanced. Sutures that are too tightly placed or too closely positioned eventually result in wound disruption because of necrosis of the tissue encompassed by the suture material.

Because sutures combine the undesirable effects of foreign bodies and interference with blood supply, as few sutures as possible should be used to close or approximate the wound. Sutures should be as fine as possible, monofilament, and nonreactive and are tied as loosely as approximation will allow.

No single technical complication is as frequently associated with infection as is the presence of a hematoma (implying poor hemostasis). Electrocautery must be very skillfully used. Wounds made with a scalpel heal better and are less susceptible to infection than those made with an electrosurgical knife.

If a hollow viscus is to be opened or other sources of contamination are to be exposed, protective towels, gauze, or plastic is used to shield the adjacent clean tissues. Dead space is eliminated and devitalized tissue removed, because these are potential areas of bacterial growth.

Postoperative Care (see Chapter 22)

The key to successful home convalescence is an informed owner. The veterinarian must provide the necessary explanation and information to allow the owner to function as a medical support unit. The owner must know what to observe and when to contact the veterinarian.

If postoperative wound infection occurs, local signs consist of pain, swelling, warmth, and erythema. If no more than 7 to 10 days has elapsed since the operation, the incision may simply be spread open with a hemostat and drained. A drain left in place for 24 to 72 hours may be desirable if properly maintained.

If systemic evidence of infection persists after drainage, either the local drainage was inadequate or other sources of infection exist and must be identified. Blood, pus, and urine specimens are cultured for bacterial isolation and identification. Initial antimicrobial therapy is instituted based on the usual susceptibilities of the most likely pathogens.

NOSOCOMIAL INFECTIONS (pp. 120–123)

Infections that are acquired by patients during the course of hospitalization are known as *nosocomial infections*. The most common nosocomial infections are of the urinary tract, lower respiratory tract, and surgical wounds. Most nosocomial infections can be associated with overuse of antimicrobials, therapeutic medical devices, diagnostic procedures, surgical procedures, advanced age, and chronic disease.

Individual risk factors include (1) an animal's susceptibility to infection, (2) the virulence of the infectious agent, and (3) the nature of exposure to the agent. The incidence of nosocomial infections can be reduced by limiting the spread of the agents and controlling the sources of exposure to patients.

Nosocomial Infectious Agents

Bacteria are the most common agents involved in nosocomial infection. The bacteria commonly implicated tend to be environmentally resistant, and the increasing use of antibiotic therapy precedes an increased antibiotic resistance in nosocomial agents.

Epidemiology

The source of most agents is the endogenous flora of the patient or exogenous agents of the hospital microflora.

Colonization of body surfaces by nosocomial bacterial pathogens is often a prerequisite to infection. Direct contamination of exposed tissues, which results in infection, occurs less frequently. Therefore, a patient is its own major reservoir of these agents.

Prevention of Nosocomial Infections

Total prevention is unrealistic. Surveillance and control procedures must be adopted to identify nosocomial infections and reduce their incidence.

Surveillance

An efficient surveillance system defines the endemic level and type of nosocomial infection. It also must quickly identify epidemics and clusters of infections as they occur. Precise identification of the agent is required. In addition, an accurate antibiogram is essential.

Scheduled or periodic microbiological sampling of the hospital environment to monitor the level of contamination with potential nosocomial agents may not be cost-effective or rational. However, microbiological sampling is an important epidemiological tool when used to detect a specific agent that is responsible for a cluster of nosocomial infections.

Control

A control program must include systematic evaluation of the problem, application of sound management techniques, and integration of a productive educational program for all hospital personnel.

1. Appointment of an Infection Control Committee or Infection Control Officer
2. Development of written standards for medical asepsis and hospital sanitation
3. Development of a practical system of surveillance, identification, and accurate reporting of infections
4. Facilities for the isolation of infected patients
5. An adequate microbiology service
6. A periodic review of the use of antimicrobial agents

Veterinarians should be encouraged to evaluate their use of antimicrobials to determine if the medical condition requires antimicrobial treatment, to choose the most effective and least expensive drug, and to prescribe the correct dosage and duration of therapy.

The key components of successful nosocomial infection control and prevention programs include an attitude of awareness of potential risk factors and willingness to comply with recommended procedures, use of barrier protection procedures to prevent cross-infection in the hospital, and rational use of antimicrobials.

CHAPTER 11

Sterilization (pages 124–129)

Sterilization is the complete elimination of microbial viability, including both the vegetative forms of bacteria and spores.

The methods of sterilization can be divided into physical and chemical. Although sterility can be achieved with certain chemicals, physical methods are generally more reliable. Heat, filtration, and radiation are the most commonly used physical methods of sterilizing medical and surgical materials. Chemical sterilization is usually accomplished with ethylene oxide.

STEAM STERILIZATION (pp. 124–127)

Principles of Steam Sterilization

Bacteria are destroyed by either wet or dry heat, although when moisture is present, death occurs at a lower temperature and in a shorter time. Although the ultimate cause of death due to both wet and dry heat is protein denaturation, it appears that moist heat causes death by the coagulation of critical cellular proteins, whereas death by dry heat is primarily an oxidation process.

Saturated steam under pressure is the most dependable medium known for the destruction of all forms of microbial life. For sterilization, steam is maintained under pressure for the sole purpose of attaining a higher temperature. The pressure itself has no direct effect on the antimicrobial properties of steam.

Steam is unique as a thermal sterilizing agent in its ability to permeate porous substances by condensation. For sterilization, supplies must be arranged to allow rapid and complete penetration of steam. Steam penetrates each pack to be sterilized, heats the pack through condensation, and leaves the entire contents slightly moistened. Because steam sterilization depends on direct steam contact, certain materials such as oils and greases should not be sterilized using this technique. Similarly, needles and fine instruments cannot be sterilized in test tubes with stoppered ends; the tubes must be sealed with cotton plugs.

Types of Steam Sterilizers

The word *autoclave* means self-closing—that is, the door of the sterilizing chamber is held closed by the pressure within the chamber.

The autoclaves in use in most veterinary institutions and private practices today are *gravity displacement* or *downward displacement* sterilizers. In these autoclaves, steam is introduced under pressure into the top of the sterilizing chamber. Because the steam is considerably less dense than air, it "floats" to the top of the chamber, compressing the air to the bottom. Most gravity displacement sterilizers are also equipped with condensers, vacuum pumps, and ejector systems, which assist in the removal of air.

Prevacuum steam sterilizers have recently come into general use. In these autoclaves, air is evacuated from the chamber by means of a vacuum pump before steam is admitted to the chamber. In prevacuum sterilizers, steam penetrates the load almost instantly, permitting the use of a high sterilization temperature and a reduced holding time.

Finally, *steam pulsing systems* decrease the need for the development of a high prevacuum. A steam pulse increases the chamber pressure to a set pressure, whereupon the chamber is vented to a minimal pressure preceding the next pulse.

The Steam Sterilization Procedure

Cleaning Surgical Supplies Before Sterilization. Gross contamination must be removed from surgical instruments before sterilization. Instruments may be cleaned manually, with washer-sterilizers, or with ultrasonic cleaning equipment as soon as possible after use.

Manual cleaning is best achieved with a hand brush with stiff bristles. The best cleaning agents are moderately alkaline, low-sudsing detergents. After washing, the instruments are rinsed in hot water and dried thoroughly.

Ultrasonic cleaners use vibratory waves to clean through *cavitation.*

Preparation of Surgical Packs and Loading of the Autoclave. Steam must be able to thoroughly penetrate the material in which the pack is wrapped, as well as the contents of the pack. The ideal wrapping material is permeable to steam but not microbes, resistant to damage when handled, flexible, and easily returned to a flat position. Cotton muslin wraps are more durable and flexible than other wraps and have the best handling properties. Cotton muslin has a thread count of 140 threads per square inch. The main disadvantage of muslin is that it provides a shorter safe storage time than do other wraps. Muslin wraps should be double layered, and two wraps used for each pack. A number of different types of paper are also available for the preparation of surgical packs. Regardless of the number of layers used, paper provides storage time superior to fabrics.

Materials are positioned in packs to allow complete steam penetration. To ensure that all surfaces of instruments are exposed to steam, they are sterilized with the box locks open. Complex instruments such as Balfour retractors are disassembled if possible unless they are specifically designed for steam penetration. Containers such as saline pans are positioned in the pack so that the open end is facing either down or horizontally when the pack is in the sterilizer.

Linen packs are limited in size to $12 \times 12 \times 20$ inches and should not weigh more than 6 kg. Drapes are wrapped singly and are not packaged with other equipment.

Instrument packs are positioned vertically (on edge) and longitudinally in the sterilizer. In this position, they are oriented with the direction of steam flow and do not trap air. A slight amount of empty space should be present between each pack. Linen packs are loaded so that their layers are oriented vertically.

Autoclave Operation. A number of minimum time–temperature standards have been established for routine sterilization of surgical packs. Most authorities agree that 13 minutes' exposure to saturated steam at 120°C (250°F) is a safe minimum standard. In general, 5 to 10 minutes at this temperature will destroy most resistant microbes, and the additional 3 to 8 minutes provides a margin of safety.

Emergency sterilization of instruments is usually performed in prevacuum sterilizers. The recommended exposure time is 3 minutes at 270°F (131°C). The instruments are sterilized in perforated metal trays that may be carried to the operating field.

Large linen packs require 30 minutes at 121°C (250°F) in gravity displacement sterilizers and 4 minutes at 131°C (270°F) in prevacuum sterilizers. All instrument and linen packs are allowed to dry for a minimum of 20 minutes after the sterilization cycle.

Chemical indicators most commonly are paper strips impregnated with a chemical that undergoes a color change when a certain temperature is reached.

Biological indicators are superior to chemical indicators, because they provide absolute proof that sterilizing conditions have been met. All systems use a heat-resistant organism that is many more times resistant to the sterilization process than the organisms likely to be present as natural contaminants. The most commonly used organism is the spore of *Bacillus stearothermophilus*.

Sterile Pack Storage. If possible, sterile packs should be stored in closed cabinets rather than on open shelves. All packs are dated, preferably with an expiration date. Safe storage times for packs wrapped in commonly used materials are given in Table 11–1.

TABLE 11–1. SAFE STORAGE TIME FOR STERILE PACKS

Wrapper	Closed Cabinet	Open Shelves
Single-wrapped muslin (two layers)	1 week	2 days
Double-wrapped muslin (each two layers)	7 weeks	3 weeks
Single-wrapped crepe paper	At least 8 weeks	3 weeks

CHEMICAL STERILIZATION (pp. 127–129)

Ethylene Oxide

Ethylene oxide is capable of destroying all known microorganisms, including bacteria, spores, fungi, and at least the larger viruses. It is flammable and explosive except when mixed with carbon dioxide.

Physical and Chemical Properties of Ethylene Oxide

Ethylene oxide is a simple cyclic ether. It is a colorless gas that liquefies at 51.6°F (10.9°C) and freezes at -168.3°F (-111.3°C). Ethylene oxide–air mixtures are flammable and explosive. Ethylene oxide diffuses rapidly and penetrates easily so that objects may be packaged before sterilization. It also rapidly diffuses from the object after sterilization.

Effects of Concentration, Temperature, Time, and Humidity

The effectiveness of ethylene oxide as a sterilizing agent depends on (1) gas concentration, (2) temperature, (3) exposure time, and (4) humidity. Doubling the ethylene oxide concentration decreases the sterilization time by approximately one-half. The activity of ethylene oxide is slightly more than doubled with each 10°C (20°F) increase in temperature. Exposure time varies from 48 minutes to several hours. Twelve hours exposure is allowed when sterilizing at room temperature.

Equipment and Technique

At the end of the exposure time, the ethylene oxide gas is removed from the chamber. A period of aeration is allowed for diffusion of ethylene oxide gas from sterilized objects. Recommended minimum aeration times for different materials are listed in Table 11–2.

TABLE 11–2. AERATION TIMES FOR VARIOUS SURGICAL SUPPLIES AFTER ETHYLENE OXIDE STERILIZATION

Material	Natural Aeration (Hours)	Mechanical Aeration (Hours)
Absorbent anesthesia equipment	120–168	5–8
Conductive rubber	30	16
Gloves, catheters	168	—
Items sealed in plastic	96	—
Internal pacemakers	500	—
⅛-inch-thick polyvinylchloride	300	—
Polyethylene	48	12
Polypropylene	48	12
Red rubber	55	18
Thick rubber	24	4
Thin polyvinylchloride	168	12
Thin rubber	6	1
Vinyl plastic	76	32

Toxicity

Exposure to ethylene oxide gas and its by-products should be avoided. Ethylene oxide sterilizers and aerators should be located in a room that has at least ten air changes per hour.

Cold Sterilization

Cold sterilization refers to soaking instruments in disinfectant solutions. A disinfectant is an agent that destroys pathogenic organisms on inanimate objects. Spores and viruses may not be destroyed by disinfectants, and for this reason cold sterilization should not be used for critical instruments; critical instruments are those that potentially may be introduced beneath the surface of the body.

Alcohols. Ethyl alcohol and isopropyl alcohol kill bacteria by the coagulation of protein. Ethanol is generally used as a 70 per cent solution, and isopropyl alcohol is effective in concentrations of up to 99 per cent. Alcohols should generally not be used as cold sterilants.

Aldehydes. Formaldehyde is available as formalin. Glutaraldehyde in dilute concentrations is less toxic than formaldehyde and is the liquid disinfectant of choice for lensed instruments.

Chlorhexidine. This is an antiseptic agent available in detergent, tincture, and aqueous formulations. It is now widely used as an agent for the preparation of surgical patients and for surgical hand scrubs because it is nonirritating to skin.

Iodines. Inorganic iodines are effective bactericidal agents but stain fabrics and tissue. The main disadvantage of iodines as cold sterilants is that they corrode instruments.

Iodophors have less tendency than inorganic iodines to stain fabric and tissue and are less irritating to skin. As with inorganic iodines, long-term use of iodophors may produce corrosion of instruments.

Phenols. Phenol or carbolic acid is the oldest known germicidal agent. Unlike many disinfectants, they are not adversely affected by organic materials. Phenols are commonly used as cold sterilants in combination with detergents or soaps to increase the spectrum of their activity.

Quaternary Ammonium Compounds. Compounds such as benzalkonium chloride are synthetic cationic detergents. These are surface-active agents that dissolve lipids in bacterial cell walls and membranes. They are nontoxic to tissues and are therefore popular. They are selectively absorbed by fabrics such as gauze.

C H A P T E R 1 2
Preparation of the Surgical Team (pages 130–137)

SCRUB SUITS (p. 130)

A scrub suit is an occlusive but not impermeable barrier to microorganisms. Because routine laundering of a suit does not eliminate pathogenic organisms, a suit may act as a source of seeding of pathological bacteria and may need to be steam sterilized periodically.

When a surgeon leaves the operating room, the scrub suit is protected by a coat to reduce contamination from higher microorganism counts in the hallways and kennels. Scrub suits are not worn to change bandages, apply cast materials, or examine patients when additional surgery is scheduled that day. The scrub suit is discarded and laundered after wearing and changed when wet or soiled.

SURGICAL HEAD COVERS (p. 130)

Hoods rather than caps are recommended for all operating room personnel. Although there is no statistical difference in environmental contamination in the wearing of caps, hoods, or bouffants, hoods that cover the head and neck permit significantly less contamination of the shoulder area.

Head covers should cover occipital and temporal hair completely, be durable and comfortable to wear, and not shed lint into the wound. If cloth head covers are used, they must be laundered daily.

SHOE COVERS (p. 130)

When properly worn, shoe covers effectively block bacteria from street shoes, reduce the possibility of contaminating the operating room, and protect the wearer's own shoes from contamination by hospital bacteria.

FACE MASKS (p. 131)

Of all traditional surgical articles worn to promote asepsis in the operating room, the face mask contributes the least. The major function of face masks in surgery is to protect the wound from droplets of saliva expelled by the surgical team members when talking, but they do not reduce environmental contamination.

PREPARATION OF THE SURGEON'S SKIN (pp. 131–133)

The objectives of the surgical scrub are (1) mechanical removal of gross dirt and oil from the hands, (2) reduction of the transient microorganism count to as close to zero as possible, and (3) a prolonged depressant effect on the resident microflora of the hands and forearms. Transient flora are organisms isolated from the skin but not demonstrated to be consistently present in the majority of persons. Transient bacteria do not multiply and are presumed to be deposited on the skin from the mucous membranes or the environment. Resident flora are organisms persistently isolated from the skin of most people. These organisms are permanent residents of the skin and are able to multiply within the skin. Washing with bar soap removes most of the transient bacteria by mechanical friction, and the resident population is killed by antiseptic solutions. Three common surgical scrub solutions used are hexachlorophene, povidone-iodine, and chlorhexidine gluconate.

The surgical scrub protocol is based on either an anatomical timed scrub procedure or the counted brush stroke method. Either method ensures sufficient exposure of all skin surfaces to friction and the antimicrobial solution. Numerous studies have found no significant difference in bacterial populations after 5- or 10-minute timed scrubs.

Hexachlorophene

Hexachlorophene is a polychlorinated bisphenol that in high concentrations acts by disruption of microbial cell walls and precipitation of cell proteins. In low concentrations, it probably acts by inactivating essential enzyme systems within microorganisms. It is bacteriostatic for gram-positive cocci but has little activity against gram-negative bacteria, fungi, or viruses. Hexachlorophene is not fast acting, and one scrub with it does not reduce cutaneous flora.

Hexachlorophene has a cumulative antibacterial action after subsequent application because it is not metabolized by skin enzymes and is bound to keratin.

Iodophors

Iodophors are complexes that consist of iodine and a carrier such as polyvinylpyrrolidone. The amount of free iodine in these complexes is less, but their antimicrobial effects are similar to those of iodine and are less irritating. The iodophors act by cell wall penetration, oxidation, and replacement of microbial contents with free iodine. They are effective against both gram-negative and gram-positive bacteria, fungi, and viruses. They have some activity against bacterial spores. The presence of organic material does affect the efficiency of the iodophors. Iodophors require at least 2 minutes of skin contact time to allow release of free iodine. The use of iodophors results in a greater immediate reduction in bacteria counts than hexachlorophene and comparable or slightly less reduction than chlorhexidine gluconate.

Chlorhexidine Gluconate

Chlorhexidine is a cationic bisdiguanide that derives its antimicrobial action by causing disruption of microbial cell membrane and precipitation of cell contents. It is more effective against gram-positive than gram-negative bacteria, is only a fair fungicide, but is active against many viruses. Its speed of killing is classified as intermediate. Its strong affinity for the skin makes it chemically active for at least 6 hours after surgical scrub. Its persistent effect is greater than any other skin antiseptic.

GOWNS (pp. 133–136)

Surgical gowns should be made of material that establishes a barrier, eliminating the passage of microorganisms between sterile and nonsterile areas. Criteria to meet in establishing an effective barrier are as follows:

1. Blood and aqueous fluid resistance.
2. Resistance to the stresses of stretch, pressure, and friction.
3. Freedom from lint to reduce particles in the air.
4. Fire resistance, wearing comfort, economy, and accessibility.

Gowns are *woven* and *nonwoven*. Woven fabric is produced by interlacing two yarns or similar material so that they cross each other at right angles.

A popular material for cloth gowns is loosely woven all-cotton fabric type 140 muslin. This muslin has 140 threads per square inch of material and is used in single or double layers. Type 140 muslin is not an ideal material and is instantly permeable to bacterial penetration when wet.

Reusable barrier gowns made of Gore-Tex are also available. An expanded film of polytetrafluoroethylene (PTFE) is laminated between two layers of polyester fabric in combination with nonbarrier portions of a 50/50 polyester/cotton blend. This barrier portion inhibits liquid and bacterial migration but allows the wearer's perspiration to pass to the environment for greater comfort.

Nonwoven gowns are not made from yarn but are made directly from fibers. Nonwoven materials have interstices that are so closely joined or are in such a random pattern that bacteria and fluids are prevented from passing through.

Disposable nonwoven gowns are folded and sealed in sterilized packages. Used disposable gowns should not be laundered and recycled for use in sterile surgery, because individual fibers may break; these defects are difficult to detect grossly, but the material becomes porous. Unused disposables should not be resterilized unless the manufacturer provides instructions for reprocessing.

Lengthy surgical operations during which surgical gowns are subjected to the stresses of stretch, shear, and pressure and come in contact with blood and other fluids have a greater risk of moisture strike-through contamination. A gown should be considered a sterile field only from the surgeon's shoulders to the waist, including the sleeves.

GLOVES (p. 136)

Gloves do provide a barrier but are not completely impermeable, particularly when in use. When unused gloves were filled with water, leaks were observed in 4.1 per cent of the vinyl and 2.7 per cent of the latex gloves tested. Glove manufacturers use magnesium silicate (talcum) as a glove mold-release agent. This talc is difficult to remove and may be shed into surgical wounds, resulting in a foreign body reaction.

Washing the gloved hands may not be sufficient to remove powder from the exterior surface, and the gloves should be wiped on a lint-free towel to remove powder.

CHAPTER 13

Assessment and Preparation of the Surgical Patient (pages 137–147)

Preoperative care of surgical patients is as important for ensuring a successful outcome of surgery as the procedure itself. Preoperative stabilization and preparation of surgical patients minimize risk and the potential for complications after surgery.

ASSESSMENT OF PATIENTS (pp. 137–139)

Preoperative evaluation is performed to thoroughly assess an animal's general health and evaluate the system affected by the primary disease. A surgeon uses this information to decide if surgery is warranted, to determine a prognosis, and to select the best procedure for the patient. The minimum data base for potential surgical candidates is a complete history and thorough physical examination.

History

Collecting a complete history from the owner is an important part of evaluating prospective surgical candidates. Because this is often the first meeting between the surgeon and the client, the impressions formed are the foundation of the future professional relationship. It is important to establish rapport with the owners and to determine their expectations and financial restrictions.

General information about signalment, general health, diet, environment, and past medical problems is collected. Specific questions on the nature, duration, and course of the presenting problem aid in formulating differential diagnoses and selecting diagnostic tests.

Physical Examination

The physical examination should be a systematic evaluation of the entire animal despite natural enthusiasm to concentrate on the presenting problem.

The examination is completed by evaluating the affected area and related systems. For example, fractures are assessed for associated skin wounds, soft-tissue trauma, swelling, vascularity, and peripheral nerve deficits. When the examination is completed, a physical status is assigned (Table 13–1).

Supplemental Testing

The tests selected should be the minimum necessary to evaluate the presenting problem and its systemic manifestations as well as to determine the significance of concurrent disease conditions detected during the initial examination. Preoperative tests may also be performed to establish baseline values for postoperative monitoring.

Specific Tests

Hematology. The minimum data base for surgical candidates is determination of packed cell volume and total serum protein. These are rapid, economical parameters that provide a baseline for monitoring of hemorrhage and fluid balance.

Biochemistry. See Table 13–1.

Urinalysis. Complete urinalysis is indicated in patients with a physical status of III or more, or in patients that are older than 7 to 10 years and are undergoing major surgery.

Other Tests. In geographic areas with a high incidence of heartworm or intestinal parasites, Knott's testing and fecal flotation are a recommended part of preoperative evaluation.

DETERMINATION OF SURGICAL RISK (pp. 139–141)

Many factors are used to determine surgical risk, such as a patient's general health status and primary disease or reason for surgery. Surgical risk also considers the invasiveness of the procedure, the potential for complications, and the quality of life for the patient both with and without the recommended procedure.

Cardiopulmonary System

Thoracic radiographs and electrocardiography are recommended by some for all trauma and geriatric patients because of a high incidence of asymptomatic dysrhythmias and valvular insufficiencies, but significant abnormalities are generally detected by physical examination. Compensated heart disease does not contraindicate surgery, but it is an important consideration when determining anesthetic protocol and formulating plans for fluid therapy.

Pre-existing lung disease increases the potential for fatal complications, and animals with conditions like laryngeal paralysis, collapsing trachea, elongated soft palate, everted lateral ventricles, and stenotic

TABLE 13–1. PHYSICAL STATUS AND RECOMMENDED LABORATORY TESTS

Physical Status	Definition	Examples	Recommended Laboratory Tests		Prognosis
			Minor*	Major†	
I	Healthy	Elective procedures, e.g., ovariohysterectomy	PCV, TP, urine sp gr	CBC, U/A, surgical panel‡	Excellent
II	Local disease, no systemic signs	Nonelective surgery in healthy patients, e.g., skin laceration, simple fracture	PCV, TP, urine sp gr	CBC, U/A, surgical panel‡	Excellent
III	Disease causes moderate systemic signs	Heart murmur, anemia, fever	CBC, U/A, biochemical panel§	CBC, U/A, surgical panel‡	Good
IV	Disease causes severe systemic signs	Ruptured bladder, gastric torsion	CBC, U/A, biochemical panel§	CBC, U/A, biochemical panel§	Guarded
V	Moribund	Endotoxic shock	CBC, U/A, biochemical panel§	CBC, U/A, biochemical panel§	Poor
E	Emergency	Qualifier of above classes	PCV, TP, urine sp gr	Depends on facilities available	Variable

*Minor = duration <60 min.
†Major = duration >60 min or patients >7 years.
‡Surgical panel = urea, creatinine, alkaline phosphatase, alanine aminotransferase.
§Biochemical panel = full panel.
CBC, complete blood cell count; PCV, packed cell volume; TP, thromboplastin time; U/A, urinalysis.

nares have more complications during recovery. Asymptomatic pulmonary contusions and pneumothorax are relatively common in patients suffering acute trauma, and preoperative chest radiographs are recommended to evaluate their significance.

Urinary Tract

A major concern in animals with compromised renal function is causing further deterioration, although abnormalities in coagulation and wound healing may also be observed. Risk is minimized by administering appropriate fluid therapy, avoiding significant blood loss or hypotension, and ensuring careful monitoring and early therapy. Postoperative renal failure is most commonly associated with failure to recognize and appropriately treat patients with subclinical disease.

Liver

Animals with liver disease have an increased surgical risk because of decreased ability to metabolize drugs, increased sensitivity to protein-bound drugs, decreased or defective synthesis and degradation of clotting factors, delayed wound healing, and poor nutritional status. Risk in these patients may be lessened by improvement of nutrition through hyperalimentation, careful fluid therapy, and plasma or blood transfusions to increase supplies of albumin and clotting factors.

Endocrine Disorders (pp. 140–141)

Hyperadrenocorticism affects a number of body functions to various degrees depending on the severity of disease. Ventilation during anesthesia may be compromised by respiratory muscles weakened by protein catabolism and fat accumulation within the thoracic and abdominal cavities. Surgical risk is also increased by delayed wound healing. Affected animals have decreased tissue tensile strength, so tissues tear easily and sutures have an increased tendency to pull out. Fibrous tissue formation is decreased, and dehiscence is more common. An increased potential for wound infections, hyperglycemia, and acid-base and electrolyte disturbances is noted in patients with hyperadrenocorticism.

Thyroid diseases increase surgical risk primarily because of altered cardiac function. Abnormalities in cats with hyperthyroidism include tachycardia, gallop rhythms, systolic murmurs, hypercontractility, ventricular hypertrophy, and congestive heart failure. Surgical risk is reduced by treatment with propranolol and antithyroid drugs for 2 to 4 weeks before surgery.

Animals with diabetes mellitus have a higher incidence of surgical complications. Diabetic patients are also more susceptible to infection.

Other

Animals with poor preoperative nutritional status may have insufficient reserves to meet their needs. They have a significantly higher rate of complications because of abnormal cell-mediated and humoral immunity, delayed wound healing, and increased susceptibility to shock, multiple organ failure, and death.

Obesity also increases the risk of complications. Ventilation is depressed as a result of intrathoracic fat accumulations, especially when a patient is positioned in dorsal recumbency or for perineal surgery.

CLIENT COMMUNICATION (p. 141)

Once assessment of a patient is complete and surgical risk has been determined, the surgeon should discuss the findings with the client.

The discussion should include an explanation of the disease, its course and prognosis both with and without treatment, options for treatment, the recommended procedure, its prognosis and potential complications, aftercare, and an estimate of the immediate and follow-up costs.

PATIENT STABILIZATION (pp. 141–143)
Fluid Therapy

It is important to ensure that surgical patients have normal fluid balance before surgery, because peripheral vasodilation is frequently associated with anesthetic induction, and losses in excess of maintenance result from hemorrhage, tissue drying, and shifts in fluid compartments.

The volume of fluid to be administered is the sum of fluid deficit, maintenance fluid requirements, and estimated future losses. Fluid deficit (in liters) equals the per cent of dehydration multiplied by body weight (in kilograms). Maintenance requirements for healthy dogs and cats are 40 to 60 ml/kg over 24 hours. Fluids may be administered at a rate of up to 100 ml/kg/hr in hypovolemic patients without evidence of cardiopulmonary disease.

Acid-Base Disorders

Specific therapy is usually not necessary for abnormalities in pH between 7.2 and 7.4. Outside this range, specific treatment of the acid-base disorder may be required. Abnormalities should be corrected before the induction of anesthesia.

Electrolyte Disturbances

Sodium is the major extracellular cation and the most important determinant of serum osmolality. Isotonic saline solutions are generally used to replenish sodium levels, although more concentrated solutions may be needed in patients with severe deficiencies.

The majority of potassium is contained within the intracellular fluid space, so serum values must be interpreted with caution because severe total body deficits may exist without changes in serum concentration.

Blood and Blood Component Therapy

Oxygen-carrying capacity of the blood during anesthesia should be sufficient if the packed cell volume is greater than 25 per cent.

The amount of blood needed may be calculated by the following formula, in which PCV is packed cell volume:

$$\text{Volume of blood required (ml)} = \text{body weight (kg)} \times$$

$$\frac{PCV_{desired} - PCV_{patient}}{PCV_{donor}} \times \frac{70 \text{ ml/kg (cat)}}{90 \text{ ml/kg (dog)}}$$

Surgical patients with plasma protein levels less than 45 g/l or albumin concentrations less than 15 g/l should receive plasma transfusions before surgery to avoid complications associated with low plasma oncotic pressure, diminished protein binding of anesthetic drugs, and delayed wound healing. The volume required may be calculated as follows:

$$\text{Plasma volume (ml)} = \text{body weight (kg)} \times \frac{TP_{desired} - TP_{patient}}{TP_{donor}},$$

in which TP is total protein.

Nutritional Status

Resting energy requirements in healthy individuals may be calculated by the following formula: kcal/24 hours = $70 \times 1.25 \times$ body weight $(kg)^{0.75}$. Values are adjusted according to the estimated increase in metabolic rate for the patient.

The oral route is preferred because it is easier to maintain, is economical, and is associated with fewer complications. It can be accomplished by nasal, pharyngostomy, gastrostomy, or jejunostomy tubes. Parenteral nutrition is recommended for gastrointestinal diseases that prevent sufficient nutrient use and for patients who are anorectic for more than 10 days regardless of the cause.

Infection

Infection detected preoperatively should be controlled before surgery to prevent local or systemic spread. Antibiotics used in these situations are therapeutic and accepted practice. Antibiotic prophylaxis is the practice of administering antibiotics to prevent establishment of an infection. Routine antibiotic use in this fashion is to be avoided because it establishes resistant bacterial strains and is not effective (see Chapter 6).

GENERAL PREPARATION OF PATIENTS (p. 143)

Excessively soiled patients should be bathed before surgery to avoid contamination of the operating room and surgical site. Food is withheld for 12 hours before surgery to minimize vomiting and aspiration during anesthesia. When this is not possible, vomiting may be induced. Water should be restricted for 3 to 4 hours before premedication, and animals should be walked to encourage voiding.

SURGICAL SITE PREPARATION (pp. 143–146)

Skin preparation techniques kill surface bacteria but do not sterilize the skin because approximately 20 per cent of bacteria reside within deeper skin structures inaccessible to disinfectant solutions.

Hair Removal

Because the incidence of postsurgical wound infections increases with the time interval between hair removal and surgery, hair should be removed just before surgery.

Clipping is the most recommended technique of hair removal for animals. It causes less skin trauma and is associated with lower postoperative infection rates than other techniques. A minimum of 15 cm on each side of the proposed incision is clipped.

Skin Disinfectants

Quaternary ammonium compounds, including benzalkonium chloride (Zephiran), benzethonium chloride, cetyldimethylbenzylammonium chloride, and cetylpyridinium chloride, are cationic surface agents that have been used in various antiseptic and disinfectant solutions. On the skin, they form a film underneath which microorganisms may survive. Because more effective agents are available, use should be restricted to the cleaning of nonsterile areas.

Hexachlorophene (pHisoHex). Single applications have little advantage over plain soap. Its residual action is less than that of chlorhexidine, and repeated applications may favor overgrowth of gram-negative organisms.

Aliphatic alcohols are effective, economical antiseptics with defatting and drying actions. Ninety per cent isopropyl alcohol is slightly more effective than 70 per cent ethyl alcohol, but it causes more skin irritation.

Povidone-iodophor compounds allow slow, continuous release of iodine. Rapid destruction of 99 per cent of accessible bacteria is reported 30 seconds after application. Povidone-iodophors have minimal residual activity, and effectiveness is reduced by organic materials such as blood, fat, and necrotic debris. They are inactivated by alcohol. Iodophors are less irritating than iodine tinctures, but skin irritation is commonly associated with use.

Chlorhexidine. Bacterial kill rates of 99 per cent are observed 30 seconds after application. Chlorhexidine has excellent residual activity and remains effective when exposed to organic matter, alcohol, and soaps. Skin reactions are uncommon.

Preparation Technique

Initial site preparation is performed outside the operating room with the animal positioned for easy access to the proposed surgical site.

Antibacterial detergents are commonly applied to skin by wet gauze sponges, although a gloved hand may be more effective in reducing bacterial numbers. Scrub brushes are avoided because they cause excessive skin trauma. The clipped area is scrubbed by applying gentle pressure in a circular motion. Beginning at the proposed incision site, the scrubbing action continues outwardly, in enlarging concentric circles, until the outer margins of the clipped area are reached. The sponge is then replaced with a clean one, and the process is repeated until dirt is absent on discarded sponges.

The detergent's lather and scrubbing action are important for mechanical removal of debris and bacteria. Sufficient water to ensure production of a good lather is used, but excess volumes are avoided because wetting the animal increases both heat loss during surgery and moist contamination of surgical drapes.

Transporting and Positioning Patients

Contamination of the prepared area is avoided while a patient is moved to the operating room and placed on the surgery table.

The surgical site is wiped with an antiseptic to complete the preparation. If contamination occurs during transport or positioning, the entire site preparation procedure is repeated.

Draping
(see also Chapter 12)

Draping isolates the surgical site from nonsterile areas and provides a sterile working area for the surgeon. The first layer of drapes isolates a central area containing the proposed incision site. If necessary, additional drapes are placed to ensure complete coverage of the animal and surgical table.

The second drape layer consists of a large single sheet with a central opening. The slit should be slightly larger than the maximum incision size anticipated. The slit is positioned at the incision site and opened outward from this point. Additional drapes are used, as necessary, to ensure that the animal and table are covered by two layers of drapes.

For orthopedic procedures involving long bones and joints, access to the entire limb is necessary. The limb is suspended above the surgery table or elevated by an assistant. The limb is isolated at its base by four drapes. Before release, the distal limb is grasped through a drape by the surgeon. The drape is wrapped around the distal limb and secured with a towel clamp. The entire limb may be covered by a double-layered orthopedic stockinette and secured to the corner drapes by towel clamps. The limb is inserted through the slit drape, and the drape is opened to cover the animal and table with a second layer.

Techniques of Skin Draping (p. 146)

CHAPTER 14
Surgical Facilities and Equipment (pages 147–153)

The surgery suite should be in a location convenient to the work and intensive care areas of the hospital but out of the general traffic flow. The operating room should have a single door, prohibiting the room from becoming a high-traffic area. The door should connect the preparation room, which may double as a treatment room, and the operating room.

Room temperature of approximately 21°C (70°F) with a relative humidity of approximately 50 per cent provides a comfortable environment. Lower ambient room temperatures make it more difficult to maintain a patient's normal body temperature. Airflow should move from areas of least to greatest potential contamination. Air within the operating room is under a mild positive pressure so that when the surgery room door is opened, air flows out of the room rather than into it.

ANESTHESIA AND SURGICAL PREPARATION ROOM (pp. 148–149)

CONTAMINATED SURGERY ROOM (p. 149)

To minimize the spread of infection and cleaning and disinfecting of the surgical suite, a surgery room outside the sterile surgery area for operating on contaminated patients is most beneficial. It may also be used for emergency cases such as a gastric torsion, which may cause gross contamination of the surgical suite. Dental procedures may also be performed here.

STERILE OPERATING ROOM (pp. 149–150)

Microfilm dust pads applied to the floor outside the sterile corridor collect much of the dust from patient transport table rollers and other such equipment. All individuals in the sterile surgery suite should change out of street clothes or cover them. Caps, masks, and shoe covers must be worn. Anyone approaching the surgical field must wear a gown and gloves.

The patient's body temperature must be maintained during surgery. This is best accomplished with a circulating water blanket between the patient and the operating table.

SURGICAL RECOVERY (pp. 150–151)

Intermediate Care

When the surgery case load is high, postoperative patients can be readily observed in a separate recovery ward yet kept separate from sick patients. Cages in this ward are easily cleaned and disinfected. It is of considerable advantage for these cages to have interchangeable oxygen doors. Alternatively, oxygen can be piped to each cage, and nasal oxygen can be delivered through flowmeters and moisturizers mounted above the cages. The entire room should be kept several degrees warmer than the other wards.

Patients requiring continuous monitoring should be taken directly to the intensive care ward from surgery or transferred there, as the condition of the patient dictates.

Intensive Care

Patients requiring continuous monitoring should be taken directly to the intensive care ward. Monitoring equipment, including electrocardiographic, arterial and central venous pressure, and respiratory arrest alarms should be immediately available for use as needed. True intensive care requires continuous supervision, and the intensive care unit must be staffed accordingly.

SUPPORT AREAS (p. 151)

FACILITY AND EQUIPMENT CLEANING AND MAINTENANCE (p. 152)

In-house control of cleaning personnel, whereby specific individual accountability can be defined for specific areas of cleaning, usually results in optimal performance of duty. Surgery rooms must be cleaned superficially between each surgery and thoroughly on a daily basis. The entire room should be disinfected at least once weekly or immediately after a contaminated operation has been performed.

Cleaning equipment and solutions must be kept clean. Mop heads as well as the disinfectant solution used to clean the floors must be changed as soon as they appear dirty (at least daily). The specific disinfectant solution used should be virucidal as well as bactericidal, nonstaining, and noncorrosive. Surfaces to be disinfected should be cleaned well before the disinfecting procedure.

STAFFING THE SURGERY AREA (pp. 152–153)

Whether working in a small facility or a larger one, each individual staff member needs to have a written job description that includes major responsibilities, as well as the organizational structure of the area and the clinic. Employees must know to whom they are expected to answer and, as accurately as possible, their duties. Scheduled periodic evaluations should be made of all staff.

Operating Room Supervisor

An operating room supervisor is essential regardless of the size of the operation. The supervisor is responsible for ordering and stocking all supplies. A relatively constant inventory should be maintained, and as items are used, they should be entered on a reorder list. A surgery log should be maintained, and it may be separate or combined with an anesthetic log. Accurate records on inventory of all controlled substances and their use *must* be maintained.

Surgical Assistant

An invaluable aid to the surgeon is a surgical assistant who anticipates the needs of the surgeon and provides for them accordingly. Technicians with the proper basic training, skills, and attitude should be able to attain an acceptable level of proficiency in a relatively short time with minimal additional training.

Anesthetist

A properly trained anesthetist allows the surgeon to concentrate entirely on the surgical procedure. The anesthetist must have the necessary monitoring and therapy equipment, however, as well as the laboratory support to properly carry out these ends. Flowcharts of the vital parameters should be maintained, and all medications used should be recorded along with their time, amounts, and routes of administration.

CHAPTER 15

Surgical Instruments (pages 154–168)

NEEDLE HOLDERS (p. 154)

The Mayo-Hegar needle holder is the most common type used in veterinary surgery. Selecting too large a needle for a delicate needle holder can result in breakage or damage to the box lock or shank if the instrument is tightly closed. Large needle holders can damage small needles and are often difficult to control when placing delicate sutures.

Better-quality needle holders can often be identified by tungsten carbide inserts, which provide excellent grip and durability. They offer the added advantage of being replaceable.

SCISSORS (pp. 154–155)

Many different types, sizes, and shapes of surgical scissors are available; most are classified by the configuration of their tips.

The Mayo are very sturdy operating scissors that can be used for cutting connective tissue and tough fascial planes. Metzenbaum dissecting scissors are delicate and are reserved for finer tissues. Both of these surgical scissors are available with tungsten carbide inserts.

Specialized scissors are available for many uses. The Potts-Smith, with their various angled blades, are excellent for cardiovascular work. Lister bandage scissors are used for removing large bandages and dressings.

Removal of surgical sutures is best performed with suture scissors. The Littauer scissors are long and sturdy. The smaller Spencer suture scissors are more delicate. Specialized wire-cutting scissors are used for wire skin suture removal.

HEMOSTATIC FORCEPS (pp. 155–156)

Halsted mosquito hemostatic forceps are primarily used to control point bleeders. Larger pedicle or stump ligations that include additional tissue are not appropriate for these instruments.

Kelly and Crile hemostatic forceps are sturdier than the Halsted and can stand more aggressive use. The Kelly have transverse grooves on the distal half of their gripping surface, whereas the Crile have transverse grooves over their entire jaw surface.

Rochester-Carmalt hemostatic forceps are used primarily for ligation of stumps and pedicles. Their grooves run longitudinally, making removal easier during tying of the ligature.

Ochsner hemostatic forceps are sturdy and can stand aggressive use. Their gripping surface has deep cross-grooves and sturdy 1×2 teeth at the tip.

TISSUE FORCEPS (pp. 156–157)

Tissue forceps of various sizes, shapes, and uses are available. Allis tissue forceps are sturdy and can be traumatic to tissue, and should be applied to connective tissue or fascial planes only. Babcock intestinal forceps are similar to Allis but are less traumatic to tissue. The gripping surface on the jaws has fine longitudinal striations. Noyes alligator tissue forceps have many uses. These forceps work well for removing foreign bodies from ear canals and have been used for thoracolumbar disc fenestration. Doyen intestinal forceps are constructed with thin, bowed jaws. The tips of the jaws meet at about the same time as the ratchet's first teeth engage, giving a delicate, nontraumatizing grip. The grooves in the gripping surface are generally longitudinal. Lahey bile duct forceps (right-angled tissue forceps) have jaws with longitudinal grooves and a blunt tip. They are most suitable for blunt dissection in hard-to-view areas and for mobilizing vascular structures for ligation.

THUMB FORCEPS (pp. 157–158)

Thumb forceps are so named because they are generally held between the thumb and first finger. Dressing forceps generally do not have teeth, and their jaws are either smooth or have delicate cross-striations. They are used to grasp sponges or gauze during surgery. Tissue forceps are of similar design to dressing forceps, except that the tips are designed to hold tissue, hence they have teeth that intermesh.

TOWEL CLAMPS (p. 158)

Towel clamps are used for securing drapes to the skin. Towel clamps are also used to secure suction lines, electrocautery cables, and power equipment lines to drapes. Nonpenetrating towel clamps are more appropriate for securing equipment to drapes because they do not create a hole in the drape and thus prevent contamination of the surgical field once the clamp is removed.

BULLDOG CLAMPS (pp. 158–159)

RETRACTORS (pp. 159–161)

Finger-Held Retractors (p. 159)

Hand-Held Retractors (pp. 159–160)

Self-Retaining Retractors (pp. 160–161)

CHAPTER 16

Basic Operative Techniques
(pages 168–191)

All operative procedures, regardless of complexity, involve four basic techniques: (1) incision and excision of tissues; (2) maintenance of hemostasis; (3) handling and care of exposed tissues; and (4) use of sutures, knots, and other materials to restore anatomical structure and support tissues during healing.

INCISION AND EXCISION OF TISSUES (pp. 168–174)

Steel Scalpel

The sharp scalpel with disposable steel blades is the standard soft-tissue cutting instrument against which all others are compared. Properly used, it allows a surgeon to divide tissues with the least trauma.

Three basic grips have been advocated for holding the scalpel: the pencil grip, the fingertip grip, and the palm grip. Each grip has specific characteristics associated with precision of cut, incision length, required cutting force, and angle of the blade.

The *pencil grip* facilitates steadying the hand by allowing it to rest on the patient and uses finger rather than arm movement to incise with the scalpel. This grip is best suited for short, precise incisions.

The *fingertip grip* uses arm motion rather than finger motion to cut tissue and maximizes contact of the cutting edge of the blade with the tissue being incised. The index finger is placed on the upper edge of the blade for stability.

The *palm grip* is advantageous when great pressure must be applied to incise tissue and is more applicable to other cutting instruments, such as the periosteal elevator, than to the scalpel.

Four motions of the cutting edge of the scalpel blade have been described for incising and excising tissues: pressing, sliding, sawing, and scraping.

Press cutting uses the pencil grip and application of increasing pressure in the same direction as the proposed motion of the blade. A stab incision results when the bursting threshold of the tissue is exceeded. This technique is used to initiate gastrotomy, cystotomy, and ventral midline celiotomy incisions.

Slide cutting is the safest and most common method of incising tissues with a scalpel. The increased safety of slide cutting is attributable to application of pressure at a right angle to the motion of the blade. This facilitates precise control of incisional depth as the blade is drawn through tissue.

Sawing or *push-pull slide cutting* uses the pencil grip and allows a short incision to be continued deeper than a single slide cut without removal and reinsertion of the blade into the wound.

High-Energy Scalpels

High-energy cutting instruments include the electrosurgical scalpel, the plasma scalpel, and various forms of lasers (see Chapter 18). Although their energy sources differ, they share a common cutting mechanism.

Advantages reported for electrosurgical incision over the steel scalpel include (1) reduction of total blood loss, (2) decreased need for ligatures, thus reducing the amount of foreign material left in the wound, and (3) reduction of operating time. These advantages are acquired at the expense of delayed wound healing and decreased resistance of wounds to infection.

Electrosurgery uses radiofrequency current to produce one or more of the following effects: incision, coagulation, desiccation, or fulguration of tissues. The predominant effect depends on the waveform of the current. Continuous undamped sine waves provide maximal cutting and minimal coagulation. Conversely, interrupted damped sine waves maximize coagulation and minimize cutting capability. Modulated, pulsed sine waves enable simultaneous cutting and coagulation, or "blended function."

Scissors

Efficient scissor cutting depends on three forces: (1) closing force, which causes the blades to come together; (2) shearing force, which pushes one blade flat against the other during closing; and (3) torque, which rolls the leading edges of each blade inward to touch the other. The grip that best uses scissor design to maximize these forces is the *wide-based tripod grip*, in which the tips of the right thumb and third finger are placed through the rings to grasp the scissors, and the right index finger is placed on the shanks near the fulcrum for support.

Scissor cutting, push cutting, and blunt dissection are the three basic methods of incising and excising tissues with scissors.

Scissor cutting is most applicable to short incisions. Only the tips are used for cutting and the blades are nearly but not completely closed as the scissors are advanced through the tissue with a series of consecutive short cuts.

Long incisions are often initiated with a scissor cut and continued by pushing the nearly closed scissor blades forward to cut the tissue in one continuous motion. This technique, termed *push cutting,* is especially useful for incising sheets of tissue such as pleura, peritoneum, pericardium, and light fascia.

Blunt dissection is accomplished by inserting the closed scissor blades between tissue layers to be separated and opening the handles to spread the blades. Scissors are withdrawn from the wound before closing the blades, preventing inadvertent transection of vital structures within the deeper portion of the wound.

ALTERNATIVES TO CONVENTIONAL METHODS OF EXCISION (p. 174)

Alternatives to standard methods of excision (electrosurgery and cryosurgery) offer the potential advantages of reduced trauma, hemorrhage, and operative time. These techniques also have the potential to inflict extensive damage to surrounding normal tissues, thus negating any advantage over sharp excision.

HEMORRHAGE AND HEMOSTASIS (pp. 174–181)

Hemostasis is important because (1) bleeding obscures the surgical field, reducing operative accuracy and efficiency; (2) blood on the field, gloves, instruments, and drapes provides an ideal medium for bacterial growth and increases the likelihood of infection; (3) postoperative hemorrhage prevents proper coaptation of wound edges, delays healing, and encourages infection; and (4) severe or protracted hemorrhage may result in shock, progressive hypoxemia, and death of the patient.

Primary hemorrhage (which occurs immediately after traumatic disruption of blood vessels) is a predictable consequence of even the most skilled surgical dissection. Experienced surgeons practice ''preventive hemostasis'' through careful planning of approaches, ligation or coagulation of vessels before transection, and gentle accurate dissection to minimize primary hemorrhage.

Delayed hemorrhage, termed *intermediate* if it occurs within 24 hours of injury and *secondary* if it occurs thereafter, is often the result of ineffective treatment of primary hemorrhage.

Pressure Hemostasis

Control of low-pressure hemorrhage from small vessels can often be obtained by applying pressure to the bleeding points for several minutes with gauze sponges or similar material. The success of this method depends on maintaining pressure long enough for effective thrombus formation to occur, followed by careful removal of the pressure pad to avoid disruption of blood clots.

Hemostatic Forceps

When bleeding vessels are to be sacrificed rather than repaired, they can be clamped with hemostatic forceps. Various lengths, shapes, and types are available, including Halsted mosquito and Kelly forceps for small vessels and Crile, Ochsner, and Carmalt forceps for large tissue bundles and vessels.

Basic principles for application of hemostatic forceps are summarized (p. 176).

Cautery

Vascular cauterization can be used for hemostasis for arteries up to 1 mm and veins up to 2 mm in diameter. It is most often performed with a highly damped radiofrequency current from an electrosurgical unit.

Monopolar coagulation, the more commonly used mode, involves flow of current from the handpiece (active electrode) through a patient's body to a ground plate. When using this mode, it is important that current enter a small volume of tissue and leave through a large volume of tissue to prevent pathway burns.

Bipolar coagulation generally uses a bayonet tissue forceps as the active electrode or handpiece. In contrast to monopolar coagulation, the current pathway is much shorter for bipolar coagulation. When tips of the forceps handpiece are held about 1 mm apart, current passes from one tip through the tissue being held to the opposite tip.

Bipolar has advantages over monopolar coagulation: (1) less current is required for a similar coagulative effect because current passes through a much smaller volume of tissue; (2) the risk of unintentional injury to surrounding tissues is greatly decreased, and alternate pathway burns of distant tissues are precluded; and (3) effective coagulation can be obtained in a wet surgical field.

The major advantage of monopolar cautery is its ability to coagulate as well as cut tissues. Regardless of whether monopolar or bipolar coagulation is used, the minimum intensity and duration of current capable of producing hemostasis are selected to minimize trauma.

Vascular Clips and Ligatures

The most secure method of hemostasis for severed vessels that do not require primary repair is application of ligatures or vascular clips. The major disadvantage of clips or ligatures is the foreign material left in the wound.

Vascular clips are usually bent pieces of metal (silver, tantalum, or stainless steel) that can be easily applied to vessels using an applicator similar in design to a needle holder.

Metal vascular clips offer several advantages over ligatures. They can be applied more rapidly and can be securely placed in locations that are virtually inaccessible to ligation. The disadvantages of metal vascular clips are that they are more frequently dislodged by continuing surgical manipulations than are ligatures and they persist in the wound as foreign material, which can interfere with subsequent radiographic studies or radiation treatments.

Ligation, the use of suture material and surgical knots to occlude blood vessels, is used most commonly. Ligatures offer increased security over most hemostatic clips and are better suited for the occlusion of multiple vessels and vascular tissue pedicles. The major disadvantage of ligatures is increased application time.

Ligatures are tied with square knots, which are the least likely to loosen or untie. The simple knot, a *half-hitch,* is the basic component of three different types of knots. Depending on how they are thrown, two consecutive simple knots can result in a square knot, a granny knot, or a half-hitch. *Square knots* are produced by reversing direction on each successive simple knot and maintaining even tension on both strands parallel to the plane of the knot as each throw is tightened.

A *surgeon's knot* is similar to a square knot except that one strand is passed through the loop twice on the first throw. This additional twist of the suture around itself produces increased friction. This knot can be used to advantage for ligation of vascular pedicles with synthetic sutures when tissue tension precludes adequate tightening of the first throw of a square knot. The increased bulk and asymmetry of the surgeon's knot make it less suitable for general ligation than the square knot. Additionally, its security is often less if it is not covered by a square knot.

Basic methods of tying knots include one-hand, two-hand, and instrument tying techniques. *Two-hand tying* is the most reliable technique for consistently producing square knots. Disadvantages of this method are that it is awkward for deep ligatures and it is the most time-consuming method of producing a knot. *One-hand tying* promotes rapid tying, allows a surgeon to carry an instrument in one hand, and is more adaptable to application of deep ligatures. One-hand ties, however, are more susceptible to loosening of the first throw and inadvertent conversion to half-hitch knots. *Instrument tying* uses less suture material and is a reliable technique for producing square knots. Complete tightening of each throw is somewhat less consistent with instrument ties, because a surgeon receives less tactile feedback than with hand ties.

The following *general principles of knot tying* apply to all sutures but especially to ligatures.

1. Knot security is inversely proportional to suture diameter; thus, the smallest suture material providing adequate strength is used.

2. Inadequate tightening of each throw results in a bulkier and less secure knot.

3. To minimize foreign body reaction, the completed knot is small with the ends cut short.

4. Inclusion of a frayed portion of material within a suture weakens it.

5. Extra knots result in unnecessary bulk. Only the minimum throws needed to produce a secure knot are used.

Additional Hemostatic Techniques

Topical hemostatic agents, such as fibrin adhesives, oxidized cellulose, microfibrillar collagen, sponge, and gelatin sponge alone or in combination with thrombin, have been effectively used to control hemorrhage from the cut surfaces of liver, spleen, cancellous bone, and other tissues.

Bleeding from cut bone surfaces, sometimes encountered in decompressive spinal operations, can also be controlled by gently pressing small amounts of *bone wax* into the cancellous bone at hemorrhage points.

Another means of controlling diffuse hemorrhage involves applying pressure by various techniques. Umbilical tape wound packing in the nasal cavity and gauze tampons in the vaginal region have been used to reduce postoperative hemorrhage from these areas. Wound closure and external pressure bandages are additional examples of limiting hemorrhage by pressure.

HANDLING AND CARE OF TISSUES (pp. 181–184)

Gentle manipulation of tissues with respect for blood supply, innervation, and hydration are prerequisites to ''atraumatic'' surgical technique. Optimal surgical results are possible only with continual attention to careful tissue handling.

Tissue Forceps

Tissue forceps are usually held in a surgeon's nondominant hand. When in use, they are grasped with a pencil grip. When temporarily not in use, tissue forceps may be carried in the palmed position, leaving the thumb, index finger, and middle finger free. Tissue forceps are used to stabilize tissues for incision or suturing, to retract tissues for exposure or excision, and to grasp vessels for electrocoagulation. When using tissue forceps, grasp the minimum amount of tissue and apply the minimum amount of pressure necessary to produce a secure hold. Grasping too much tissue or repeated regrasping of tissue produces unnecessary trauma.

Stabilization and Retraction of Tissues

Numerous forceps with box locks are available for stabilizing tissues or occluding hollow organs during surgery. These instruments may be applied with impunity to tissues that are to be excised. They must be used judiciously on tissues that are to remain, because they are capable of producing crushing trauma.

Self-retaining retractors are indispensable when working without an assistant. The major hazard of self-retaining retractors is trauma or ischemia at the point of contact. During lengthy procedures, it is advisable to release self-retaining retractors periodically to prevent devitalization of wound edges.

Wound Irrigation and Suction

Operative wound lavage has been associated with reduced rates of postoperative infection for both clean and contaminated wounds in direct proportion to the volume of the irrigating solution used. This phenomenon has been attributed to removal of surface bacteria and debris from contaminated wounds, dislodgment and removal of bacteria and exudate from infected wounds, and dilution and removal of toxins associated with infection.

Antibiotics and antiseptics have been added to lavage solutions and may be effective in contaminated wounds; however, conclusive evidence that this technique is superior to saline lavage with concurrent administration of systemic antibiotics is lacking.

Simple flooding followed by suctioning is commonly used for lavage of the peritoneal and pleural cavities. Complete removal of the lavage fluid is essential to avoid dilution of opsonins required for phagocytosis, especially if the peritoneal cavity is being lavaged. More superficial wounds may benefit from treatment using moderate- or high-pressure lavage, especially if bacteria or foreign debris is present.

WOUND CLOSURE (pp. 184–191)
Needle Holder

Inefficient use of the needle holder accounts for more wasted time than poor technique with any other instrument. Its proper use in placement of a suture involves ten basic steps:

1. *Positioning the needle*—generally grasped perpendicular to the long axis of the needle holder and near the tip of the needle for greatest driving force (dense tissue), near the midpoint of the needle for general purpose suturing and near the eye of the needle when suturing delicate tissues.

2. *Properly grasping the needle holder.*

3. *Positioning the free end of the suture,* generally on the far side of the field.

4. *Placing the needle point*—introduction of the needle to permit forehand sewing is easiest (toward the surgeon or from right to left depending on the orientation of the wound).

5. *Driving the needle*—a single rotating motion of the hand with an arc similar to that of the needle is most efficient.

6. *Releasing the needle*—use of tissue forceps to stabilize the tissue layer being sutured during release of the needle holder decreases the chance of needle dislodgment.

7. *Regrasping the needle*—perpendicular regrasping is most efficient.

8. *Extracting the needle*—extraction with the hand supinated often allows the next suture of a continuous pattern to be placed without having to reposition the needle; extraction with the hand pronated facilitates more precise extraction.

9. *Pulling the desired length of suture through the wound*—one

uninterrupted motion with the needle holder away from the wound is preferable to hand-over-hand pulling of the suture by the assistant.

   10. *Tying the knot or repositioning the needle for the next suture.*

Suture Patterns

A vast number of suture patterns have been described, categorized according to the following factors: (1) anatomical areas in which they are placed; (2) tendency to promote apposition, inversion, or eversion of tissues; (3) ability to overcome tension forces that may disrupt accurate approximation of tissues; and (4) whether they are placed in a continuous or an interrupted fashion.

   The major advantage of interrupted patterns is the ability to precisely adjust tension at each point along the wound. The major advantage of continuous patterns is suturing speed.

   Each suture is a separate entity in interrupted patterns, and failure of one suture is often inconsequential. Suture breakage in a continuous pattern, however, may lead to disruption of the entire line of closure. Disadvantages of interrupted patterns include increased time needed to tie multiple knots, increased volume of foreign material left in the wound when sutures are buried, and poor suture economy. In contrast, continuous patterns use less suture material and minimize knots, reducing both operative time and the amount of foreign material left in the wound. In addition, continuous patterns form a more air- or watertight seal. Disadvantages of continuous patterns include less precise control of suture tension and wound approximation and the potentially disastrous effects of suture breakage.

CHAPTER 17

Cryosurgery (pages 191–196)

Cryosurgery is the controlled destruction of unwanted tissue by the application of cold temperature.

CRYOBIOLOGY (pp. 191–192)

Cooling to a temperature of $-20°C$ ($-4°F$) destroys almost all unprotected mammalian cells. The destruction of tissue is either direct or early, or indirect or delayed. Direct injury begins with the formation of ice crystals, both intracellular and extracellular. Intracellular crystals cause rupture of a cell's outer membrane. Extracellular ice formation causes dehydration of the cellular environment, resulting in lethal electrolyte concentrations and pH shifts.

   Indirect or delayed injury from freezing is mostly the result of vascular stasis. The permeability of the vessels is increased, and loss of plasma results in local hemoconcentration. Damage to the endothelium of the arterioles and venules causes adherence of red blood cells and platelets to the vessel wall. Thrombosis of the vessels and infarction of the frozen tissue occur within hours of freezing.

   Rapid freezing causes the greatest development of intracellular ice. Slow thawing of the tissue permits the phenomenon of recrystallization, during which small crystals grow to a larger, more damaging size.

   Tissues react to cold differently depending on their water content, cellularity, and vascularity. Relatively "dry" tissues, such as corneal stroma, are somewhat resistant to damage by freezing because their low water content limits ice formation. Cortical bone, although weakened by loss of the cellular components, remains as a mineral scaffold for revascularization. Because of their continuous heat input, major blood vessels and highly vascular tissues are difficult to freeze rapidly and tend to thaw quickly without loss of function.

During a single freeze-thaw cycle, it is possible that some unwanted tissue within the ice ball will be positioned near the periphery or close enough to a major artery that the treatment will not be lethal. Because precooled tissue freezes faster than normal tissue, repeating the rapid-freeze–slow-thaw cycle helps ensure the entire tissue mass is destroyed.

CRYOGENS (p. 192)

Liquid nitrogen is probably the most versatile cryogen available. It has a boiling point of $-195.8°C$ ($-320.4°F$) and can be used by spray or probe.

Although it can be used as a spray, nitrous oxide is most commonly used to cool cryosurgical probes. The gas is released under high pressure through a small orifice inside the probe, and the rapid expansion of the gas (Joule-Thomson effect) produces probe temperatures of $-89°C$ ($-128.2°F$).

CRYOSURGICAL INSTRUMENTATION (pp. 192–193)
Sprays

Self-pressurizing spray guns are designed to deliver a combination of vapor and droplets of liquid cryogen onto the target surface. All liquid nitrogen spray units must be able to withstand increased internal pressures and low temperatures without damage; the use of homemade thermos bottle sprayers is extremely dangerous.

Probes

Freezing temperatures can be achieved in cryosurgical probes by either circulating liquid nitrogen through them or by releasing a high-pressure gas through a small orifice within the tip of the probe. Probe freezing is generally easier to control than spray but is less lethal to tissues than direct application of the cryogen.

Probes can be used for either contact or penetration freezing. Contact freezing involves placing the cold probe against the moist surface of the tumor to form a cryoadhesion. Penetration freezing is usually performed in larger lesions. A core biopsy specimen is removed from the center of the tumor, and the cryoprobe placed directly within the mass.

METHODOLOGY (pp. 193–194)
Preparation of Patients

Clipping the hair from the area immediately surrounding the target tissue permits easier visual inspection of the expanding ice ball and recognition of potential problems with runoff of liquid nitrogen. It also prevents postoperative accumulation of debris in the hair around lesions and decreases odors. Sterility is not needed.

Anesthesia

Freezing the surrounding normal tissue does cause pain, and animals are sometimes startled by the hissing noise made by the cryosurgical units. Sedation is usually all that is required to perform minor cryosurgery on a calm patient in a quiet environment. If infiltration with local anesthetic is elected, the use of lidocaine with epinephrine not only helps to obtund the pain of the treatment but facilitates a rapid-freeze–slow-thaw cycle by creating local vasoconstriction.

Biopsy Samples

Biopsy samples should usually be taken from all neoplasms or tumors.

Monitoring the Frozen Area

Monitoring the depth of freezing can be done either subjectively or objectively. Subjective assessment is by visual inspection and palpation of the ice ball as it spreads from the edge of the tumor. Approximately 75 per cent of the tissue within the ice ball is destroyed by freezing. Fixation of frozen tissue to deeper fascial planes can also be used to estimate the depth of the ice ball when freezing a cutaneous tumor. Objective monitoring requires the use of pyrometers to measure the temperature achieved beyond the limits of the target tissue.

POSTOPERATIVE SEQUELAE (pp. 194–195)

Swelling. Swelling of the treated area occurs within hours of freezing because of local vasodilation and increased vascular permeability. This local swelling is self-limited and resolves within 48 hours of treatment.

Bleeding. If the lesion was ulcerated or underwent biopsy and was not treated with some form of styptic or sutures, postfreezing vasodilation can cause excessive bleeding.

Necrosis. As frozen cutaneous tissue undergoes necrosis, it forms a dry eschar that protects the underlying healing wound. Treatment is neither needed nor recommended, and the scab sloughs in 10 to 14 days.

Depigmentation. Because of their relative cryosensitivity and superficial location, melanocytes and hair follicles are destroyed by freezing.

Odor. If freezing involved a mucous membrane or mucocutaneous junction or if the patient licks excessively at the site, the eschar is moist and accompanied by drainage and odor.

INDICATIONS (pp. 195–196)

Cancerous and noncancerous cutaneous lesions are common in small animals. The reduced need for general anesthesia in geriatric patients commonly afflicted with these lesions is an advantage of cryosurgery.

Because cryosurgery does not require a sterile surgical field, it is a good choice for the treatment of benign perianal and oral tumors. Cryosurgery is also a recommended method of "debulking" and treating perianal fistulas. Many ophthalmic procedures make use of the relative cryoresistance of the fibrous support tissues of the eye (see Chapters 81 and 82).

CONTRAINDICATIONS (p. 196)

Mast cells lysed by freezing release histamine and heparin locally. Local erythema and the size of the sloughing may be excessive for the size of the tumor. Tumors that have major bony involvement do not respond well and should probably not be treated by cryosurgery. Although major blood vessels and nerves are resistant to permanent damage by freezing, they can be destroyed by necrosis and sloughing of surrounding tissues.

CHAPTER 18
Surgical Lasers (pages 197–203)

HOW LASERS WORK (p. 197)

The acronym *LASER* stands for *l*ight *a*mplification by the *s*timulated *e*mission of *r*adiation. Understanding lasers requires knowledge of how stimulated emission multiplies light and produces the unique differences between coherent (laser) and noncoherent (regular) light. Three requirements for lasers are a specific medium, a photoresonator, and a way to energize the medium.

SURGICAL LASERS (p. 197)

No ideal or all-purpose surgical laser exists. An all-purpose laser would be tunable with operator-defined wavelengths from the infrared through ultraviolet, have a wide range of power, be portable, and exhibit economical and reliable performance.

LIGHT–TISSUE INTERACTIONS (pp. 197–199)

Light interaction with tissue causes tissue and surgical effects. Light may be reflected from, transmitted through, scattered by, or absorbed into the target. Reflection is angular diversion of light from the air–skin interface or the stratum corneum. Transmission is the passing of electromagnetic radiation through tissue without interaction or effect. Scatter, backscatter, diffraction, and refraction are optical phenomena that are complex in living tissue and poorly understood in terms of their cause and effects. Absorption depends on absorptive coefficients of the water and pigments in the target for a particular light wavelength. On absorption, a number of biologically relevant chemical, thermal, or mechanical effects occur.

Light Delivery

Delivery of laser output to a target is by lenses, mirrors, and optical fibers. An internally mirrored, articulated delivery arm is used to "turn corners" for some infrared lasers and will be required until economical and practical optical fibers are available. An autoclavable handpiece contains the final focusing lens that configures the optical spot size and working distance.

Energy Delivery

Power output (watts), power density (watts/cm^2), total energy (joules = power × time), the geometric mode of the beam, lens focus, and angle of incidence influence energy delivery. Other variables in thermal damage in wounds are water vaporization, flow of molten collagen within the wound, rate of heat conduction into adjacent tissue, and local blood perfusion.

WOUND HEALING (p. 199)

Healing time of primarily closed laser skin wounds is 5 days longer than with cold-blade incisions. Ultimate tensile and bursting strength, cicatrix formation, dehiscence, and other aspects of wound healing are normal after the increased lag phase.

SURGICAL INDICATIONS FOR CARBON DIOXIDE LASERS (pp. 199–200)

The high absorption of far infrared light by intracellular water confines the thermal effects of carbon dioxide (CO_2) lasers to the target's surface. The CO_2 laser is especially well suited for efficient, excisional photovaporization of infected, dysplastic, or neoplastic lesions on skin or mucous membranes.

NEODYMIUM:YTTRIUM-ALUMINUM-GARNET LASERS (p. 200)

The near-infrared light (1,064 nm) of the neodymium:yttrium-aluminum-garnet (Nd:YAG) laser is not well absorbed by either water or tissue pigments. The absorption ''window'' causes irregular thermal effects in tissue proteins in a three-dimensional volume. The surgeon always considers potential injury to normal adjacent structures when planning an Nd:YAG laser approach.

OPHTHALMIC Nd:YAG LASERS (p. 200)
ARGON LASERS (p. 201)
"TUNABLE" DYE LASERS (p. 201)
LOW-POWER LASERS (p. 201)

Milliwatt lasers are popular in sports medicine and produce light in the visible red and near-infrared spectrum. These lasers purport to facilitate pain relief, wound healing, and repair of ligament and tendon injury. Conclusive evidence for laser effects is not currently available.

SURGICAL TECHNIQUE (p. 201)

The operative techniques of laser surgery are simple but different from mechanical surgery. Changing power output changes the general working speed. Focus versus defocus, continuous versus pulsed mode, angle of incidence, and projected beam versus contact probe also modify surgical effects. Use the highest available power for the shortest possible duration, increase the handpiece ''drag rate,'' and use painting patterns in continuous-wave lasing. To drill a hole, one maintains focus as the hole deepens. For hemostasis, the bleeder must be seen and blotted dry before photocoagulation. As with other forms of thermal surgery, traction and countertraction across the proposed incision are effective in improving the efficiency of cutting.

LASER SAFETY (pp. 201–203)

Preoperative Precautions

Before surgery, the laser is tested to validate control function, focus, and power output. Equipment for fighting a possible fire is kept available, and a laser emblem logo is always posted outside the operating room door as a safety warning.

As the eye captures and focuses light, a major safety objective is to prevent ocular damage to the patient and operating team. Visible light and YAG lasers, however, require full-coverage goggles having specific and rigid transmittance specifications.

Endotracheal tubes require special preoperative preparation if laser light has any conceivable access to the tube. For maximum protection, the endotracheal tube is removed during critical lasing periods in oral, laryngeal, or tracheal procedures.

Operative Precautions

The primary safety objective is that a laser never fire by accident or at an unintended target. During an operative procedure, the standby mode is always selected to disable output when the machine is not needed.

Photofulguration and photovaporization often produce large quantities of noxious smoke. Evacuation of smoke is a strict requirement for safety and aesthetic reasons.

Hand burns to the operative team result from reflections off of shiny surgical instruments. Obtain blackened or "pitted" instrument finishes for those instruments frequently brought into a laser surgical field.

CHAPTER 19

Suture Materials, Tissue Adhesives, Staplers, and Ligating Clips (pages 204–212)

Many different types of suture materials are currently available. Suture selection should be based on knowledge of the physical and biological properties of suture materials, an assessment of local conditions in the particular wound, and the healing rate of wounds in various tissues.

CLASSIFICATION (pp. 204–208)

Sutures are either absorbable or nonabsorbable. Absorbable sutures undergo degradation and rapid loss of tensile strength within 60 days. Nonabsorbable sutures retain tensile strength for longer than 60 days. Sutures are also either natural or synthetic.

Natural Absorbable Sutures

Surgical Gut (Catgut)

Surgical gut is prepared from the submucosa of sheep or cattle small intestine and is composed of formaldehyde-treated collagen. Surgical gut is a capillary multifilament suture that is machine ground and polished to yield a relatively smooth surface that resembles a monofilament.

Absorption of surgical gut after implantation is a two-stage process primarily involving macrophages. First, molecular bonds are broken by acid hydrolysis and collagenolysis. Second, digestion and absorption by proteolytic enzymes occur during the later stages of removal.

Because of its collagenous composition, surgical gut stimulates a significant foreign body reaction in implanted tissue.

Surgical gut is available in plain and chromic forms. Treatment with chromium salts increases intermolecular bonding, tensile strength, and resistance to digestion and decreases tissue reactivity. Surgical gut generally exhibits good handling characteristics. When wet, surgical gut swells, weakens, and has poor knot security. Disadvantages of surgical gut include its variability in loss of tensile strength, capillarity, the inflammatory reaction it induces, and the occasional sensitivity reaction.

Collagen (p. 204)

Synthetic Absorbable Sutures

Synthetic absorbable sutures were introduced to reduce variability in absorption and loss of tensile strength associated with natural products.

Polyglycolic Acid

Polyglycolic acid (PGA) is a braided multifilament polymer of glycolic (hydroxyacetic) acid. It is absorbed by hydrolysis, not phagocytosis, presumably through esterase activity. Absorption is minimal until 14 days after implantation, complete within 120 days, and associated with a markedly reduced inflammatory process compared with surgical gut. PGA is relatively strong and ductile, similar to polyglactin 910 and monofilament nylon. Loss of tensile strength is 33 per cent by 7 days of implantation and approximately 80 per cent within 14 days. Disadvantages of PGA sutures include their tendency to drag through the tissues, to cut friable tissue, and possibly to have poorer knot security than surgical gut.

Polyglactin 910

Polyglactin 910 is a braided synthetic fiber composed of glycolic and lactic acid in a ratio of 9:1. It is both more hydrophobic and more resistant to hydrolysis than PGA suture. Absorption is by the same mechanism (i.e., hydrolysis) and with a similar pattern of tensile strength loss as PGA. Both polyglactin 910 and PGA sutures have no detectable strength by 21 days. Polyglactin 910 is stronger than PGA up to 21 days after implantation.

Polydioxanone (PDS)

PDS is a polymer of paradioxanone; it is extruded into monofilaments of variable size. PDS, like PGA and polyglactin 910, is degraded by hydrolysis but at a slower rate. PDS suture loses 26 per cent of its tensile strength after 14 days, 42 per cent after 28 days, and 86 per cent after 56 days. Absorption is essentially complete at 182 days after implantation. Tissue reactivity is similar to that with PGA and polyglactin 910.

Polyglyconate

Polyglyconate, a monofilament suture, is a copolymer of glycolic acid and trimethylene carbonate. Polyglyconate is capable of supporting healing wounds for long periods and has similar tensile strength to PDS. The pattern of loss of tensile strength is similar to that of PDS.

Natural Nonabsorbable Sutures

Silk

Silk is available as a twisted or braided multifilament. Although classified as a nonabsorbable suture, silk slowly loses tensile strength and is absorbed within approximately 2 years of tissue implantation. Silk is inexpensive and has excellent handling characteristics, having the best "feel" of any available suture material.

One of the disadvantages of silk is the tissue reaction that it incites. Silk's limitations include the potential to produce gastrointestinal ulceration if the suture protrudes into the lumen and to serve as a nidus for calculus formation in the lumen of the urinary bladder or gallbladder.

Silk should also be avoided in contaminated wounds. The interstices between its fibers permit serum and blood to penetrate and form a refuge for bacteria.

Cotton (p. 206)

Stainless Steel

Stainless steel is available as a monofilament or twisted multifilament suture. It is biologically inert, noncapillary, and easily sterilized by autoclaving. It has the highest tensile strength and greatest knot security of all the suture materials, and it maintains this strength when implanted in tissues. Stainless steel incites virtually no inflammatory reaction on implantation, except for that caused by tissue movement against the inflexible ends of the suture. The monofilament form can be used effectively in contaminated and infected wounds, because it does not support infection. Disadvantages of stainless steel include its tendency to cut tissues, poor handling characteristics, and diminished ability to withstand repeated bending without breaking.

Nonabsorbable Synthetic Sutures

Nylon

Nylon causes minimal tissue reaction. After implantation, monofilament nylon loses about 30 per cent of its original tensile strength by 2 years as a result of chemical degradation. Multifilament nylon loses 100 per cent of its tensile strength after 6 months in tissue.

The main disadvantages of nylon are its poor handling characteristics and knot security. It possesses "memory," which is a tendency to revert to its original configuration. This characteristic may be overcome by careful placement of knots with four or five throws.

Polymerized Caprolactam (Vetafil, Supramid)

Polymerized caprolactam is a twisted multifilament polyamide suture of the nylon family that is commonly used in veterinary surgery. It has superior tensile strength compared with nylon. It has relatively poor knot security, and autoclaving increases the difficulty in handling. Polymerized caprolactam is intermediate in tissue reactivity.

Polyester Fibers

Polyester is a braided multifilament available in plain and coated forms. Coatings, including polybutylate, Teflon, and silicone, add a lubricant-like quality that decreases suture drag when drawn through tissue. This suture is one of the strongest nonmetallic suture materials available and undergoes little or no loss of tensile strength after implantation in tissues. Once properly placed, polyester sutures offer prolonged support for slowly healing tissues.

Polyester causes the most tissue reaction of the synthetic suture materials. It produced a reaction equal to chromic gut when implanted for 4 weeks in a canine tendon. Shedding of the Teflon coat in tissues increases the inflammatory response.

Polybutester

Polybutester possesses many of the advantages of both polypropylene and polyester, because it is slippery and plastic, yet has good tensile strength and knot security characteristics.

Polyolefin Plastics

Polypropylene. Polypropylene is a polymer of propylene and is available as a monofilament. It has greater knot security than all other monofilament nonmetallic synthetic materials. It retains its strength on implantation. It is not weakened by tissue enzymes and is the least thrombogenic suture. Because of its high flexibility, it is suitable for closing tissues having great elongation capability, such as skin and cardiac muscle. Advantages of polypropylene are its strength, inertness, retention of strength after implantation, minimal tissue reactivity, and resistance to bacterial contamination. The only disadvantages are its slippery handling and tying characteristics.

Polyethylene. Polyethylene is similar to polypropylene in its minimal tissue reactivity and resistance to bacterial contamination. The major disadvantage of polyethylene suture is its poor knot security.

Polytetrafluoroethylene. Polytetrafluoroethylene is a new nonabsorbable monofilament suture material that has favorable characteristics including relatively high strength, flexibility, and good knot security when four throws are used. Its primary disadvantage is its high cost.

SELECTION OF SUTURE MATERIALS (p. 208) (Table 19–1)

SUTURE MATERIALS FOR DIFFERENT TISSUES (p. 209)

Skin. Monofilament nylon and polypropylene are the preferred sutures for skin.

Subcutis. Synthetic absorbable sutures are preferred because of their low tissue reactivity.

Fascia. Synthetic nonabsorbable suture materials are recommended for closure of fascia if prolonged suture strength is required. Surgical gut and synthetic absorbable sutures have also been used effectively in fascia.

TABLE 19–1. PRINCIPLES OF SELECTING A SUTURE MATERIAL

Sutures should be at least as strong as the normal tissue through which they are placed.

The relative rates at which suture loses strength and the wound gains strength should be compatible.

If the suture biologically alters the healing process, these changes must be considered when selecting a suture.

The mechanical properties of the suture should closely match those of the tissue to be closed.

Muscle. Synthetic absorbable or nonabsorbable sutures may be used effectively in muscle.

Hollow Viscus. Surgical gut, synthetic absorbable sutures, and monofilament nonabsorbable sutures may be used in viscera.

Tendon. Nylon and stainless steel are usually recommended for tendon repair.

Blood Vessel. Because it is the least thrombogenic suture, polypropylene is probably the material of choice in vascular repair.

Nerve. Low reactivity is the most important consideration in peripheral nerve repair. Nylon and polypropylene are recommended.

SELECTION OF THE APPROPRIATE SUTURE SIZE (p. 209)

Proper suture selection involves the choice of both the appropriate type and size. Suture is sized as either United States Pharmacopoeia (USP) or metric. Guidelines for the selection of appropriately sized suture in small animal surgery are listed in Table 19–2.

SELECTION OF SURGICAL NEEDLES (pp. 209–210)

Important factors to be considered in needle selection are the characteristics of the needles, the wound to be sutured, and the tissue being sutured. There are two categories of surgical needles: swaged (eyeless) needles and eyed needles. Swaged needles are immediately available, are less traumatic to the tissue, are always sharp, and are guaranteed sterile. Eyed needles are reusable and less expensive than swaged needles.

The common shapes are straight, half-curved, and parts of a circle (e.g., three-eighths circle, one-half circle). Straight needles are best used near the surface of the body. One-half circle needles are convenient for small wounds and wounds deep within a cavity.

The type of point is another consideration in needle selection. Noncutting needles are round (taper) needles with no edges. They are generally used for parenchymatous organs, fat, and muscle. Cutting needles are ground and honed to produce an edge that penetrates dense tissues. Three types of cutting needles are available: conventional, reverse, and tapered. Conventional curved cutting needles have the cutting edge along the concave surface. Reverse curved cutting needles have the cutting edge along the convex surface. They have two advantages over conventional cutting needles: minimized risk of cutting out of the tissue and increased needle strength. Tapered cutting needles

TABLE 19–2. GUIDELINES FOR SELECTION OF SUTURE IN SMALL ANIMAL SURGERY

Tissue	Suture Size (USP)
Skin	4-0 to 3-0
Subcutis	4-0 to 3-0
Fascia	3-0 to 0
Muscle	3-0 to 0
Hollow viscus	5-0 to 2-0
Tendon	3-0 to 0
Vessel (ligatures)	4-0 to 2-0
Vessel (sutures)	6-0 to 5-0
Nerve	6-0 to 5-0

combine a round shaft with a cutting point. They are used when both delicate and dense tissue need to be penetrated.

TISSUE ADHESIVES (p. 210)

The cyanoacrylates have been used most extensively. Monomers of cyanoacrylate are converted from a liquid to a solid state by polymerization, catalyzed by minute amounts of water on the tissue surfaces.

Tissue toxicity is a problem with some of the cyanoacrylates. Other problems that have been reported with the use of cyanoacrylate tissue adhesives are granuloma formation, severe wound infections when used in contaminated wounds, delayed healing if the wound edges are separated, poor adhesion on excessively moist surfaces, and interference with normal cortical fracture union.

SURGICAL STAPLERS (pp. 210–211)

LIGATING CLIPS (p. 211)

Ligating clips often offer improved efficiency for achieving hemostasis when compared with other surgical methods such as ligation. They are currently available as metallic or absorbable clips. Metallic clips are widely used in surgery, are V shaped, and have minimal reactivity in tissues, appropriate strength, and proper malleability. Absorbable clips have an integral locking mechanism to prevent reopening. Potential disadvantages of ligating clips are the relative instability of the clip in the applicator, insecurity of a clip that is inadequately applied to the vessel, and permanence of metallic clips in tissue.

CHAPTER 20
Monitoring the Surgical Patient (pages 212–224)

Monitoring of important physiological functions allows awareness of a patient's homeostatic state, response to adverse changes, and prevention of compensatory failure.

GENERAL VARIABLES (pp. 212–214) (Table 20–1)

Monitoring of surgical patients centers on assessment of cardiovascular and pulmonary function and the status of body fluid compartments. Assessment of these physiological variables is done directly by specific observation and indirectly by measurement or observation of variables strongly influenced by the one of interest. Measurement of body temperature is a direct observation, whereas measurement of urine output is a reflection of tissue perfusion.

General Condition

The overall appearance of a patient is used as a nonspecific parameter of health status. Deviation from normal can be detected by simple observation, and although the information it relates lacks specificity

TABLE 20-1. Normal Values for Some Physiological Variables in Dogs and Cats*

Variable	Dog	Cat†	Variable	Dog	Cat†
Ventilatory variables			*Circulatory variables*		
Breaths per minute	16–30		Heartbeats per minute	80–140	60–140
Tidal volume	10–15 ml/kg		Arterial pressure		
PaO_2	85–105 mm Hg		Systolic (direct)	105–156 mm Hg	
PvO_2	35–40 mm Hg		Systolic (indirect)	110–158 mm Hg	
$PaCO_2$	26–38 mm Hg		Mean (direct)	85–130 mm Hg	
$PvCO_2$	29–44 mm Hg		Mean (indirect)	80–110 mm Hg	
Arterial pH	7.33–7.45	7.29–7.40	Central venous pressure		
Venous pH	7.30–7.40	7.24–7.38	(mean)	1–4 mm Hg	
Hemoglobin saturation (%)	Arterial 95–97		(mean)	1–6 cm H_2O	
	Venous 65–75		Pulmonary artery pressure		
			(systolic)	20–35 mm Hg	
Blood and fluid variables			(diastolic)	8–15 mm Hg	
Sodium mEq/L (serum)	140–160		(mean)	10–16 mm Hg	
Potassium mEq/L (serum)	3.7–5.8	4.0–4.5	Pulmonary wedge pressure	6–10 mm Hg	
Chloride mEq/L (serum)	100–115	115–123	(mean)	7–14 cm H_2O	
Bicarbonate mEq/L (serum)	16–23		(mean)		
Total protein g/dl	5.0–7.6	5.2–6.6	Cardiac index	1.8–3.5 L/m²	
Hemoglobin g/dl PCV	12–18	8–15	Tissue pH	7.31–7.42	
	35–49	27–45	Capillary refill time	1–2 seconds	
Urine output	1.0–1.7 ml/kg/min	0.8–1.5 ml/kg/min			
Urine specific gravity	1.015–1.045	1.020–1.060			

*These variables have been gathered from many sources, the data from which have been averaged and rounded to clinically useful ranges.
†Data for cats are presented only if they differ from those for dogs. Data for some variables are not available.

and objectivity, observation of the overall condition is valuable for interpreting the significance of changes in other variables.

Body Temperature

Anesthetics depress the thermoregulatory center, making environmental exposure an important cause of heat loss during surgery and recovery. During procedures in which body cavities are open, evaporative heat loss may be dramatic, particularly in small animals.

Elevations in body temperature during anesthesia may signal the onset of malignant hyperthermia or heat gain from a heating pad. Patients kept in oxygen cages or incubators, under heating lamps, or on heating pads may also have elevations in temperature. Elevations in body temperature during the first 24 hours after surgery are usually benign and due to tissue injury.

Monitoring

Intraoperative monitoring is most conveniently done using a thermistor probe and an electronic thermometer. Core temperature is not accurately reflected by a rectal or esophageal probe if the abdominal or thoracic cavity, respectively, is open during surgery.

VENTILATORY VARIABLES (pp. 214–216)
Breathing Pattern

Many conditions induce changes in the rate of breathing. During surgery, tachypnea can indicate a lightening of anesthesia, pain, or, if anesthesia is being delivered in a closed system, saturation of the carbon dioxide (CO_2) absorber or malfunction of the oxygen delivery system. Bradypnea can be due to deepening of anesthesia, stimulation of the vagus nerve, alkalosis, or hypocarbia. In the postoperative period, tachypnea can signal hemorrhage, pneumothorax, pulmonary edema, pain, pneumonia, or increased body temperature.

Monitoring

Assessing ventilatory efficiency requires thoughtful observation, stethoscopy, ventilometry, and, when indicated, radiography.

Changes in the rate, character, and sounds of breathing and in tidal volume do not correlate directly with changes in blood gas values and are only presumptive evidence of impaired ventilation. However, they are important signs and should be monitored routinely.

Blood Gases

Pa_{CO_2} is used to characterize ventilatory status, elevated Pa_{CO_2} indicating hypoventilation and decreased Pa_{CO_2} indicating hyperventilation. Blood CO_2 in conjunction with blood pH is used to determine a patient's acid-base balance. Respiratory acidosis is encountered with accumulation of CO_2 through hypoventilation. Conversely, respiratory alkalosis accompanies excessive elimination of CO_2 through hyperventilation. Metabolic acidosis is due to accumulation of nonvolatile acids such as lactic acid. Metabolic alkalosis evolves through loss of nonvolatile acids when hydrochloric acid is lost through vomiting. Mixed states are created when the body attempts to compensate for acidosis or alkalosis by decreasing or increasing elimination of CO_2.

Pa_{O_2} is used to assess the efficiency of ventilation. It is only slightly influenced by the rate and depth of breathing. It is more strongly influenced by the balance between pulmonary blood flow and alveolar ventilation.

Oxygen saturation gives information about the amount of oxygen held by hemoglobin. Therefore, the oxygen saturation of arterial and mixed venous blood are used to assess tissue oxygenation.

Monitoring

Blood samples are drawn under anaerobic conditions into heparinized syringes. The sample should be analyzed immediately because gas exchange between the blood and the atmosphere proceeds through the plastic syringe.

Capnography (p. 215)
Pulse Oximetry

Pulse oximetry provides continuous noninvasive *in vivo* measurement of arterial hemoglobin saturation by determining the color of the blood between a light source and a photodetector.

Monitoring

Monitoring is carried out by placing a sensor on the skin or a mucous membrane. The per cent arterial saturation, heart rate, and, with some machines, pulse contour are displayed continuously.

Packed Cell Volume

Changes in packed cell volume (PCV) commonly occur in surgical patients and are usually associated with blood loss and dehydration. Low PCVs are tolerated well if they develop slowly so that physiological compensation can occur. However, patients with PCVs less than 20 per cent do not tolerate stress as well as those with normal PCVs.

If PCV is concurrently reduced by half, cardiac output must double to meet baseline requirements and triple to meet the postoperative demand for oxygen. Such increases in cardiac output may not be possible for very ill or hypovolemic patients. Additionally, myocardial oxygenation is inadequate if PCV is acutely lowered to 20 per cent or less.

Monitoring

PCV is conveniently monitored using capillary tubes and a micro-hematocrit centrifuge.

CIRCULATORY VARIABLES (pp. 216–219)
Heart Rate

Rates outside the normal range, both high and low, are associated with reduced cardiac output. A continuously high resting rate or a rate that is gradually increasing with time indicates hypoxemia, deteriorating myocardial function, or hypovolemia. Bradycardia is caused by vagal stimulation during surgery, deep planes of anesthesia, and hypothermia.

Monitoring

Palpation of either the apex impulse or the arterial pulse detects cardiac activity but can be unreliable in obese patients and those in shock.

Auscultation provides accurate assessment of rate and also provides some indication of the strength of cardiac activity.

Electronic heart rate meters that trigger on the R wave can be used for continuous monitoring. Their usefulness is limited because no information about mechanical activity of the heart is obtained. A disadvantage of Doppler flow probes is the probe's sensitivity to position and movement.

Direct recording of arterial pulse waves is a highly accurate means of monitoring heart rate. Its disadvantages include its invasiveness and the expense of the necessary equipment.

Arterial Pulse

Palpation of the pulse is a time-honored way to quickly and easily make a subjective evaluation of cardiovascular function. A small stroke volume ejected rapidly into a vascular tree having increased tone, as encountered in patients in early shock, produces a sharp, high-amplitude, short-duration pulse in the femoral artery and an imperceptible pulse in a distal artery. Conversely, a normal volume ejected weakly into a low-tone vascular tree, as may exist during anesthesia, produces a soft, low-amplitude, long-duration pulse in the femoral artery and a weak distal pulse.

Monitoring

Arterial pulse is most readily monitored by palpating a peripheral artery. The femoral artery is most commonly used, but the lingual, labial, brachial, distal ulnar, cranial tibial, plantar, and median coccygeal arteries can also be used.

Arterial Pressure

Arterial pressure depends on cardiac output and vascular tone. If arterial pressure is below a mean pressure of about 60 mm Hg, blood flow within organs becomes pressure dependent, perfusion is inadequate, and organ function begins to fail.

Monitoring

Arterial pressure can be estimated by palpation of the pulse or measured directly or indirectly. Direct measurement is best accomplished using a saline-filled catheter, transducer, signal processer, and recorder.

Direct arterial pressure measurement is accurate and has the advantage of allowing access to arterial blood for blood gas analysis. However, direct measurement has the distinct disadvantage of being invasive and having complications such as thrombosis, embolization, hemorrhage, and infection.

Blood pressure is indirectly measured most conveniently using either of two types of ultrasonic detectors. One is a flow detector (Doppler) that detects the movement of red blood cells; the other (oscillometry) detects movement of the arterial wall as it moves during the pulse wave. Two disadvantages of indirect measurement are that measurements may not be as accurate at low pressures, and at low pressure, it may be difficult to find a peripheral artery over which to place the sensor. Nonetheless, indirect pressure measurement is relatively inexpensive, easy, noninvasive, and safe.

Central Venous Pressure

Blood pressure in the cranial vena cava and intrathoracic portion of the caudal vena cava depends on intrathoracic pressure, tone of the capacitance vessels, blood volume, rate of venous return, and right ventricular function. The ability of changes in venous tone to compensate for changes in volume makes monitoring trends in central venous pressure (CVP) during volume replacement a more reliable guide than making isolated measurements.

Monitoring

CVP is measured using a large-bore catheter inserted into the vena cava near the right atrium. The catheter is commonly connected to a saline-filled manometer, and CVP is read in centimeters of saline. The system is flushed to remove all air bubbles. Pressure readings are made during several breathing cycles to ensure accuracy.

Pulmonary Arterial and Wedge Pressure (p. 218)

Cardiac Output (p. 218)

Capillary Refill Time

Capillary refill time is a simple method for assessing tissue perfusion. It reflects local vasomotor tone more closely than it reflects systemic blood pressure. When arterial and arteriolar vasoconstriction are present or when arterial pressure is reduced, perfusion of a capillary bed is diminished and slower than normal.

Monitoring

Digital pressure is applied for a short time (1 to 2 seconds) and rapidly released. The time needed for the blanched area to return to the color of the surrounding membrane is the capillary refill time.

BODY FLUID VARIABLES (pp. 219–222)

Fluid Balance

The volume and distribution of fluid in the three major body compartments must be normal to maintain a constant and adequate exchange of nutrients and metabolic products throughout the body. Osmotic forces maintain the volume of these compartments in a closed relationship. Water is translocated from the extracellular to the intracellular compartment and back again as it is lost or gained by the body.

Monitoring

Fluid balance can be monitored by assessing a number of volume-dependent variables and measuring input and output. Weighing patients twice daily is a method of monitoring fluid balance. Changes in physical signs of hydration, such as skin turgor and moistness of the mucous membranes, when assessed carefully, can provide information about fluid balance. In the absence of renal tubular disease, urine specific gravity within the normal range suggests adequate hydration; elevated specific gravity indicates conservation of water and suggests dehydration, and low specific gravity suggests the converse. In the absence of ongoing red blood cell or plasma protein loss, PCV and serum total solids are inversely related to intravascular water concentration — that is, elevated PCV and solids indicate decreased water concentration of plasma (dehydration).

Serum Protein

Surgical patients lose protein owing to pre-existing diseases, hemorrhage, and tissue injury and from inflamed and traumatized mesothelial membranes and tissue surfaces during surgical procedures.

Monitoring

Total protein and albumin can be measured by colorimetric methods. Total protein can also be measured by a refractometer using the plasma obtained by determining PCV.

Urine Output

Intravascular volume is an extremely important stimulus for changes in urine output. Decreases in intravascular volume cause an increase in antidiuretic hormone secretion with a decrease in urine volume. As volume is further decreased, glomerular filtration pressure is decreased and further reduction in urine volume occurs. If mean arterial pressure decreases to about 60 mm Hg, renal autoregulation fails, glomerular filtration stops, and urine production ceases. Because of these renal responses to intravascular volume and pressure changes, measuring urine output provides information about fluid volume and intravascular pressure and, by inference, tissue and organ perfusion.

Monitoring

Urine output is collected and measured during a preselected interval. Measurement of the specific gravity of urine as well as the volume collected provides additional information about intravascular volume and fluid balance.

Acid-Base Balance

Acid-base abnormalities are common in surgical patients. They may occur before surgery as part of the disease problem requiring treatment or may develop during anesthesia and surgery and the postoperative period. The most important effects of acid-base changes are on the heart and oxygen transport. Acidosis depresses ventricular function when severe (pH 7.2), and alkalosis (pH 7.5) inhibits oxygen delivery to tissues by shifting the oxygen-hemoglobin dissociation curve to the right. Acid-base changes also influence the distribution of electrolytes, which may also adversely affect cardiac function.

Monitoring

Acid-base balance is most rapidly and accurately assessed by measuring blood pH and CO_2 tension with a blood gas analyzer.

Electrolytes

Sodium is the major extracellular cation and is the electrolyte primarily responsible for maintaining the tonicity of extracellular fluid. Sodium is lost through vomiting and diarrhea and when extracellular fluid is sequestered in injured tissues or body cavities. In these instances, sodium is lost with water and the serum or plasma concentration of sodium is normal.

Potassium is the other major cation. Its concentration in the extracellular fluid is low and must be kept within a narrow range to ensure normal neuromuscular and cardiac function. Potassium concentration in the extracellular fluid is affected by acid-base balance, being elevated during acute acidosis and depressed during alkalosis. Hyperkalemia can also occur transiently after massive tissue trauma.

Hypokalemia may be the most common electrolyte abnormality to develop in surgical patients.[57] Potassium is not conserved as avidly by the kidneys as is sodium. Therefore, patients that are not eating and that have conditions predisposing to potassium loss deplete their potassium pool and develop hypokalemia, as in the case of patients with vomiting due to gastrointestinal obstruction.

Chloride is the major extracellular cation, and its movements are associated with those of sodium.

PATHOPHYSIOLOGICAL BASIS FOR MONITORING
(pp. 222–224)

All surgical patients require some monitoring during their treatment to detect complications associated with anesthesia, emergence from anesthesia, and the surgical procedure. Even normal patients presented for minor elective procedures must have their vital functions monitored during anesthesia and recovery. It is obvious that patients with pre-existing abnormalities need diligent care because of the superimposition of additional stresses of anesthesia and surgery.

Particular monitoring for a patient depends on (1) the physiological abnormalities and the severity of their deviation from normal as detected on preoperative evaluation; (2) the changes expected as a result of anesthesia and surgery; and (3) the magnitude of physiological changes expected in the postoperative period.

Standard Monitoring

Three groups of patients and their general needs can be described.

Category I (Low Risk)

The first category includes patients with minor tissue injury, no injuries within a major body cavity, and no pre-existing diseases affecting major organs or organ systems.

The variables to be monitored include general condition, pulse rate and quality, ventilatory rate and character, capillary refill time, and body temperature. Surveillance is frequent during surgery and recovery from anesthesia.

Category II (Moderate Risk)

Patients in category II have a disease problem affecting a major body system or have moderate tissue injury with a large volume of tissue involved. Blood and fluid losses are significant but are rapidly replaced, and hypovolemia and hypotension are short-lived. A major body cavity may be entered during surgery, and the chance of invasive infection is present. The anticipated period of starvation does not exceed 72 hours. Variables such as CVP, urine output, and arterial blood pressure are measured in addition to basic variables. Blood sampling for laboratory analysis of PCV and total serum solids is also often necessary. Patients are monitored frequently during surgery and in the postoperative period for up to 48 hours, because restoration of a normal internal environment may take several days.

Category III (High Risk)

This third category contains patients with massive tissue injury or severe illness with signs of stressed vital functions. Invasion of a body cavity has occurred or is necessary in these patients. Hypovolemia and hypotension are present, and the chance of invasive infection is greater than 50 per cent. Prolonged (longer than 72 hours) starvation is anticipated. Patients with severe preoperative illness or multiple trauma are included in this category. For these patients to survive surgery and the recovery period, they require intensive and frequent operative and postoperative monitoring. In addition to monitoring basic variables, variables of greater specificity are needed, such as blood gases, CVP, arterial pressure, and electrolytes. These patients need comprehensive, continued surveillance for up to several days after they are stabilized.

CHAPTER 21
Bandages and Drains (pages 225–230)

BANDAGES (pp. 225–228)

The two general functions of bandages are dressing of open wounds and the support or protection of body parts.

The components of bandages are the primary or contact layer, which directly contacts a wound or lesion; the secondary or intermediate layer, which overlies the primary layer and absorbs wound fluids and provides various degrees of support and pressure to the bandaged structure; and the tertiary or outer layer, which covers and protects the bandage and provides additional support.

Wound Dressings

Contact Layer

The primary layer of a wound dressing can be either adherent or nonadherent. The purpose of an adherent contact layer is to facilitate mechanical débridement during the early stages of wound healing. This layer usually consists of a wide-meshed gauze, which allows the desiccation and adherence of necrotic tissue, foreign debris, and exudate on the wound surface. The adhered material is removed with the gauze when the dressing is changed.

Adherent bandages can be applied as dry-to-dry dressings, wet-to-dry dressings, or wet-to-wet dressings. The terminology refers to the condition of the dressing when it is applied and at the time it is removed. Adherent dressings have several disadvantages. They can impede wound healing if not used properly. A dry, adherent bandage can be difficult and painful to remove. In addition, deeper tissues may become desiccated if the bandage becomes too dry.

Nonadherent dressings are indicated in wounds in the early stages of repair. Nonadherent dressings should also be used early in the treatment of acute wounds. Nonadherent dressings can be subdivided into semiocclusive and occlusive categories. Semiocclusive dressings allow absorption of wound fluids into the intermediate bandage layer but retain sufficient moisture at the wound surface to prevent desiccation of tissues.

Occlusive dressings are impermeable to wound fluids, although they vary in permeability to gases. Many of these dressings are adhesive and rely on the accumulation of fluid under the dressing to loosen them physically and allow atraumatic removal.

The four basic types of occlusive dressings are films, foams, hydrocolloids, and hydrogels. Films are made of transparent adhesive polyethylene, which is able to transmit water, oxygen, and carbon dioxide. Foam dressings are constructed of polyurethane, which is nonadhesive and must be taped in place over the wound. They absorb minimal amounts of wound fluid. Hydrocolloid dressings are opaque, absorbent, and impermeable to oxygen and carbon dioxide. The hydrocolloid adheres to surrounding dry surfaces, but it interacts with fluid in the wound to form a nonadhesive gel. Hydrogel dressings consist of a semitransparent, nonadhesive, absorbent polyethylene oxide membrane covering a gelatinous matrix.

Secondary Layer

The main function of the secondary or intermediate layer when applying a bandage for the purpose of dressing a wound is absorption of blood, serum, exudate, and necrotic debris. The secondary layer also serves to secure the contact layer to the wound, provide support to the bandaged part, and perhaps provide some pressure to obliterate dead space or prevent edema. The secondary layer must have sufficient capillarity to draw fluids away from the wound surface and should be thick enough to allow absorption of fluid. The intermediate layer should conform to the contact layer covering the wound surface, but it should not be under excessive tension, which would compromise the absorptive capacity of the bandage.

Tertiary Layer

The main function of the tertiary layer is to secure the other components of the bandage. The tertiary layer can also supply support and pressure to the bandaged part, but the need for pressure must be balanced against the need to absorb wound fluids. This layer is usually composed of gauze, surgical tape, or a combination of both.

Protection/Support Bandages

In addition to dressing wounds, bandages can provide protection, support, or pressure to underlying soft tissues or skeletal structures. Examples include obliteration of dead space using a pressure bandage or immobilization of a skin graft using a nonadherent padded bandage. Coaptation of fractures is discussed in Section 15. When bandages are used to support or immobilize structures, the secondary and tertiary layers assume added importance.

Pressure Bandages

Pressure bandages are the most common type of bandage used to hold soft tissues together. They function to control hemorrhage, prevent edema, obliterate dead space, and prevent excessive granulation tissue. Controlled even pressure is achieved by applying an elastic gauze or tape layer under tension over a padded intermediate layer.

The pressure generated by these bandages must be distributed evenly across the bandage surface, avoiding circumferential areas of concentrated pressure caused by bunching or slipping of the bandage material. Second, the two center toes should remain exposed when applying a pressure bandage to a limb. These toes serve as an indicator of blood flow under the bandage. The bandage must be removed if the animal is actively traumatizing the bandage.

SURGICAL DRAINS (pp. 228–230)

Surgical drains are implants placed, usually on a temporary basis, to channel away unwanted fluid or gas from a wound or body cavity.

Principles of Drain Usage

The most common complication of drain use is the increased risk of ascending infection. Local tissue resistance to infection is decreased by drain placement. The most likely mechanisms for this are foreign body reaction, pressure ischemia, and tissue trauma at the time of removal.

Incisional dehiscence is another complication associated with drain placement. Placing the drain through a separate stab incision that is slightly larger than the diameter of the drain minimizes the risk of wound dehiscence. The drain must never be placed through the primary incision or suture line.

Classification of Drains

Passive drains function by using naturally occurring pressure gradients, gravity, and overflow. Active drains rely on artificial pressure gradients created by applying negative pressure to the egress port of a drain tube.

Passive Drains

Passive drains are constructed of either soft latex (Penrose drain) or more rigid materials. Penrose drains are the most common type used. Drainage occurs both within and outside the lumen of this type of flat drain. Efficiency is directly related to the surface area of the drain.

Tube drains are more rigid than the flat latex drains, providing a consistent lumen. Tube drains can be either single or multiluminal, and they can be used actively or passively.

Sump drains are double-lumen tube drains. Drainage of wound fluid occurs through the large outer lumen. The smaller inner lumen provides an air vent.

Active Drains

Active drains are created by applying negative pressure to tube drains. Active drains increase the efficiency of dependently placed drains and can remove fluid against gravity if necessary. Open suction drains are constructed by applying a vacuum to the drainage lumen of a sump drain. The influx of room air introduces bacteria from the environment, thereby increasing the risk of nosocomial infection.

Closed suction drains are constructed by applying negative pressure to a tube drain that does not have an air vent. These drains are particularly useful in areas where dependent drainage is difficult to establish or where a patient's posture frequently alters the point of dependency.

Removal of Drains

All drains incite a foreign body reaction, and the production of fluid results from this reaction. Therefore, some fluid is always present at the exit port of any drain. Drains placed in small potential cavities to evacuate capillary bleeding may usually be removed within 24 hours. When a drain is placed to evacuate exudate from bacterial infection, 48 to 72 hours often elapses before the exudate subsides. Drains that are placed in large cavities to facilitate union of local tissues, such as after excision of large tumors, may be left in place for 1 to 2 weeks. In most patients, when the fluid from the drain diminishes to a small, consistent volume and is serosanguineous in consistency, the drain can be removed.

Patient Aftercare (pages 230–240)

This chapter deals with aftercare but does not address specific surgical complications unless they threaten homeostasis during recovery.

VENTILATION (pp. 230–232)

Hypoventilation is frequently encountered and may be caused by depression of the central nervous system, reduction in ventilation, or changes in the airway that interfere with ventilation.

Central Nervous System Depression

Causes of Central Nervous System Depression

The clinical signs of hypoventilation caused by CNS depression are shallow tidal volumes, bradypnea, and cyanosis. CNS depression immediately after surgery is most likely the result of anesthetics. The inhalants on their own do not generally cause serious hypoventilation but may impair the response of the animal to other causes of hypoventilation. Opioids commonly cause central respiratory depression. In several studies of postoperative opioid use in dogs, ventilatory depression was minimal ($Paco_2$ did not exceed 45 mm Hg). This lack of serious depression may be related to the stimulating effect these drugs have on the thermoregulatory center, which increases ventilation, thus counteracting the depressive effects. This same stimulation of the thermoregulatory center is not observed in cats, but opioids can have a marked CNS stimulatory effect in cats.

Diagnosis and Therapy of Central Ventilatory Depression

Clinical diagnosis is based on the findings of a depressed animal taking small, inadequate breaths. Hypoventilation can be confirmed by measuring arterial blood gases ($Paco_2$ >60 mm Hg, accompanied by a Pao_2 of ≤75 mm Hg). Cyanosis is a serious sign, but its absence should not deter a diagnosis of hypoxemia because many factors can interfere with the appreciation of cyanosis.

If an animal is sufficiently depressed after inhalation anesthesia, it can be reintubated, and some form of positive-pressure ventilation instituted. Once CNS depression is reduced, the animal can be removed from the ventilator, but the endotracheal tube is left in to allow further ventilatory support if needed. If opioids have been used and there is some suspicion that these are the cause of the ventilatory depression, a small test dose of naloxone (Narcan) can be given (0.01 to 0.02 mg/kg) intravenously. A response should occur within 2 to 3 minutes. Because the action of naloxone is short, the patient is monitored for "re-narcosis." A mixed opioid agonist/antagonist, such as nalbuphine (Nubain), can be used (0.03 to 0.1 mg/kg), with the advantage that this does not totally abolish the opioid-induced analgesia, and re-narcosis is less likely.

Residual Neuromuscular Blockade

Clinical signs of residual neuromuscular blockade vary from complete apnea to shallow respiration associated with diaphragmatic movement

101

but little or no intercostal involvement. It is easy to reverse the effects of muscle relaxants using an anticholinesterase (neostigmine or edrophonium) combined with an anticholinergic drug (atropine or glycopyrrolate).

Interference with the Airway

Inspiratory dyspnea or stridor is associated with extrathoracic upper airway obstruction and is commonly noted in brachycephalic breeds because of anatomical abnormalities. Expiratory dyspnea is associated with intrathoracic airway obstruction and is noted in dogs with a collapsing trachea. An increased resistance results in fewer breaths with prolonged inspiration and expiration. Alteration in compliance causes rapid, shallow ventilation.

Therapy for Interference with the Airway

Hypoxemia is treated with 100 per cent oxygen. Administration varies according to the facilities available and the degree of abnormality present. The simplest technique is to use a face mask or a nasal catheter, which allows more freedom and can achieve adequate oxygen delivery for most small animals. If an oxygen cage is available, the animal can be placed in an oxygen-enriched environment. In severe upper airway obstruction, it may be necessary to bypass the upper airway and place a transtracheal catheter or a tracheostomy.

In animals with atelectasis, the most effective therapy may simply be a change in posture without oxygen therapy. The dog or cat is encouraged to sit or is supported in a sternal position. This change in posture rouses the animal and also improves ventilation. If hypoxemia persists despite the change in posture, the application of positive end-expiratory pressure or continuous positive airway pressure may be necessary.

HYPERVENTILATION (p. 232)

Hyperventilation is uncommon in the recovery period and is not serious. Therapy is aimed at treating the underlying disorder.

HYPOTENSION (p. 232)

Clinical signs related to hypotension include pale mucous membranes, slow capillary refill time, poor peripheral pulse, depression, oliguria or anuria, and cool peripheral tissues. The causes and treatment of hypotension are outlined in Chapter 23.

ARRHYTHMIAS (pp. 232–233)

Arrhythmias are common during recovery because of interactions between the autonomic nervous system and the effects of residual anesthetic drugs. These arrhythmias are usually benign and do not cause lasting damage. Sinus tachycardia, sinus bradycardia, and premature ventricular contractions are discussed in Chapter 23.

Tachycardia

Pain is the most likely cause of sinus tachycardia during recovery, and analgesics may be necessary. Hypotension, hyperthermia, hypoxemia, and pre-existing diseases may also cause tachycardia.

Bradycardia

Hypothermia is the most common cause of bradycardia during the recovery period. A sinus bradycardia that persists despite restoration of body temperature is treated only if cardiovascular function is depressed. Temporary atrioventricular blocks are usually benign and can be treated with anticholinergics; if this treatment fails, it may be necessary to increase the heart rate with isoproterenol or to insert a temporary pacemaker.

Premature Ventricular Contractions

Premature ventricular contractions are common during recovery and may be the result of catecholamine release or hypoxia. They are usually benign, and therapy is instituted only if there are more than 20 premature ventricular contractions per minute, if they are multifocal, or if they occur immediately after the T wave. Lidocaine (Xylocaine, 1 to 2 mg/kg) is used, followed by an infusion of 50 to 70 μg/kg/min if the initial bolus eliminates the problem. Procainamide (Pronestyl, 1 to 5 mg/kg IV or IM) is also useful. In cats, the therapeutic ratio for lidocaine is lower than in dogs, and elimination of lidocaine takes longer.

HYPOTHERMIA (p. 233)

Hypothermia is the most common complication occurring during recovery. Hypothermic animals have a decreased rate of drug metabolism and a slow recovery.

Treatment of Hypothermia

The most effective form of therapy for hypothermia is prevention of heat loss. Covering with a warm blanket or wrapping with plastic reduces heat loss, but a patient may take a long time to return to normothermia if external heat is not provided. It is particularly important that this heat be supplied with no risk of burning. The safest techniques are warm air and circulating water blankets.

HYPERTHERMIA (pp. 233–234)

Hyperthermia is uncommon in the postoperative period.

POSTOPERATIVE PAIN (pp. 234–238)

Damaged tissue releases several chemical mediators that affect local circulation and nociceptors in the area. The administration of cyclo-oxygenase inhibitors (nonsteroidal anti-inflammatory drugs) helps to reduce prostaglandin production and therefore the degree of facilitation of nociceptors. Because tissue damage occurs during surgery, these drugs are more effective if given preoperatively.

Assessment of Pain

Because veterinary patients cannot describe their postoperative discomfort, assessment of pain depends on observation of their behavior. Cats and dogs tend to respond in different ways: A cat in pain is more likely to crawl to the back of the cage and curl up into a ball, whereas a dog is much more likely to bark and draw attention to its discomfort. Many animals recovering from anesthesia go through a period of "emergence delirium" and may cry out and be restless. If it is thought that adequate analgesia has been provided, it may be best to comfort the animal with soft words and a soothing hand or to provide extra sedation. The restlessness may occasionally be due to gastric dilation or a full urinary bladder, so the abdomen is palpated and the animal treated appropriately.

Treatment of Pain

It is better to prevent pain than to treat it. We know that *every* surgical procedure causes some pain and that some procedures are more painful than others. When considering prevention, we must first do everything possible to reduce factors that potentiate pain perception. To allay a patient's anxiety before surgery, we need to provide gentle care and handling. Phenothiazines do not provide analgesia, but they do tranquilize an animal and reduce anxiety. Traumatized animals may need to be started on analgesics ahead of the operation to reduce the nociceptive facilitation caused by injury.

At the end of an operation, an analgesic is more effective when given before the animal wakes up than after the animal regains consciousness and is in pain. Pain is much harder to control once a patient has become conscious of it.

Local Anesthetics

A local anesthetic can provide total analgesia to the affected area. Local anesthetics can be used topically on mucous membranes but afford only temporary relief (e.g., 20 minutes). They can also be infiltrated into the area of the operation, but again, the analgesia is brief and there may be some risk of affecting wound healing.
   Intercostal Nerve Blocks (p. 235)
   Interpleural Analgesia (p. 235)
   Epidural and Subarachnoid Analgesia (pp. 235–236)

Opioid Analgesics

Opioid analgesics have provided the most consistent and effective analgesia and are still the best drugs available for pain control in small animals. The opioids can be used by systemic administration or can be applied more directly to the spinal receptors by injecting the drug epidurally or intrathecally (Table 22–1).
   Systemic Injection. This route of administration produces variable degrees of analgesia depending on the dose and the agent used. The most common side effects include respiratory depression, nausea and vomiting, histamine release, constipation, and central excitement. Cats are particularly prone to central excitement, and reduced doses must be given.
   Morphine. This is a mu agonist with 3 to 4 hours' duration of action. It is a very effective analgesic and produces some sedation. When given with no other drugs, panting, bradycardia, and vomiting are common. The panting is due to action at the thermoregulatory center, causing the animal to cool itself. Morphine can produce significant release of histamine when given to dogs intravenously.
   Meperidine (Demerol). Meperidine is less potent than morphine. It produces less sedation but has similar side effects. It has a short duration of action and provides 1 to 2 hours of pain relief.
   Oxymorphone (Numorphan). Oxymorphone is about ten times more potent than morphine and has a similar duration of action. When given at the end of an operation, it delays recovery because it produces sedation. This technique usually allows a smooth transition from anesthesia to recovery.

TABLE 22–1. OPIOID DOSES FOR POSTOPERATIVE PAIN

Drug	Dose	Species	Route	Duration
Morphine	0.5–1.0 mg/kg	Canine	IM, SC	3–4 hours
	0.5 mg/kg plus 0.1–0.2 mg/kg/hr	Canine	IV	As long as infusion lasts
	0.1 mg/kg preservative-free morphine	Canine/feline	Epidural	12–24 hours
Meperidine	0.05–0.1 mg/kg	Feline	IM, SC	3–4 hours
	3–5 mg/kg	Canine/feline	IM, SC	1–2 hours
Methadone	0.1–0.2 mg/kg	Canine	IM, SC	4 + hours
Oxymorphone	0.05–0.1 mg/kg	Canine, IV, SC	IM, IV, SC	3–4 hours
	0.03–0.05 mg/kg	Feline	IM, SC	3–4 hours
Butorphanol	0.1–0.2 mg/kg	Canine/feline	IM, IV, SC	3–4 hours
Pentazocine	1–3 mg/kg	Canine/feline	IM, IV, SC	2–4 hours
Nalbuphine	0.03–0.1 mg/kg	Canine/feline	IM, IV, SC	2–4 hours
Buprenorphine	5–10 μg/kg	Canine/feline	IM, IV, SC	8–12 hours

Methadone. Methadone is about 1.5 times more potent than morphine and has similar analgesic properties.

Butorphanol (Torbugesic). Butorphanol is an agonist/antagonist, and its actions are slightly different from the other opioids. This drug causes mild sedation and has a duration of at least 2 hours. It is about seven to ten times more potent than morphine but does not seem to be as effective in patients with severe pain.

Pentazocine. Pentazocine is another agonist/antagonist that is less potent than morphine and does not work well as a mu antagonist.

Nalbuphine. In trials as a postoperative analgesic in humans, nalbuphine was as effective as pentazocine or meperidine. This drug does not produce much sedation and has minimal effects on respiration.

Buprenorphine. The main advantage of buprenorphine is that it has 8 to 12 hours of action. Buprenorphine produces moderate sedation when used in the postoperative period.

Epidural or Intrathecal Administration. Because there are opioid receptors in the spinal cord, these drugs can be applied directly to these receptors. Smaller doses can be used and the systemic effects are minimized. Morphine (0.1 mg/kg diluted to 0.3 ml/kg with sterile saline to a maximum volume of 6 ml) on its own or in combination with local anesthetics can be used during surgery in dogs and cats. Morphine should be preservative free. The epidural injection is given as soon after induction as possible. It takes approximately 60 minutes to reach peak effect. It provides postoperative analgesia, with one dose lasting for approximately 12 to 24 hours.

Nonsteroidal Anti-Inflammatory Drugs

NSAIDs may be useful for analgesia for more minor procedures; they are given preoperatively for maximum benefit. The drugs most commonly used are aspirin, phenylbutazone, flunixin, meclofenamic acid, and dipyrone. Indomethacin, naproxen, and ibuprofen are not recommended for use in dogs and cats. Cats are very sensitive to NSAIDs, and great care needs to be taken when using them in this species; aspirin can be used, but acetaminophen must be avoided. Given the possible toxic side effects, the chance of interactions with anesthetics, and the sparse information about NSAIDs in dogs and cats, their routine use is *not recommended*.

HEMOSTASIS (pp. 238–239)

One of the keys to detecting postoperative hemorrhage is a high index of suspicion that it is possible or even probable. Some of the simplest and most reliable monitors are the color of mucous membranes and capillary refill time. Checking the packed cell volume may help to confirm blood loss if it has been occurring slowly over a period of hours, but if the hemorrhage is acute there will be little or no change in hematocrit. Gradual swelling of a body cavity or a wound area is investigated as soon as it is discovered because it is unlikely to be noticed until serious blood loss has occurred.

Management of Hemorrhage

If bleeding is from a specific large vessel, the vessel must be exposed and ligated or pressure applied over the vessel for sufficient time to allow a strong clot to form. If the bleeding is a result of general oozing, a number of other avenues must be investigated. If stored blood or crystalloid fluids were transfused during the operation, a coagulopathy due to thrombocytopenia and dilution of existing clotting factors may be present. Both can be treated by administering fresh compatible whole blood. A citrate overdose after massive transfusion can be reversed by administration of calcium. Disseminated intravascular coagulation may be a cause of hemorrhage in the postoperative period and is a grave sign.

NEUROLOGICAL DYSFUNCTION (p. 239)

Raised Intracranial Pressure

After anesthesia, a patient should recover steadily to the level of consciousness exhibited before anesthesia. Loss of a palpebral response, dilated or constricted unresponsive pupils, or papilledema may be seen with progressing CNS edema. Care must be taken to avoid anything that further raises intracranial pressure, such as occlusion of venous return from the head, raised intrathoracic pressure, coughing, or rough handling. Measures that can lower intracranial pressure include hyperventilation to reduce the $PaCO_2$ to 20 to 25 mm Hg and the use of mannitol (1 to 2 g/kg IV), furosemide (1 to 2 mg/kg IV), or corticosteroids (e.g., dexamethasone phosphate, 1 to 2 mg/kg IV).

Seizures

Seizures may occur postoperatively as a result of drugs used during anesthesia or physical injury during surgery. Anesthetic drugs most commonly associated with seizure activity include methohexital, ketamine, tiletamine, etomidate, and althesin. The nonionic water-soluble radiographic contrast media used for myelography are also commonly associated with seizure activity.

Treatment of Seizures

Ketamine or tiletamine seizure-like activity is best treated with a tranquilizer such as acepromazine. If seizures occur after myelography, a bolus of 5 to 20 mg of diazepam is given, and a similar amount is added to the maintenance fluid to be given during the next hour (0.3 to 0.5 mg/kg/hr).

CHAPTER 23

Operating Room Emergencies (pages 240–259)

ANESTHETIC DEPTH (pp. 240–243)

As patients awaken from general anesthesia or anesthesia becomes too light, a complex of signs is manifested: increase in mandibular muscle tone; a strong palpebral reflex; central position of the eye with a midsize pupil; increased ventilation rate and volume; increased heart rate, cardiac output, and blood pressure; and spontaneous muscular movement. It is important to evaluate the available signs of anesthetic depth so that adequate warning of light levels of anesthesia can be recognized. Care is taken not to attribute too much significance to any one sign.

Causes of Premature Awakening

Hypoventilation following barbiturate induction is common, and the gaseous anesthetic is not taken up in sufficient quantities to keep the patient anesthetized once the barbiturates are redistributed from the brain to other tissues. If postinduction hypoventilation is suspected, the lungs should be inflated once every 30 seconds, with normal induction settings on the vaporizer, until the patient regains adequate spontaneous ventilation.

Inspired anesthetic concentrations may be too low. Inadequate administration may occur if (1) the vaporizer is set too low, (2) the setting is decreased before adequate loading of the visceral and muscular tissues, or (3) if gas flows are too low with vaporizer-outside-the-circuit systems.

Esophageal intubation prevents anesthetic uptake. Coughing is good evidence of proper placement, but many anesthetized animals do not cough when the tube is placed. The only way to ensure that the endotracheal tube is properly placed is to see it pass through the glottis, using a laryngoscope.

Bronchial intubation reduces the lung surface area for anesthetic uptake. Bronchial intubation may be indicated by inability to keep the patient anesthetized, by tachypnea and hyperventilation, hypoxemia and cyanosis, decreased tidal volume and pulmonary compliance, and hypercapnia. If bronchial intubation is suspected, withdraw the tube until its position is verified by palpation of the trachea, or withdraw it entirely and replace it.

Insufficient cuff inflation allows inspiration of room air around the tube, diminishing inspired anesthetic concentration. The cuff is inflated to stop leakage of air from around the tube during the application of positive airway pressure (15 cm H_2O). Care must be taken not to overinflate the cuff because this predisposes to avascular necrosis of the tracheal wall.

Refilling the rebreathing bag with the oxygen flush bypasses the vaporizer and decreases anesthetic concentration. If the rebreathing bag needs to be filled rapidly with anesthetic-containing gases, use high flowmeter settings. The oxygen flush is used to fill the bag rapidly to decrease anesthetic concentrations, when terminating the anesthetic, or in cases of anesthetic overdose or cardiac arrest.

Excessive Anesthetic Depth

Physical signs of excessive anesthetic depth include flaccid muscle tone and absence of all reflexes; centrally positioned eyes, dilated pupils, and dry corneas; absence of the pupillary light reflex; and bradycardia, hypotension, and bradypnea.

Causes of Excessive Anesthetic Depth

1. Excessive administration of anesthetic.
2. Individual variations in anesthetic requirements—some patients require less than others.
3. Synergistic events such as hypothermia, hypotension, shock, hypoxia, hypercapnia, hypothyroidism, preanesthetic exhaustion, acid-base and electrolyte disorders, toxemias, or brain disease depress the central nervous system (CNS) and decrease the amount of anesthetic necessary to maintain anesthesia.
4. Nonrebreathing circuits are more efficient than large reservoir circle systems; inhaled anesthetic concentrations are similar to those leaving the vaporizer. Vaporizer settings that work satisfactorily with circle systems can easily result in overdose with nonrebreathing systems, particularly during positive-pressure ventilation (PPV).

5. Anesthetic overdose is also likely to occur when PPV is used with a nonrebreathing circuit, with in-circuit systems, and when PPV is used to deepen the level of anesthetic (especially if the vaporizer setting is simultaneously increased).

6. A vaporizer may function improperly and deliver anesthetic even though turned off.

Delayed Recovery

1. Prolonged recoveries are often attributed to excessive anesthetic administration. Re-reversal or temporary supportive care may be necessary if CNS or ventilatory depression becomes severe.

2. Synergistic disorders such as hypothermia, hypotension, or shock prolong recovery from any anesthetic.

3. Delayed metabolism and elimination of anesthetic drugs may result from diffuse kidney or liver disease or portocaval shunts.

4. Many drugs are sufficiently fat soluble that redistribution from the brain to other tissues has an important role in the early termination of the drug's clinical effects. Accumulation of anesthetic in these redistribution sites, associated with repeated doses, diminishes this mechanism of recovery.

5. Pentobarbital recovery is always prolonged because it relies on hepatic metabolism. Repeated administrations of ultrashort-acting barbiturates are associated with prolonged recovery due to "saturation" of redistribution sites. Administration of large amounts of glucose toward the end of barbiturate anesthesia prolongs recovery.

6. Sight hounds, such as greyhounds, Italian greyhounds, Salukis, and Afghans, may exhibit prolonged recovery when standard anesthetics are used. The barbiturates, especially the thiobarbiturates, are metabolized slowly in these breeds, which also exhibit a smaller volume of distribution than similar-sized mixed-breed dogs.

7. Postoperative administration of analgesics or tranquilizers causes CNS depressant effects that are additive to anesthetic drugs.

8. Prolonged recovery from a gas anesthetic usually can be attributed to a simple overdose and the saturation of aqueous tissue stores where blood flow and anesthetic reabsorption is sufficient to cause CNS depression.

TACHYPNEA, HYPERVENTILATION, AND EXAGGERATED BREATHING EFFORTS (pp. 243–244)

Tachypnea is rapid breathing without regard to volume. Hyperventilation is a higher than normal alveolar minute ventilation without regard to breathing rate. Exaggerated breathing efforts are identified in a patient that appears to be working hard to breathe or is having difficulty breathing effectively and may be tachypneic or bradypneic.

Causes of Tachypnea and Exaggerated Ventilation
(Table 23–1)

BRADYPNEA, HYPOVENTILATION, AND APNEA
(pp. 244–245)

Bradypnea is slow breathing without regard to volume. Hypoventilation is a low alveolar minute ventilation without regard to breathing rate.

Causes of Bradypnea

Carbon dioxide is the primary stimulant of the respiratory center, and hypocapnia in an anesthetized patient results in apnea. Most anes-

TABLE 23–1. CAUSES OF TACHYPNEA AND EXAGGERATED VENTILATORY EFFORTS

Too lightly anesthetized	Pleural space filling defects
Too deeply anesthetized	Excessive obesity
Hypercapnia	Abdominal enlargements
Hypoxemia	Pulmonary parenchymal disease
Hypotension	Atelectasis
Hyperthermia	Drug-induced
Upper or lower airway obstruction	Idiopathic

thetics are potent respiratory depressants, and many are given as loading doses to induce anesthesia. Most patients hyperventilate just before induction because of excitement and apprehension, and intubated patients are often artificially ventilated to ensure proper cuff inflation. This hypocapnia, associated with anesthetic-induced respiratory center depression, results in apnea after anesthetic induction, even though the patient may be lightly anesthetized.

Neuromuscular interference may occur preoperatively with disc prolapse, vertebral fractures, myasthenia gravis, or polyradiculoneuritis and during operation with spinal cord edema secondary to needle tap or surgical trauma. Neuromuscular blocking agents may be a residual problem if they are not adequately reversed, and aminoglycoside antibiotics may cause neuromuscular blockade when administered with a neuromuscular blocking agent, gas anesthetics, or alone.

HYPERCAPNIA (p. 245)

Hypercapnia ($Paco_2$ >45 mm Hg) is caused by alveolar hypoventilation. $Paco_2$ should not be allowed to exceed 60 mm Hg because it causes respiratory acidemia, increases cerebral blood flow and intracranial pressure, is associated with hypoxemia if a patient is breathing room air, and may enhance CNS narcosis.

Causes of Hypercapnia

Hypercapnia may result from hypoventilation due to bradypnea, airway obstructive diseases, restrictive diseases such as chest wall problems (flail chest, open pneumothorax, restrictive bandages), pleural space filling defects, abdominal enlargements, and severe pulmonary parenchymal disease.

Hypercapnia may also be caused by increased inspired carbon dioxide associated with excessive dead space or exhausted soda lime within the anesthetic circuit. Hypercapnia may occur as a compensatory response to metabolic acidosis. The extent of the hypoventilatory compensation is limited by the concurrent hypoxemia; Pco_2 is not likely to exceed 60 mm Hg by compensation alone.

HYPOXEMIA (pp. 245–246)

Hypoxemia is defined as low blood oxygen content and is usually identified by cyanosis or Pao_2 less than 80 mm Hg.

Causes of Hypoxemia

Hypoventilation causes hypoxemia if a patient is breathing air. When hypoxemia is due to hypoventilation, improvement of ventilation is the treatment of choice.

Low ventilation/perfusion ratio is another cause of hypoxemia. Disease associated with diminished ventilation of the lower regions of the lung or diseases associated with enhanced ventral distribution of blood flow upset the balance between ventilation and perfusion and decrease the ventilation/perfusion (V/Q) ratio. The P_{CO_2} and P_{O_2} of the blood passing through these areas is increased and decreased, respectively.

Physiologic shunting is a common cause of hypoxemia in pulmonary parenchymal disease. It occurs when the small airways or alveoli collapse; the blood flowing through these areas is not oxygenated. Enriching inspired oxygen concentration does not provide much benefit because of the inability of collapsed airways to conduct the oxygen to the capillary level. PPV reinflates collapsed airways and alveoli and dramatically improves P_{O_2}.

Intrapulmonary (pathologic arteriovenous shunts) or extrapulmonary (right-to-left shunting, patent ductus, or septal defect) anatomical shunts cause hypoxemia that is unresponsive to oxygen or PPV.

Diffusion hypoxia may occur if a patient breathing nitrous oxide is not allowed to breathe 100 per cent oxygen for 3 to 5 minutes after the nitrous oxide has been turned off.

UPPER AIRWAY OBSTRUCTION (p. 246)

PULMONARY EDEMA (pp. 246–247)

Pulmonary edema may develop as a result of excessive capillary hydrostatic pressure or increased capillary permeability.

Central venous pressure or pulmonary capillary wedge pressure should be monitored with pulmonary edema or congestive heart failure, and fluid therapy is conservative. Once pulmonary edema has developed, oxygen and PPV are started.

ASPIRATION OF GASTRIC CONTENTS (p. 247)

Vomiting and regurgitation are minimized by preoperative withholding of food. If a patient has a full stomach, surgery is postponed. If this is not possible, preoperative vomiting is induced with apomorphine (0.04 mg/kg) or morphine (0.2 to 0.4 mg/kg). If induction of vomiting is undesirable, the patient is induced and intubated rapidly. Patients with an esophagus full of fluid are induced and intubated in a sternal position with the head elevated.

Postoperatively, the endotracheal tube is maintained in place for as long as possible. The patient is extubated in a head-up sternal position after return of the swallowing reflex. Oxygen and broad-spectrum antibiotics are indicated if aspiration occurs. Tracheal lavage or steroids are of little value in the treatment of aspiration.

POSITIVE-PRESSURE VENTILATION (p. 247)

PPV is indicated when a patient is unable to maintain adequate alveolar ventilation as determined by clinical judgment, a minute volume less than 100 ml/kg/minute, or a Pa_{CO_2} greater than 60 mm Hg. Normal lungs can be ventilated with proximal airway pressures of approximately 15 cm H_2O; an inspiratory time of about 1 second, or just long enough to achieve a full tidal volume, without an inspiratory hold; and a ventilatory rate of about 10 to 12 times per minute.

Routine settings may not be completely effective in severe pulmonary disease. An increase in mean airway pressure may be accomplished by increasing the peak inspiratory pressure, prolonging the inspiratory time, or increasing the breathing rate. Positive end-expiratory pressure (PEEP) may be applied by careful hand bagging, by adjustable ventilators, or by submerging a tube leading from the pressure relief valve under water. The optimal amount of PEEP varies between 5 and 15 cm H_2O, depending on the severity of the pulmonary disease.

CARDIAC ARREST (pp. 247–251)

Cardiac arrest is characterized by absence of heartbeat or pulse, mucous membranes that are gray or blue, dilated pupils, and absence of breathing. If cardiac arrest is questionable, the resuscitation procedure should commence.

Airway and Breathing

The airway is secured by endotracheal intubation, PPV with 100 per cent oxygen is started, and the vaporizer is turned off. One ventilation is delivered every 3 to 5 chest compressions but twice per 15 compressions if the resuscitation is being conducted by one person.

External Circulation Techniques

External chest compression is accomplished by applying pressure directly over the heart with a force that is appropriate for the size of the patient, at 80 to 120 times per minute. The compression is held for a brief time to maximize the elimination of blood from the heart and the chest. Time must be allowed between compressions for adequate diastolic filling of the ventricles. If the initial technique does not generate palpable pulses or an improvement in mucous membrane color, an alternate technique is used. Compression force, rate, duration of systole, and position of the hands or the animal can be changed. Additional procedures that may help maximize artificial circulation include fluids, alpha-agonist drugs, an abdominal tourniquet, abdominal counterpressure, intermittent abdominal compression, and simultaneous ventilation.

Exogenous fluid administration (such as lactated Ringer's) in aliquots of approximately 40 ml/kg (dogs) and 20 ml/kg (cats) is used to establish an effective circulating blood volume.

Peripheral vasoconstriction by the administration of an alpha-agonist redistributes blood into the central circulation and diminishes the loss of central blood volume into the periphery.

Abdominal counterpressure splints the abdomen and decreases posterior displacement of the diaphragm when the chest is compressed. By preventing dissipation of the pressure of external chest compression through the abdomen, it increases intrathoracic pressure and improves cerebral blood flow.

Intermittent abdominal compression, alternating with external chest compression, improves venous return to the chest and improves arterial blood pressure and cerebral and myocardial perfusion.

Internal Circulation Techniques

Internal cardiac compression techniques are associated with better cardiac output, cerebral and coronary perfusion, resuscitation rates, and neurological recovery compared with external compression. If external techniques do not generate a peripheral pulse with each compression, or if the mucous membrane color does not improve in 5 minutes, or if the heart has not started beating spontaneously in 10 minutes, a thoracotomy and internal heart compression are indicated.

When the chest is open, the adequacy of diastolic filling can be assessed between each compression; the heart should fill as rapidly as it is released. The descending aorta can be depressed with the index finger of the opposite hand or clamped, directing essential blood flow to the brain and heart.

Drugs

When basic procedures have not restarted the heart after 2 to 3 minutes, additional drugs may be useful.

Excessive vagal tone and the lack of an idioventricular rhythm may cause and maintain asystole. Atropine may reverse this phenomenon. A dose of atropine (0.04 mg/kg) is recommended.

Catecholamines with only alpha-agonist activity (e.g., phenylephrine) or with alpha- and beta-agonist activity (e.g., epinephrine) are beneficial in cardiopulmonary resuscitation (CPR). Beta-agonist activity stimulates pacemaker activity and enhances contractility and cardiac output if the heart starts beating. Epinephrine may be associated with better cerebral and myocardial blood flow and more successful resuscitation rates than occur with phenylephrine.

Sodium bicarbonate combats metabolic acidosis generated by anaerobic metabolism in hypoxic tissues. Sodium bicarbonate is associated with generation of carbon dioxide and hypercapnia if a patient is not well ventilated. The current recommendation for sodium bicarbonate is none for the first 5 to 10 minutes and then 0.5 mEq/kg/5 min of cardiac arrest thereafter.

The use of calcium during CPR may contribute to diminished coronary and cerebral blood flow secondary to vasoconstriction following an otherwise successful resuscitation. Calcium does not improve the success of resuscitation and is not currently recommended in the routine management of cardiac arrest.

Routes of Drug Administration

Intracardiac injections were previously recommended, but this route may cause myocardial trauma, pericardial tamponade, lung laceration and pneumothorax, or ventricular fibrillation. A central venous catheter is the best route of administration. Peripheral venous drug administration is associated with significant delays in the arrival of the drugs to the heart and with lower blood levels compared with the central venous route.

Electrical Activity of the Heart

ECG monitoring during resuscitation is important because it defines the type of cardiac arrest and guides therapeutic interventions (Table 23–2). Direct-current defibrillation is indicated as soon as possible when ventricular fibrillation is identified (Table 23–3).

Postresuscitation Monitoring and Support

Cardiovascular and pulmonary function are monitored closely for several hours after successful resuscitation. It is important to monitor (1) the electrical activity of the heart, (2) the mechanical activity of the heart, (3) the adequacy of peripheral perfusion, (4) the rate, rhythm, and nature of the breathing efforts, (5) auscultatory and radiographic findings in the thorax, and (6) the adequacy of oxygenation.

Consciousness should return shortly after restarting the heart. If not, or if resuscitation exceeds 15 minutes, cerebral edema should be assumed. Corticosteroids may be beneficial in the support of membrane integrity and as an anti-inflammatory (dexamethasone, 0.5 mg/kg IV; prednisolone sodium succinate, 2 mg/kg IV). Mannitol (0.5 g/kg IV

TABLE 23–2. DIFFERENT TYPES OF CARDIAC ARREST

Type	Electrical Activity	Coordinated Mechanical Contraction	Visual Appearance of the Heart	Treatment
Ventricular asystole	None	No	Standstill	Beta-agonists stimulate pacemaker activity
Ventricular fibrillation	Chaotic	No	Fine to coarse myocardial ripping	Defibrillation to create simultaneous asystole
Cardiovascular collapse due to excessive vasodilation	Normal	Yes	Normal contractions	Rapid fluid administration: alpha-receptor agonists
Electrical-mechanical dissociation	Normal	No	Standstill	Corticosteroids (?)

administered slowly) osmotically decreases cerebral edema. Furosemide (5 mg/kg) is a weak vasodilator and redistributes blood away from the brain. Both diuretics remove fluids from the body.

BRADYCARDIA (p. 251)

Bradycardia requires definitive therapy when it causes the mean blood pressure to decrease below 50 to 60 mm Hg or when the heart rate decreases below 50 to 60 beats per minute.

Causes of Bradycardia

Excessive anesthetic depth may cause bradycardia. Excessive vagal tone may cause bradycardia and atrioventricular conduction blocks. Many anesthetics and some muscle relaxants cause bradycardia by either increasing vagal tone or decreasing sympathetic tone.

Hypothermia decreases tissue oxygen demands, resulting in a proportionate decrease in heart rate, cardiac output, and blood pressure. Direct cold-induced myocardial depression does not occur until the core temperature decreases to $<78.8°F$ ($<26°C$).

TABLE 23–3. DEFIBRILLATION METHODS

	Power Settings (Watt-Seconds)	
	External	*Internal*
Direct-current defibrillation		
Small patient	100 to 150	10 to 25
Large patient	400	100 to 150
or		
<7 kg	2/kg	0.2 to 0.4/kg
8 to 40 kg	5/kg	0.2 to 0.4/kg
>40 kg	5 to 10/kg	0.2 to 0.4/kg
Pharmacological defibrillation		
Potassium chloride (1 mEq/kg) followed by 10% calcium chloride (0.2 ml/kg)		

Exogenous toxemias and endogenous metabolic disturbances such as hypoxia, acidosis, digitalis intoxication, hypothyroidism, visceral organ failure, hyperkalemia, hypocalcemia, and end-stage shock may also cause bradycardia.

Prevention and Treatment of Bradycardia

Atropine (0.04 mg/kg IM) is often given before induction to prevent vagus-mediated bradycardia. Repeat doses can be administered (0.02 mg/kg IV) if bradycardia develops.

If the specific cause of the bradycardia cannot be determined, is judged to have deleterious effects on blood pressure, and has not responded to atropine, the administration of beta-receptor stimulants may be indicated. Dopamine, dobutamine, mephentermine, or a combination of these supports blood pressure without causing excessive peripheral vasodilation or vasoconstriction.

SINUS TACHYCARDIA AND HYPERTENSION (pp. 251–253)

PREMATURE VENTRICULAR CONTRACTIONS (p. 253)

Premature ventricular contractions (PVCs) signify an underlying complication that may lead to serious arrhythmias or cardiac arrest. PVCs should be suspected whenever auscultation reveals a triple heart sound followed by a compensatory pause. The diagnosis should be confirmed by an ECG: a bizarre QRS complex; no preceding P wave or a shortened PR interval; or the abnormal complex following the preceding complex too closely followed by a compensatory pause.

Causes of Premature Ventricular Contractions

PVCs may be caused by endogenous catecholamine release as well as exogenous catecholamine therapy.

PVCs may also be caused by endogenous or exogenous toxemias such as severe acidosis or alkalosis, hypokalemia, hypercalcemia, hypoxia, hypotension, visceral organ failure, severe hypothermia, digitalis toxicity, and some anesthetics. Another cause of PVCs is direct endocardial, myocardial, or epicardial stimulation.

Treatment of Premature Ventricular Contractions
(pp. 253–254)

Specific therapy should be considered whenever PVCs occur frequently, when their occurrence is increasing in frequency, when the ectopic beat overrides the T wave of the preceding beat, or when the rhythm causes detectable cardiovascular deterioration. Discontinue the administration of agents that may cause or lower the threshold to the arrhythmias. If the PVCs persist, administer an antiarrhythmic agent such as lidocaine (1 to 5 mg/kg IV), procainamide (1 to 5 mg/kg IV), or propranolol (0.05 to 0.3 mg/kg IV).

HYPOTENSION (pp. 253–254)

Blood pressure is a function of blood volume, cardiac output, and peripheral vasomotor tone. Alteration of one of these factors is usually compensated for by the other two to maintain adequate blood pressure.

Causes of Hypotension

Decreased cardiac output may be due to decreased venous return, decreased contractility, bradycardia, severe tachycardia, or severe arrhythmias. Decreased venous return may be caused by surgical packing, PPV, gastric torsion, or pericardial tamponade. Decreased contractility may be due to acute or chronic intrinsic heart failure, anesthetic drugs, or toxemias and electrolyte disturbances (potassium, calcium, magnesium).

Vasodilation may be caused by propofol, acepromazine, gaseous anesthetics, epidural or subarachnoid deposition of local anesthetics, and vasodilator drugs. Hypoxia, hypercapnia, hyperthermia, surface rewarming of hypothermic patients, and sepsis cause peripheral vasodilation. Hypoxia and the accumulation of noxious metabolic products in tissues that have been inadequately perfused cause peripheral vasodilation.

Treatment of Hypotension

1. When hypotension occurs during general anesthesia, the first treatment is to decrease the quantity of anesthetic administered.

2. Replacement fluids, such as lactated Ringer's, are administered if the hypotension is not due to heart failure. Patients with heart failure, pulmonary edema, or cerebral edema may be sensitive to fluid loading. Central venous pressure or pulmonary capillary wedge pressure should be monitored in these patients to enable more careful titration of the fluids.

Crystalloids

Any solution with electrolyte concentrations similar to normal extracellular fluid is economical, can be administered fairly rapidly, and is a good extracellular fluid volume expander. A suggested rate of fluid administration during routine surgery is 10 ml/kg/hr plus a volume two to three times that of the estimated blood loss. The fluid administration rate is increased to 20 ml/kg/hr in patients with large fluid transudations (extensive thoracotomies, laparotomies, or fracture repairs), when active diuresis is desirable, and when signs of mild hypovolemia or hypotension develop.

When the packed cell volume decreases below 20 per cent and further volume therapy is needed, infusion of red blood cells is indicated. When the total plasma proteins decrease below 3.5 g/dl and further volume therapy is needed, the infusion of plasma or dextran 70 is indicated.

Plasma

Plasma is a more effective fluid for restoring blood volume than crystalloids because a larger percentage of it is maintained within the vascular space (50 per cent) after equilibration has taken place.

Dextran

High-molecular-weight dextran (MW 20,000) is commercially available as a 6 per cent solution and is used when plasma is not available. Blood volume is increased by about 0.75 times the volume actually administered. The duration of the volume expansion by dextran 70 is about 12 to 24 hours.

Dextran decreases platelet adhesiveness and has an antithrombotic effect, which may cause a hemorrhagic diathesis if given too rapidly or in excessive amounts.

DECREASED CARDIAC OUTPUT (p. 254)

ANESTHETIC-INDUCED VASODILATION (p. 254)

PERIPHERAL VASOCONSTRICTION (pp. 254–255)

METABOLIC ACIDOSIS (see also Chapter 2) (p. 255)

HYPOTHERMIA (p. 255)

Hypothermia during anesthesia is the consequence of decreased basal metabolic rate and muscular activity and increased heat loss associated with depilation, the application and evaporation of antiseptic solutions, exposure to cold table surfaces, and open body cavities.

Consequences of Hypothermia

At 96°F (36°C) and above, there is no effect except for postanesthetic shivering. Shivering increases oxygen consumption and decreases ventilatory capacity.

At 90° to 94°F (32° to 34°C), anesthetic requirements are reduced. Recovery may be prolonged and thermoregulation may be impaired.

At 82° to 86°F (28° to 30°C), little or no anesthetic is required to maintain anesthesia; recovery is prolonged; patients often must be artificially rewarmed; ventilatory support should be instituted; and metabolic acidosis due to inadequate tissue perfusion occurs on rewarming.

At 77° to 79°F (25° to 26°C), cold-induced ECG changes begin to occur; arrhythmias such as PVCs or fibrillation appear; bradycardia causes insufficient cardiac output; and microcirculatory sludging due to excessive blood viscosity may occur.

At 72°F (22°C) and below, spontaneous ventilation ceases. Ventricular fibrillation and coagulation disorders occur.

Prevention of Heat Loss

Heat loss may be reduced by minimizing duration of preparation of the surgical site, by protecting the animal from its cool environment with blankets or towels, by minimizing the duration of the surgical procedure, and by actively warming the animal or its immediate environment.

In recovery, a patient's environment can be warmed by infrared heat lamps, surgical lamps, electric floor heaters, forced-air hair dryers, heating blankets, or hot water blankets. Care should be taken to avoid excessive environmental temperatures and overheating the patient.

HYPERTHERMIA (pp. 255–256)

Skin and Adnexa (pages 260–369)

CHAPTER 24
The Integument (pages 260–268)

FUNCTIONS OF THE SKIN (p. 260)

Functionally, the integument serves as the body's first line of defense against microorganisms. The stratum corneum provides protection against desiccation and hydration. The skin produces vitamin D and serves as a reservoir for electrolytes, water, fat, carbohydrates, and protein. The total cutaneous circulation has a considerable volume and can affect blood pressure. The skin is a sensory receptor for touch, pressure, vibration, heat, cold, and pain. The skin and its overlying haircoat provide a barrier against chemicals and radiation and, in combination with subcutaneous fat, provide a cushion against mechanical trauma as well as insulation against heat and cold.

SKIN STRUCTURE (pp. 260–261)

Epidermis

The epidermis of hairy skin consists of three major layers: the stratum cylindricum (stratum basale), the stratum spinosum (stratum malpighii, prickle cell layer), and the stratum corneum.

Dermis (Corium)

The dermis consists of collagenous, reticular (precollagen), and elastic fibers surrounded by a mucopolysaccharide ground substance. This ground substance, composed of hyaluronic acid and chondroitin sulfuric acid, is the major component of the dermis.

The most pliable skin regions (axilla, flank, dorsum of the neck) have smaller and more loosely woven collagen bundles in the dermis. Elastic fibers in these areas are more numerous. Areas where the skin is least mobile (tail, ear, digital pads) have wider, more closely packed collagen bundles with fewer elastic fibers.

APPENDAGES OF THE SKIN (pp. 261–263)

Hair

The basic unit of hair production is the hair follicle. The wall of the hair follicle is continuous with the epidermis and is divided into inner and outer root sheaths. Germinative cells eventually give rise to the inner epithelial root sheath and the hair shaft. Epidermal cells encircling the shaft become the outer epithelial root sheath, which is a continuation of the stratum cylindricum.

Compound follicles contain a main, or guard, hair surrounded by a number of finer, woolly lanugo, or underhairs. Although the hair shafts share the same external follicular orifice at the epidermal surface, they branch into their respective hair follicles below the level of the sebaceous glands.

Siamese cats have a temperature-dependent coat color owing to an enzyme that converts melanin precursors to melanin at lower temperatures. As a result, haircoats grow back darker after clipping.

Hair growth rates vary seasonally among breeds. Hair growth is more rapid in the winter. As a rule, short canine haircoats take approximately 130 days to regrow. However, as long as 18 months is required for regrowth of the haircoat in long-haired breeds.

Glandular Structures of the Skin

The major cutaneous glands include the sebaceous glands, sweat glands, supracaudal (tail) glands, anal sacs, circumanal glands, and mammary glands. Like the hair follicles, these glands are ectodermally derived by downgrowth of epidermal cells into the dermis during embryonic development.

Sebaceous glands most frequently originate from the external root sheath. The oily secretion produced exits through the pilosebaceous canal to keep the skin and hair soft and pliable and to protect them from excessive moisture and drying.

Circumanal glands (superficial sebaceous glands) and perianal glands (deep sebaceous glands) are modified sebaceous glands located at the mucocutaneous junction of the anus. Perianal glandular tissue can also be found in the skin of the prepuce and groin. The mammary glands of the skin are compound tubuloalveolar apocrine glands resembling sweat glands in their mode of development.

Anal sacs contain both sebaceous and apocrine sweat glands and have a thin, stratified squamous epithelial lining. Sebaceous glands tend to line the neck of the sac, whereas the apocrine glands are concentrated in the fundus.

THE HYPODERMIS (SUBCUTIS) (p. 263)

The hypodermis is composed primarily of fat with loose collagenous trabeculae and elastic fibers. It varies in thickness in various regions of the body, being poorly developed beneath the eyelids, ears, scrotum, and other areas where the skin is closely attached to underlying structures.

Panniculus Muscle

The panniculus muscle (panniculus carnosus) is a collection of thin cutaneous muscles in the hypodermis in dogs and cats. The panniculus muscles in the head and neck regions are the platysma, sphincter colli superficialis, and sphincter colli profundus. The cutaneous trunci is the major cutaneous muscle of the body, extending from the gluteal region cranial and ventral to the pectoral region.

Panniculus muscle fibers are very irregular, tend to run transversely, penetrate the dermis, and allow voluntary movement of the skin. The cutaneous trunci is used to shake the skin in response to irritating or noxious stimuli.

VASCULAR SUPPLY TO THE SKIN (pp. 264–265)

The cutaneous vascular system is divided into three interconnected levels: (1) the deep, subdermal, or subcutaneous plexus, (2) the middle, or cutaneous, plexus, and (3) the superficial, or subpapillary, plexus.

The subdermal plexus is the major vascular network to the overlying skin. Where there is a layer of cutaneous muscle, the subdermal plexus lies both superficial and deep to it.

The middle plexus shows developmental and positional variations according to the distribution of the hair follicles in the skin. Radicals from the middle plexus ascend to supply the superficial plexus. The superficial plexus lies in the outer layer of the dermis. Capillary loops from this plexus project into the dermal papillary bodies to supply the epidermal papillae and adjacent epidermis.

Segmental vessels arising from the aorta deep to the body muscle mass give off perforator branches, which traverse the skeletal muscles to supply the subdermal plexus.

SURGICAL CONSIDERATIONS (pp. 265–267)

Partial-thickness skin losses, in which the epidermis and a variable portion of the dermis are tangentially removed or destroyed, often heal by adnexal re-epithelialization. As previously noted, the hair follicles, apocrine sweat glands, and sebaceous glands have a common ectodermal origin. The epithelial components of these adnexa may remain viable and serve as a source of epithelial cells to resurface the exposed dermal surface. This is in contrast to full-thickness skin losses, which rely on wound contraction and epithelialization from the viable bordering skin.

Preservation of the cutaneous microcirculation and the feeding of direct cutaneous arterial/venous vasculature are critical to skin survival. The following six points can be used by clinicians as general guidelines for undermining skin in small animals:

1. Skin should be undermined below the panniculus muscle layer when present to preserve the subdermal plexus and associated direct cutaneous vessels.

2. Skin without an underlying panniculus muscle layer (middle and distal portion of the extremities) should be undermined in the loose areolar fascia beneath the dermis to preserve the subdermal plexus.

3. Preserve direct cutaneous arteries and veins whenever possible during undermining.

4. Skin closely associated with an underlying muscle should be elevated by including a portion of the outer muscle fascia with the dermis rather than undermining between these structures.

5. Avoid direct injury to the subdermal plexus by using atraumatic surgical technique.

6. Avoid or minimize the surgical manipulation of skin recently traumatized until circulation improves.

CONGENITAL SKIN DISORDERS (pp. 267–268)

Cutaneous Asthenia

Cutaneous asthenia is a congenitohereditary skin disorder reported in man and other animals. In animals, this condition is analogous to the Ehlers-Danlos syndrome (EDS) in man, a group of collagen disorders characterized by unduly fragile connective tissue. The disease is considered autosomal dominant with incomplete penetrance in mink, dogs, and cats. Increased skin fragility with hyperelasticity and laxity is the outstanding clinical feature of cutaneous asthenia in dogs and cats. Affected animals usually have a history of lacerations, abscesses, and tissue-paper–thin scars (onion skin scars). Pseudotumor formation due to injury to fragile blood vessels may be noted. The skin tears easily with minor trauma, but little bleeding usually is noted.

Surgical problems associated with EDS are proportional to the severity of the connective tissue abnormality. Clipping the hair and preparation for any surgical procedure must be performed gently. Use of tissue forceps should be minimized. Round-bodied atraumatic suture needles may be advisable to prevent skin tears during suturing. Tension suture patterns may be necessary if simple interrupted sutures pull through the delicate tissue. Although wounds are susceptible to dehiscence from tearing of the thin dermis, the stages of healing appear similar to unaffected skin. Once healed, the tensile strength of the scar may be comparable to the surrounding dermis.

Epitheliogenesis Imperfecta (p. 268)

CHAPTER 25
Management of Superficial Skin Wounds (pages 269–280)

A wound is an injury characterized by disruption of the normal continuity of body structure. The cause of a wound often determines the amount of tissue damage. Regardless of the type of injury, wound closure can be performed immediately or delayed until the risk of infection and subsequent dehiscence is decreased. In some wounds with tissue loss, delayed skin reconstruction using skin flaps or grafts may be required.

WOUND CLASSIFICATION (pp. 269–270)

There is no inclusive classification for wounds. In simple terms, wounds may be open or closed. Open wounds include lacerations or skin loss. Closed wounds include crushing injuries and contusions.

By etiology, open wounds are classified as follows:

1. Abrasion: Damage to the skin consisting of loss of the epidermis and portions of the dermis.
2. Avulsion: A wound characterized by tearing of tissue from its attachments.
3. Incision: A wound created by a sharp object.
4. Laceration: An irregular wound created by tearing of tissue.
5. Puncture wound: A penetrating wound of the skin caused by a missile or sharp object.

Another classification of open wounds relates strictly to degree of contamination. *Clean wounds* are surgically created under aseptic conditions. *Clean contaminated wounds* have minimal contamination, and the contamination can be effectively removed. *Contaminated wounds* have gross contamination with foreign debris. *Dirty* and *infected wounds* are characterized by an existing infectious process.

In the absence of objective data (quantitative wound bacteriology), the wound is regarded as infected if doubt exists.

LOCAL WOUND FACTORS AND WOUND INFECTION (p. 270)

Local wound factors that impair resistance to infection include foreign bodies, necrotic or ischemic tissue, closure of the wound under tension, irradiation, hematoma formation, wound dead space, and excessive or inappropriate suture material. The method of suture placement and local wound environment are as important to wound closure as the type of suture material selected.

SYSTEMIC FACTORS AND WOUND INFECTION (p. 270)

Host resistance to infection may be impaired by systemic disease such as uncontrolled diabetes mellitus, Cushing's disease, and hypoproteinemia. Pharmacological agents such as corticosteroids and cancer chemotherapeutic agents impair host resistance and potentiate wound infection.

THEORY OF WOUND CLOSURE (p. 270)

Primary closure is usually performed when the wound is classified as clean or clean contaminated. Delayed primary closure is performed 48 to 72 hours after the wound has occurred, before the formation of granulation tissue. It is a proven method for decreasing the incidence of wound infection when contamination cannot be removed or when judgment of tissue viability or definitive surgical débridement cannot be performed initially. Secondary closure consists of wound closure in the presence of granulation tissue. Second intention healing by epithelialization and contraction is successful in small animals because of abundant highly elastic skin.

WOUND CARE (pp. 270–271)

At this time, no available pharmacological agent can augment or significantly increase the rate of healing or strength of repaired wounds.

In general, there should be minimal interference with a wound before definitive treatment is performed. Topical agents including harsh antiseptics, ointments, solutions, and powders may inhibit normal wound healing and cause chemical injury to tissue.

WOUND CLEANING (p. 271)

Further contamination of the wound should be avoided. The simplest method of protecting an open wound is with sterile gauze or nonadherent sponges. Sterile water-soluble ointments may also be applied temporarily and removed by lavage during definitive surgical management.

A wide area surrounding the wound is clipped of hair with number 40 clipper blades. The area surrounding the wound should be prepared using an effective surgical scrub solution. Both povidone-iodine and chlorhexidine gluconate are effective scrub solutions for skin preparation.

Bacterial numbers within the open wound may be reduced by surgical débridement, wound lavage, and antimicrobial chemotherapy. Large volumes of irrigants provide some dilutional effects to bacteria, but the concept that large-volume wound lavage by itself provides effective wound irrigation is erroneous. Irrigants should be delivered at a pressure of 8 psi to be maximally effective. This pressure may be generated by use of a 35-ml syringe and a 19-gauge needle.

The ideal wound antiseptic is bactericidal without harming healing tissues. Chlorhexidine diacetate when used as 0.05 per cent solution (1:40 dilution of stock chlorhexidine solution to water) significantly reduces bacterial population in contaminated wounds in dogs without increasing tissue inflammation.

Povidone-iodine has been widely used as a 1 per cent wound lavage solution (1:10 dilution of stock povidone solution to saline) and has good antimicrobial activity. Povidone-iodine has limited residual activity because of inactivation of free iodine by organic matter in the wound.

Hydrogen peroxide has been used as a wound irrigant. It has little or no value as an antiseptic and causes injury to the capillary bed. Because it may delay healing, this agent has no positive value in wound management.

WOUND DÉBRIDEMENT (pp. 271–272)

Débridement is the process of removing devitalized tissue from a wound. The objective is to convert the wound to a clean status, containing tissue with adequate blood supply for normal healing. Wound débridement may be surgical, enzymatic, mechanical, or hydrodynamic (lavage).

Sharp excision by scalpel blade is preferred over scissors. Evaluation of skin viability in the acute period after wounding may be difficult because of temporary vasospasm or edema. Under these circumstances, viable skin may not bleed. If doubt exists, especially where skin is sparse, skin débridement may be delayed 48 to 72 hours until obvious color demarcation occurs.

Trypsin and chymotrypsin have been used topically for wound débridement. Disadvantages of enzymes include expense, time required, and insufficient débridement.

Mechanical wound débridement may be accomplished by use of bandages. The use of wet-to-dry wound dressings is indicated for wounds with necrotic or devitalized tissue, foreign material, or viscous exudate. Sterile saline-soaked gauze sponges are applied directly to the wound surface, followed by application of a second absorbent layer of bandage material. The wound is débrided of necrotic tissue and foreign material, which adheres to the bandage as it dries.

TOPICAL ANTIBIOTICS (p. 272)

The use of topical antimicrobials is controversial. Epithelialization may be slowed by some topical agents, especially those with a petroleum base. Topical antibiotic ointments should be handled aseptically and used in *limited* amounts on wounds.

SYSTEMIC ANTIBIOTICS (p. 272)

Systemic antibiotics may be used prophylactically or therapeutically. Antibiotics selected for antimicrobial prophylaxis should be effective against the microorganism most likely to cause postoperative wound infection and should be present in adequate concentrations in tissue at the time of contamination or within hours afterward. When used prophylactically, antibiotics are not continued postoperatively.

CLOSURE OF ACUTELY CONTAMINATED WOUNDS
(pp. 272–273)

Factors to be considered include degree of contamination, time interval since injury, presence of devitalized and damaged tissue, adequacy of blood supply, adequacy of hemostasis, availability of tension-free closure, overall status of the patient, and client compliance with wound management. The wound is better left unsutured if a surgeon doubts the success of primary wound closure. Premature closure predisposes to wound dehiscence and infection.

Most wounds caused by sharp objects have low levels of bacteria and minimal soft-tissue damage and are amenable to primary closure. Crush wounds have a higher incidence of infection from more extensive damage and possible induction of foreign material.

DELAYED PRIMARY CLOSURE OF ACUTELY CONTAMINATED WOUNDS (p. 273)

Delayed primary closure is indicated under the following conditions: the presence of gross contamination, purulent exudate, extensively devitalized or necrotic tissue, edema, erythematous wound edges, lymphangitis, or skin tension. Under these circumstances, wound closure is performed 3 to 5 days after injury, based on the time interval usually required to control local infection.

The advantage of delayed primary closure is that it permits evaluation of the progression of wound healing and serial débridement of devitalized tissue that was either missed during initial débridement or had questionable viability. Bandaging the wound is essential during the interval of open management. Wet-to-dry dressings are probably most appropriate.

CLOSURE OF CHRONIC CONTAMINATED WOUNDS (p. 273)

Chronic contaminated wounds are candidates for secondary closure.

The wound is initially treated as described for delayed primary closure. Once wound cleaning and débridement are complete and granulation tissue starts to form, closure over drains may be considered. To provide mobility, excess granulation tissue is usually excised, together with a thin rim of skin at the wound margin. Excessive undermining of adjacent skin, however, is avoided.

SECOND INTENTION HEALING (pp. 273–274)

When indicated, wounds can be allowed to heal completely by second intention or wound contraction and epithelialization. Although healing time is protracted and cosmetic and functional results may be less than optimal, wounds are frequently treated in this manner with favorable results. If necessary, disfiguring scars can be revised once healing is complete.

CONTAMINATED WOUND CLOSURE WITH GRAFTS OR FLAPS (p. 274)

MANAGEMENT OF SPECIFIC WOUNDS (pp. 274–278)

Dog Bites

Dog bite wounds are "iceberg" wounds in which a major component of tissue damage frequently resides beneath the relatively benign appearance of the cutaneous puncture wound. Large areas of devitalized tissue, ischemia, and dead space below the skin facilitate bacterial colonization.

Bite wounds involving the thorax may cause rib fractures, pyothorax, hemothorax, and pneumothorax. Bite wounds involving the abdomen are evaluated for penetration of the peritoneal cavity and for evidence of visceral damage or abdominal herniation. Penetrating bite wounds warrant a mandatory exploratory laparotomy to assess the integrity of the abdominal viscera.

Surgical débridement of all devitalized muscle and fat is essential to prevent or control infection; however, fascia, nerves, tendons, and ligaments are preserved if viable. Copious wound lavage is recommended. Active or passive drains are used to obliterate extensive dead space.

Ideally, all drains should be covered with sterile dressings to reduce contamination, with dressings changed as frequently as indicated by the quantity of drainage. Drains are removed once they have served their purpose.

Once necrotic skin is excised, the wound is frequently treated by delayed primary closure or second intention healing.

Pressure Sores

Every effort is made to prevent pressure sores (decubitus ulcers) in patients that have to remain recumbent for prolonged periods. The following considerations may aid in their prevention:

1. Change the position of the animal frequently, ideally every 2 hours.
2. Provide sufficient padding. Water mattresses are particularly useful.
3. Maintain adequate nutrition.
4. Maintain skin health. The skin should be kept clean and dry.
5. Avoid dragging the patient.

The basis of nonsurgical treatment of pressure sores is the use of topical wound therapy, usually wound lavage and topical medication. Surgical treatment of pressure sores follows general principles—débridement followed by wound therapy and delayed closure.

Footpad Wounds

The use of nonabsorbable monofilament suture material in a tension-apposition suture pattern is recommended. Strong, absorbable subcutaneous sutures are placed in the footpads to help support tissues. It is advisable to prevent the animal's weight from splaying the pad outward by bandaging the limb, preferably in a non-weightbearing position or with the incorporation of a firm splint.

Degloving Injuries (p. 277)

Rotational forces applied to the skin and supporting tissues frequently result in a low-velocity avulsion injury referred to as a *degloving injury*. The general principles of wound management are followed, with particular attention to débridement of devitalized tissues.

Nonhealing Wounds

The failure of a wound to heal may be an indication of a local or systemic disorder. Poor suturing techniques, including excessive tension, improper suture material, and poor knot-tying techniques, can interfere with healing. The presence of microorganisms, foreign material, necrotic tissue, seroma or hematoma, and poor circulation also may result in wound dehiscence.

Systemic factors also may delay wound healing. Endocrine imbalances, nutritional deficiencies, senility, obesity, anemia, and "wasting" diseases all are considered as potential causes. Lesions being treated as open wounds may occasionally represent areas of tumor infiltration or infection by fungal elements or resistant bacteria. In such cases, biopsy samples and bacterial and fungal cultures aid in selecting therapy.

Radiation Ulcers (pp. 277–278)

Chemical Ulcers (p. 278)

Chemotherapy and Wound Healing

Experimental investigations show that alkylating agents, antimetabolites, antitumor antibiotics, and corticosteroids cause complicated wound healing. Clinical data do not support these experimental findings. Deferment of chemotherapy until wound healing has become established and the risk of wound complications has passed (usually 7 to 10 days) is justifiable.

WOUND HEALING COMPLICATIONS (pp. 278–279)

Wound Dehiscence

Impending wound disruption is often preceded by necrosis of the skin edges, extensive cutaneous bruising, the presence of serum beneath the skin, and serosanguineous discharge from the suture line.

If infection and underlying disease have been ruled out, primary wound closure can be attempted, using Penrose or closed suction drains to obliterate dead space. If infection is present, the wound is treated open, allowing healing to proceed by second intention, or by secondary closure when appropriate.

Hematoma and Seroma Formation

Fluid that collects between tissue layers can delay healing by preventing apposition of the tissues, by interfering with blood supply to the area, and by inhibiting the influx of phagocytic cells into the area, encouraging bacterial growth.

Small accumulations of fluid usually resolve without treatment. Larger seromas that interfere with function may require needle aspiration under strictly aseptic conditions, followed by compression bandaging, or the removal of skin sutures to permit drainage and to allow healing by second intention. In some cases, drains may be required to prevent recurrence.

Wound Contracture (p. 279)

The deleterious consequences of contraction and excessive scar tissue, including deformity and loss of function, are referred to as *wound contracture*.

Infection

Infection delays wound healing by the physical separation of wound surfaces from exudative processes and the production of necrotizing enzymes that destroy tissues, impair fibroblastic activity, and decrease wound strength. The treatment of infected wounds follows the general principles of débridement, lavage, delayed closure or second intention healing, and appropriate systemic antimicrobial therapy.

CHAPTER 26

Principles of Plastic and Reconstructive Surgery

(pages 280–294)

BASIC INSTRUMENTS (p. 280)

SUTURES (pp. 280–283)

Principles of Suturing (see Chapter 19)

Placement of Sutures

The goal in skin closure is square skin edges accurately apposed with no overlapping. Slight eversion of the wound edges helps ensure good dermal apposition and avoids inversion of the wound edges.

There are four ways to even up skin edges that do not lie on the same level.

1. Manipulation of the suture knot from one side of the wound to the other may help even up the edges, usually the low side.
2. Place the suture in the skin at the same depth from the surface on both sides of the wound.
3. A half-buried horizontal mattress suture is placed with the intradermal portion on the low side of the wound.
4. A slight elevation of one side of a wound between two sutures can be corrected by placing a piece of stiff suture material from high on the high side to low on the low side without tying it. This evens the edges, and the suture can be removed in 2 to 3 days.

Place as many sutures as close together as necessary to satisfactorily appose the wound edges. The distance between sutures varies with the wound type and location and requires judgment for the best and most cosmetic closure.

Suture Knots

The square (reef) knot is the most common knot used in surgery. For additional knot security and when using suture material with a low coefficient of friction, additional half-knots may be placed on the knot. After the knot is tied, the surgeon should be able to pull it up gently and see a space between the suture loop and tissue, indicating that allowance has been made for normal postoperative swelling.

The smallest suture bite that apposes wound edges both superficially and deeply without crimping or cutting through the tissues is used. This keeps the amount of tissue under tension to a minimum and reduces scarring from sutures.

Basic Suture Patterns

Subcuticular and Intradermal Sutures. Subcuticular sutures are placed in the subcutaneous tissues. They have three roles: (1) elimination of dead space, (2) reduction of tension across the wound margin before placing skin sutures, and (3) approximation of wound margins.

Simple Interrupted Sutures. The most common pattern for skin closure is the simple interrupted suture. Each suture is a single loop of

127

suture material passed perpendicular to the plane of the tissues, with the ends emerging on opposite sides of the wound.

Simple Continuous Sutures. The simple continuous suture pattern is a progressive series of sutures inserted perpendicular to the plane of the tissues without interruption, with only two ends of the suture tied.

Vertical Mattress Sutures. A vertical mattress suture is a loop of suture material placed perpendicular to the tissue plane with both suture ends emerging on the same side of the wound. It is useful as both a tension suture and an everting skin suture.

Interrupted Horizontal Mattress Sutures. These sutures are placed in the same plane as the tissue, with both ends of the suture emerging on the same side of the wound. They evert skin edges, close dead space, and relieve tension. Due to their geometric configuration, they may tend to cut through the skin and impair the blood supply to the wound edges.

Continuous Lock Sutures. The continuous lock suture pattern is a progressive series of sutures inserted in the same plane as the tissue, with the needle passing over the unused suture material after each suture. These sutures may cause tissue inversion, and tension adjustment along the suture line may be difficult.

STAPLES (p. 283)

Staples provide a rapid, everted, and accurate skin closure that is more convenient than conventional suturing. There is less likelihood of wound infection and tissue strangulation from this strong, nonreactive type of closure. The higher cost is a disadvantage.

UNDERMINING AND ADVANCING SKIN (pp. 283–284)
Undermining Techniques

Undermining is indicated when a wound is too large to close with tension sutures and stents alone but is not large enough for a skin flap.

Skin is undermined deep to the panniculus muscle layer where it is present. Skin without a panniculus muscle layer is undermined in the loose areolar fascia deep to the dermis.

Walking Sutures

The skin is undermined around the wound, leaving intact any large blood vessels coming from underlying tissues to the dermis. Each suture is placed by passing the needle in the deeper dermis first, followed by a second bite in the underlying tissue *toward* the center of the wound. Tying the suture advances the skin slightly toward the wound's center. Walking sutures are placed in rows, which gradually advance the skin over the wound. Walking sutures have the advantages of (1) moving skin from the area around the defect to cover the defect, (2) obliterating dead space, and (3) evenly distributing tension to the tissues around the wound rather than concentrating tension at the wound's edge.

Presuturing

Presuturing refers to skin around a skin lesion being sutured over the lesion 12 to 14 hours before its removal. This technique is based on the biomechanical properties of skin that allow the skin to stretch beyond its inherent extensibility. I believe the same effect is gained by using one procedure with walking sutures.

Tissue Expanders (p. 284)

COSMETIC CLOSURE OF VARIOUSLY SHAPED WOUNDS
(pp. 284–288)

Fusiform Defects

Most skin lesions can be corrected by fusiform excision. The proposed excision is outlined around the lesion so that the sides are of equal length and in a 4:1 length/width ratio.

Fusiform excisions are made parallel to skin tension lines if possible. When direction of tension lines is uncertain, the lesion is excised in a circular pattern. After noting the direction of the long axis of the defect created by the pull of adjacent tension lines, the defect can be remodeled to a fusiform shape with its long axis in the direction of tension.

Crescent-Shaped Defects

Closure of crescent-shaped defects entails suturing two skin edges of unequal length. Sutures are placed closer together on the short side of the wound and farther apart on the long side of the wound. Another technique is the rule of halves; one suture is placed in the center of the wound, and the resulting defects are halved progressively by sutures until the wound is closed.

Triangular, Rectangular, and Square Defects

When located in an area where there is movable skin on all sides of a triangular, rectangular, or square defect, the defect is closed from the corners toward the center. Suturing progresses around the defect from corner to corner. The result is a Y-shaped scar for triangular closure, a double Y-shaped scar for rectangular closure, and an X-shaped scar for square closure.

Chevron-Shaped Defects

With V-shaped wounds, part of the skin flap may have been lost or trimmed with débridement. The defect is closed as a Y. Starting at the point of the chevron, suturing is continued until wound tension begins to develop; then the two arms of the Y are closed.

Circular Defects

A technique for closing circular defects to avoid dog-ears involves converting the defect to a fusiform shape by removing two triangular pieces of skin on opposite sides of the circle with the base of each triangle incorporated into the circle's edge. The defect is then closed as a fusiform defect. Several other techniques are available for closing circular defects that do not require the removal of additional tissues.

TENSION-RELIEVING TECHNIQUES (pp. 288–292)

Simple Relaxing Incision

A simple relaxing incision is made parallel and adjacent to a wound to advance the skin between the wound and the incision over the defect. Because of the lack of loose elastic skin in the area, the relaxing incision is left to heal as an open wound. When relaxing incisions are created on both sides of a defect, the width of each flap equals the widest part of the defect.

Multiple Punctate Relaxing Incisions

Parallel staggered rows of punctate relaxing incisions adjacent to a wound may release tension for closure.

Bipedicle Flap

A bipedicle flap is similar to a relaxing incision, but the defect left after closing the original wound is closed because it is in loose, elastic skin (see Chapter 27).

V-Y–Plasty

A V incision is made in the loose elastic skin adjacent to the area where relaxation is needed, with the point of the V away from this area. The skin between the V and the area of needed relaxation is undermined and advanced. The remaining chevron-shaped defect is closed in the shape of a Y.

Z-Plasty

Dynamics and Design of a Z-Plasty

Z-plasty is the transposition of two interdigitating triangular flaps of skin.

When the flaps of a Z-plasty are transposed, there is a gain in length in the original direction of the central limb of the Z as a result of shortening of the skin along the opposite sides of the Z-plasty. There is also a rotation of the axis of the tissues included in the flaps of the Z and a change in the direction of the central limb of the Z.

Use of a Z-Plasty

Z-plasty can release tension along a linear scar across a curved flexor surface, which limits extension of the surface. Z-plasty can be used also as a relaxing incision to aid closure of large defects.

TENSION SUTURES (pp. 292–294)

Simple Interrupted Tension Sutures

Simple interrupted tension sutures are indicated for closing wounds with minimal tension. The size of the bite of tissue is alternated when placing the skin approximation sutures (i.e., wide bite, narrow bite, wide bite).

Horizontal Mattress Sutures

Horizontal mattress sutures are placed well away from the skin edge as previously described to serve as tension sutures. Placing stents of rubber tubing or buttons under the sutures helps to overcome the tendency of these sutures to cut through the skin and impair circulation at the wound edges.

Vertical Mattress Sutures

Vertical mattress sutures are placed at a distance from the wound margin as tension sutures. When wound closure results in significant tension, stents of firm or soft rubber or buttons can be placed under the suture loops. These sutures have less tendency to reduce circulation at the wound edges than do horizontal mattress sutures and can be used with simple interrupted skin apposition sutures.

Cruciate Sutures

Cruciate sutures provide strength and prevent eversion of the wound edges. The needle is inserted from the wound edge on one side and is directed to the opposite side of the wound like a simple interrupted suture. The needle is passed a second time through the tissue parallel to the first passage. The suture ends, which are on opposite sides of the wound, are tied together to form an X on the skin surface.

"Far-Near-Near-Far" Sutures (p. 294)

"Far-Far-Near-Near" Sutures (p. 294)

CHAPTER 27
Pedicle Grafts (pages 295–325)

A pedicle graft is a portion of skin and subcutaneous tissue with a vascular attachment moved from one area of the body to another.

Properly developed flaps survive because of their intact circulation, unlike free grafts, which depend on revascularization from the recipient bed. Pedicle grafts can be used to cover defects with poor vascularity, areas difficult to immobilize, holes overlying cavities, and areas where padding and durability are essential. They are equally valuable for immediate coverage and protection of nerves, vessels, tendons, and other structures susceptible to exposure and trauma.

When used properly, flaps can bypass many of the potential problems associated with contraction and epithelialization, including prolonged healing time and wound care, nonhealing, excessive scarring, a fragile epithelialized surface more prone to reinjury, wound contracture, compromised venous return distal to the injury, and the direct exposure of important underlying structures until healing occurs.

FLAP CLASSIFICATION (pp. 295–297)

Flap Classification Based on Blood Supply

Most pedicle grafts used in dogs and cats are elevated without including a direct cutaneous artery and vein. Flap survival depends on the deep or subdermal plexus entering the base of the flap. This is termed a *subdermal plexus flap*.

A pedicle graft incorporating a direct cutaneous artery and vein is termed an *axial pattern flap*. Axial pattern flaps have an excellent blood supply and a surviving area approximately 50 per cent greater than that of subdermal plexus flaps of comparable dimension in dogs.

Compound and Composite Flaps

A *compound flap* or *composite flap* denotes the elevation and transfer of flaps that incorporate skin with other tissues, including muscle, fat, bone, and cartilage.

Flap Classification Based on Location with the Recipient Bed

Pedicle grafts developed adjacent to the recipient bed are termed *local flaps*, whereas flaps transferred from a distant region are termed *distant flaps*.

Local flaps are both simple and economical. They are more able to maintain a similar pattern of hair growth and color than distant flaps. Distant flaps are used almost exclusively for major skin losses involving the extremities.

PLANNING THE FLAP: GENERAL CONSIDERATIONS
(pp. 297–299)

Ideal donor areas have ample skin available to elevate a flap without creating a secondary defect (donor bed) unamenable to simple closure. It is best to avoid donor sites subject to excessive motion and stress to avoid wound dehiscence or decreased local mobility.

Factors that maximize the circulation to a pedicle graft should be considered during flap planning. The cutaneous circulation differs regionally, and a set length/width ratio is not applicable. I recommend (1) flaps with a base slightly wider than the width of the flap body to avoid inadvertent narrowing of the pedicle and (2) flaps limited to the length required to cover the recipient bed without excessive tension.

Skin is best undermined below the panniculus carnosus, when present, to preserve the subdermal plexus and adjacent direct cutaneous vasculature (see Chapter 24). Large flaps should include a direct cutaneous artery and vein when possible.

The Delay Phenomenon

Large flaps raised in two or more stages before transfer are more likely to survive than pedicle grafts transplanted at the first operation. This method of augmenting flap survival is called the *delay phenomenon*. Although the exact delay mechanism is unclear, sustained vasodilation is currently believed to be the cause of improved flap survival.

PREPARING THE RECIPIENT BED (pp. 299–300)

The recipient bed should be free of debris, necrotic tissue, and infection. Distant flaps require the establishment of circulation from the defect to eventually divide the pedicles for completion of flap transfer. Vascular tissue, such as healthy muscle, periosteum, and the paratenon, is capable of vascularizing an overlying skin flap. Chronic granulation tissue can be excised to re-establish a healthy granulation bed within 3 to 5 days.

GUIDELINES FOR LOCAL FLAP DEVELOPMENT AND TRANSFER (pp. 300–304)

Rotating Flaps

Rotation Flap

A rotation flap is a semicircle sharing a common border with a triangular defect. In veterinary practice, a curved incision is usually created in a stepwise fashion, and the flap is undermined until it covers the wound without excessive tension. Properly planned rotation flaps in dogs and cats rarely create a donor defect that cannot be closed.

Transposition Flap

A transposition flap is a rectangular pedicle graft usually created within 90° of the long axis of the defect. It is a rotational pedicle graft. An edge of the defect comprises a portion of the flap border.

Secondary defects (donor bed) usually are closed directly after the cutaneous borders are undermined.

Interpolation Flap

An interpolation flap is a rotating rectangular flap lacking a common border with the skin defect. As a result, a portion of the flap must cross the skin between the donor and recipient beds. The donor bed is closed directly, and the redundant portion of the flap can be excised after healing is complete.

Advancement Flaps

Advancement Flap (Single Pedicle)

A single-pedicle advancement flap is one of the local flaps most commonly used in animals. Advancement is accomplished by taking advantage of the elasticity of the skin. Two single-pedicle advancement flaps (H-plasty) may be more effective than a longer single advancement flap to close a large square or rectangular wound.

To create a single-pedicle advancement flap, two skin incisions equal to the width of the defect are made in progressive fashion. The distant edge of the flap borders the defect. The flap is undermined and is advanced into the defect.

Bipedicle Advancement Flap

Bipedicle advancement flaps are constructed by making an incision parallel to the long axis of a defect, the width of the flap being equal to the width of the adjacent defect.The flap is undermined and sutured into the defect.

GUIDELINES FOR DISTANT FLAP DEVELOPMENT AND TRANSFER (pp. 304–307)

Direct Flap

Direct flaps include the single-pedicle flap (hinge flap) and the bipedicle flap (pouch flap). The affected limb is elevated to the flap and secured beneath it until each pedicle can be divided to complete the transfer.

The donor area is generally located over the lateral surface of the thorax or abdomen. The width of the flap equals the width of the defect, whereas the length of the flap is determined by the length of the defect plus that additional portion required to position the flap over the recipient bed.

Division of the pedicle necessitates revascularization between the recipient bed and overlying dermal surface of the flap. Pedicles are divided 10 to 14 days after the initial transfer in stages.

Indirect Flap: The Delayed Tube Flap

The length and width of tubed flaps are determined by the size of the defect and the additional portion of flap required to reach the recipient bed without tension. Tubing the flap is easily accomplished by elevating the bipedicle flap and suturing its edges together. The donor bed is undermined and closed directly. Delays of 2 or 3 weeks are most commonly used to improve flap circulation before the staged division of one pedicle to complete the transfer. Tubed flaps are moved by migration in dogs and cats by one of three techniques: "caterpillaring," "waltzing," or "tumbling." Of the three, tumbling is the most direct method of transfer.

To cover the recipient site, the flap is divided along its original seam and opened by careful blunt dissection. The remaining pedicle is divided in stages once the flap has healed to the area, 10 to 14 days after its application.

GUIDELINES FOR AXIAL PATTERN FLAP DEVELOPMENT AND TRANSFER (pp. 307–318)

Axial pattern flaps enable transfer of large skin segments in a single stage safely without the need for a delay procedure.

Axial pattern flaps can be rotated into adjacent defects or to distant sites of the lower trunk and extremities. A portion of the flap can be tubed to traverse the skin between the donor and recipient beds, or a bridge incision may be used to avoid tubing the flap.

Omocervical Axial Pattern Flap

The omocervical axial pattern flap incorporates the superficial cervical branch of the omocervical artery and its associated vein. The vessels originate adjacent to the prescapular lymph node and arborize dorsally just cranial to the scapula. The omocervical axial pattern flap has potential use for large skin defects within its arc of rotation, including wounds involving the face, head, ear, shoulder, neck, and axilla.

Thoracodorsal Axial Pattern Flap

The thoracodorsal axial pattern flap is based on a cutaneous branch of the thoracodorsal artery and associated vein. This moderately sized direct cutaneous artery arborizes in a dorsal direction behind the scapula. As a result, thoracodorsal axial pattern flaps of considerable length can be developed to cover defects involving the shoulder, forelimb, elbow, axilla, and thorax.

Superficial Brachial Axial Pattern Flap

The superficial brachial artery branches from the brachial artery 3 cm proximal to the elbow joint. This small, direct cutaneous artery lies medial to the cephalic vein. The vessel is capable of supporting an axial pattern flap of sufficient size to cover major defects involving the antebrachium and elbow.

Caudal Superficial Epigastric Axial Pattern Flap

The caudal superficial epigastric axial pattern flap is a highly versatile pedicle graft for closure of major skin defects of the caudal abdomen, flank, inguinal area, prepuce, perineum, thigh, and rear limbs. The flap includes the last three or four mammary glands and skin nourished by the caudal superficial epigastric vessels arising at the inguinal canal.

The cranial superficial epigastric vessels could be used in a similar way. However, the origin of the cranial superficial epigastric vessels precludes its effective use for most cutaneous defects in small animals. It has potential use for defects involving the ventral thorax.

Deep Circumflex Iliac Axial Pattern Flap

The deep circumflex iliac artery (and paired vein) exits the lateral abdominal wall, cranioventral to the wing of the ilium. It divides to form a dorsal and ventral branch. Each branch can be used independently for axial pattern flap development. The shorter dorsal branch has greater general application for defects involving the ipsilateral flank, lateral lumbar area, caudal thorax, lateral thigh, and pelvic area. The ventral branch extends down the lateral flank and craniolateral thigh. Perhaps its greatest use is for creating an island arterial flap for closure of major sacral and lateral pelvic skin wounds that preclude the use of the dorsal branch of the deep circumflex iliac artery for axial pattern flap development.

Genicular Axial Pattern Flap

The genicular axial pattern flap originates over the short genicular branch of the saphenous artery and medial saphenous vein. The genicular artery extends cranially over the medial aspect of the stifle and terminates over its craniolateral surface. It is sufficient to support a flap that has potential use in closing many skin wounds of the lateral or medial tibial region.

Reverse Saphenous Conduit Flap

The reverse saphenous conduit flap incorporates branches of the saphenous artery and medial saphenous vein, which in turn supply and drain the overlying skin by means of direct cutaneous vessels. By division of vascular connections with the femoral artery and vein, blood flow is maintained in reverse by distal anastomotic connections between the cranial branch of the saphenous artery with the perforating metatarsal artery by way of the medial and lateral plantar arteries, the cranial branch of the medial saphenous vein, the cranial branch of the lateral saphenous vein, and other venous connections with the cranial and caudal branches of the medial saphenous veins distal to the tibiotarsal joint.

The resultant flap with a distally based pedicle has potential for use in major cutaneous defects at or below the tarsus, especially wounds overlying the metatarsal surface.

Secondary Axial Pattern Flaps (p. 316)

Island Arterial Flap (p. 316)

Free Flaps (pp. 316, 318)

COMPOUND AND COMPOSITE FLAP DEVELOPMENT AND TRANSFER (pp. 318–319)

Myocutaneous flaps (primary and secondary) have limited clinical use in dogs and cats owing to the generous amount of loose skin available for wound closure and axial pattern flap development. They may be useful in adding bulk or padding to wound depressions or bony prominences after trauma or tumor removal.

Latissimus Dorsi: Myocutaneous Flap

Although the latissimus dorsi myocutaneous flap is thicker, less pliable, and less elastic than the adjacent cutaneous trunci myocutaneous flap and adjacent thoracodorsal axial pattern flap, it is capable of extending down the forelimb to various degrees, depending on the patient's body conformation. The thoracodorsal axial pattern flap and cutaneous trunci myocutaneous flap are better suited for skin defects, whereas the latissimus dorsi myocutaneous flap with its greater bulk is better suited for thoracic defects, in which the simultaneous replacement of muscle and skin is highly desirable.

Cutaneous Trunci Myocutaneous Flap

Although flap size and coverage are similar to those in the thoracodorsal axial pattern flap, I have safely developed longer thoracodorsal axial pattern flaps in dogs when necessary.

FLAP CIRCULATION (pp. 319–323)

Flap Revascularization and Pedicle Division

When a skin flap is raised, the inherent vascular supply may be insufficient to maintain flap viability. Revascularization from the wound bed is of greater importance than from the wound edges. Beds with high vascular density vascularize a flap more rapidly, especially in ischemic areas of the flap. Staged division of pedicles in axial pattern flaps or distant flaps without direct cutaneous vessels can avoid sudden ischemia and enhance revascularization of the flap by staged ischemia.

Causes of Flap Necrosis

Although flap necrosis can result from infection and toxic agents, an inadequate blood supply is the cause in most cases.

Sufficient perfusion pressure is necessary to drive blood into the distant portion of the flap to avoid necrosis. As little as 10 per cent of the total circulation is necessary for nutrient support of the skin.

Pure arterial obstruction caused pale flaps in experimental rabbits without obvious signs of necrosis for more than 3 days. Pure venous obstruction resulted in venous engorgement, ecchymosis, and cyanosis within 24 hours, with variable degrees of necrosis. Combined arterial and venous occlusion is the most common cause of flap necrosis, with cyanosis in the rabbit flap by 1 hour and a clear demarcation of necrosis by 3 days. Canine flap necrosis may not be visually apparent for 5 or 6 days in some flaps, and a minimum of 1 week was required to determine whether all of a flap survived.

Excessive wound tension is one cause of flap necrosis. A skin tension of 25 g applied to each side of experimental skin flaps is sufficient to cause an elevation of interstitial fluid pressure resulting in flap necrosis from circulatory blockage.

Underlying hematomas have been implicated as a cause of flap necrosis from pressure beneath the flap. Evacuation of the hematoma within 12 hours of its formation may improve flap survival.

Infection is more likely to occur in tissue with poor circulation. Studies of germ-free rats suggest that endogenous bacterial flora may play a part in flap necrosis. An obstruction to blood reflow in peripheral tissues, caused by various periods of tourniquet ischemia, has been called the *no-reflow phenomenon*.

Subjective Assessment of Flap Circulation

Skin color after trauma is deceptive. Contused skin often survives if no additional circulatory compromise occurs. Pigmented skin may initially show no obvious color changes. Portions of flaps pass from red to lavender with eventual resolution without necrosis.

Temperature measurements of skin flaps under controlled conditions are necessary to accurately assess circulation. Because most flaps are partially denervated when elevated, a lack of pain sensation in a responsive animal is not an accurate reflection of flap survival.

Objective Assessment of Flap Circulation

Fluorescein dye has been used to assess circulation in skin, bowel segments, and areas compromised by peripheral vascular disease. Fluorescein is currently the most widely accepted agent for predicting flap survival. Repeated fluorescein dye studies are required to assess circulatory compromise in the postoperative period.

Salvaging the Failing Flap

Controlling the diameter of blood vessels may be a major determinant in blood flow and its distribution. If so, chemical vasodilators may be used to salvage failing flaps. Various drugs have been used in experimental animals and human clinical patients with variable results.

Corticosteroids have variable benefit in improving flap survival in rabbits and pigs. They may be useful in sustaining anoxic cells, may have a vasodilating action, and may stimulate alternate metabolic pathways. Minimizing postoperative edema may be valuable in preventing circulatory compromise due to swelling. Prednisolone is best given preoperatively to reach compromised tissues after the blood supply has shut down.

Prostaglandin inhibitors increase flap survival in rats and may be beneficial by causing vasodilation with increased blood flow, decreased thrombus formation, decreased inflammation, and stabilization of lysosomes. Both steroidal and nonsteroidal (aspirin, ibuprofen, indomethacin) anti-inflammatory drugs are nonspecific inhibitors of prostaglandins and thromboxane synthesis at different stages of metabolic pathways of arachidonic acid.

Topical dressings (antibiotic creams) improve the surviving length of rat flaps by diminishing the depth of tissue loss from desiccation of the deeper ischemic portions of the flap until revascularization can occur. Application of ointments is a simple and practical technique until further studies better define chemical alternatives to modulating blood flow to compromised skin.

Hypothermia can prolong survival of free flaps. Delayed flaps can withstand only 4 hours of normothermic ischemia, apparently due to depleted metabolic stores. At 37.4° to 39.2°F (3° to 4°C), skin grafts can tolerate up to 3 weeks of complete ischemia.

MANAGEMENT OF NECROTIC FLAPS (p. 323)

CHAPTER 28
Skin Grafts (pages 325–340)

INSTRUMENTATION (pp. 325–326)

Split-thickness skin grafts can be harvested freehand using a knife, scalpel blade, or safety razor. However, these blades are hard to control, and holes may be cut in the skin. The electric or pneumatic Brown dermatome has been described for cutting split-thickness grafts in veterinary surgery. Although expensive, it requires less skill or experience to use and can rapidly yield a uniform split-thickness graft.

A piece of skin can be meshed with a scalpel blade, or a split-thickness segment of skin can be laid on an aluminum block that contains numerous staggered parallel rows of notched cutting blades. As a Teflon roller is passed over the graft, numerous slits are cut in the skin, producing a mesh graft.

DEFINITION, CLASSIFICATION, INDICATIONS, AND FACTORS TO CONSIDER (pp. 326–327)

A skin graft is a segment of epidermis and dermis that is completely removed from the body and transferred to a recipient site. Its survival at that site depends on absorption of tissue fluid and development of a new blood supply. Grafts may be either full thickness (composed of epidermis and the entire dermis) or split thickness (composed of epidermis and varying thicknesses of the dermis).

In dogs, skin grafting is primarily indicated for injuries to the skin of the extremities, where skin immobility precludes tissue shifting and the construction of local flaps for repair. They are occasionally used to resurface full-thickness burns after major thermal injuries.

GRAFT BEDS (p. 327)
Where Grafts Will Take

A graft "take" is a successful skin transplant in which the transplant heals in its new location. Grafts are placed on either healthy granulation tissue or a fresh surface that is vascular enough to produce granulation tissue. The wound must appear free of infection, and provision for drainage from beneath the graft is indicated if there was any doubt about the condition of the tissues.

Where Grafts Will Not Take

Grafts will not take over stratified squamous epithelial surfaces. Bone, cartilage, tendon, or nerve denuded of overlying connective tissue cannot support a skin graft. Infected wounds, crushed tissues, heavily irradiated tissues, avascular fat, long-standing granulation tissue, hypertrophic granulation tissue, and chronic ulcers provide poor graft beds.

ACCEPTANCE OF GRAFTS (pp. 327–328)
General Factors

Degeneration begins in a skin graft immediately after it is taken from the donor site, and regeneration begins after graft placement on the recipient bed. Graft survival depends on early re-establishment of sufficient circulation to provide nutrition and dispose of metabolic waste products.

Adherence

Early after placement, a fibrin network adheres a graft to its bed, and the fibrin strands contract to pull the graft into close apposition with the bed. Gain in adherent strength continues with conversion of fibrin network to fibrous tissue until a complete union is present by the tenth postoperative day.

Plasmatic Imbibition

Serum containing erythrocytes and polymorphonuclear cells accumulates between the graft and graft bed as a result of leakage of plasma from graft bed venules. Capillary action pulls the cells and serum into dilated graft vessels, keeping the graft vessels dilated until the graft revascularizes and providing nourishment for graft tissues.

Inosculation

Inosculation is the anastomosis of graft vessels with recipient bed vessels of approximately the same diameter. This takes place as early as 22 hours after graft placement but it is more commonly noted between 48 and 72 hours. Blood flow is sluggish in the graft vasculature on the third or fourth day, but it continues to improve until normal velocity is present by the fifth or sixth day.

Penetration and Ingrowth of New Vessels

Grafts are also revascularized by the ingrowth of new vessels from the bed into the graft. These vessels may grow into the dermis or into pre-existing graft vessels, which serve as nonviable conduits for new ingrowing vessels.

TYPES OF GRAFTS (pp. 328–340)

Split-Thickness Grafts

Definition and Indications

A split-thickness skin graft is composed of epidermis and a variable quantity of dermis. The main indication for this type of graft in dogs is for reconstruction of defects with extensive skin loss. Because the skin of a cat is so thin, split-thickness grafts are not indicated.

Technique (pp. 328–330)

Aftercare

After placement of the graft, hematomas may be removed from under the graft by swirling a cotton-tipped applicator under the graft.

Antibiotic ointment may be placed around the graft edges, and a nonadherent dressing pad or a gauze pad impregnated with petrolatum may be placed over the graft. An absorbent conforming mesh gauze is wrapped over the area, followed by application of an immobilizing splint and tape or a split cast and tape that can be removed periodically for dressing changes. Immobilization is necessary until fibrous tissue anchorage is strong enough to withstand shearing strain without capillary rupture. Immobilizing splints are usually necessary for 10 to 14 days after surgery.

The frequency of bandage changes depends on an animal's temperament and bandage cleanliness. The first bandage is usually changed 48 hours after surgery. Because of the risk of contamination or graft movement, the longer the intervals between bandage changes, the better.

Advantages and Disadvantages

Split-thickness grafts have the advantage of better viability than full-thickness grafts. Their success is attributed to the more abundant capillary network on the exposed dermal surface of the grafts compared with full-thickness grafts.

If wound contraction may cause problems, a split-thickness graft may be advantageous in dogs. These grafts result in expansion of the graft size after healing.

Split-thickness grafts have several disadvantages. The grafts may be less durable and more subject to trauma, making them of questionable use on canine limbs. The hair growth may be absent or sparse on a split-thickness graft. Grafts may have a scaly appearance and lack sebaceous glands.

Full-Thickness Mesh Grafts

Definition and Indications

A full-thickness mesh graft is a piece of full-thickness skin into which numerous slits have been cut in parallel, staggered rows to allow the graft to expand in two directions to increase its size. There are three indications for mesh grafts: (1) to cover a wound that is less than ideal; (2) to cover a large skin defect when there are inadequate donor sites, such as in extensively burned patients; and (3) to reconstruct irregular surfaces that are difficult to immobilize.

Technique (pp. 332–333)

The graft is further immobilized by placing simple interrupted sutures between the slits in the graft at strategic points (i.e., places where the graft lies over a convex or concave part of the wound surface) and other intermittent places but not through all adjacent slits.

Aftercare

A sterile, nonadherent absorbent dressing pad with a thin coating of antibiotic ointment is placed over the graft. This is followed by an absorbent secondary wrap and porous adhesive tape or elastic bandage material as the tertiary bandage. In general, splints are needed only during the first 10 to 14 days after grafting; bandaging is usually continued for 21 days. Bandages are usually changed daily during the first week. As healing takes place and wound drainage decreases, the bandage is changed less frequently.

Advantages and Disadvantages

Mesh grafts have several advantages over other types of grafts. The slits in the graft provide flexibility for the graft to conform to convex or concave surfaces. The graft is stable because it can be fixed to the wound surface by sutures through the slits. Exudate, serum, and blood can drain from the wound surface through the slits, allowing the graft to contact the wound for revascularization. A possible disadvantage is that excess granulation tissue may grow up through the slits and over the top of the graft.

Modifications

Split-Thickness Mesh Graft. Mesh grafts can also be prepared from split-thickness skin. These grafts may be meshed by hand as described earlier or may be meshed by placing the graft dermal side down on an aluminum block that contains many staggered parallel rows of small cutting blades. When expanded to cover a large wound, this type of graft covers a defect three times the width of the original wound.

The aftercare of these grafts is like that for full-thickness mesh grafts. These grafts have the same advantages as a full-thickness mesh graft, with the additional advantage of being thin skin that revascularizes rapidly.

Full-Thickness Unmeshed Graft. A full-thickness unmeshed graft is prepared just as a full-thickness mesh graft, but no slits are cut in the graft. The graft is placed on the wound so the direction of hair growth is like that on the surrounding skin. Several nonabsorbable stay sutures are placed at key points around the graft, with definitive suturing using a simple interrupted or continuous suture pattern.

For drainage from beneath the graft, a closed suction drain may be placed before placing the graft on the bed. Bandaging of the graft is performed as described for split-thickness grafts.

Full-thickness unmeshed grafts become pliable and movable over subcutaneous tissues, resist trauma, and are more like normal skin in color, texture, elasticity, and hair growth than split-thickness grafts.

Full-thickness unmeshed grafts have certain disadvantages. They do not survive well in the presence of infection. This is primarily true when there is no provision for drainage.

Seed Grafts

Definition and Indications

Seed grafts are small pieces of skin placed in a granulation tissue bed with regular spacing between the grafts. These grafts may be harvested by elevating a piece of skin and cutting it free (pinch graft) or by cutting it as a plug with a biopsy punch (punch graft).

Technique (pp. 336–338)

Aftercare

The grafts are covered with a nonadherent contact layer such as an antibiotic ointment and gauze. The area is wrapped with an absorbent conforming mesh gauze, followed by application of a splint if the wound is on a limb. The first bandage is usually changed 3 to 4 days after surgery, taking care not to disturb or pull off any grafts adhered to the dressing.

Advantages and Disadvantages

Seed grafts are simple to perform and require no special equipment. The grafts revascularize well from their deep surface and from the dermal circumference.

Seed grafts have disadvantages. Excessive bleeding of the graft bed may float the plug out of its recipient hole or delay graft revascularization. The grafts generally have a poor cosmetic appearance with sparse hair growth, and the epithelium covering the granulation tissue between grafts may lack durability.

Strip Grafts

Definition and Indications

Strip grafts are 5-mm-wide strips of skin that are placed in parallel grooves cut in a granulation tissue bed.

Technique (pp. 338–339)

Aftercare

The grafts are covered as for seed grafts. Daily bandage changes are usually necessary during the first 7 days and then less often as the drainage abates.

Advantages and Disadvantages

Strip grafts are easily accomplished without expensive equipment. As the grafts heal, epithelium grows over the remaining wound from the edges of the grafts, and the grafts widen as they heal. Hair growth and final cosmetic appearance are not good.

Stamp Grafts

Definition and Indications

Stamp grafts (chess board grafts) are usually made from split-thickness skin that is cut into square patches. The patches are placed on a healthy bed of granulation tissue.

Technique (p. 339)

CHAPTER 29
Surgical Management of Specific Skin Disorders
(pages 341–354)

LIP SURGERY (pp. 341–344)

Lip Fold Excision

Redundant lip folds occur most commonly in breeds such as Saint Bernards, spaniels, schnauzers, English bulldogs, and other brachycephalic breeds. Intertriginous dermatitis occurs within these folds, and secondary pyoderma results in irritation and a foul odor.

The lip fold margins are identified, and then an elliptical incision is made just outside these margins so the fold and infected skin can be excised *en bloc*. Subcutaneous tissue and skin are closed routinely.

Lip Tumor Excision and Restoration of Lip Defects (pp. 341, 343)

Cheiloplasty

The major indications for cheiloplasty are to improve appearance and to decrease drooling, whether it be caused by droopy lips characteristic of certain breeds, by facial nerve paralysis, or by loss of lip support after hemimandibulectomy. In any of these situations, modification of the commissure of the lip is done to decrease drooling and in the latter situation to provide support so that the tongue does not hang from the side of the mouth.

TAIL SURGERY (pp. 344–346)

Caudectomy

Cosmetic tail docking is usually performed at 3 to 5 days of age and is carried out in compliance with breed standards. It is important to preserve enough skin to cover the bone adequately. If closure of the skin over the bone results in excessive incisional tension, wound dehiscence may occur or the resultant scar will be large and nonhaired and may require corrective surgery.

Tail Fold Excision

Skinfold pyoderma (intertriginous dermatitis) occurs commonly in brachycephalic breeds and Manx cats, in which the tail fold created by corkscrewing of the terminal coccygeal vertebrae causes retention of moisture and cutaneous secretions and becomes macerated from contacting skin surfaces. Medical treatment consisting of local cleaning of the affected area with topical wound irrigants and systemic antibiotics is helpful before surgery and results in clinical improvement, but it cannot control relapses of pyoderma because of the abnormal tail conformation. Amputation of the tail and the folds is usually necessary to resolve tail fold pyoderma.

Ingrown Tail

Surgical correction of ingrown tail (''screw-tail'') requires a caudectomy and an *en bloc* débridement of the infected tail fold region.

VULVAR FOLD EXCISION (p. 346)

Skinfold pyoderma may occur in old, obese female dogs that have a pronounced vulvar fold or in young dogs that have a juvenile vulva. Excision of the redundant skinfold (episioplasty) is performed to improve ventilation and lessen the predisposition to pyoderma. The goal is to remove enough skin and excessive subcutaneous tissue to eliminate the fold but not so much to create undue tension on wound closure.

PRINCIPLES OF SKIN TUMOR EXCISION (pp. 346–347)

The goal of tumor removal is to remove all neoplastic cells; therefore, an adequate surgical margin of normal tissue around neoplasm is necessary to ensure that no neoplastic cells are left at the primary location. If it is not possible to leave a proper thickness of normal tissue underneath the neoplasm, an attempt is made to remove an anatomical mesodermal barrier, such as fascia, periosteum, or perichondrium, with the neoplasm. The recommended surgical margin (all sides of the excision) for tumors that tend to recur locally is 2 to 3 cm.

Planning excision should take into consideration the tension lines in the area of the excision, the amount of skin or normal skin tension, and the potential for mobilization of skin in the area of excision.

MASTECTOMY (pp. 347–349)

Mastectomy is defined as the removal of one or more mammary glands. The indication for mastectomy is usually mammary neoplasia but may include septic mastitis refractory to medical treatment.

Mammary tumors account for nearly half of all neoplasia in female dogs. Of these, 41 to 53 per cent are malignant. In cats and male dogs, the majority of mammary tumors are malignant.

Surgical excision of mammary tumors should be recommended for all dogs and cats except when distant metastatic disease is evident or when inflammatory carcinoma is present. Local tumor excision is a palliative measure only when distant metastases are noted.

There are several ways to resect mammary tumors: excisional biopsy, local mastectomy, regional mastectomy, unilateral mastectomy, staged bilateral mastectomy, and simultaneous bilateral mastectomy. Because aggressive surgery has not been shown to prolong survival, excisional biopsy seems the most prudent method for resection of small mammary tumors. A margin of normal tissue is removed with the tumor, and the wound is closed in two layers. Excisional biopsy is quick, is associated with minimal postoperative morbidity, and removes the tumor. Wider excision can be performed later, if biopsy results warrant. Because most feline mammary tumors are malignant, less radical procedures are associated with local recurrence. Wide excision is advisable.

Unilateral mastectomy is performed by removing one entire mammary chain. This procedure is commonly used when multiple mammary masses involve two or more glands on one side.

Bilateral mastectomy can be performed simultaneously in many breeds. It requires one anesthetic period and removes all mammary tissue. Close inspection of skin margins is warranted to ensure that all peripheral mammary tissue is excised. This procedure is reserved for dogs and cats with many glands affected by mammary tumors or with necrotizing septic mastitis. Adequate skin must be present for closure to prevent deliberately retaining glandular tissue for fear that wide margins may preclude adequate wound closure.

PILONIDAL SINUS (pp. 349–350)

SPECIAL SURGERY INVOLVING LIMBS (pp. 350–354)

Elbow Hygroma

An elbow hygroma is a fluid-filled cavity that has a dense wall of fibrous tissue surrounding it. It develops in large or giant breeds of dogs secondary to repeated trauma or pressure over a bony prominence. Hygromas are pseudocysts rather than true cysts because they have no epithelial or synovial lining.

The primary treatment for hygroma is elimination of the cause: repeated trauma to the elbow. This trauma can be ameliorated by applying a padded bandage or providing a well-padded surface for the animal to lie on. Conservative methods, such as aseptic needle drainage and bandaging, are successful only if the repeated trauma ceases.

Surgical treatment of elbow hygroma is indicated when conservative management fails, in truly chronic hygromas, and for those that are secondarily infected. Surgical treatment is by establishing drainage or by excision or both.

Acropruritic Lick Granuloma (pp. 350–351)

Footpad Surgery

Footpad lacerations are common in dogs. Because walking causes periodic pressure and tension on the pad, impaired wound healing may result if the injury is not protected by a support bandage. Splint bandaging alone allows wounds in footpads to heal at nearly the same rate as sutured wounds that are splinted. Footpad wounds that heal solely by second intention may have exposed granulation tissue between wound edges, and chronic ulceration may occur if the pad is unprotected. Suturing footpad lacerations also results in a better cosmetic appearance.

Footpad injuries that result in tissue loss are allowed to heal by second intention. If chronic ulceration of a portion of a footpad results from denervation (trophic ulcer), a neurovascular island flap can be transposed over the ulcerated area to provide epithelial coverage that is innervated. Alternatively, defects involving the metacarpal or metatarsal pads may be closed by digital pad transplantation.

Interdigital Cysts

Interdigital cyst lesions are chronic inflammation rather than true cysts. Clinical signs include pain resulting in lameness, licking, and chewing at the interdigital space. Although foreign bodies are sometimes causative, the etiology is usually undetermined.

Lesions that fail to respond to medical and conservative surgical therapy can be excised. The entire web and cyst are removed. The interdigital wound is closed in two layers by apposing soft tissues with fine interrupted absorbable sutures and skin with simple interrupted sutures of nonabsorbable suture. After surgery, the foot is placed in a padded bandage, which is changed periodically until the incision heals.

Despite removal of the interdigital lesion, recurrence of the lesions in the same area or in another digital web is common.

Cosmetic Surgery
Onychectomy

Onychectomy is the surgical removal of the third phalanges and claws.

The horny claw, a modified layer of epidermis, arises from the ungual crest and ungual process. Most of the germinal cells that produce the claw are situated in the dorsal aspect of the ungual crest. This region must be removed completely, or regrowth of a vestigial claw and abcessation result.

Bandages are applied after surgery to control hemorrhage and to keep the paws clean until blood clots form in the surgical wounds. The bandages are left in place for 24 hours and then removed. Extreme caution is warranted to avoid tight bandages that result in ischemic necrosis of the paw. Cats are kept away from clay litter for 1 week. Physical activity is kept to a minimum for 7 to 10 days.

Deep Digital Flexor Tenectomy (p. 352)
Dewclaw Removal

Rear dewclaws often have no first or second phalanges, leaving the third phalanx to dangle on a soft-tissue "stalk" and predisposing them to traumatic injury. In some dogs, rear dewclaws are absent, whereas Great Pyrenees and briard breeds must have double rear dewclaws to satisfy breed standards. Dewclaws are removed most commonly in toy breeds to prevent clipper trauma in dogs groomed frequently, and in some larger hunting breeds to prevent traumatic injury.

Digit Amputation

Amputation of a digit is usually required after a traumatic injury has resulted in damage that reduces function, including fractures, sprains, luxations, or severe wounds. Other indications for digit amputation are chronic osteomyelitis, arthritis, and neoplasia. Digit amputation in which the third and fourth toes are preserved results in good function, often without resultant lameness. If more than two toes are removed or if the third or fourth toe is removed, various degrees of lameness result.

After surgery, a well-padded bandage is applied to the entire foot and changed as needed for several days. Sutures are removed 10 days after surgery.

CHAPTER 30
Burns: Thermal, Electrical, Chemical, and Cold Injuries
(pages 355–369)

CLASSIFICATION OF BURNS (p. 355)

Burns are described as first, second, or third degree, but the terms *partial thickness* and *full thickness* are more commonly used now and are more appropriate for animals. First-degree burns are superficial partial-thickness injuries involving only the epidermis. Second-degree burns are deeper partial-thickness injuries resulting in complete destruction of the epidermis and variable depths of the dermis. In deep partial-thickness burns, healing can be prolonged and cause significant scarring. Third-degree burns are full-thickness injuries. *Fourth degree* is sometimes used to indicate extension of the injury into the subcutaneous tissue, muscle, fascia, and bone. In the alternate system, partial-thickness burns are classified as superficial or deep, and full-thickness burns include the full thickness of the skin and any structures beneath.

THERMAL BURNS (pp. 355–361)

The causes of thermal burns in small animals include fires, scalding injuries from hot water or grease, direct contact with hot objects such as automobile exhaust pipes and hot stoves, and iatrogenic burns caused by placing anesthetized or debilitated animals on heating pads for prolonged periods and by improper use of hair dryers.

Pathophysiology of the Burn Wound

The extent of the injury is influenced by (1) the temperature of the heat source, (2) duration of contact, and (3) heat conductance characteristics of the tissue contacted.

When heat energy is applied at a rate that exceeds the tissue's ability to absorb and dissipate it, injury occurs. In the outermost zone closest to the heat source *(zone of destruction or coagulation)*, the excessive heat results in denaturation of cellular proteins and coagulation of blood vessels. The area adjacent to this irreversibly damaged tissue, the *zone of stasis*, is characterized by reduced blood flow, intravascular sludging, and potentially reversible tissue damage. In the innermost zone *(zone of hyperemia)*, minimal tissue damage occurs and complete healing follows.

Thermal injury results in an immediate but transient decrease in blood flow to the damaged tissue. This is followed by pronounced arteriolar vasodilation in the remaining microcirculation. The capillaries and venules become highly permeable, resulting in the movement of large volumes of fluid, electrolytes, and proteins from the vascular to the extracellular space.

The movement of protein into the extracellular space of the burn wound rapidly exceeds the capacity of the lymphatic system to return it to the general circulation. Severe hypoproteinemia develops as the protein-rich fluid becomes trapped in the extracellular space. The hypoproteinemia is further magnified during fluid resuscitation and results in generalized edema.

Loss of protein into the extracellular space is greatest during the first 8 to 12 hours after injury. The rate of plasma volume loss decreases substantially by 18 to 24 hours if adequate perfusion is maintained. In dogs, partial-thickness burns of 20 per cent of body surface area resulted in loss of 28 per cent of the plasma volume during the first 6 hours.

Inhalation Injury

Inhalation injury can occur as a single entity or in conjunction with cutaneous burns. Inhalation injury causes thermal burns of the upper airway, carbon monoxide poisoning, and smoke inhalation.

Thermal injury causes progressive edema in the oropharynx and larynx, leading to upper airway obstruction. Thermal injury extending farther down the airway to the distal trachea and primary bronchi causes bronchospasm and bronchorrhea.

Carbon monoxide is one of the most common poisonous gases generated during a fire, as a result of imperfect combustion of wood. Because of its greater binding affinity for hemoglobin, carbon monoxide displaces oxygen from hemoglobin, resulting in tissue hypoxemia. Tissue hypoxia occurs in all end-organs, with arrhythmias being the most common cause of death. Besides its direct effects, carbon monoxide may favor the development of pulmonary injury by reducing the normal reflex decrease in breathing when heated air is inhaled.

Systemic Effects of Thermal Burns

Cardiac Abnormalities

Cardiac output decreases soon after injury, even before major fluid shifts lead to hypovolemia. The decrease in cardiac output is due to a combination of peripheral vascular responses and direct myocardial effects. Peripheral vascular resistance doubles within minutes in dogs with 50 per cent burns and remains high unless adequate fluid therapy is instituted. In untreated dogs, blood viscosity rises to two to three times normal within hours of burning.

Direct myocardial depression occurs in the early postburn period. The depressed contractility was attributed to hypoxia arising from decreased oxygen uptake and altered carbohydrate metabolism.

Anemia

Coagulation necrosis caused by excessive heat results in the immediate destruction of erythrocytes in destroyed vessels. The decrease in erythrocyte mass is usually clinically inapparent because of the fluid shifts that maintain the hematocrit above normal levels.

Thermal injury causes morphological changes in erythrocytes that result in their early removal from the circulation. Younger erythrocytes are more susceptible to injury, resulting in an overall decrease in life span of the remaining erythrocyte population.

Bone marrow suppression and inhibition of erythropoiesis contribute to the anemia, which continues for weeks after burning. The anemia is normocytic and normochromic and is accompanied by low serum iron and iron-binding capacities similar to anemia in chronic disease.

Electrolyte Abnormalities

Alteration of membrane potentials and the affinity of sodium for denatured collagen in the burn wound result in a shift of sodium and water from the vascular space to the interstitial and intracellular spaces. Hyperkalemia is common in the early postburn period because of the thermal destruction of erythrocytes and tissue, which releases intracellular potassium into the circulation. Hypokalemia can occur in the postresuscitation period as a result of the diuresis induced by the fluid therapy and later as a result of mobilization and excretion of burn wound edema fluid.

Renal Function (p. 360)

Hepatic Function (p. 360)

Immune System (pp. 360–361)

Gastroduodenal Ulceration (p. 361)

Multiple Organ-Failure Syndrome (p. 361)

Burn Toxins (p. 361)

INITIAL ASSESSMENT AND TREATMENT (pp. 361–363)

An estimation of the size and depth of the burn wounds is made during the initial examination to guide therapy and establish a prognosis. If the injury occurred in a closed space, the possibility of inhalation injury is considered.

First Aid

Immediate cooling of the affected areas limits further extension of the thermal damage, but when extensive burns are present, overzealous treatment can cause hypothermia.

Fluid Resuscitation

Hypovolemic shock due to sequestration of massive amounts of fluid in the burn wound is the most critical problem in the initial management of patients with extensive burn wounds.

As in other forms of hypovolemic shock, a patient's response to treatment can be monitored using various techniques. Vital signs, mental status, hematocrit, total protein, urine output, and central venous pressure are easily measured parameters.

An isotonic crystalloid fluid such as lactated Ringer's solution is the fluid of choice for initial resuscitation. Colloid-containing fluids are not indicated for at least the first 8 hours after injury. Colloids administered during this period add to accumulation of edema fluid. By 6 to 8 hours, stabilization of membrane permeability and increased lymph return decrease the loss of protein into the tissue. If hypoproteinemia is present, a colloid-containing fluid can be added without adding significantly to burn wound edema. In the postresuscitation period, evaporation from the surface of deep wounds becomes a major source of water loss.

Treatment of Inhalation Injuries

Temporary tracheostomy is indicated for animals with progressively worsening stridor and dyspnea. In most instances, the damage caused by direct thermal injury resolves by 2 to 5 days.

The most reliable clinical sign of carbon monoxide poisoning is cherry-red mucous membranes and blood. Although the oxygen content of the blood is reduced, the PaO_2, which measures dissolved oxygen, remains normal. The half-life of carboxyhemoglobin in human patients breathing room air is more than 4 hours. With supplemental oxygen supplied by mask or nasal tube, the half-life is reduced to 45 to 60 minutes.

NUTRITIONAL REQUIREMENTS OF BURNED PATIENTS
(pp. 363–364)

Burns involving less than 10 to 15 per cent of total body surface area rarely cause increased metabolic rate. Severe burns (>50 per cent) cause the greatest increase in metabolic demands of all types of injuries, with the resting metabolic rate reaching levels up to twice the basal rate.

Alterations in normal hormonal balance after injury are responsible for many of the physiological changes noted. Circulating levels of catecholamines, glucocorticoids, and growth hormone increase dramatically. This stress response results in a relative glucose intolerance and preferential use of fat and protein. Excess glucose is converted to triglycerides and results in fatty infiltration of the liver.

MANAGEMENT OF BURN WOUNDS (pp. 364–365)

Immediately after injury, the wound is sterile, but the dead tissue of burn eschar is ideal for bacterial growth. Endogenous skin and intestinal flora are the most common sources of bacterial contamination.

The use of topical antimicrobial agents has resulted in an approximately 50 per cent reduction in the death rate, yet infection remains the primary cause of death in human patients surviving the initial resuscitation period. Meticulous wound care must still be used for effective topical therapy.

Silver sulfadiazine is the most frequently used topical agent in human hospitals and is probably the agent of choice for veterinary patients. Silver sulfadiazine (1 per cent) is available as a water-soluble cream. It can be applied once or twice daily with or without dressings. A thin proteinaceous gel several millimeters thick often forms on the surface of the wound. This ''pseudoeschar'' is removed.

Silver nitrate and mafenide are also commonly used in man. Silver nitrate is used as a 0.5 per cent aqueous solution. Mafenide has a wide spectrum of antibacterial activity but little antifungal activity.

Systemic antibiotics are reserved for treatment of established infections in the burn wound and infections disseminated to distant organs. Because most invasive burn wound infections are caused by gram-negative organisms, particularly *Pseudomonas* spp., an antimicrobial with activity against these organisms is administered empirically until results of culture and sensitivity testing are available.

Débridement

Débridement of the burn wound can be accomplished by épluchage, enzymatic débridement, or surgical débridement. Épluchage is serial piecemeal removal of loose or obviously devitalized tissue by using a gauze sponge or forceps and scissors. It is usually performed with daily hydrotherapy. Although it results in minimal blood loss and removal of viable tissue, épluchage is tedious and time-consuming.

Chemical débridement using various enzyme preparations offers theoretical advantages in burn wound management, but results are inconsistent. The primary advantage of chemical débridement is removal of necrotic tissue early after injury without removing additional viable tissue. Decreased blood loss and elimination of multiple anesthetic and surgical episodes are potential advantages.

In animals, eschar excision followed by immediate reconstruction by local movement of skin is indicated if sufficient donor skin is available. If immediate reconstruction is impossible, the wound is managed open until healthy granulation is present and then a skin graft is applied.

ELECTRICAL INJURIES (pp. 365–367)

Electrical burns are primarily the result of heat generated as current passes through a solid conductor (tissue). Because blood offers low resistance to its flow, low-voltage current preferentially moves along blood vessels, producing damage that can lead to thrombosis and further tissue destruction.

The most common electrical injury in small animals results from chewing electrical cords. This low-voltage type of injury usually causes local injury to the mouth but rarely causes an exit wound. Immediate death can result from respiratory paralysis or ventricular fibrillation. Many animals are found unconscious or in a tonic state with the electrical cord in their mouth. Burn lesions may be apparent on the lips, gums, palate, or tongue, but the extent of the injury may not be clearly demarcated for 2 to 3 weeks.

Dogs and cats have pulmonary edema as a common complication of low-voltage electrical injury. Electrical stimulation of the central nervous system causes acute fulminating pulmonary edema, which may be attributed to a massive outburst of sympathetic activity resulting in constriction of both resistance and capacitance vessels. The increase in preload and afterload causes pulmonary hypertension resulting in movement of fluid and blood into the interstitial space and ultimately the airways.

Treatment

In low-voltage injuries, pulmonary edema is the most life-threatening complication in animals that survive the initial shock. The treatment for pulmonary edema includes the use of diuretics such as furosemide, morphine to allay anxiety and to produce a sympatholytic and vasodilatory effect, and bronchodilators such as aminophylline, which also causes vasodilation. Patients who fail to respond to medical therapy may benefit from ventilatory support.

Surgical repair of the oral lesions is delayed until the full extent of injury can be determined. Minor lesions can be allowed to heal by second intention. Second intention healing of lip injuries, particularly those involving the commissures, can limit opening of the mouth. Chronic exposure and drying of teeth and gingiva predispose to periodontal disease. Cheiloplasty is indicated to correct these problems.

CHEMICAL BURNS (pp. 367–368)

FROSTBITE (p. 368)

Body Cavities and Hernias (pages 370–482)

CHAPTER 31

Thoracic Wall (pages 370–381)

ANATOMY (p. 370)

PHYSIOLOGY AND PATHOPHYSIOLOGY (pp. 370–371)

The thoracic wall is composed of passive elastic structures and an active musculature. Together, these passive and active elements produce the bucket-handle motion of the ribs allowing expansion and contraction of the thoracic cavity. The passive elements of the thoracic wall possess a characteristic compliance defined as the change in thoracic volume over the change in pressure across the thoracic wall (pleural pressure).

The lung volume at which the passive elastic structures of the pulmonary system are in equilibrium is the functional reserve capacity (FRC). At FRC, the inward elastic recoil of the lungs exactly balances the passive outward elastic recoil of the relaxed thoracic wall.

The thoracic wall and diaphragm form the active respiratory bellows. Contraction of the diaphragm and inspiratory thoracic muscles generates a negative transthoracic pressure resulting in airflow into and expansion of the lungs. Transthoracic pressures generated by the inspiratory musculature must be sufficient to overcome both airway resistance and inward elastic recoil of the lungs and thoracic wall. Passive expiration is driven by the elastic recoil of the lungs and thoracic wall.

Paradoxical movement of the thoracic wall may result from paralysis of the thoracic wall musculature. Negative pleural pressures generated by the contracting diaphragm overcome passive outward recoil of the thoracic wall, resulting in inward movement of the thoracic wall during inspiration.

PREOPERATIVE DIAGNOSIS (p. 371)

Diagnosis of diseases involving the thoracic wall is based on history and physical examination. Additional information is gained by radiographic examination, aspiration cytology, and limited pulmonary function testing.

SURGICAL APPROACHES TO THE THORAX (pp. 371–374)

Intercostal Thoracotomy

An intercostal thoracotomy is the standard approach when exposure of a defined region of the thorax is desired. This approach affords good access to structures in the immediate area of the thoracotomy; however, access to structures not in the immediate area of the thoracotomy is limited. A lateral thoracic radiograph helps determine the intercostal space that best exposes a desired thoracic structure.

Rib Resection Thoracotomy

A rib resection thoracotomy offers increased exposure over an intercostal thoracotomy. Rib resection is associated with fewer postoperative lung adhesions to the thoracotomy site and may be preferred if multiple thoracotomies are anticipated.

Median Sternotomy

Median sternotomy is the only thoracic approach that provides access to the entire thoracic cavity and is therefore the approach of choice when exploratory surgery of the thorax is indicated. Structures in the dorsal thoracic cavity such as the great vessels and bronchial hilus are more difficult but not impossible to access in deep-chested dogs when using this approach. Median sternotomy may be combined with a ventral midline celiotomy or a ventral midline cervical incision if a combined approach to the abdomen or neck, respectively, is desired.

Trans-sternal Thoracotomy

The exposure provided by an intercostal thoracotomy may be dramatically increased by extending the thoracotomy through the sternum to connect it with an intercostal thoracotomy on the opposite side of the chest. A trans-sternal thoracotomy is indicated when extensive exposure of a specific region of the thorax is desirable.

SURGICAL CONDITIONS OF THE THORACIC WALL
(pp. 374–378)

Pectus Excavatum (p. 374)

Rib Deformities (p. 374)

Infections

Basic treatment principles of surgical drainage, débridement, and antibiotic therapy are applicable to infections of the thoracic wall. Pyothorax should be ruled out before commencing treatment.

Trauma

The resilient nature of the thoracic wall renders it resistant to injury by blunt trauma. For this reason, absence of injury to the thoracic wall does not rule out significant injuries to internal organs of the thorax and cranial abdomen after blunt trauma to the thorax. The primary concern in penetrating thoracic injuries is the status of internal structures.

Open wounds that are continuous with the pleural cavity are immediately sealed with a sterile petroleum-based ointment and gauze pack. Definitive management of open chest wounds should follow pleural evacuation and stabilization of the patient.

Rib fractures are usually associated with contusion of thoracic musculature and laceration of intercostal vessels. Laceration of an intercostal vessel usually produces an extrapleural hematoma or a hemothorax. Simple nondisplaced rib fractures can be managed conservatively with rest. Multiple unstable rib fractures usually require internal fixation.

Multiple rib fractures producing a free-floating segment of thoracic wall result in a *flail chest*. The paradoxical movement of the flail chest segment causes significant reductions in ventilation. Initial management of flail chest is directed at elimination of paradoxical ventilation and medical management of pulmonary contusion. An external splint eliminates paradoxical motion without restricting ventilation. The flail segment may be secured to an aluminum frame or polyvinyl splint using percutaneously placed circumcostal sutures and local anesthesia.

Neoplasia

Benign cutaneous neoplasms commonly arise from subcutaneous tissues and skin of the thorax. Benign neoplasms of the thorax are managed by local excision, ensuring that a sufficient margin of normal tissue is removed with the neoplasm to prevent recurrence.

Malignant neoplasms of the thoracic wall include chondrosarcoma, osteosarcoma, fibrosarcoma, mast cell sarcoma, and hemangiosarcoma. Thoracic radiographs usually provide strong evidence of primary bone sarcoma involving the ribs, with the most common findings being osteolysis, intrathoracic and extrathoracic soft-tissue masses, and mineralization. Malignant neoplasms of the thoracic wall are removed by *en bloc* resection of the involved thoracic wall.

THORACIC WALL RECONSTRUCTION (pp. 378–380)

A defect involving six ribs is generally considered the upper limit that can be adequately reconstructed. A thoracic wall reconstruction must be rigid to prevent paradoxical movement during respiration, as well as airtight to prevent pneumothorax. In resections involving the caudal thoracic wall, the diaphragm can be transposed cranial to the defect, reducing the requirement for a rigid and airtight reconstruction. The latissimus dorsi and external abdominal oblique muscles may be mobilized and sutured over the defect to seal the reconstruction. Defects in the skin and subcutaneous tissues that are too large to close by mobilizing local tissue may be closed by a thoracodorsal or deep circumflex iliac axial pattern flap.

POSTOPERATIVE MANAGEMENT (p. 380)

Hypoventilation, hypothermia, acid-base disorders, shock, and oliguria are among the problems that may arise after thoracic surgery. Ventilation may be depressed by anesthetic drugs, postoperative pneumothorax, or somatic pain arising from the thorax wall.

Hypothermic animals are slowly surface warmed with warm water bottles or circulating water blankets. Urine production is monitored to ensure adequate renal function. Hypothermia and hypotension perpetuate oliguria and are corrected early in the postoperative period.

Selective intercostal nerve blocks provide analgesia and avoid some of the undesirable side effects of high doses of narcotics, such as hypoventilation and bronchoconstriction. The accuracy of placement of the nerve block is enhanced by performing the block before closure of the thorax.

Chest bandages aid in sealing the thoracotomy incision and reduce the development of incisional emphysema. However, chest bandages should be placed loosely in thoracic surgery patients because they can restrict ventilation. Routine placement of a thoracostomy tube during thoracic surgery is strongly recommended because it allows a surgeon to closely monitor the pleural space for the presence of air or blood during the recovery period.

CHAPTER 32

Pleura and Pleural Space
(pages 381–399)

ANATOMY (p. 381)

The thoracic cavity is lined entirely by a serous membrane known as the *pleura.* The pleura is divided into the *visceral pleura,* which covers the lungs, and the *parietal pleura,* which covers the remaining thoracic cavity.

PHYSIOLOGY AND PATHOPHYSIOLOGY (pp. 381–382)

Under normal conditions, the pleural space is a potential cavity. The visceral and parietal pleurae are separated by a thin layer of pleural fluid. There is a net pressure of 9 cm H_2O encouraging fluid movement from the parietal pleura into the pleural space. The net pressure (10 cm H_2O) favors fluid absorption from the pleural space by the visceral pleura.

Pleural fluid and protein are also absorbed from the pleural space by parietal pleural lymphatics. Lymphatic drainage of the pleural space is particularly important when the protein content of the pleural fluid increases, because an increase in the colloid osmotic pressure of the pleural fluid reduces absorption by pulmonary capillaries.

The total gas pressure of atmospheric air within the pleural space is approximately 70 cm H_2O greater than the total gas pressure of venous blood, producing a constant gradient that removes gas from the pleural space. This gradient keeps the pleural space free of gas under physiological conditions and explains the spontaneous resolution of a closed pneumothorax.

Right-sided congestive heart failure increases parietal capillary hydrostatic pressure and pleural fluid formation, whereas left-sided congestive heart failure increases visceral capillary hydrostatic pressure and reduces pleural fluid absorption. Hypoproteinemia increases formation and decreases absorption of pleural fluid by reducing capillary colloid osmotic pressure. Lymphatic absorption of pleural fluid and protein is reduced by inflammatory thickening of the pleura, neoplastic obstructions of the thoracic duct or lymph nodes, or lymphatic hypertension associated with right-sided congestive heart failure.

DIAGNOSIS (pp. 382–384)

Physical Findings

Small quantities of noninflammatory effusion are difficult to detect clinically, whereas patients with moderate to large quantities of pleural fluid or air usually are in acute respiratory distress.

The presence of pleural fluid or air reduces functional reserve capacity (FRC). Patients may exhibit increased respiratory distress in lateral recumbency (orthopnea), preferring to remain in a sternal recumbent or sitting position. In severe cases, elbows are abducted and the head and neck are extended. Stress associated with handling may cause respiratory arrest as a result of limited respiratory reserve.

Auscultation of animals with pleural effusion usually reveals muffling of heart sounds. Percussion is an invaluable diagnostic tool for evaluation of the pleural space. Dull, flat, hyporesonant percussion suggests the presence of pleural fluid. Pleural air produces a characteristic hyper-resonant ping on percussion.

Radiographic Findings (pp. 383–384)

Clinical Pathological Findings

Once pleural effusion is demonstrated either clinically or radiographically, thoracentesis is indicated to remove fluid for diagnostic and therapeutic purposes. Diagnostic procedures performed on the pleural fluid include (1) preparation of direct smears for cytological examination, (2) submission of fluid for aerobic and anaerobic bacterial culture and sensitivity tests, (3) determination of physical and biochemical characteristics, and (4) determination of total cell counts and preparation of centrifuged cell concentrate smears.

MANAGEMENT (pp. 384–390)

Pleural Drainage

Needle thoracentesis carries an inherent risk of lung laceration that is minimized only by careful and proper technique. Advancement of the needle is stopped immediately on entering the pleural space. An extension tube placed between the syringe and needle allows the needle to be held steady while the syringe is manipulated. Substitution of a teat cannula for the hypodermic needle also greatly reduces the risk of lung laceration.

A thoracostomy tube (chest tube) is indicated if accumulation of pleural effusion is sufficient to warrant repeated pleural drainage, and it is often necessary to accomplish complete evacuation of the pleural space. Tubes for thoracostomy should be flexible but resistant to collapse. The size of a thoracostomy tube should approximate the diameter of a mainstem bronchus as estimated from a thoracic radiograph.

Intermittent pleural drainage is generally adequate when accumulation of a pleural effusion or air is not life threatening. Intermittent pleural drainage permits measurement of both fluid and air volumes and allows the thoracostomy tube to be incorporated entirely into a bandage, reducing the chance of removal by the patient.

Continuous closed suction is indicated when the accumulation rate of pleural effusions or air becomes life threatening. Continuous suction has the advantage of keeping pleural surfaces in contact, aiding in sealing pleuropulmonary fistulas or hemorrhage.

Pleurodesis

Pleurodesis is the obliteration of the pleural space by the induction of diffuse pleural adhesions. The traditional indication for this procedure has been chronic pleural effusions that are refractory to treatment. Pleurodesis has been reported in dogs for the management of refractory chylothorax, neoplastic effusion, and recurrent spontaneous pneumothorax. Pleurodesis may be induced by either *chemical* or *mechanical* methods.

Pleuroperitoneal Shunting

Pleuroperitoneal shunting can be used to manage refractory chylothorax, nonseptic inflammatory effusions, or persistent transudates but is contraindicated with septic effusions and less contraindicated with neoplastic effusions. The rationale behind pleuroperitoneal shunting is to transfer the effusion from the pleural space, where it causes respiratory distress, to the peritoneal cavity, where more surface area is available for resorption. Pleuroperitoneal shunting may be either *active* or *passive*.

HYDROTHORAX (p. 390)

Hypoproteinemia reduces capillary colloid osmotic pressure, causing fluid to remain in interstitial compartments including the pleural space. Hydrothorax due to hypoproteinemia is often accompanied by ascites and dependent edema. Right-sided, left-sided, or biventricular congestive heart failure may cause hydrothorax by disturbing pulmonary or systemic capillary hydrostatic pressures. Hydrothorax may result from obstruction of venous and lymphatic drainage such as occurs with lung lobe torsion or incarcerations of liver through a diaphragmatic herniation. These effusions result from transudation of fluid through the liver capsule. The treatment of hydrothorax consists of pleural drainage if respiratory distress is present and correction of its underlying cause.

PLEURITIS AND PYOTHORAX (pp. 390–391)

Pleuritis and pyothorax frequently have an insidious course, and presentation is often delayed. Moderate to severe respiratory distress is usually present. Patients show signs of systemic infection characterized by anorexia, weight loss, malaise, and fever. Physical and radiographic findings are those of pleural effusion. Diagnosis of pleuritis or pyothorax is suggested by the presence of an inflammatory exudate. *Inflammatory exudates* characteristically exhibit a total protein greater than 3 g/dl, a specific gravity greater than 1.018, and a total cell count greater than 3×10^9 cells per liter. Gram stains may give an early indication of the types of bacteria present. Fluids are cultured for aerobic and anaerobic bacteria.

Treatment of pyothorax must be prompt and aggressive. The prognosis is guarded but not hopeless. Dramatic results may be obtained with proper therapy. The initial goal of therapy is relief of respiratory embarrassment by thoracentesis. Supportive care with intravenous fluids is necessary to correct dehydration and acid-base and electrolyte imbalance. Systemic antibiotics are started once fluid is collected for aerobic and anaerobic bacterial culture. Pleural drainage and lavage by tube thoracostomy constitute the most appropriate initial therapy for pyothorax.

Lack of significant clinical improvement within 48 to 72 hours or radiographic demonstration of undrained encapsulated fluid is an indication to surgically explore the thoracic cavity. Exploratory thoracotomy should be by median sternotomy, which gives access to both hemithoraces.

CHYLOTHORAX (pp. 391–395)

Chylothorax develops when chyle from the cisterna chylothoracic duct system enters the pleural space. The etiology of chylothorax is poorly understood in dogs and cats.

Trauma is an often-cited cause of chylothorax in dogs and cats. Thoracic duct rupture might result from blunt or penetrating injuries. Rupture of the thoracic duct has been reported in conjunction with traumatic diaphragmatic herniation in cats. Experimental ligation of the cranial vena cava produces a lymphangiectasia-like condition of the thoracic duct and a high incidence (>50 per cent) of chylothorax in dogs and cats. It is speculated that lymphangiectasia allows extravasation of chyle through the lymphatic vessel wall. Malignancies that occlude the cranial vena cava might induce chylothorax by such a mechanism. Invasion and subsequent erosion of the thoracic duct by the malignancy might also be a cause.

Lymphangiectasia of the thoracic duct similar to that observed with cranial vena cava ligation has been demonstrated in dogs and cats with spontaneous idiopathic chylothorax. The underlying cause of lymphangiectasia in dogs and cats with idiopathic chylothorax is unclear.

Diagnosis of chylothorax is based on recognition of characteristic clinical and radiographic findings of pleural effusion, followed by demonstration of a chylous effusion on fluid analysis (pp. 393–394).

Treatment of chylothorax may be medical or surgical. Formation of a therapeutic plan for chylothorax is based on a consideration of its etiology, an evaluation of the nutritional status of the patient, and an understanding of the advantages and limitations of various treatments available. Because spontaneous closure of a thoracic duct fistula is possible, initial medical management of chylothorax is usually recommended. Medical management is directed at draining the pleural space and reducing the formation of chyle.

Surgical management of chylothorax involves transthoracic ligation of the caudal thoracic duct. The following indications for surgery are suggested: (1) failure to significantly diminish the flow of chyle after 14 days of medical management, (2) losses of chyle exceeding 20 ml/kg/day during a 5-day period, or (3) imminent protein-calorie malnutrition and hypoproteinemia.

Despite vigorous attempts at medical and surgical management, a significant number of patients with chylothorax fail to respond. Chemical pleurodesis has been successfully used to palliate refractory chylothorax in dogs.

HEMOTHORAX (pp. 395–396)

Pleural effusions often have a sanguineous component; however, the term *hemothorax* is usually reserved for effusions resulting from direct hemorrhage into the pleural space. The most common cause of hemothorax is trauma, particularly blunt thoracic trauma involving fractured ribs.

Hemorrhagic effusions within the pleural space generally do not clot because of mechanical defibrination and activation of fibrinolytic mechanisms. Hemorrhage associated with severe thoracic trauma occasionally clots within the pleural space as a result of release of tissue thromboplastin.

Treatment of hemothorax depends on the volume and flow of hemorrhage in the pleural space. Dogs are capable of complete resorption of 30 per cent of their blood volume from the pleural space within 90 hours. Because 70 to 100 per cent of the red blood cells are absorbed intact without hemolysis, hemothorax that does not induce significant respiratory distress is managed without pleural drainage. Pleural hemorrhage occasionally is sufficient to require pleural drainage for relief of respiratory embarrassment.

Surgical decortication may be required if a chronic hemothorax organizes to form a fibrous coat. Decortication is ideally performed within 5 weeks of the inciting injury before fibrous infiltration of the visceral pleura has occurred.

NEOPLASTIC EFFUSION (pp. 396–397)

Neoplastic effusions may have either an exudative or a transudative pattern and are identified by the presence of neoplastic cells on cytological examination. Differentiation of neoplastic cells from reactive mesothelial cells is often difficult even for experienced cytologists.

Cytological findings should be correlated with other findings on physical and radiographic examination.

PNEUMOTHORAX (pp. 397–398)

Pneumothorax results when atmospheric air gains access to the pleural space by a pleurocutaneous, pleuroesophageal, or pleuropulmonary leak.

Diagnosis of pneumothorax is based on characteristic physical and radiographic findings (see the sections on physical and radiographic findings) and on thoracentesis of air from the pleural space. Pneumothorax caused by traumatic rupture of a large airway is often associated with subcutaneous emphysema and pneumomediastinum. Pneumothorax resulting from esophageal perforation is likely to show a concurrent inflammatory pleural effusion. Open pneumothorax is readily recognized by the presence of a ''sucking'' thoracic wound.

Management of traumatic pneumothorax depends on the source, volume, and flow of air into the pleural space. Open thoracic wounds should be quickly sealed with an occlusive dressing, and the pleural space promptly evacuated of air. A closed pneumothorax that is not causing hypoventilation can often be managed conservatively, because pleural air is eventually absorbed.

Severe pneumothorax often resolves rapidly when managed by continuous suction. Failure to significantly reduce the flow of a pleuropulmonary fistula after 5 days of continuous suction is an indication for exploratory thoracotomy.

CHAPTER 33
Abdominal Wall (pages 399–406)

ANATOMY (pp. 399–400)

Median-Paramedian Area

The linea alba is evident in dogs as a trough between the slightly elevated, paired rectus abdominis muscles. The linea alba in dogs is rarely more than 2 or 3 mm wide; its widest part is found around the umbilicus. In cats, the linea alba may be as much as 4 mm wide and is seen as a definite flat, white band on the ventral midline.

An understanding of the arrangement of the aponeuroses of the abdominal muscles in conjunction with the rectus abdominis muscle and linea alba is fundamental to secure midline and paramedian closure.

Flank-Paracostal Area

On the lateral abdominal wall lie the fleshy elements of the oblique abdominal muscles. The fibers of the external abdominal oblique muscle originate from the 4th or 5th to the 12th rib and from the last rib and thoracolumbar fascia and extend in a caudoventral direction. The fibers of the internal abdominal oblique muscle arise from the thoracolumbar fascia caudal to the last rib and particularly from the tuber coxae. They extend cranioventrally, thus crossing the fibers of the external abdominal oblique muscle approximately at right angles. The transverse abdominal muscle fibers extend in a dorsoventral direction. The transverse fascia and peritoneum cover its inner surface.

CELIOTOMY (pp. 400–404)

Celiotomy is an incision into the abdominal cavity. *Laparotomy* strictly refers to flank incisions, although used similar to *celiotomy*.

General Surgical Principles

The surgical site should always be prepared so that extension of the incision is possible. After skin incision, excessive undermining of the subcutaneous tissues is avoided because the fascia of the linea alba receives some blood supply from overlying subcutaneous and adipose tissue.

Once the abdominal cavity has been entered, saline-moistened laparotomy sponges are placed around the edges of the wound to protect the soft tissues and exposed organs. Lavage is used to protect exposed viscera from desiccation.

Ventral Midline Approach

The ventral midline celiotomy is the standard access route for almost all the abdominal contents. In only a few cases it is not the superior technique. Midline cesarean section does not interfere with nursing of puppies.

Access

The aim is to incise precisely through the linea alba and avoid the rectus abdominis muscle on each side.

Closure

The midline incision is closed in three layers: rectus abdominis and its sheaths, subcutaneous tissue, and skin. Closure of peritoneum formerly was an integral part of celiotomy closure; this is now not the case. Serosal defects heal rapidly without formation of adhesions or evidence of cellular proliferation of the margins of the serosal wound. Leaving the peritoneum unsutured does not reduce the tensile strength or bursting strength of abdominal wounds in experimental animals.

Suture Materials and Patterns (see Chapters 16 and 19)
Paramedian Approach

Paramedian approaches have little to commend them in dogs and cats. One indication for a paramedian incision is unilateral cryptorchidectomy, in which a prepubic paramedian incision gives direct access to the abdominally located cryptorchid testis and obviates the need for reflection of the penis and prepuce. Bleeding from the incised rectus abdominis muscle is often observed. The internal leaf and rectus muscle and the external leaf of the rectus sheath generally require separate closure.

Flank Approach

Flank approaches to the abdominal cavity provide good access to dorsally located abdominal organs, including the adrenals, kidneys, and ovaries; however, access to both ovaries and the whole of the uterus is somewhat limited, and in recent years the flank approach to ovariohysterectomy has received less favor. Flank incisions are also used for placement of gastrostomy feeding tubes and for gastric decompression.

Each of the three muscles encountered—external abdominal oblique, internal abdominal oblique, and transverse abdominal—are separated in the direction of their fibers. The individual layers of the flank abdominal wall are closed separately with simple continuous sutures of synthetic absorbable suture.

Paracostal Approach

A paracostal approach provides access to the cranial and ventral part of the abdominal cavity, including organs such as the stomach, spleen, and cecum.

Combined Midline Paracostal Approach

Increased access to the cranial abdomen can be obtained by adding a paracostal incision to an already completed ventral midline incision.

Combined Paralumbar Paracostal Approach

This approach can be combined with a transdiaphragmatic incision to give access to both thoracic and abdominal cavities.

The incision commences in the flank and is carried cranial to the last rib in a ''lazy S'' pattern or ventrally to the xiphoid if necessary.

POSTOPERATIVE EFFECTS AND PAIN CONTROL
(pp. 404–406) (See Chapter 22)

CHAPTER 34
Peritoneum and Peritoneal Cavity (pages 407–430)

ANATOMY (pp. 407–410)

Gross Anatomy

Caudally, the abdominal cavity is continuous with the pelvic cavity; the division between them is a transverse plane through the pelvic inlet. Cranially, the abdominal cavity is limited by the diaphragm. The lateral and ventral walls are formed by the abdominal muscles and the 8th through the 13th ribs. It is lined internally by the *transverse fascia*, which is covered by the parietal peritoneum.

A more practical division separates the abdomen into four quadrants by one transverse and one sagittal line through the umbilicus, thus creating the cranial right, cranial left, caudal right, and caudal left quadrants. The terms *right* and *left paravertebral gutters* are used to designate the troughlike regions in the dorsal abdominal cavity to the right and left of the vertebral column.

Natural Openings

In cats and dogs, there are three unpaired openings leading into the abdominal cavity through the diaphragm: the *esophageal hiatus*, the *vena caval hiatus*, and the *aortic hiatus*. Paired slitlike openings, dorsal to the diaphragm, are formed ventrally by the dorsal edge of the diaphragm and dorsally by the psoas muscles. At these sites, the pleura and peritoneum are separated only by a thin layer of fused endothoracic and transverse fascia. The proximity of the pleura to the peritoneum has clinical importance in the understanding of how certain disease processes in the thoracic cavity can lead to similar entities within the abdominal cavity by direct extension.

Umbilicus

After the umbilical cord is disrupted at birth, the umbilical aperture rapidly closes, forming a faint *umbilical scar* on the ventral midline. In an undetermined percentage of dogs and cats, the umbilical scar remains incomplete with a small aperture (at maximum only 1 to 3 mm in diameter).

Inguinal and Pelvic Canals

The fissures between abdominal muscles and their aponeuroses on each side of the caudal ventral abdominal wall are called the *inguinal canals*. These contain the vaginal processes and associated intraperitoneal structures. Another pair of abdominal openings in the caudal part of the abdominal wall are the right and left *vascular lacunae*. The femoral artery and vein, lymphatics, and saphenous nerve surrounded by a short projection of transverse fascia pass through each lacuna.

Transverse Fascia

The abdominal and pelvic cavities are lined by a fascia throughout. The fascia can be named according to the region or parts covered. The term *transverse fascia* is used to include all of these fascial divisions.

Retroperitoneum

Retroperitoneal organs lie against the walls of the abdominal or pelvic cavities and are covered on only one surface by parietal peritoneum. In dogs and cats, these structures include the kidneys, ureters, aorta, adrenal glands, lumbar (para-aortic) lymph nodes, vena cava, and diaphragm.

Greater and Lesser Sacs

The peritoneal cavity is divided into the general peritoneal cavity, or greater sac, and the lesser sac, which has the epiploic foramen as its only natural opening. The lesser sac, also known as the *omental bursa* or *lesser peritoneal cavity*, is completely collapsed *in vivo*.

PHYSIOLOGY (pp. 410–412)

The surface area of the peritoneum is roughly one to one and one-half times that of the skin. Most of this membrane behaves as a passive semipermeable lining for the *diffusion* of water and low-molecular-weight solutes.

Contraction of the diaphragm empties the lymphatic fluid containing the erythrocytes and other materials into efferent ducts. A simultaneous reduction in intrathoracic pressure during inhalation assists in the process of ''pulling'' lymphatic fluid from the peritoneal cavity.

Increased capillary permeability, increased capillary pressure, decreased plasma osmotic pressure, and blockage of the peritoneal lymphatics can lead to accumulation of fluid within the peritoneal cavity (ascites).

Lymphatic Drainage

Sternal lymph nodes receive about four-fifths of the total lymphatic effluent arising from the peritoneal cavity. The lymphatic vessels extend cranially through the ventral portion of the diaphragm to lymph nodes in the region of the second rib. Mediastinal lymph nodes receive lymphatic vessels from the cranial part of the peritoneal cavity, especially the peritoneal surface of the diaphragm. Dorsal abdominal lymphatic vessels empty into the cisterna chyli and thoracic duct. The mesenteric lymphatics primarily drain the intestine and not the peritoneal cavity.

Intraperitoneal Circulation

Regardless of the site of injection, a common tendency is movement of fluid along the ventral abdominal wall in a cranial direction toward the diaphragm and dorsally along the diaphragmatic surface of the liver.

Capillary-Peritoneal Pressure

The peritoneal cavity is more susceptible to accumulation of excessive quantities of fluids than most of the other body cavities, because the pressure in the capillaries of the visceral peritoneum is higher than elsewhere owing to resistance to portal blood flow through the liver. When the portal system is blocked or even partially occluded, the return of blood from the intestines, stomach, pancreas, and spleen to the systemic circulation is impeded.

Innervation of the Peritoneum

Although the visceral peritoneum has little sensory innervation, the afferent fibers may detect stimuli that are strong or prolonged, particularly in the presence of inflammation. *The root of the mesentery is quite sensitive to traction.*

HEALING OF PERITONEAL INJURY AND DEFECTS
(pp. 412–413)

The mesothelium of the peritoneal cavity is so easily damaged that it sloughs even after exposure to air or saline. Regeneration is rapid, and the healing of denuded or débrided peritoneum is usually complete within 5 to 7 days regardless of the defect's size.

Healing of débrided parietal peritoneum without adhesion formation occurs by (1) mesothelial cell deposition onto the denuded surface or (2) proliferation of mesothelial cells from the *depths* of the wound. Because peritoneal healing occurs with equal speed regardless of the size of the original defect, healing by epithelial cell migration from the edges of the defect alone, like that of full-thickness skin defects, does not occur.

With diseases or injury involving large defects in the deep abdominal fascia and parietal peritoneum, omental covering speeds reperitonealization and prevents adherence of other intra-abdominal visceral structures. The omentum also produces significant vascular ingrowth and assists in treatment of ischemic tissues.

ADHESIONS (pp. 413–415)

Adhesions are fibrinous or fibrous bands that form abnormal unions between two or more surfaces that are normally covered with serosa and are not "attached" to each other. After peritoneal injury, fibrinous adhesions can be observed within 24 to 48 hours during the inflammatory stage of healing. The attachment may break down in 48 to 72 hours as the inflammatory phase dissipates.

Clinically, only restrictive adhesions are important, because they are generally those prone to cause visceral strangulation or obstruction. Nonrestrictive adhesions involve more compliant connections between structures.

Postoperatively, adhesions may result from excessive drying of serosal surfaces, infection, traumatic handling of serosal tissues, and contamination with foreign materials such as gauze lint, glove powder, talc (magnesium silicate) crystals, and antibiotic powders. Excessive use of electrocautery and suture materials or the use of reactive or contaminated suture materials may also cause adhesions.

In untreated peritonitis, adhesion formation may be lifesaving by sealing a perforated viscus or by isolating bacteria from the abdominal lymphatics, where they would be absorbed and cause bacteremia. Individuals that are hypoproteinemic and hypofibrinogenemic may have difficulty in generating enough fibrin to seal accidental or surgical wounds within the abdominal cavity.

Adhesion Prevention

There is no reliable way to prevent adhesions; consistent efforts to prevent foreign bodies from entering the peritoneal cavity decrease the incidence of adhesions. Gloving powder and lint from surgical drapes are commonly implicated as foreign bodies responsible for adhesion formation. Unretrieved threads from cotton gauze pads are important sources of irritation and may also increase adhesion formation. Suture materials are about equal in their capacity to induce adhesions.

In areas in which adhesions are inevitable or highly probable (such as intestinal anastomosis), it is advisable to cover the suture line with omentum, creating less rigid, unrestricting omental adhesions. With adhesions unrelated to surgery, formation is most effectively controlled by reducing peritoneal inflammation.

PERITONITIS (pp. 415–425)

Inflammation of the peritoneum may be classified by its extent, nature, source, and causative agents. Because of widespread peritoneal involvement and the absorption of endogenous or exogenous toxic products into the circulation, diffuse peritonitis often leads to serious systemic illness and is usually fatal without aggressive treatment.

Primary Peritonitis

Most cases are caused by a microorganism, either a specific virus or bacterium that gains access to the peritoneum by the hematogenous route. Examples include feline infectious peritonitis (FIP) and occasional bacterial peritonitis associated with a "distant" infection elsewhere. Bacteria may also gain entrance into the peritoneal cavity via the ovarian bursa from retrograde (ascending) contamination from an infected uterus. A third source is infection of the pleural cavity that spreads to the peritoneal cavity via the space at the lumbocostal arch.

A fourth possible route of infection in primary peritonitis is transmural migration of endogenous intestinal bacteria. Because this route of bacterial peritonitis is often associated with a pathological process within the peritoneal cavity, this form takes on characteristics of a secondary peritonitis and may more appropriately be considered a *secondary peritonitis.*

Secondary Peritonitis

Secondary peritonitis, which is much more common than primary peritonitis, is defined as peritoneal inflammation secondary to disruption of the abdominal cavity or a hollow viscus. It may be associated with a surgical procedure or occur after trauma or disease.

Mechanical and Foreign Body Peritonitis. Peritoneal foreign bodies may have several consequences: (1) If small enough (0.5 to 15 μm diameter), they are removed by peritoneal circulation and lymphatic absorption; or (2) phagocytosis physiologically removes the foreign material; or (3) if phagocytosis cannot remove it, an attempt to wall it off may occur, leading to a granulomatous peritonitis or localized granuloma formation; or (4) a draining fistula to the outside of the body may form to expel the material.

Clinical manifestations of an intraperitoneal foreign body vary, depending on the type and location of the foreign body and whether bacteria are present. Foreign bodies of nonreactive materials with smooth surfaces may remain undetected for years.

Granulomatous Peritonitis. Talcum powder, commonly used as a sizing agent in the process of glove manufacture, was associated with granulomatous peritonitis. Cornstarch, rice starch, and calcium carbonate powder are now used on surgical gloves, and the reaction is much less severe. Surgical gloves should always be washed and wiped before entering the peritoneal cavity.

Chemical Peritonitis. *Bile* reaches the peritoneal cavity as a result of disruption of the biliary tract or proximal small intestine. The bile salts in sterile bile are mildly irritating, and bile unassociated with cholehepatic disease is usually sterile. Death due to biliary peritonitis requires bacteria. Bacteria associated with naturally occurring bile peritonitis invade the peritoneal cavity as a result of permeability changes of the intestinal wall due to the action of bile on the intestine's serosal surface.

Gastric and pancreatic secretions are irritating and produce more intense chemical peritonitis than bile. Contact with these chemical irritants produces immediate cellular damage similar to a chemical burn.

Approximately 3 hours after the onset, intestinal bacteria and accumulated bacterial toxins cross damaged intestinal barriers and enter the peritoneal cavity. Chemical peritonitis is thus converted into both chemical and bacterial peritonitis.

Septic Peritonitis (pp. 417–425)

Ischemic intestine, either as a result of strangulation or secondary to mechanical obstruction and distension, is an important source of pathogenic bacteria commonly associated with septic peritonitis. The intestine may still be grossly intact, but enteric bacteria enter the peritoneal cavity because of altered intestinal permeability.

Septic peritonitis after an operation is usually bacterial and commonly results from breakdown of a suture line in a hollow viscus or from visceral ischemia. Bacteria may also enter through an abdominal wound or peritoneal drain.

Pathophysiology of Generalized Septic Peritonitis. Consequences of diffuse peritonitis are similar to a severe thermal burn. Significant quantities of fluid, electrolytes, and plasma proteins along with erythrocytes can be lost into the peritoneal cavity because of peritoneal vascular dilation and increased capillary permeability.

Clinical Signs. Unless an owner reports recent trauma or abdominal surgery, the history may only indicate general depression, inappetence, vomiting, or other nonspecific signs of illness. Animals may simply appear tucked up and show abdominal tenderness during palpation. Abdominal pain is not a consistent finding, however.

Physical findings suggestive of peritonitis include wounds or bruises in the caudal thorax or abdomen, abdominal discomfort or intra-abdominal mass detected by palpation, an unusual posture, vomiting during palpation, injected mucous membrane (indicative of hemoconcentration and sepsis), and slow capillary refill time.

Diagnosis. Plain radiographs may reveal free gas or fluid in the abdomen. Air is normally introduced into the peritoneal cavity during surgery and can be radiographically detectable for at least 1 week after surgery. Fluid in the abdomen is seen as a lack of normal detail or gives a ground glass appearance. Generalized intestinal ileus and intraluminal accumulation of gas are frequent radiographic observations.

Diagnostic Abdominal Paracentesis and Lavage. Most cases of septic peritonitis can be accurately diagnosed by cytological examination of fluid obtained by paracentesis or lavage. An increase in neutrophil numbers (cells $\leq 10,000/mm^3$) commonly occurs in the *lavage fluid* of animals that have had recent abdominal surgery without peritonitis as a complication. However, the abdominal leukocytes in these animals should not be degenerate or contain bacteria. Lavage fluid leukocyte counts in normal animals before surgery are usually less than $1,000/mm^3$.

Treatment. Repeated and systematic clinical examination yields the greatest amount of information and is the most important monitoring tool available. Laboratory determinations such as urine specific gravity, hematocrit, total protein, peripheral leukocyte count and differential, serum electrolytes levels, serum creatinine levels, blood glucose levels, and arterial blood gases may help in making appropriate decisions about supportive therapy.

Fluid and Electrolyte Replenishment. Diffuse peritonitis causes a rapid change in the fluid-electrolyte balance, and correction of functional hypovolemia and changes in electrolyte balance are considered first. The use of whole blood or plasma may be required for patients that are anemic or that develop a hematocrit less than 20 per cent or total plasma protein less than 3.5 g/100 ml during treatment.

Antibiotics. Antibiotics are given intravenously in high doses as soon as the diagnosis of bacterial peritonitis is made or suspected, based on knowledge of the organisms commonly involved or Gram stain results and microscopic examination of peritoneal fluid. Aerobic and anaerobic bacterial cultures of the peritoneal fluid and antibiotic sensitivity testing are recommended at the time of paracentesis, diagnostic lavage, or surgery.

Whether antibiotics should be included in peritoneal irrigating fluid has been vigorously debated. The inclusion of water-soluble antibiotics in irrigation fluids initially increases intra-abdominal levels of antibiotics; however, concomitant intravenous administration is usually necessary to maintain therapeutic levels in the serum and peritoneal fluid after surgery.

Corticosteroids. Intravenous corticosteroids in antishock doses are advocated preoperatively for their positive inotropic effect on the heart. Caution is advised in using more than one or two antishock doses, which might negatively affect an animal's immune function and gastrointestinal mucosal integrity.

Nutritional and Transfusion Support. Metabolism may increase twofold in animals with septic peritonitis. This hypermetabolic condition is generally accompanied by anorexia. Persistent hypoglycemia in dogs with experimentally induced peritonitis is an accurate predictor of mortality.

Nutritional support is critical to survival of animals. Hyperalimentation can be performed by intravenous administration of nutrients or the use of a feeding tube (nasogastric, pharyngostomy, gastrostomy, jejunostomy) (see Chapter 5).

Miscellaneous Supportive Measures (p. 422)

Surgery. After appropriate supportive measures have been instituted and a patient is hemodynamically improved, surgery is recommended to treat the inciting condition and peritonitis. The goals are to halt ongoing contamination, remove foreign and purulent material, provide drainage of peritoneal exudate, and provide a route for enteral nutritional support through a feeding tube.

Drainage. Establishing effective "global" peritoneal cavity drainage is important for successful treatment of generalized peritonitis. Local drainage is important for localized peritonitis when an accumulation of exudate occurs. Within 6 hours of placement, drains are sealed from the general peritoneal cavity by fibrin and adhesions. Adequate drainage of the peritoneal cavity can be achieved by (1) placement of multiple drains and continuous or intermittent *lavage* of the peritoneal cavity and (2) maintaining an open peritoneal cavity and using the animal's posture and movement to allow dependent drainage into sterile absorbent pads that are changed frequently.

Prognosis. The outcome of diffuse secondary peritonitis is determined by (1) the underlying cause and animal's previous health, (2) timing of the operation, (3) adequacy of repair and débridement, (4) drainage effectiveness, (5) choice and administration of antibiotics, and (6) nutritional and hemodynamic support.

The initial prognosis for patients with diffuse secondary peritonitis is guarded. Vital signs are the most reliable prognostic indicator.

OTHER PERITONEAL DISORDERS (pp. 425–429)

Urine Peritonitis

The escape of sterile urine in small amounts into the peritoneal cavity is of little consequence. Prolonged leakage causes abdominal distension and peritonitis. If a urinary tract infection is present, septic peritonitis may develop; if the urine is sterile, aseptic peritonitis occurs.

Appropriate treatment consists of surgical exploration and correction of urine leakage. A sterile multiholed catheter introduced using local anesthesia allows temporary drainage; a urethral catheter should also be passed. Most animals respond dramatically to 24 hours of fluid support and urine drainage and are better surgical and anesthetic candidates.

Chylous "Peritonitis"

Chylous peritonitis is an inflammatory process caused by chyle from (1) rupture or chylous discharge from a lymphatic-chylous mesenteric cyst, (2) intestinal obstruction with distension of lacteals, (3) injury of the cisterna chyli or major mesenteric lymphatic vessels, or (4) blockage of chyle flow with exudation through dilated lymph vessels.

We believe chylous abdominal effusion must be accompanied by other disorders for peritonitis to exist.

Treatment varies with the cause. Chyle is removed initially by centesis to alleviate dyspnea. Total parenteral nutrition is recommended.

Intra-Abdominal Abscesses (pp. 426–427)

Hemoperitoneum (p. 428)

PRIMARY NEOPLASMS (p. 429)

Primary mesotheliomas of the peritoneum are rare. They cause ascites, weight loss, and palpable abdominal masses. Abdominal mesotheliomas can also spread to the pleural cavity by direct extension through the diaphragm or by hematogenous or lymphatic routes. Pleural effusion is common.

CHAPTER 35

Hernias (pages 431–433)

DEFINITION (p. 431)

A hernia is defined as the protrusion of an organ or part through a defect in the wall of the anatomical cavity in which it lies.

CLASSIFICATION (p. 431)

Anatomical Site

The anatomical site of herniation is used for classification, such as abdominal, diaphragmatic, or perineal.

Congenital Versus Acquired Hernias

A congenital hernia is due to a defect already present at birth, although the herniation may not develop until later. The defect in an acquired hernia occurs after birth.

Reducible, Incarcerated, and Strangulated Hernias

When the protruding hernial contents are freely movable and can be readily manipulated back into the cavity, the hernia is classified as reducible. If adhesions form and the contents are fixed in the abnormal location, the hernia is classified as incarcerated (or irreducible).

Type of Herniated Tissue

Hernias may also be classified according to their contents, such as intestine or omentum.

PARTS OF A HERNIA (p. 431)

The three parts of a hernia are the ring, the sac, and the contents. The ring is the actual defect in the limiting wall.

The hernial sac consists of the tissues that cover the herniated contents. In congenital hernias, the sac includes a mesothelial covering. In the initial stages of traumatic hernias, the sac has no peritoneal lining, although peritonealization may occur later. The contents of a hernia are the organs or tissues that have moved to the pathological location.

EPIDEMIOLOGY (pp. 431–432)

PATHOPHYSIOLOGY (p. 432)

Alteration in the function of body cavities and of hernial contents may be important in herniation. These changes in function vary in severity from insignificant to lethal and can be due to a space-occupying effect, obstruction of a hollow viscus, or strangulation of hernial contents leading to tissue death.

SIGNS OF HERNIATION (p. 432)

Swelling is the classical sign of herniation. In uncomplicated hernias, no pain is elicited on palpation and the consistency of the swelling depends on the contents. Additional signs depend mainly on the nature and state of the contents of the hernia (e.g., reducible hernias compared with strangulated intestinal hernias).

PRINCIPLES OF HERNIORRHAPHY (pp. 432–433)

The four main aims of hernia repair are as follows:

1. Return of viable contents to their normal location.
2. Secure closure of the neck of the hernia, preventing recurrence.
3. Obliteration of redundant tissue in the sac.
4. Use of the patient's own tissues whenever possible.

CHAPTER 36

Abdominal Hernias (pages 433–454)

An abdominal hernia is defined as any defect in the *external* wall of the abdomen that may allow protrusion of abdominal contents.

True hernias are abdominal wall defects that have anatomically defined hernial rings and have a complete sac of peritoneum surrounding the hernial contents. "False" hernias allow protrusion of organs *outside* of a normal opening in the abdomen and usually do not contain a complete peritoneal sac.

VENTRAL ABDOMINAL HERNIAS (pp. 433–443)

Umbilical and Ventral Midline Hernias

Anatomy, Etiology, and Pathogenesis

Congenital umbilical hernias result from failure or delayed fusion of the lateral folds (principally the rectus abdominis muscle and fascia). Most umbilical hernias are inherited and are probably the result of a polygenic threshold character. Until more is learned about the inheritance and expression, affected dogs or cats should not be bred.

Cryptorchidism frequently coexists in dogs with umbilical hernias, as well as other congenital defects. Cranioventral abdominal hernias, incomplete caudal sternal fusion, and umbilical defects with concomitant diaphragmatic hernias of various types occur in dogs. Congenital heart defects and portosystemic shunts may be associated with supraumbilical defects.

Omphaloceles are large midline umbilical and skin defects that permit abdominal organs to protrude from the body. Herniated contents are initially covered by a transparent membrane (amniotic tissue) attached to the edges of the umbilical defect until minor trauma ruptures the membrane, exposing the prolapsed contents to contamination. Gastroschisis grossly appears like an omphalocele, but the defect is paramedian.

Acquired causes of umbilical hernia are uncommon. Umbilical hernias may form from excessive traction on the umbilical cord at parturition, severance, or ligation of the umbilical cord too close to the abdominal wall.

Umbilical hernias are the most common abdominal hernias in small animals. Airedale terriers, Basenjis, Pekingeses, pointers, and Weimaraners are most at risk. There is no sex predilection for umbilical hernia in the general population.

Clinical Signs

Umbilical hernias appear as soft, round masses located at the umbilical scar. The swelling may feel firm if fat becomes entrapped and irreducible. Examination of the animal in dorsal recumbency facilitates reduction of the hernia contents and hernia ring palpation.

Treatment

Most small, reducible umbilical hernias in dogs and cats contain only falciform fat and are of little clinical significance. Initially it is wise to treat puppies with small hernias conservatively, as spontaneous closure has been reported as late as 6 months of age. Affected animals are neutered because of the genetic predisposition for this disease.

Hernias approximating the size of intestine with large hernial sacs in mature animals are at greater risk for strangulation. I recommend surgical correction in this instance. Smaller defects are dealt with during other elective surgical procedures or treated conservatively and observed carefully.

Umbilical hernias containing abdominal organs may require more extensive surgery. The skin incision is made around the base of the hernia. In incarcerated hernias, the hernial sac is dissected free and the hernia ring is enlarged along the linea alba to release the contents into the abdomen. Released contents are inspected for viability. The sac is excised, and the hernial ring is débrided before the linea alba is closed. In rare situations, absence of a portion of the abdominal wall accompanies large umbilical hernias. Releasing incisions can be made to reduce tension on the primary suture line provided the rectus muscles and underlying fascia have adequate strength. Prosthetic materials may be used to span larger defects.

Animals with supraumbilical hernias and diaphragmatic defects require the diaphragmatic hernia to be repaired first so that normal pulmonary function is resumed.

Aftercare and Prognosis

Minimal postoperative care is required after uncomplicated umbilical hernia repair, and patients have an excellent prognosis. Complicated hernias have a guarded to poor prognosis depending on the patient's status before surgery, the nature of the herniated contents, and the extent of the defect.

Inguinal Hernias

Inguinal hernias result from a defect in the inguinal ring through which abdominal contents protrude. If abdominal viscera enter the cavity of the vaginal process, an *indirect* hernia exists. *Direct* hernias are less common and occur when organs pass through the inguinal rings adjacent to the normal evagination of the vaginal process. *Inguinal hernia* generally denotes direct and indirect hernias in females and direct hernias in males. Indirect hernias in males are considered separately as *scrotal hernias.* Congenital inguinal hernias in dogs and cats are rare. Acquired inguinal hernias are common and most often involve middle-aged intact bitches.

Anatomy and Pathogenesis

The vaginal process, containing the spermatic cord in males or the round ligament in females, passes through an opening in the caudoventral abdominal wall termed the *inguinal canal.* The inguinal canal is an approximately sagittal slit between the abdominal muscles connected by the external and internal inguinal rings. The close superimposition of the external and internal inguinal rings in small animals does not form a "canal," as its name implies, but a potential gap where hernial disruption may occur.

A significant heritable influence may exist in golden retrievers, cocker spaniels, and dachshunds. Affected small animals should be neutered. Enlargement of the entrance to the vaginal process, which remains open, is the most important cause of inguinal hernias in domestic animals. Bitches may be predisposed because the inguinal canal is both shorter and of larger diameter than in males. Congenital inguinal hernias may disappear spontaneously at 12 weeks of age owing to a decrease in the relative size of the inguinal rings. Traumatic inguinal hernias in dogs may be due to a pre-existing anatomical weakness in the area.

Sex hormones may have a role in the etiology of inguinal hernias, since the majority of inguinal hernias appear in estral or pregnant bitches and acquired inguinal hernias have not been reported in neutered females.

Obesity increases intra-abdominal pressure, which may force abdominal fat through the inguinal canals. Accumulation of fat around the round ligament may dilate the vaginal process and inguinal canal, allowing herniation.

Clinical Signs

Affected animals are most commonly presented with a painless, unilateral or bilateral mass with a soft, doughy consistency. In dogs, unilateral inguinal hernias occur more often on the left. Inguinal hernias may be undetectably small or very large, containing, for example, a gravid uterus (hysterocele), bladder, or jejunum. Direct inguinal hernias in male dogs may resemble scrotal hernias because of swelling and edema of the testicle and spermatic cord due to venous or lymphatic obstruction at the inguinal ring.

Diagnosis

Careful history taking and palpation are helpful for diagnosis.
Diagnosis is confirmed by reduction of the hernia and palpation of

the inguinal canal. Reduction is facilitated by elevating the hindquarters to reduce caudal intra-abdominal pressure while the animal is in dorsal recumbency. Careful palpation of *both* inguinal canals is recommended, because early inguinal hernias may be small and remain undetected.

Palpation of incarcerated hernias may not yield a definitive diagnosis. Plain and contrast radiographs can be used to confirm the nature of the hernial contents. Particular attention is paid to the caudal abdominal strip and the fascial detail of the flank musculature. A herniated gravid uterus is easily detected on plain radiograph. Pneumocystography may be used to detect bladder involvement.

Surgical Repair

Inguinal hernias are best repaired at the time of diagnosis. Uncomplicated unilateral inguinal hernias are approached over the inguinal rings. In more complicated hernias, the approach is first through the ventral midline for exploration, with hernia repair subsequently performed extra-abdominally.

For complicated inguinal hernias, an incision is made over the lateral aspect of the swelling, parallel to the flank fold. The hernial sac is exposed and the contents are reduced gently through the canal. If the hernia is not reducible, the canal is enlarged by incising through the inguinal ring in a craniomedial direction. The neck of the hernial sac is ligated and the sac is amputated. Incisions in the abdominal wall and enlarged external inguinal ring are closed with a synthetic monofilament absorbable or nonabsorbable material.

The midline approach avoids incising through mammary tissue and allows exploration of both inguinal rings. Mammary tissue is dissected directly off the external rectus fascia until the inguinal regions are exposed.

The simplest option for treating a herniated gravid uterus in a domestic pet is ovariohysterectomy. If a valuable litter is expected in a breeding bitch, successful primary repair of the hernia and replacement of the incarcerated uterus can be attempted.

In most cases, inguinal hernias can be repaired primarily. Large defects due to trauma or recurrent inguinal hernias may require reinforcement of the primary hernia repair using an onlay polyethylene mesh technique. Use of a cranial sartorius muscle flap is an alternative technique when primary repair is not possible.

Complications, Aftercare, and Prognosis

The most common complication is hematoma formation. Patients frequently are reluctant to walk for several days after surgery. Prophylactic antibiotics or bandages are generally not used. Exercise is limited until suture removal. Prognosis for uncomplicated inguinal hernia repair is good.

Scrotal Hernia

Anatomy and Pathogenesis

Scrotal hernias are indirect hernias that result from a defect in the vaginal ring, allowing abdominal contents to protrude into the vaginal process beside the contents of the spermatic cord. These hernias are rare.

Clinical Signs

The presenting signs of scrotal herniation result from the protrusion of abdominal contents through the vaginal process, causing pain, swelling, and frequently organ dysfunction. This hernia is predominantly unilateral; however, careful inspection of the contralateral inguinal ring is warranted.

Swelling is generally cordlike, extending from the inguinal ring to the caudal aspect of the scrotum.

Diagnosis

The diagnosis of a scrotal hernia can be confirmed by reducing the contents of the hernia and palpating the hernial ring; however, scrotal hernias frequently cannot be reduced. Ultrasonography may be helpful in obtaining a definitive diagnosis.

Surgical Repair

Repair of scrotal hernias is required as soon as a definitive diagnosis has been made, because strangulation is frequently present. Bilateral castration is currently recommended with scrotal hernia to reduce recurrence. In addition, an increased incidence of testicular tumors in dogs has been associated with scrotal hernias, and scrotal hernias may be inherited.

Complications, Aftercare, and Prognosis

Scrotal dermatitis and scrotal hematomas are the most common local complications after repair. In most instances, no antibiotics or bandages are used. Suture removal and exercise restrictions are similar to those after inguinal herniorrhaphy. Freely reducible hernias generally have a good to excellent prognosis. Patients with strangulated hernias have a guarded to poor prognosis but may undergo successful repair with correct treatment.

Femoral Hernias (pp. 441–443)

TRAUMATIC AND INCISIONAL HERNIAS (pp. 443–453)

GENERAL COMPLICATIONS (p. 453)

Most complications stem from technical error. Late complications are usually related to wound infection or hernia recurrence (Table 36–1).

TABLE 36–1. SUMMARY OF COMPLICATIONS ASSOCIATED WITH ABDOMINAL HERNIORRHAPHY

Operative Complications	Early Postoperative Complications
Anesthetic complications	Seroma
Hemorrhage	Hematoma
Visceral injury	Dermatitis
Strangulated hernia	Infection
Gross contamination at the operative site	Wound dehiscence and evisceration
Inability to close the abdominal wall without tension	Pain
''Loss of domain''	*Late Postoperative Complications*
Poor tissue strength at hernia margins	Skin sinus
	Hernia recurrence

CHAPTER 37

Diaphragmatic, Pericardial, and Hiatal Hernias (pages 455–470)

TYPES AND CAUSES OF HERNIAS (pp. 457–458)

Diaphragmatic hernias are generally categorized by etiology because, except for hiatus hernia, true diaphragmatic hernias are rare. Herniated viscera in false diaphragmatic hernia are not contained within a sac but lie free within the pleural cavity or pericardial sac.

Congenital Pleuroperitoneal Hernia

These defects do not involve the pericardial sac. Incomplete development or failure of fusion of the pleuroperitoneal membrane across the pleuroperitoneal canal during diaphragmatic development may be the cause of congenital pleuroperitoneal hernia.

Congenital Peritoneopericardial Hernia (pp. 457–458)

Traumatic Diaphragmatic Hernia

Trauma is the most common cause of diaphragmatic hernia in dogs and cats. Automobiles are the chief source of trauma, with kicks, falls, and fights being implicated less frequently.

Injury to the diaphragm can be either direct or indirect in origin. Direct injuries from thoracoabdominal stab and gunshot wounds are rarely encountered in animals.

The mechanism for indirect injury to the diaphragm is suspected to be a sudden increase in intra-abdominal pressure with the glottis open. Normally, during quiet inspiration, the pleuroperitoneal pressure gradient varies from 7 to 20 cm H_2O, but it rises beyond 100 cm H_2O on maximal inspiration. Application of force to the abdominal cavity with the glottis open further increases this gradient, and herniation of viscera is usually immediate after the diaphragm ruptures. Because of the nature of automobile trauma, multisystem injury and shock are potential complications in traumatic diaphragmatic hernia.

Hiatal Hernia

Hiatal hernia is defined as protrusion of abdominal contents through the esophageal hiatus of the diaphragm into the thorax.

Diaphragmatic Eventration

Although not a hernia, diaphragmatic eventration is unilateral bulging of the diaphragm into the thorax. It needs to be distinguished from diaphragmatic hernia.

PATHOPHYSIOLOGY (pp. 458–460)

Traumatic Diaphragmatic Hernia

The diaphragmatic costal muscles are more often ruptured than the central tendon, whereas the stronger crural muscles are seldom ruptured. Overall, left-to-right distribution is probably uniform in dogs and cats, with about 15 per cent being bilateral or multiple. Orientation of tears in the costal muscle at surgery in dogs was circumferential (40 per cent), radial (40 per cent), or a combination (20 per cent), whereas cats had a preponderance of circumferential tears (59 per cent) and fewer radial tears (18 per cent).

Pathophysiological events result from effects on the herniated abdominal viscera and the effects of herniated viscera on cardiorespiratory dynamics. Incarceration, obstruction, and strangulation are the chief effects on abdominal viscera. These detrimental effects on abdominal organs are often due to pressure applied by the edge of the diaphragmatic tear as the organs pass over it or result from the formation of fibrous adhesions and strictures.

Incarceration of the stomach and intestine in a diaphragmatic hernia can cause partial or complete obstruction to flow of ingesta. Gastric tympany may follow stomach herniation. Unrelieved interference with cardiorespiratory function by compression of the caudal vena cava and lungs is rapidly fatal. Severely compromised blood supply can also induce ischemic necrosis, intestinal perforation, and abscessation.

Major effects of liver herniation are hepatic venous stasis, hepatic necrosis, bilary tract obstruction, and jaundice. Normally, a gradation of pressure throughout the hepatic venous system exists. Depending on the location of the lobe, rapid accumulation of hydrothorax, pericardial fluid, ascites, or a combination occurs. Diaphragmatic rupture with concomitant biliary tract injury, bile peritonitis, and bile pleuritis has been reported.

Bacterial proliferation in devitalized traumatized liver or herniated liver with vascular obstruction, followed by systemic release of toxins after repositioning of liver lobes, may be a concern.

Dyspnea is the most common clinical sign in diaphragmatic hernia. In addition to lack of a functioning diaphragm, respiratory insufficiency can result from shock and dysfunction of the chest wall, pleural space, lungs, airway, and cardiovascular system. Compression and atelectasis of lung lobes by herniated organs, fluid, or air in the pleural cavity cause hypoventilation, ventilation/perfusion mismatch, and hypoxia. Pulmonary function deteriorates further in shock after an increase in pulmonary vasculature permeability, pulmonary edema, and hypoventilation causing further ventilation/perfusion mismatching.

DIAGNOSIS (pp. 460–464)

Congenital Peritoneopericardial Hernia (p. 460)

Traumatic Diaphragmatic Hernia

Patients with a diaphragmatic hernia due to trauma usually have a history of trauma, but failure to radiograph the thorax often results in delayed diagnosis. The interval between trauma and diagnosis has ranged between hours and 6 years, with a mean of several weeks. Acute trauma patients may have severe injuries other than the hernia and generally have signs of hypovolemic shock. A high index of suspicion needs to be maintained in trauma patients so that diaphragmatic hernia is not overlooked. Although no pathognomonic signs of diaphragmatic hernia have been identified, respiratory signs predominate, and 38 per cent of victims have dyspnea and exercise intolerance. Some animals adopt a sitting or standing position, with elbows abducted and head extended. Gastroenteric signs include vomiting, dysphagia, diarrhea, and constipation. Other signs include depression, weight loss, and difficulty in lying down.

Findings on physical examination are normal in some animals. On auscultation, heart sounds are muffled, abnormally positioned, or more intense on the side contralateral to the hernia. Pleural effusion causes a hyporesonance of the chest wall on percussion, whereas gastric tympany causes hyper-resonance. Borborygmi due to viscera in the thorax is an infrequent and unreliable finding. With experience, thoracic palpation for localization of the cardiac apex beat is 80 per cent accurate in determining the side of the hernia. A tucked-up or empty appearance of the abdomen is a rare finding.

Thoracic radiographs should be taken of all patients presented with serious trauma, especially those with any evidence of dyspnea or fractures. Radiography is the most useful test for diagnosis of diaphragmatic hernia. Undue restraint and struggling are avoided, because animals with diaphragmatic hernia may already have severe respiratory and cardiovascular dysfunction.

The finding of viscera in the thorax is diagnostic.

Thoracentesis may be performed for fluid analysis, to alleviate hypoventilation, and to improve radiographic quality.

Ultrasonography is particularly useful in animals with pleural effusion because fluid is an excellent ultrasound-transmitting medium. Using ultrasonography, viscera can be differentiated from pleural fluid.

Contrast radiography is indicated only when plain radiographs are nondiagnostic and ultrasonography is unavailable. A disadvantage is delayed transit of barium down the small intestine due to partial gastrointestinal obstruction caused by the hernia.

Hiatal Hernia (pp. 462–464)

TREATMENT (pp. 464–468)

Timing of Surgery

Surgical correction of traumatic diaphragmatic hernia is performed at the earliest opportunity in a stable patient, taking into account other injuries. Herniorrhaphy performed within 24 hours of injury has the highest mortality rate, 33 per cent, owing to shock and multiorgan failure compounded by the stress of anesthesia and surgery. Acutely injured animals are treated for shock, allowed to rest quietly, and given supplemental oxygen. Surgery is only performed on an emergency basis in the presence of life-threatening hypoventilation due to compression of the lungs by abdominal viscera. This situation can develop rapidly with herniation of the stomach in left-sided diaphragmatic rupture. Acute gastric gaseous distension effectively produces a tension pneumothorax. Emergency decompression of the stomach with a hypodermic needle inserted through the left chest wall into the stomach is performed, followed by surgery. Diaphragmatic hernia has a higher priority than definitive fracture repair. Repair of damaged abdominal organs and correction of obstruction, incarceration, and strangulation of abdominal viscera are performed in conjunction with herniorrhaphy through a laparotomy. Continuous monitoring of animals with diaphragmatic hernia in the interval between diagnosis and surgery is mandatory because of the risk of sudden respiratory decompensation.

Midline Laparotomy. This is the preferred approach for most traumatic diaphragmatic hernias and all congenital peritoneopericardial hernias. It is simple, allows inspection of all the abdominal viscera, can be extended to a sternotomy for thoracic exposure, causes less postoperative pain than a thoracotomy, and provides access to all of the diaphragm. Using this approach, it is not necessary to know the position of the diaphragmatic tear before surgery.

Median Sternotomy. A sternotomy of the caudal two to three sternebrae is rarely performed alone.

Lateral Thoracotomy. A ninth intercostal approach is simple, provides adequate exposure of herniated viscera and the tear in the diaphragm, and allows inspection of the convex pleural surface. Adhesions can be easily seen and transected, although significant adhesion formation in chronic diaphragmatic hernia is rarely a complication.

Congenital Peritoneopericardial Hernia (p. 465)

Traumatic Diaphragmatic Hernia (pp. 465–467)

After anesthetic induction, an endotracheal tube is inserted to allow control of ventilation and to maintain gaseous anesthesia. Even if the lungs are compressed by viscera or fluid, controlled ventilation usually allows adequate pulmonary expansion and oxygenation. Preparation of the thoracic wall should also extend laterally should a thoracostomy tube be needed.

An incision is initially made from the xiphoid to beyond the umbilicus. A generous incision facilitates exposure of the diaphragm and abdominal viscera. Finochietto or Balfour self-retaining retractors are inserted to provide better exposure of the cranial abdominal cavity. Traumatic hernia may be multiple, so a thorough examination of the whole diaphragm should be made. The hernia can usually be easily reduced by gentle traction. Incarcerated liver and spleen are often congested and friable and need careful handling to avoid rupture. For irreducible hernia due to relative undersize of the hernia ring, the hole in the diaphragm is enlarged with a ventrally directed radial incision, avoiding major phrenic vessels, phrenic nerves, and the vena cava. Intrathoracic adhesions are divided under direct observation. Adhesions to the caudal lung lobes may be seen through the hernia. In some cases, it is better to extend the laparotomy into a median sternotomy.

Mobile abdominal viscera are displaced to the caudal abdomen or wrapped in saline-moistened laparotomy sponges and exteriorized. The liver is held back with broad, malleable ribbon retractors. In a chronic hernia, muscle around the edges may be rolled over, atrophied, and contracted by scar tissue. Incision of fibrous tissue permits diaphragmatic musculature to be returned to its normal position. The need for freshening, resection, or débridement of the edges of chronic hernias is not essential. Resection of the edges is disadvantageous because it increases the size of the defect. Correct orientation of tissues is essential. Diaphragmatic tears that have a complex shape are approximated temporarily with a series of stay sutures inserted in the corners of each component.

Atrophy and fibrotic contraction of the torn diaphragm may produce a defect that cannot be closed with sutures. These can be patched with omentum, muscle, liver, fascia, polypropylene mesh, or silicon rubber sheeting. Double layers of omentum, supported by a scaffold of sutures, healed diaphragmatic defects with fibrovascular scar tissue. A disadvantage of omentum is that it is too weak to provide adequate support alone. However, omental pedicle grafts are used effectively to buttress sutured herniorrhaphies, particularly those involving any of the hiatuses, and promote an early fibrin seal and healing. A caudally directed rectangular flap of peritoneum and transverse abdominal muscle, with its base on the 13th rib, can be used. The flap, about 10 per cent larger than the defect, is reflected forward so that the peritoneum becomes the parietal pleura of the repaired diaphragmatic defect. Autologous fascia closure of defects results in a tough tendinous repair.

Before the final one or two sutures in the diaphragm are tightened and tied, pneumothorax is eliminated by inflation and expansion of the lungs to re-establish negative intrathoracic pressure.

All abdominal organs are carefully inspected for viability. Herniated liver is usually congested and swollen. Despite the discolored appearance of these lobes, they usually remain viable on re-establishment of normal hepatic circulation, and lobectomy is rarely necessary. In repositioning swollen, deformed, cirrhotic, or malpositioned lobes, kinking or occlusion of the caudal vena cava is avoided. Proliferation of clostridial organisms in incarcerated liver lobes and release of toxins into the circulation after repositioning displaced lobes is of concern. On this basis, for liver incarceration and biliary tract injury, prophylactic antibiotics are given before and for 2 to 3 days after surgery.

Closure of sternotomy and laparotomy incisions is routine (see Chapters 31 and 33). Before final closure of the linea alba, residual air is expelled from the peritoneal cavity by gentle pressure on each side of the abdomen to help re-establish a pleuroperitoneal pressure gradient. Closure of the laparotomy after repair of a large, chronic hernia may produce large increases in intraperitoneal pressure and impede venous return, in which case careful monitoring of cardiovascular dynamics and intravenous fluid volume loading are indicated. Although not routine, a thoracic radiograph is taken before recovery from anesthesia if there is concern about persisting pneumothorax, pleural effusion, collapsed lung lobes, or the position of the thoracostomy tube.

Hiatal Hernia (pp. 467–468)

POSTOPERATIVE CARE AND COMPLICATIONS (p. 468)

Close postoperative observation and monitoring of vital signs, mucous membrane color, respiratory pattern, and capillary refill time are essential. Pain can be severe after an intercostal or sternotomy exposure. Thoracic wall pain causes significant hypoventilation and is relieved by intercostal nerve blocks with bupivacaine, narcotic analgesics, or preferably a combination. Morphine commencing at a dose of 0.2 mg/kg IV is followed by further incremental doses of 0.1 mg/kg until pain is alleviated.

PROGNOSIS (pp. 468–469)

Congenital Peritoneopericardial Hernia (p. 468)

Traumatic Diaphragmatic Hernia

The prognosis for animals that sustain a traumatic diaphragmatic hernia is guarded. The overall survival rate for animals diagnosed as having diaphragmatic hernia is 52 to 88 per cent. Several studies have indicated that approximately 15 per cent of animals die before presentation for anesthesia and surgical correction.

Induction of anesthesia is a critical phase of anesthesia, and any undue delay in intubation and controlling ventilation can cause death. Postoperative complications that result in death fall into two groups. In the first 24 hours after surgery, death can be caused by hemothorax, pneumothorax, pulmonary edema, shock, pleural effusion, and cardiac dysrhythmias. Deaths occurring later after surgery are due to rupture, obstruction or strangulation of the gastrointestinal tract, or diseases unrelated to hernia.

Hiatal Hernia (p. 469)

Perineal Hernia (pages 471–482)

Perineal hernia results from failure of the pelvic diaphragm to support the rectal wall, which stretches and deviates. Pelvic and occasionally abdominal contents may protrude between the pelvic diaphragm and the rectum. A subcutaneous swelling occurs ventrolateral to the anus, and, in bilateral cases, caudal projection of the anus is also seen.

SURGICAL ANATOMY (p. 471)

The perineum is the part of the body wall that covers the pelvic outlet and surrounds the anal and urogenital canals. Its skeletal boundaries are the first caudal vertebra dorsally and the right and left ischial tuberosities and ischial arch ventrally. The lateral borders are formed by the sacrotuberous ligament, which extends from the lateral angle of the ischial tuberosity to the transverse process of the first caudal vertebra and the caudal end of the sacrum. The principal structure of the perineum is the pelvic diaphragm. It consists of the coccygeal and levator ani muscles, together with their external and internal coverings. These muscles are anchored to the pelvis and caudal vertebrae.

STRUCTURES OF SURGICAL IMPORTANCE FOR HERNIORRHAPHY (pp. 471–473)

ETIOLOGY (pp. 473–475)

Predisposition

The following data and discussion are confined to dogs unless otherwise specified.

Signalment

Perineal hernia has been documented in humans and dogs and rarely in cats, cows, and ewes. It is most common in dogs from 7 to 9 years of age, with few cases in those less than 5 years old. Perineal hernia occurs commonly in males and rarely in females. Reports on perineal hernia cases taken from veterinary hospital records have shown an over-representation of certain breeds, including the Boston terrier, boxer, collie, corgi, kelpie and kelpie crosses, purebred and crossbred dachshund, Old English sheepdog, and Pekingese. Both sexes of Pekingese are also predisposed to herniation at other sites.

Right Versus Left Side

Of 453 cases reported by 10 researchers, 270 (60 per cent) were unilateral and 183 (40 per cent) were bilateral. Of the unilateral cases, 183 (68 per cent) were on the right and 87 (32 per cent) on the left.

Although herniation occurs unilaterally, the contralateral side is frequently weak. The side on which herniation occurs may be related to the rate and extent of tissue deterioration on that side of the pelvic diaphragm rather than to causes affecting one side or the other preferentially.

Pathogenesis

Perineal herniation commonly occurs between the external anal sphincter and the levator ani muscle and occasionally between the levator ani and coccygeal muscles. Herniation develops after deterioration of the supporting function of the pelvic diaphragm.

CLINICAL SIGNS (pp. 475–476)

The majority of animals present with a reducible perineal swelling and one or more of the following signs: constipation (difficult defecation or defecation at prolonged intervals), obstipation (intractable constipation), tenesmus (straining to defecate or urinate without evacuation of feces or urine), and dyschezia (painful defecation). The swelling is usually ventrolateral to the anus, although in some bilateral cases ventral swelling with caudal projection of the anus becomes evident. Stranguria (painful urination, with urine being voided drop by drop) may occur in association with prostatic disease or retroflexion of the bladder and prostate.

The contents of the hernia most commonly include rectal sacculation or flexure, prostate gland, fluid, connective tissue, and retroperitoneal fat. The last two of these may resemble omentum and may contain small, firm nodules and areas of necrosis. Some investigators have used the terms *rectal sacculation, dilation, flexure, deviation*, and *diverticulation* synonymously. *Rectal sacculation* occurs when unilateral loss of support for the rectal wall enables it to expand to one side; *dilation* of the rectal lumen results from a bilateral loss of wall support; and rectal *flexure* or *deviation* occurs when the rectum herniates, resulting in a bend in the course of the rectum.

CONSERVATIVE THERAPY (p. 476)

Medical and Dietary Treatment

Medical and dietary treatment are adjuncts to surgical procedures. They may be alternatives to surgery when straining to defecate is infrequent. This form of treatment without surgical intervention was unsuccessful in permanently controlling clinical signs associated with herniation.

SURGICAL THERAPY (pp. 476–480)

Preoperative Procedures

Catheterization. Up to 20 per cent of patients with perineal hernia present with retroflexion of the bladder and partial or total urethral obstruction.

Radiographs. Radiographs that delineate anatomical structures present at the hernial site provide information that enables a surgeon to anticipate possible problems and determine the best surgical procedure for repair of the defect.

Enema. Warm water enemas to which stool softener may be added should be given to all constipated animals approximately 12 to 18 hours before surgery. This interval is required to allow total evacuation of fluid from the large intestine and avoid surgical site contamination.

Restrictions. Food is withheld 24 hours before surgery. Intravenous fluid therapy may be required during this period if the animal is dehydrated or uremic.

Surgical Procedures

The surgical area, including the scrotal and prescrotal regions, is clipped. A rectal examination allows assessment of the laxity in rectal wall support and prostate size. Feces, if present, are removed, and a purse-string suture is placed around the anus after inserting a plastic syringe case or a plug of absorbent cotton. The skin is scrubbed with povidone-iodine scrub solution.

Standard Herniorrhaphy (p. 477)

Elevation of the Internal Obturator Muscle (pp. 477–478)

Incorporation of the Sacrotuberous Ligament in Sutures Dorsolateral to the External Anal Sphincter (pp. 478–479)

Transposition of the Superficial Gluteal Muscle (p. 479)

Subcutaneous Perineal Fascia Reconstruction (p. 479)

Placement of Prosthetic Implants. Implants have been placed in position by both perineal and abdominal approaches. Critical assessments of the long-term effectiveness of any of the techniques used have been limited.

Cystopexy and Colopexy. These procedures, together with partial closure of the defect in the caudal pelvic wall, were used in the treatment of a perineal hernia involving retroflexion of the bladder.

Anal Splitting. Results have not been entirely satisfactory.

Postoperative Management

Contamination of the healing wound must be avoided. Antibiotics are not used unless there is evidence of infection. An Elizabethan collar prevents a patient from irritating the wound or removing the sutures. Conditions leading to abdominal straining are avoided. Diet regulation and medication, as discussed previously, assist in achieving this aim. Skin sutures may be removed 10 to 14 days after surgery.

Surgical Complications

Wound Infection. The incidence of infection or wound breakdown following standard herniorrhaphy has been recorded as 6, 13, 20, and 26 per cent. After superficial gluteal muscle transposition, 58 per cent experienced wound breakdown, which was primarily superficial. Routine use of antibiotics has little effect on the postoperative development of infection.

Fecal Incontinence. Damage to the pudendal or caudal rectal nerves may result in decrease or loss of external anal sphincter function. Permanent fecal incontinence generally results from bilateral nerve damage.

Tenesmus. Signs frequently resolve with time. If this problem is due to sutures inadvertently placed through the rectal wall, they are removed.

Rectal Prolapse. This may be a transient problem, responsive to temporary placement of a purse-string suture. Recurrent prolapse may necessitate resection or colopexy.

Urinary Tract Malfunction. Neurological injury may result in anuria or urinary incontinence. Signs are generally transient.

Sciatic Nerve Paralysis. Damage to the sciatic nerve may occur if sutures that are placed craniolaterally around the sacrotuberous ligament penetrate or entrap it. Temporary or permanent lameness may result. Marked pain and non-weightbearing lameness are the main clinical signs.

Positional sciatic neuropraxia may result from positioning the patient in a rectal stand with the legs tied firmly forward. Knuckling occurs, but there is no sciatic pain.

RECURRENCE OF HERNIATION AFTER SURGICAL REPAIR (pp. 480–481)

Follow-up Time. The overall recurrence rate, in surveys involving detailed postoperative follow-up investigations, ranges between 31 and

45 per cent. The recurrence, when the follow-up time was greater than 1 year, may be associated with continued deterioration of perineal tissue rather than technical factors.

Effect of Castration. Analysis of pooled data from four publications indicated that castration reduced the recurrence of herniation subsequent to perineal herniorrhaphy from 43 per cent to 23 per cent.

Gastrointestinal System
(pages 483–691)

CHAPTER 39

Functional Anatomy of the Digestive System (pages 483–502)

THE ORAL CAVITY (pp. 483–485)

Lips and Cheeks

The lips of cats and dogs have few functions. They are lean, relatively immobile, and long, with an extensive rima oris between them.

They consist mostly of flimsy strands that are difficult to see and distinguish. They all are innervated by the facial nerve. Sensory innervation is by branches of the trigeminal nerve. Blood vessels include branches of the facial and infraorbital arteries.

Tongue

Because a carnivore's tongue participates in a number of vital functions such as lapping, sucking, and swallowing, only slight dysfunction can be tolerated. There are three pairs of extrinsic muscles. All the muscles receive motor innervation from the hypoglossal nerve. The lingual nerve is the principal sensory nerve to the tongue.

The tongue is highly vascular, with about 30,000 arteriovenous anastomoses beneath the dorsal side. The large lingual arteries are sinuous to allow excursions of the mobile tongue.

Teeth

The permanent dentition of a dog is $2(I3/3\text{-}C1/1\text{-}P4/4\text{-}M2/3) = 42$, and that of a cat is $2(I3/3\text{-}C1/1\text{-}P3/2\text{-}M1/1) = 30$. The fewer cheek teeth of cats reflect their more carnivorous nature, with sectorial teeth predominating.

Hard Palate

The palate develops by the inward growth of two horizontal ledges, the palatine processes, which ultimately meet and fuse in the midline with the downwardly growing nasal septum. Abnormal growth of one or more of these processes may result in uni- or bilateral cleft palate.

THE PHARYNX (pp. 485–486)

There is a basic flaw in the design of the respiratory system of air-breathing animals—the airway arises from the ventral surface of the digestive tube, where it is in constant danger of being flooded or choked by ingesta. Dysfunction may result in such serious consequences as inability to swallow or bronchial aspiration.

Soft Palate

The soft palate stretches like a canopy across the front of the pharynx, dividing it into oral and nasal parts. Its free, curved caudal edge is formed by the right and left palatopharyngeal arches. The epiglottis usually projects through the ostium to rest on the dorsal surface of the palate, but the epiglottis may frequently be found beneath the soft palate.

Tonsils

Dogs and cats possess palatine tonsils on the lateral walls of the oropharynx (the fauces), pharyngeal tonsils on the roof of the nasopharynx, tonsils of the soft palate on its ventral surface, and occasionally paraepiglottic tonsils, but no lingual or tubal tonsils.

SALIVARY GLANDS (pp. 486–487)

Parotid Gland

The V-shaped parotid gland fits snugly behind the jaw and temporomandibular joint and beneath the conchal part of the ear. Several important structures pass deep to it (superficial temporal artery and vein, external carotid and maxillary arteries, facial nerve), and a few pass over or through it.

Mandibular Gland

It shares a common connective tissue capsule with part of the sublingual gland and is a readily palpable landmark behind the angle of the jaw. The mandibular duct emerges from the deep surface of the gland and it opens on a small papilla, the sublingual caruncle, at the foot of the frenulum of the tongue.

Sublingual Gland

The sublingual gland is smaller and pinker than the mandibular; it is clinically important because salivary mucoceles may result from leakage of saliva from a defect in its major duct.

Zygomatic Gland

The zygomatic gland is an enlarged member of the dorsal buccal gland series. It is well developed in carnivores but is relatively inaccessible, concealed deep to the rostral end of the zygomatic arch ventral to the periorbita.

ESOPHAGUS (pp. 487–489)

Capacity

A carnivore's esophagus is narrowest near its origin, near its termination, and by the thoracic inlet; an inflated esophagus also reveals a fourth constriction over the base of the heart (where it passes between the azygos vein on the right and the aorta on the left). Movement of the esophagus is most restricted at these four sites. In the caudal part of the neck, the esophagus separates from the longus colli muscle and rests on the left of the trachea; in the caudal thorax, the surrounding structures are soft and yielding, giving the esophagus maximum freedom.

The thyroid arteries and esophageal branches of the carotids supply much of the cervical esophagus, and the bronchoesophageal artery supplies most of the thoracic part. Esophageal branches straight off the aorta usually supply the terminal segment in conjunction with the esophageal branch of the left gastric.

Veins leaving the cervical esophagus drain into the external jugular veins, and those from the thoracic esophagus drain mostly into the azygos vein. Portocaval anastomoses exist at the gastroesophageal junction.

STOMACH (pp. 489–492)

Capacity

The stomach is highly distensible. The empty organ is palpably inaccessible beneath the ribs, but the laden stomach bulges beyond the costal arch, pushing and crowding the intestines behind it. A greatly distended stomach of an adult dog can extend caudal to the umbilicus.

Regions

The *fundus* of the stomach is that part dorsal to the cardiac ostium, and the cranial surface of the fundus pushes against the upper left half of the diaphragm. The *body* of the stomach is pushed against the left lobes of the liver and makes up the middle third of the organ. The *pyloric part* is found ventrally and mostly on the right and surrounds a funnel-shaped pyloric antrum, which opens into a narrower pyloric canal that ends at the pyloric ostium, the orifice into the duodenum.

Vessels and Nerves (pp. 491–492)

INTESTINES (pp. 492–494)

A carnivore's intestine is about five times the length of the trunk. The small intestine is about four times the length of the large and measures between 1 and 1.5 m in cats and between 2 and 5 m in dogs.

Knowledge of the position of the initial and terminal segments of the gut (descending duodenum and descending colon) greatly facilitates exploration of the abdomen. The descending duodenum is on the right and the descending colon is on the left. During a laparotomy, one can grasp the descending colon or descending duodenum and draw the whole intestinal mass to one side or the other, exposing the abdominal roof on the left or right.

RECTUM AND ANUS (pp. 494–496)

The rectum is the part of the large intestine within the pelvis. Its origin is often marked by a slight constriction where the circular muscle is thicker and resembles a sphincter. It reaches as far as the third coccygeal vertebra, where it is continuous with the anal canal, a short tube that typically opens beneath the fourth coccygeal vertebra. The terminal part of a dog's rectum is sometimes slightly dilated to form a rectal ampulla, which is absent in cats. Most of the rectum is within the peritoneal cavity, although a short segment some 2 cm long continues retroperitoneally before it joins the anal canal. The line of peritoneal reflection is located beneath the second coccygeal vertebra in dogs and a little farther back in cats; it slopes forward so that much of the ventral surface of the rectum lies retroperitoneally.

The anal sacs (strictly the paranal sinuses) are paired globular invaginations of the inner cutaneous zone. The anal sacs are located ventrolateral to the anus (at 4 and 8 o'clock); they are typically 8 to 10 mm in diameter and partly collapsed and are sandwiched between the pale internal and the redder external anal sphincters.

The muscle tunics of the rectum are continuous with those of the anal canal. An inner circular layer becomes slightly thickened terminally to form the internal anal sphincter. The anus is surrounded by another smooth-muscle slip, the anal part of the retractor penis muscle.

The external anal sphincter is composed of striated muscle and is much larger and thicker than the other components. The cranial division is itself partly subdivided into superficial and deep parts that overlie the anal sacs.

Innervation

The rectum is innervated by autonomic nerves from the pelvic plexus.

The anus is innervated by the pudendal nerve. Its caudal rectal branch (mainly from S2 and S3)[69] provides motor fibers to the external anal sphincter, and its perineal branch is sensory to the area.

THE LIVER AND BILIARY SYSTEM (pp. 496–498)

The vulnerable liver is housed beneath the ribs, resting on a cushion of falciform fat and molded to the soft dome of the diaphragm. It is fissured to allow it to adapt to the changing form of the diaphragm or the arching of the back and to allow the lobes to slide over one another like a stack of saucers.

The seven major lobes or processes are as follows: right and left lobes, each subdivided into lateral and medial parts; the quadrate lobe between them; and the caudate and papillary processes of the caudate lobe.

Biliary Tree

Intralobular ducts form within the liver parenchyma from bile canaliculi. These become the tributaries of the lobar ducts, which on emergence from the liver surface are called *hepatic ducts*. Once the hepatic ducts receive the cystic duct from the gallbladder, the single vessel is known as the (common) bile duct (ductus choledochus), and in dogs it runs a fairly straight course for some 5 cm within the lesser omentum from the porta to the duodenum.

The gallbladder is a flattened piriform sac lodged between the quadrate and the right medial lobes of the liver.

Blood Vessels

The hepatic arteries (vasa privata) may be regarded as the liver's principal maintenance vessels, supplying about 20 per cent of the blood and about 50 per cent of its oxygen needs. The portal vessels (vasa publica) supply the remaining 80 per cent of blood.

Portosystemic Communications (pp. 497–498)

Only during fetal life is it proper for the portal and systemic venous systems to be in free communication with each other except at the capillary level. A persistent ductus venosus, one of the more common portal anomalies in dogs, allows portal blood to bypass the liver sinusoids. Four other congenital portal anomalies have been reported. Two of them involve an anastomosis between the portal and azygos veins (the original venous pathway of the embryo), another between the portal and caval veins directly, and the fourth between the portal vein and a number of smaller mesenteric, splenic, or renal veins.

Acquired portocaval communications develop as a result of portal hypertension and occur in sites other than those of the congenital anomalies.

Hepatic veins are found exclusively within the substance of the liver, where the stiff parenchyma guarantees they remain patent. They open by many orifices directly into the vena cava as it courses through the dorsal border of the liver.

THE PANCREAS (pp. 498–499)

Ducts

The exocrine portion of the pancreas is a compound tubuloacinar gland whose ducts are totally concealed within the substance of the organ. Large interlobular ducts extend longitudinally in the middle of the gland and terminate in the duodenum without ever becoming visible.

Vessels

The celiac artery supplies most of the gland, with the cranial mesenteric artery supplying only the caudal part of the right limb. Two of the three branches of the celiac artery contribute radicles to the pancreas: Branches of the splenic artery enter the end of the left limb, and branches from a distal segment of the hepatic (gastroduodenal) artery supply the body of the pancreas.

CHAPTER 40
Physiology of the Digestive System (pages 502–510)

SECRETION OF SALIVA (p. 502)

Saliva has several important functions, including lubricating food for swallowing and dissolving food so it can react with taste chemoreceptors. Saliva contains a number of bactericidal agents that help prevent oral infections. Saliva evaporates from the mouth and pharynx during panting and is important in the control of body temperature.

SWALLOWING AND ESOPHAGEAL MOTILITY (p. 502)

Swallowing is initiated when a bolus of food is pushed backward by the tongue toward the pharynx. This action initiates a reflex by stimulating afferent impulses, which pass along cranial nerves V, IX, and X to the swallowing center, located in the reticular formation of the medulla and pons. Efferent impulses pass from the swallowing center along cranial nerves IX and X to stimulate and coordinate activities of structures involved in swallowing. As the bolus of food moves toward the pharynx, the soft palate is elevated to cover the posterior nares. The larynx closes by apposition of the arytenoid cartilages and vocal cords, and the epiglottic cartilage covers the entrance into the glottis. Contractions of the pharyngeal muscles propel the food toward the esophageal opening. The cricoesophageal sphincter relaxes, and the food passes into the esophagus. Primary esophageal contractions occur as continuations of the pharyngeal contractions and propel food toward the stomach. As the bolus of food approaches the stomach, the lower esophageal sphincter and the cardiac region of the stomach relax to allow food to pass into the stomach. If food lodges somewhere along the esophagus, secondary esophageal contractions are initiated at that point to propel the food distally.

GASTRIC FUNCTION (p. 502)

The stomach holds food after a meal and regulates its delivery into the small intestine to maximize the efficiency of digestion and absorption. While food is in the stomach, it is mixed with gastric secretions and physically broken down into small particles by contractions of the stomach wall.

VOMITING (pp. 503–504)

Vomiting is forceful expulsion of gastrointestinal contents through the mouth. It is a reflex act integrated in the medulla oblongata. Afferent impulses that stimulate vomiting arise from many areas, and many are transmitted to the vomiting center by sensory fibers in the vagus or sympathetic nerves. Efferent impulses from the vomiting center stimulate a coordinated sequence of events, including closure of the glottis, elevation of the larynx, and contraction of the thoracic wall to increase intrathoracic pressure. Impulses to the abdomen cause relaxation of the stomach and esophagus and then a sharp contraction of the abdominal muscles to expel the gastric contents.

PHYSIOLOGY OF THE SMALL INTESTINE (pp. 504–506)

When food enters the duodenum, it is mixed with secretions from the pancreas, liver, and intestinal mucosa. These secretions contain enzymes and compounds, such as bile salts and colipase, that are essential for digestion and absorption.

The digestive enzymes hydrolyze dietary components to small molecules that can be readily absorbed. Salivary, gastric, and pancreatic enzymes act within the gastrointestinal lumen. Enzymes bound to the brush border membranes of the intestinal mucosal cells act when substrates come into close association with the membranes.

Water and Electrolyte Absorption and Secretion

About 2.7 L of water enters the small intestine of a 20-kg dog each day from ingested fluids and gastrointestinal secretions. More than 85 per cent of this is absorbed by the small intestine, about 300 ml is absorbed in the colon, and less than 40 ml is passed in the feces.

Motility

Peristaltic and segmental contractions mix the ingesta and propel it along the intestine. Peristaltic contractions consist of circular contraction of the intestinal wall progressing along the intestine. As the contraction progresses, the segment in front of the contraction relaxes to accommodate the ingesta being pushed along. Peristaltic contractions usually occur over a few centimeters of the intestine, but they may occasionally traverse its entire length. The vast majority of peristaltic contractions progress distally, but reverse peristalsis occasionally occurs. Peristaltic contractions propel ingesta along the intestine and spread it out over the mucosa.

PHYSIOLOGY OF THE LARGE INTESTINE (pp. 506–507)

The large intestine receives material from the ileum, dehydrates it, and then stores it before it is eliminated. Absorption of water from the fecal material occurs in the proximal colon and cecum, and the dried material is stored in the distal segment of the colon.

LIVER FUNCTION (pp. 507–509)

The main functions of the liver are to metabolize endogenous and foreign compounds, to secrete bile, and to store blood and some nutrients.

Metabolic Functions of the Liver

The liver metabolizes nutrients, endogenous compounds, and many foreign compounds. A host of hormones and drugs are metabolized by enzyme systems located in the endoplasmic reticulum and cytosol of the hepatocytes.

Metabolism of bilirubin by the liver is of considerable clinical interest not only because unconjugated bilirubin is toxic but because the measurement of bilirubin and its metabolites in body fluids is used in the diagnosis of some liver diseases.

Secretion of Bile

Bile is formed by secretion of fluid from the hepatocytes and the cells lining the bile ductules. Bile salts such as cholic acid and chenodeoxycholic acid are synthesized in the liver from cholesterol and then conjugated to taurine and glycine before being secreted. The volume and the electrolyte composition of bile are modified by secretion of fluid from the epithelial cells of the bile ductules.

Functions of the Gallbladder

The gallbladder stores bile between meals, and it concentrates organic compounds in bile by absorbing water and electrolytes. The major stimulus to gallbladder contraction is the gastrointestinal hormone cholecystokinin, which is released from the wall of the small intestine when ingesta enters the duodenum.

Enterohepatic Circulation

Bile salts are transported to the intestine, actively reabsorbed in the ileum, and pass in the portal blood to the liver, where they are resecreted into bile. The amount lost is replaced by synthesis of new bile salts by the liver, so that the bile salt pool remains constant.

PANCREATIC EXOCRINE FUNCTION (p. 509)

Pancreatic juice is secreted into the duodenum by the exocrine portion of the pancreas. It contains several important digestive enzymes or their precursors, including trypsinogen, chymotrypsinogen, procarboxypeptidase, prophospholipase A, proelastase, lipase, amylase, cholesterol hydrase, and nucleases. Pancreatic secretion is stimulated by the vagus nerves and the gastrointestinal hormones cholecystokinin and secretin.

CHAPTER 41

Oral Cavity (pages 510–530)

Tongue, Lips, Cheeks, Pharynx, and Salivary Glands (pages 510–520)

Healing of incisions in the oral mucosa (lining of the tongue, lips, and gingiva) is more rapid than in skin: Phagocytic activity is greater, occurs earlier, and is mostly due to monocytes rather than polymorphonuclear leukocytes; epithelial migration occurs earlier; and epithelialization is completed earlier.

TONGUE (pp. 510–511)

Repair of lateral protrusion of the tongue, without hypoglossal nerve damage, has limited success. Macroglossia has been treated by resection of the rostral section of the tongue, with good clinical results. A short frenulum causing difficulty in eating and drinking in a dog was treated by incising the frenulum for 2 cm.

Trauma

The injuries most frequently observed are lacerations caused by licking sharp surfaces, penetrating foreign bodies such as chicken bones or wood splinters, electrical cord burns, and mucosal ulceration due to infection or ingestion of caustics. Clean lacerations are sutured with absorbable material to control hemorrhage and appose epithelial edges.

Dogs with electrical cord burn injury rarely require definitive management, and the tissue is best left to slough so that the maximum amount of tongue tissue is retained. Use of a pharyngostomy or gastrostomy tube may be necessary for feeding for several days.

Surgical resection of part of the tongue is likely to be a bloody procedure; electrosurgery is useful, and temporary occlusion of both carotid arteries through an incision in the neck should be considered if extensive surgery is likely. Ideally, tongue tissue is removed as a wedge.

LIPS AND CHEEKS (pp. 511–513)

Congenital Abnormalities

The most obvious abnormality affecting the lips is harelip, in which the two sides of the primary palate fail to fuse normally (see Chapter 52). The most frequent congenital abnormality affecting the lips and cheeks is abnormal lip fold conformation in some spaniels. The lips and tight rostrolateral frenulum form a channel causing saliva to flow onto the skin of the lip. Treatment is by resection of the folds, making a V-shaped incision through the skin and mucosa.

Giant breeds of dogs have loosely attached lower lips and may slobber a great deal. These dogs can be treated by bilateral mandibular-sublingual duct ligation, gland resection, or cheiloplasty. In this latter technique, a flap of the lower lip is isolated and sutured to a defect created in the upper lip, thus eliminating the channel or pocket that allows saliva to accumulate.

Trauma

Simple lacerations are sutured with separate layers on the mucosal and skin surfaces.

THE PHARYNX (pp. 513–515)

Pharyngotomy-Pharyngostomy

Incision into the pharynx from the skin of the neck is a useful technique for several purposes, particularly for placement of an esophageal feeding tube or an endotracheal tube that bypasses the oral cavity.

Under general anesthesia, an index finger is inserted through the mouth into the pharynx then flexed to palpate and deflect the hyoid arch and mandibular salivary gland. The skin is incised directly over the fingertip, and a large hemostat is pushed through the incision, intervening muscle, and the mucosa, guided by the finger in the mouth. A flexible feeding tube (or endotracheal tube) of suitable size is placed between the jaws of the hemostat and pulled through the incision. The tube is turned in the mouth and inserted into the esophagus or trachea.

The pharyngotomy incision is left to heal by granulation after removal of the tube.

Mandibular Symphysiotomy (p. 515)

SALIVARY GLANDS (pp. 515–519)

Examination

Swelling is the most common sign of diseases of the salivary glands, owing to swelling of the gland itself or to accumulation of salivary secretions in an abnormal area.

Plain film radiography is rarely useful in investigating salivary gland disease, except for rare sialoliths. Contrast radiography (sialography) is performed under anesthesia. A water-soluble radiopaque dye such as is used for intravenous urography is injected into a salivary duct through a blunt small-gauge needle at 1 ml/10 kg per injection.

Salivary Gland and Duct Injury

If a salivary gland or duct is injured, resulting in stenosis of the duct or diversion of salivary flow to a new opening into the mouth, there will be no long-term clinical consequences. For this reason, limited injury of the salivary glands does not require treatment. Long-term consequences of salivary gland or duct injury are sialocele or fistula formation.

Parotid Gland and Duct Injury

The parotid gland or duct may be injured by bites or blunt trauma, by surgery on the side of the face, or by adjacent disease such as carnassial abscess. The fistula typically leaks a clear thin fluid. Treatment may be to divert or reconstruct the duct, although simple ligation of the duct is quick and effective.

Sublingual Gland and Duct Injury

Salivary Mucocele

The most common clinical condition of the salivary glands of dogs and cats is salivary mucocele, which is a collection of mucoid saliva that has leaked from a damaged salivary gland. The most common sites for collection of the extravasated saliva are the subcutaneous tissues of the intermandibular or cranial cervical area (cervical mucocele) or the sublingual tissues on the floor of the mouth (ranula). The cause of the damage, which can occur anywhere in the gland or duct, is rarely known. Cervical mucoceles and ranulas occasionally occur in cats. A pharyngeal mucocele can cause more clinically significant disease by obstructing the pharyngeal airway.

Diagnosis is by palpation and aspiration of the swelling, which may require sedation if the lesion is oral or pharyngeal. Gray-gold or blood-stained mucus is obtained. The mucus is invariably viscid enough to form strings when exuded from the syringe through a needle.

Treatment of Salivary Mucocele. Definitive treatment includes removal of the salivary gland that is damaged to prevent further accumulation of mucus, as well as drainage of the mucocele.

Resection of the sublingual gland without resection of the mandibular gland is impractical because of the close apposition of the two glands; thus, even though the sublingual gland is almost always the gland affected, treatment is removal of the mandibular-sublingual gland complex.

Mandibular-Sublingual Gland Resection (for technique, see pp. 517–518)

Prognosis and Management of Recurrence. Occasional dogs show slight, usually temporary, swallowing abnormalities after surgery. Recurrence after mandibular-sublingual gland resection is less than 5 per cent in reported series of cases.

Maxillectomy and Mandibulectomy
(pages 521–530)

MAXILLECTOMY (pp. 521–524)

Partial maxillectomy involves excision of portions of the maxilla, incisive bone, or palatine bone. Portions of the zygomatic and lacrimal bones also may be included. Partial maxillectomies are described according to areas excised. Unilateral and bilateral premaxillectomy involve excision of the incisive bone and possibly the rostral maxilla. In central maxillectomy, the maxilla and portions of the hard palate are excised. Caudal maxillectomy involves excision of the caudal maxilla, hard palate, and possibly the zygomatic and lacrimal bones forming the ventral portion of the bony orbit. Hemimaxillectomy is excision of one entire side of the upper jaw, including the premaxilla, maxilla, and hard palate. It may extend as far dorsally as the ventral bony orbit.

Indications

Partial maxillectomy is indicated for excision of malignant oral tumors and benign oral tumors that involve bone or periosteum, such as the epulides and ameloblastoma. Application of this technique is limited by tumor extension into the labial or buccal mucosa or across the midline of the central or caudal hard palate. Sufficient normal labial or buccal mucosa and hard palate mucoperiosteum must be available to allow closure of the oronasal defect that results.

Preoperative Evaluation

Thorough evaluation of patients is essential before surgery because many of these patients are old and may have concomitant diseases. A vital step in the preoperative evaluation is definitive diagnosis of the mass.

Surgical Technique (pp. 521–523)
Postoperative Management and Results

The animal is watched carefully during recovery from anesthesia. Some dogs become very anxious when they are unable to nose breathe during anesthetic recovery. If this occurs, light sedation with acepromazine usually calms the dog. Analgesics such as oxymorphone or butorphanol are given.

The day after surgery, the animal is offered water and soft food. An Elizabethan collar is necessary to prevent trauma to the surgery site. Intravenous fluid therapy is continued until the animal is eating and drinking well enough to maintain hydration. The degree of facial deformity following partial maxillectomy depends on the extent of excision. Unilateral premaxillectomy causes minimal deformity if the ipsilateral canine tooth is preserved.

Complications

Oronasal fistula formation may occur after partial maxillectomy. Factors that predispose animals to wound dehiscence and oronasal fistula formation include the use of electrocoagulation along the wound edges, tension on the oral suture line, and inadequate suture placement.

MANDIBULECTOMY (pp. 524–529)

Tumors located on the lower jaw may be widely excised by partial mandibulectomy. Partial mandibulectomies are classified according to the area of the mandible that is excised: (1) unilateral rostral hemimandibulectomy, (2) bilateral rostral mandibulectomy, (3) central hemimandibulectomy, (4) caudal hemimandibulectomy, (5) total hemimandibulectomy, and (6) three-quarter mandibulectomy. Three-quarter mandibulectomy is a combination of a total hemimandibulectomy and a contralateral rostral hemimandibulectomy.

Indications

Malignant oral tumors and benign tumors that involve the mandible or its periosteum require wide excision by partial mandibulectomy.

Preoperative Evaluation

The extent of the tumor is accurately assessed by physical and radiographic examination to determine if wide resection is possible while maintaining oral function.

Surgical Technique (pp. 526–528)
Postoperative Management and Results

Analgesics such as oxymorphone or butorphanol are administered before recovery from anesthesia. Water is offered after recovery from anesthesia, and soft food is offered the next day. Most animals eat within 1 to 2 days after surgery. Some animals may require an Elizabethan collar to prevent them from scratching at the tension sutures at the lip commissure. After the surgical site is well healed, the animal may be gradually changed back to its normal diet.

Unilateral rostral hemimandibulectomy in which the canine tooth is preserved is virtually unnoticeable. If the canine tooth is removed, the tongue hangs from that side of the mouth, particularly when the dog pants. Total hemimandibulectomy causes a mild concavity on the side of the face, and the contralateral hemimandible shifts toward the midline. Bilateral rostral mandibulectomy causes an obviously shortened lower jaw. Excessive drooling is common.

Complications

Swelling, ranulas, and wound dehiscence occasionally occur after mandibulectomy. Excessive drooling is common. If the mandibular symphysis has been disrupted, some degree of malocclusion occurs.

LONG-TERM RESULTS (p. 529)

Partial mandibulectomy and maxillectomy have been very successful in the treatment of invasive benign oral tumors, such as the epulides and ameloblastoma. Most animals can be cured of these tumors. Metastatic disease continues to be the major cause of treatment failure in dogs with oral malignant melanoma. Canine fibrosarcoma and feline squamous cell carcinoma results have been disappointing because of the high incidence of local tumor recurrence.

CHAPTER 42

The Esophagus (pages 530–561)

Neuromuscular Swallowing Disorders
(pages 530–534)

Swallowing is a complex process requiring functional integrity of the tongue, muscles of mastication, soft palate, pharyngeal constrictors and larynx, pharyngoesophageal sphincter (cricopharyngeal and caudal part of the thyropharyngeal muscles), esophagus, and gastroesophageal sphincter. As a result of a series of well-coordinated sequential contractions and relaxations, food and liquids are transported from the mouth to the stomach. Any structural or functional disturbance of this *precisely timed* process results in dysphagia.

The swallowing process is divided into oropharyngeal, esophageal, and gastroesophageal phases based on cineradiographic findings. The oropharyngeal phase is further subdivided into oral, pharyngeal, and cricopharyngeal stages. All phases of swallowing, except the oral stage of the oropharyngeal phase, are under involuntary reflex control.

DIAGNOSIS (pp. 530–532)

The underlying cause of the dysfunction often is not determined. Clinical signs referable to dysphagia include regurgitation through the mouth or nares, increased drooling or salivation, and repeated attempts at swallowing with extension or twisting of the head and neck.

Physical examination includes a complete neurological evaluation because swallowing disorders may be a manifestation of a systemic neuromuscular disease. The gag reflex is evaluated by placing a finger in the pharynx. Tongue tone is evaluated. Localization of the problem to either the oral, pharyngeal, or esophageal areas can usually be based on the history and physical examination. Precise definition of the various pharyngeal and esophageal disorders is a prerequisite to surgical intervention.

Diagnostic Techniques

Radiology (p. 531)

Endoscopy

Endoscopy is an important tool in evaluating esophageal diseases.

PRIMARY DISORDERS OF NEUROMUSCULAR JUNCTION AND MUSCLE (pp. 532–533)

Myasthenia Gravis

Myasthenia gravis is a disorder of neuromuscular transmission in which autoantibodies result in a reduction of nicotinic acetylcholine receptors at the neuromuscular junction and muscle weakness. Although generalized canine acquired myasthenia gravis has been well documented, a focal form has now been recognized, in which megaesophagus with regurgitation in the absence of recognizable muscle weakness is the principal clinical sign.

The diagnosis of the focal form of canine acquired myasthenia gravis is made by demonstration of antibodies against acetylcholine receptors by immunoprecipitation radioimmunoassay.

An important part of therapy for dogs with focal myasthenia gravis is alteration of feeding procedures, offering a high-calorie diet in an elevated position. In generalized myasthenia gravis, the esophagus also does not respond as favorably to anticholinesterase drugs but limb muscle strength shows marked improvement. Immunosuppressive doses of prednisone, in the absence of aspiration pneumonia, may be of some benefit.

Central and Peripheral Neuropathic Disorders

Peripheral neuropathic disorders may result in dysphagia and megaesophagus and are diagnosed by complete neurological evaluation, electrophysiological examination, and nerve and muscle biopsies.

SECONDARY NEUROMUSCULAR DISORDERS (p. 533)

Underlying metabolic disorders can result in dysphagia and megaesophagus. Only a small percentage of patients with acquired dysphagia/megaesophagus are surgical candidates, and the dysfunction must be demonstrated by dynamic radiographic studies before surgical correction is attempted.

Surgical Diseases of the Esophagus (pages 534–539)

ESOPHAGEAL OBSTRUCTION (pp. 534–544)

Obstructions may be partial or complete. Partial obstructions, regardless of cause, may result in mild, absent, or intermittent clinical signs. Complete obstructions usually result in clinically evident dysfunction.

The hallmark of esophageal obstruction is regurgitation. It is important to differentiate this clinical sign from vomiting, which is an active movement of gastric contents in an oral direction accompanied by abdominal contractions. Regurgitation is more passive, although an animal may be in distress and make efforts to expel swallowed contents that have become blocked in their passage. Acute obstructions usually result in regurgitation that occurs immediately after ingestion of any additional material. Regurgitation may be delayed by minutes to hours in patients with chronic partial obstructions. The level of the obstruction also influences the interval between ingestion of food and regurgitation. The higher the obstruction, the sooner regurgitation occurs. It is important to distinguish a high cervical esophageal obstruction, where regurgitation may occur during or shortly after deglutition, and true dysphagia.

Another common sign of esophageal obstruction is salivation, which in some patients can be prominent, with copious amounts of thick saliva appearing at the mouth.

A frequent sequel to chronic partial obstruction is dilation (megaesophagus) of the esophagus proximal to the lesion. As the esophagus begins to dilate chronically, the ability of the muscles to contract properly may be irreparably damaged. A vicious circle ensues, the net result being permanent megaesophagus of the affected region and poor esophageal motility even after the obstruction is relieved.

The diagnosis of esophageal obstruction is based on the history, physical examination, and ancillary studies. Radiography is important for viewing the esophagus (which can be enhanced by adding a contrast agent), evaluating the respiratory tract and lungs for evidence of aspiration pneumonia, and detecting the presence of an intraluminal or extraluminal cause of the obstruction. Endoscopy, when available, is also a valuable tool for diagnosis and, in many cases, for treatment of esophageal obstruction. Evaluation of regurgitated ingesta may be helpful. Regurgitated material is usually undigested and propelled in a tube shape, and in patients with large dilations, food may be fermented. The fermented food has a foul, sour, or putrid smell.

Intraluminal Obstruction

Esophageal Foreign Bodies

The most important cause of intraluminal esophageal obstruction is ingestion of foreign bodies. Obstruction occurs because of factors relating to the character of the foreign object itself and also because of esophageal anatomy. If bones are very sharp or are trapped for a prolonged time, perforation of the esophagus may occur.

The normal esophagus has three distinct anatomical narrowings where ingested foreign bodies are likely to become lodged. The *cervical constriction* is at the level of the cricopharyngeal sphincter. The bronchoaortic constriction occurs over the base of the heart, behind the tracheal bifurcation, where the left mainstem bronchus and aortic arch cross the esophagus. The diaphragmatic constriction occurs at the level of the *hiatus,* where the esophagus penetrates the diaphragm. In addition to these, a fourth site where foreign bodies tend to lodge is at the *thoracic inlet.*

Many foreign objects produce only partial obstruction. It is possible for these objects to be present for prolonged periods before illness ensues. Other long-term complications can develop, including ulceration of the mucosa and esophagitis, frank perforation of the esophagus as the overlying esophageal wall suffers pressure necrosis, mediastinitis, pleuritis, empyema, and tracheoesophageal fistula. Esophageal foreign body obstruction is an emergency. The longer the duration of the obstruction, especially with a large or sharp foreign body, the more prone to complications is a patient.

Nonsurgical management of esophageal foreign bodies in general is the treatment of choice. The owner and veterinarian should be prepared for surgical intervention, either because endoscopic manipulation is not possible or because a gastrotomy is required to remove an indigestible foreign body pushed into the stomach.

Surgical management of esophageal foreign bodies is indicated when more conservative measures have failed or are unavailable. It is the goal of the surgeon to avoid opening the esophagus if possible, especially in the thorax, but not to hesitate if it is the only means of quickly retrieving the offending foreign body. Because of the location and potential contamination, thoracic esophagotomy is more hazardous than cervical esophagotomy (see the later section on surgical techniques).

Penetrating esophageal foreign bodies, such as fishhooks and needles, present a special problem sometimes necessitating a combination of endoscopic and surgical treatment.

If the foreign body is a bone and it is pushed into the stomach rather than retrieved orally, removal via gastrotomy is not automatically required. Most bone foreign bodies, even if covered with gristle, are quickly digested in the gastric acids and excreted in the feces within 7 to 10 days. Radiographs may be obtained over several days to ensure that complications associated with the bone are not developing.

Mural and Extraluminal Obstruction

Cicatricial Strictures

Luminal narrowing and functional obstruction of the esophagus may result from acquired severe transmural scarring. Acquired esophageal strictures can result from any insult to the wall that produces injury in the submucosal and muscular layers.

Surgical management of esophageal strictures is problematic. The length of the strictured segment can be extensive and is frequently longer than the radiographic appearance suggests. The best treatments involve mechanical dilation (bougienage, balloon catheters) and pharmacological intervention with agents that reduce fibroplasia and collagen cross-linking, as discussed in the section on conservative management.

Vascular Ring Anomalies (pp. 538–544)

Vascular ring anomalies are among the most common causes of extraluminal esophageal obstruction. They result in a wide range of clinical problems due to chronic partial obstruction. Typical complications include proximal dilation, loss of motility in the dilated segment (regional megaesophagus), ulcerative esophagitis (owing to prolonged contact with fermenting ingesta and possible addition of gastric acid from reflux), cachexia, and aspiration pneumonia.

Vascular ring anomalies are the result of abnormal development of definitive vascular structures derived from embryonic aortic arches. Clinical signs result from partial or complete entrapment of the esophagus, and possibly the trachea, between the base of the heart and the offending vessels. Not only is mechanical obstruction produced by the vascular ring itself, but concurrent fibrosis of the underlying esophageal wall develops. Hence, treatment is not only directed at correcting the vascular malformation but at releasing the stenosed esophagus.

Several patterns of vascular ring anomalies have been reported. These include persistent right aortic arch with left ligamentum (ductus) arteriosus, aberrant left subclavian, double aortic arch, aberrant right subclavian, persistent right ligamentum (ductus) arteriosus with a normal left aorta, and aberrant intercostals. Of these, only double aortic arch usually results in significant tracheal stenosis and accompanying signs of cough, stridor, or dyspnea.

By far the most common vascular ring anomaly in dogs and cats results from persistence of the right fourth aortic arch as the definitive aorta (rather than the left fourth aortic arch). Persistent right aortic arch accounts for 95 per cent of all reported vascular ring anomalies.

Ninety-two per cent of dogs with persistent right aortic arch are 15 kg or less. It seems likely that vascular ring anomalies in general and persistent right aortic arch in particular are familial/heritable problems, and affected animals should not be used for breeding.

The clinical signs reflect the severely stenotic esophagus at the vascular ring anomaly. Affected animals are usually considered normal until weaning. Liquids bypass the esophageal obstruction without difficulty. As an animal ingests solid foods, postprandial regurgitation occurs. Although the majority of affected patients are presented early in life because of regurgitation that commences with weaning, several cases of late-onset regurgitation in dogs with persistent right aortic arch have been reported.

Diagnosis of vascular ring anomalies is based on signalment, history, physical examination, radiography (including, in some cases, angiography), and endoscopy. Megaesophagus may often be appreciated on physical examination by observing and palpating a bulge in the ventral cervical and thoracic inlet after swallowing. Plain radiographs of the thorax may reveal an air- or ingesta-filled cranial thoracic esophagus. The pulmonary fields are closely inspected for evidence of aspiration pneumonia. Endoscopic examination is useful in several ways. First, confirmation of persistent right aortic arch may be made by actually observing the aortic pulsations on the right and seeing the indentation of the left dorsal esophageal wall by the ligamentum arteriosum. Passing the endoscope beyond the stenotic area permits examination of the remainder of the esophagus for signs of reflux esophagitis or dilation. The endoscope may also be used for performing percutaneous tube gastrostomy, which may be indicated pre- or postoperatively for alimentation. It is better to be certain of the specific anomaly before attempting surgical intervention, because not all vascular ring anomalies are best approached from the left side.

Other diagnostic tests are performed as part of the routine evaluation. A complete blood count is indicated to determine leukocytosis, which may be severe in patients with coexisting aspiration pneumonia, and to evaluate for anemia, which can accompany malnutrition. A biochemical profile may provide clues to associated complications such as electrolyte imbalances. A radiographic finding of esophageal dilation caudal to the heart base indicates careful screening for disease processes other than mechanical obstruction of the esophagus by a vascular ring.

Treatment of vascular ring anomalies requires division of the appropriate portion of the ring to relieve esophageal stenosis. This requires identifying the least important vessel contributing to the ring. In cases of persistent right aortic arch, this entails division of the ligamentum arteriosum on the left.

Preoperative management with vascular ring anomalies is mainly directed at controlling any secondary complications already present. If cough and pneumonia are present, surgery is delayed until the severity of these conditions is reduced. Treatment usually entails broad-spectrum antibiotics or more specific antimicrobial therapy based on culture and sensitivity testing of exudate. Cachexia and negative nitrogen balance may adversely affect a patient's ability to withstand anesthesia and surgery and to combat pneumonia. All animals with megaesophagus should be trained to feed from an upright position; many patients are able to swallow semiliquid gruels. Tube gastrostomy is an effective means of feeding patients and is usually well-tolerated.

PERIESOPHAGEAL MASSES (p. 544)

Mechanical obstruction of the esophagus may occur secondary to lesions in surrounding tissues. Such lesions may or may not actually infiltrate the esophagus itself. Complete obstruction is extremely unlikely, but signs related to partial esophageal obstruction and problems with deglutition may be the presenting complaint. Diagnosis depends on radiography, possibly including contrast esophagography to demonstrate the level of esophageal impingement.

Preoperative endoscopy is indicated to determine whether infiltration through the esophageal wall has occurred.

NEUROMUSCULAR DISEASES (pp. 544–545)

Most of these conditions are best managed medically, but surgery may in some instances be beneficial as a primary or adjunctive mode of therapy.

Megaesophagus

A more detailed discussion of neuromuscular disorders of the esophagus is presented elsewhere in this chapter.

Cricopharyngeal Achalasia

Disorders of the oropharyngeal stage of swallowing are addressed elsewhere in this text.

Gastroesophageal Achalasia

The surgical procedures are described in the techniques portion of the chapter and may be considered in some patients as an adjunct to other forms of treatment, but they are not endorsed as the primary treatment for gastroesophageal swallowing disorders.

ESOPHAGEAL DIVERTICULA (pp. 545–546)

A diverticulum is a focal outpouching of the esophageal wall. These saccular dilations may be congenital or acquired. They are not common in small animals.

Pulsion (False) Diverticulum

A pulsion diverticulum is an outpouching of mucosa through a defect or tear in the overlying muscularis. It is called a ''false'' diverticulum because not all layers of the esophagus are represented in the protruding sac. These diverticula presumably develop after focal pathological pressure is applied to the esophageal wall from within the lumen. Diverticula are a rare complication of esophageal foreign body obstruction. Clinical signs are dysphagia, regurgitation, gagging, gulping, weight loss, and possibly respiratory signs.

Traction (True) Diverticulum

True diverticula are composed of all layers of the esophageal wall (adventitia, muscularis, submucosa, and mucosa). They are termed "traction" because of their presumed pathogenesis, involving the adhesion and contraction of a fibrous band to the esophageal wall, resulting in the outpouching. The incidence of traction diverticula is unknown.

ESOPHAGEAL DISEASES WITH LEAKAGE (pp. 546–548)

Esophageal Perforation and Laceration

Perforation or laceration of the esophagus may occur from inside or outside the esophagus. Neither is common. Iatrogenic perforation can occur during endoscopy, as a result of instruments passed down the esophageal lumen, and during the retrieval or pulsion of foreign bodies.

Clinical signs depend on the location, extent, and duration of the perforation and associated leakage. The health of surrounding tissues also influences the clinical course, because a small leak into an otherwise normal tissue plane may be adequately confined and healed, whereas inflammation, hypoxia, and necrosis in local tissues may predispose to massive infection. The majority of clinical signs may reflect the effects of leakage and infection on the surrounding tissues and structures. Cervical perforations may lead to infection that spreads along fascial planes into the mediastinum, resulting in mediastinitis. Perforations or lacerations of the thoracic esophagus can incite inflammation and introduce infection into the mediastinum and pleura, which might ultimately result in pleural or pulmonary abscess formation or empyema. Confirmation of esophageal perforation is made with esophagoscopy or with contrast esophagography using water-soluble iodinated contrast agents.

Conservative management includes antibiotics, withholding of food and water for several days, and parenteral fluid replacement to maintain hydration and electrolyte balance. Pharyngostomy tubes are contraindicated. If enteral alimentation is required, tube gastrostomy is much preferred. If leakage is confirmed, surgery is warranted. Regardless of the timing of surgery, postoperative care includes a minimum of 3 to 5 days of esophageal rest, using parenteral or gastric alimentation.

Esophageal Fistula

An esophageal fistula is an abnormal communication between the esophagus and the trachea, bronchus, or lung parynchema or, less commonly, the skin. Congenital fistulae probably share an etiology similar to congenital diverticula. Acquired fistulae are more common than congenital ones. The site of the fistula depends on where the esophageal perforation occurs.

Respiratory signs predominate in patients with esophageal-airway fistulae. Diagnosis heavily depends on radiography, particularly positive-contrast studies, to demonstrate direct communication between the esophageal lumen and respiratory tract. Successful treatment involves thoracotomy to expose the esophagus, fistula, and affected portion of the respiratory system. Anesthesia may present a special challenge in patients with esophageal-airway fistula, because inhalant anesthetics may escape into the esophagus through the fistula if the defect is distal to the end of the endotracheal tube. Alternatively, an "escape valve" may be created by performing a tube gastrostomy. Postoperative care is the same as for thoracotomy, esophagotomy, and lung lobectomy complicated by infection.

GASTROESOPHAGEAL INTUSSUSCEPTION (p. 548)

Surgical Techniques for Esophageal Disease (pages 549–559)

GENERAL PRINCIPLES OF ESOPHAGEAL SURGERY
(pp. 549–552)

Esophageal surgery can potentially lead to surgical or postoperative complications. Contamination is one of the most important. Contamination may be gross or microscopic. Precautions include use of suitable prophylactic antibiotics and maintenance of a sterile operating field by drapes and pads to isolate the esophagus from the surgical site. The major elements implicated in the increased relative risk of leakage or dehiscence by the esophagus include the absence of a complete serosal covering; the absence of omentum; the possibly inadequate blood supply to the esophagus; tension, motion, and distension of the surgical site; the movement of saliva and ingesta past the surgical site; and debilitation of the patient.

The combined effects of absence of serosa and omentum, plus a potentially vulnerable blood supply, may make the esophagus more prone to wound healing complications. Each of these factors may be mitigated by application of basic surgical techniques—gentle tissue handling, minimization of contamination, appropriate selection and application of suture materials, minimal use of electrocautery, and accurate apposition of tissues.

Tension and motion are two additional factors that may complicate esophageal healing. If tension is present at the surgical site, *circumferential myotomy* is the most useful clinical technique for reducing it. It is critical that the myotomy include only partial thickness of the muscularis (i.e., incising the outer longitudinal layer but leaving the inner circular muscle layer intact). Myotomies are performed 2 to 3 cm proximal and distal to the anastomosis.

Postoperative management, particularly in terms of patient feeding, is important in avoiding complications of esophageal surgery. For procedures that do not invade the esophageal lumen (e.g., esophagomyotomy), a prolonged period of fasting is not required. Animals should be kept off food and water for 24 to 48 hours, depending on the amount of esophageal handling. When esophageal surgery requires resection, anastomosis, or patch grafting or when integrity of the surgery site is in doubt because of tension, ischemia, infection, or other factors, nothing is allowed *per os* for at least 7 days after surgery.

Suture Selection and Suturing Techniques

The most widely recommended pattern is a two-layer closure: The first layer incorporates the mucosa/submucosa, and the second layer apposes the muscularis. For an anastomosis or when tension is present, a simple interrupted pattern is used. It is helpful to preplace the last two sutures to make it easier to bury the knots in the lumen. Simple continuous patterns are acceptable for esophagotomy closures but are not recommended for anastomoses because they may impede esophageal dilation during bolus passage. Regardless of pattern, sutures are placed 2 to 3 mm apart and approximately 3 mm from the incised edge.

In dogs, the submucosa alone has the same tensile strength as the mucosa and submucosa together, and these are much stronger than the muscularis alone. It may be possible to modify esophageal suturing and consider such techniques as single-layer closures that incorporate the muscularis and submucosa (but not the mucosa), using one of the newer absorbable materials. Besides choice of material and pattern, the most important factor is atraumatic technique. Again, fine (3-0 or 4-0) monofilament sutures with a swaged-on needle are advantageous. Reverse cutting needles are preferred for easy penetration with minimal slicing of the tissues.

Suture Line Reinforcement Techniques and Patch Grafting

A vascularized omental pedicle graft may be transposed across the diaphragm from the abdomen to help support the esophagus. Experimentally, this technique has been successfully used to allow healing of incompletely closed esophageal anastomoses and to close full-thickness esophageal defects.

Surgical Approaches to the Esophagus

The cervical esophagus is exposed by a ventral midline approach between the paired sternothyroid muscles. Caudal to the third rib, the esophagus is best exposed by right intercostal thoracotomy. Caudal to the heart, the esophagus may be approached either from a left- or right-sided thoracotomy.

ESOPHAGOTOMY AND DIVERTICULECTOMY (p. 552)

The site of esophagotomy is well isolated from the surrounding tissues. The esophagus is incised longitudinally, making the incision in the muscularis slightly longer than the mucosal incision. Closure is performed using one of the techniques described earlier. The most traditional closure is the two-layer procedure.

Resection of a single small diverticulum is straightforward. The pouch is resected to the point that closure restores a normal diameter to the esophageal lumen. With very large or multiple diverticula, esophageal resection and anastomosis are performed.

ESOPHAGEAL RESECTION AND ANASTOMOSIS (p. 552)

The esophageal lumen cranial and caudal to the resection is occluded using atraumatic clamps or tourniquets. The desired portion of the esophagus is clamped off cranially and caudally, and the esophageal segment is excised sharply outside the area defined by the clamps.

The anastomosis is begun by reapposing the two cut ends by placement of full-thickness stay sutures dorsally and ventrally in each portion. The first layer of the sutured anastomosis approximates the mucosa-submucosa with a simple interrupted pattern using 3-0 or 4-0 suture material. The sutures are placed approximately 2 mm apart and penetrate 2 to 3 mm from the cut edges. Suturing commences on the far side of the esophagus, halfway between the dorsal and ventral stay sutures. Subsequent sutures are placed in an alternating fashion dorsal and ventral to the midpoint, so that the closure progresses evenly around the circumference until nearly meeting on the near side. When only two or three more sutures are needed, these are preplaced so that their knots can be buried in the lumen. To test for leakage, the esophagus is occluded cranially and caudally, and saline is injected in the lumen until the anastomotic zone is distended. If leaks are observed, additional simple interrupted sutures are placed. One or two conventionally tied knots in the submucosa do not significantly increase the risk of postoperative stricture. The second layer reapposes the muscularis with 3-0 simple interrupted sutures of a minimally reactive material.

ESOPHAGEAL REPLACEMENT AND RECONSTRUCTION
(pp. 552–554)

Skin Tube Substitution

Gastric Substitution

Intestinal Substitution

CORRECTION OF VASCULAR RING ANOMALIES
(pp. 554–557)

Persistent Right Aortic Arch

Persistent right aortic arch results in entrapment of the esophagus between the base of the heart, the aorta (on the right), and the ligamentum arteriosum crossing from the pulmonary artery on the left to the aorta. The goals of surgery are to transect the ligament and to ensure that the esophagus is not also restricted by bands of fibrous tissue.

The approach is via lateral thoracotomy through the left fourth or fifth intercostal space. The mediastinal pleura over the esophagus is opened longitudinally using blunt and sharp dissection. The vagus nerve is identified and avoided during incision and retracted dorsally with the divided mediastinum.

The pulmonary artery, aorta, and connecting ligamentum arteriosum are identified. Mixter right-angle forceps are used to bluntly dissect the ligamentum from the underlying esophagus. Once the ligament is completely free, two ligatures of 2-0 or 1-0 surgical silk are preplaced at either end, close to the aorta and pulmonary artery. After division of the ligament, releasing the esophagus from the vascular ring, the esophagus does not immediately re-expand at the stenosis. Secondary fibrotic bands are important in obstruction of the esophagus. These restrictive bands must be dissected. It is helpful to have an assistant pass a Foley catheter *per os* to the stenosis. The bulb is inflated with saline and drawn back and forth across the stricture. This enables observation of any remaining fibrous tissue.

For the dilated portion of the esophagus, one option is plication of the redundant tissue. Although plication may make the esophagus look better, it is unlikely to produce any clinical benefits to the patient. Once the esophagus is completely freed, the thorax may be closed. A thoracic drainage tube may be preplaced at the discretion of the surgeon and is probably indicated in larger patients (>7 kg).

Postoperative care includes antibiotics, upright feedings of gruel, and possible continued use of a gastrostomy tube. The goal is to have patients return to normal feeding habits. Cats often respond better to surgery than dogs, returning to normal food eaten in a nonelevated position within weeks, without complication. Some dogs may also achieve these results, although many continue to require some feeding modification.

SURGICAL PROCEDURES FOR NEUROMUSCULAR SWALLOWING DISORDERS (pp. 557–559)

When medical management fails to adequately control regurgitation associated with the disease, surgical therapy can be considered.

Cricopharyngeal Myotomy

The goal of cricopharyngeal myotomy is to make swallowing easier in dogs with *cricopharyngeal* dysphagia. Because *pharyngeal* dysphagia can be worsened by this operation, it is important to differentiate between these two swallowing disorders.

A ventral midline incision is made from a point cranial to the larynx to about 4 to 5 cm caudal to the larynx. The larynx and its extrinsic musculature are exposed. The larynx is rotated 180° on its longitudinal axis to expose its dorsal surface. The median raphe between the paired cricopharyngeal muscles is identified, and an incision is made through it down to the mucosa of the pharynx and cranial esophagus but not penetrating it. The larynx is allowed to return to its normal position, and the sternohyoid muscles are reapposed on the midline.

Distal Esophagomyotomy (Modified Heller Procedure)

The modified Heller procedure involves a single myotomy along the ventral or lateral wall of the esophagus. The operation reduces relative obstruction caused by a nonrelaxing lower esophageal sphincter zone. In dogs, the operation is strictly palliative and is reserved for dogs with otherwise unmanageable frequency or severity of regurgitation.

Surgery is performed via a left lateral thoracotomy through the ninth intercostal space. Esophagomyotomy is performed by longitudinally incising the outer and inner muscle layers down to the submucosa. The incision is continued caudally from a point 1 to 2 cm cranial to the attachment of the phrenicoesophageal ligament through the oblique muscle fibers of the cranial 1 to 2 cm of the cardiac portion of the stomach. Abdominalizing the distal esophagus and cardia helps prevent reflux and may obviate the need for a separate antireflux operation.

Cardioplasty

Cardioplasty, like the modified Heller myotomy, is designed to promote easier passage of ingesta into the stomach by expansion of the esophageal lumen through the lower esophageal sphincter zone and cardia.

CHAPTER 43

Stomach (pages 561–593)

Chronic Gastric Outflow Obstruction
(pages 561–568)

PATHOGENESIS AND ETIOLOGY (pp. 561–562)

Differential diagnosis includes congenital and acquired antral pyloric hypertrophy, gastric neoplasia, granulomatous fungal disease (e.g., histoplasmosis, phycomycosis), eosinophilic granuloma, and chronic pyloric foreign bodies. External lesions such as pancreatic neoplasia or abscessation can obstruct the pylorus, causing delayed gastric emptying. Gastric motility disorders (e.g., gastric atony) can cause delayed gastric emptying and are considered in the differential diagnosis. Antral hypertrophy and neoplasia are the two most common causes of chronic pyloric dysfunction.

Antral pyloric hypertrophy is obstruction of the pyloric canal caused by hypertrophy of the pyloric circular smooth muscle, mucosal hyperplasia, or both. The cause and pathogenesis of either congenital or acquired disease are unknown.

Surgical treatment is directed at correcting the outflow obstruction using the least radical procedure that adequately eliminates the obstruction and allows normal gastric emptying.

CLINICAL SIGNS AND LABORATORY FINDINGS
(p. 562)

The majority of animals with chronic gastric outflow obstruction have a history of *chronic vomiting.* The vomitus varies from undigested to partially digested food and may contain blood.

Chronic vomiting can cause electrolyte and acid-base imbalances. Prerenal azotemia, hypochloremia, metabolic alkalosis or acidosis, anemia, and dehydration can potentially occur secondary to chronic outflow obstruction.

DIAGNOSIS (p. 562)

Hematological and biochemical tests are useful in ruling out metabolic or concurrent diseases that cause chronic vomiting. Abdominal ultrasonography is helpful in diagnosing abdominal metastatic disease.

Radiography and fluoroscopy provide the most definitive method of diagnosing gastric outlet obstruction. Positive-contrast studies are usually necessary to definitively diagnose outlet obstruction. Delayed gastric emptying, pyloric intraluminal filling deficits, and thickening of the pylorus are radiographic signs useful in confirming outlet obstruction. Endoscopy is helpful in preoperatively assessing the pylorus and antrum for ulceration, mucosal hyperplasia, masses, or other abnormalities.

SURGICAL CORRECTION (pp. 562–568)

Fredet-Ramstedt Pyloromyotomy

Fredet-Ramstedt pyloromyotomy is the least invasive gastric outflow corrective procedure and is usually recommended for animals with minor pyloric outflow obstruction not requiring tissue resection. Healing and fibrosis of the pyloromyotomy incision may actually lessen the initial clinical improvement.

Surgical Technique

A longitudinal incision is made along the ventral pylorus in an avascular area. The depth of the incision is to the mucosal layer.

The most common technical mistake is partial incision through the muscularis layer. Another potential mistake is inadvertent penetration into the gastric lumen. If this occurs, the mucosa can be sutured or the Fredet-Ramstedt pyloromyotomy can be converted to a Heineke-Mikulicz pyloroplasty.

Pyloroplasty Techniques

The different pyloroplasty techniques have numerous advantages, including exposure of the mucosal surface, full-thickness biopsy specimen retrieval, resection of localized lesions (i.e., focal hypertrophied rugal folds), and a low prevalence of postoperative complications.

Experimentally, the smallest cross-sectional area of the gastrointestinal opening results after Heineke-Mikulicz pyloroplasty, followed by the Finney and Jaboulay procedures. Increasing the size of the luminal diameter may increase the risk of enterogastric reflux.

Heineke-Mikulicz Pyloroplasty

Surgical Technique. A longitudinal incision is made through all layers of the pylorus. The resulting transverse incision is closed using a single-layer closure of simple interrupted crushing or appositional sutures placed through all four layers of the stomach and duodenum.

Important technical points are not to make the longitudinal incision too long, avoid excessive tension on the incision, and place the sutures carefully to ensure correct alignment of tissues.

Y-U Antral Advancement Flap Pyloroplasty

This technique is not as affected by decreased tissue pliability as other pyloroplasty techniques. The technique provides excellent intraluminal exposure, allowing easy removal of hypertrophic mucosal folds. Experimentally, it increases pyloric diameter by 30 to 100 per cent.

Surgical Technique. A pedicle advancement flap is harvested from the pyloric antral region. A longitudinal serosal incision is made in the pyloric region, approximately 2 to 3 cm below the pylorus and extending to just above the proximal aspect of the pylorus. The antral flap is advanced distally to the end of the pyloroduodenal incision and sutured. A full-thickness simple interrupted crushing or appositional suture pattern can be used for closure. Technically, it is important to produce a short, rounded antral flap to prevent damaging the blood supply to the tip of the flap.

Inverted Side-to-Side Pyloroplasties

The Finney pyloroplasty and Jaboulay procedure are infrequently used in small animals because they are more technically difficult than the Heineke-Mikulicz or Y-U pyloroplasty techniques. Additionally, few advantages are gained with the use of the Finney or Jaboulay procedures.

Surgical Technique. The pylorus and duodenum are gently apposed side to side. A full-thickness U-shaped incision (Finney procedure) or parallel incisions (Jaboulay procedure) are made into the duodenum and stomach.

Resection Techniques

Pylorectomy and gastroduodenostomy or gastrojejunostomy are indicated if full-thickness resection of tissue is required (e.g., with neoplasia, granulomatous tissue, or a perforated gastric ulcer). Several potential complications or disadvantages can be associated with pylorectomy and a reconstruction procedure.

Pylorectomy and Gastroduodenostomy (Billroth I)

A section of hepatogastric ligament can be partially transected to increase caudoventral retraction of the pylorus. The common bile duct is identified and protected to prevent iatrogenic damage. The area of pylorus to be resected is excised. Everted mucosa from the cut edges of stomach and duodenum are resected to allow serosa-to-serosa apposition. A one-layer end-to-end anastomosis is performed. A simple interrupted appositional or crushing pattern can be made. A two-layer closure has no advantage.

Gastrojejunostomy (Billroth II)

When extensive resection of the pylorus, antrum, and proximal duodenum is required, a gastrojejunostomy procedure may be required. Excessive tension across the incision line may prohibit an end-to-end gastroduodenostomy. Concurrent disease involving the choledochoduodenal junction or common bile duct may require a biliary redirection procedure. If pancreatic resection is also required, treatment for pancreatic acinar insufficiency may be necessary.

After transection of the duodenum and pyloric antrum, the resulting stumps are oversewn using a two-layer closure. The mucosa and submucosa are closed with a simple interrupted or continuous suture pattern. An inverting suture material (e.g., Lembert) is placed in the seromuscular layer.

An area between the gastric incision and greater curvature is identified, and a short loop of proximal jejunum approximated. The stomach and jejunum are joined at that location with a side-to-side anastomosis using a two-layer suture closure. The mucosal and submucosal layers of the stomach and jejunum are closed using a simple interrupted or continuous suture pattern. Simple interrupted sutures are placed in the gastrojejunal seromuscular layer.

COMPLICATIONS (p. 568)

Postoperative complications associated with gastric outlet corrective procedures include incisional leakage and dehiscence, hemorrhage, pancreatic or common bile duct injury, persistent gastric outflow obstruction, and marginal ulceration.

Gastric Foreign Bodies (pages 568–571)

INCIDENCE (p. 568)

Gastric foreign bodies are found in dogs and cats of all breeds and ages.

CLINICAL SIGNS (p. 568)

The most characteristic sign is vomiting, which may be intermittent because the vomiting reflex is triggered when the foreign body is located in the pyloric antrum.

LABORATORY FINDINGS (p. 568)

Laboratory findings vary with severity and duration of vomiting and may include dehydration and electrolyte and acid-base imbalances.

RADIOGRAPHIC FINDINGS (p. 569)

Plain films are adequate in diagnosing radiopaque foreign bodies. If contrast studies are necessary, use of air or carbon dioxide as a negative-contrast medium is preferable to positive-contrast agents, which tend to mask foreign bodies. Administering a small amount of barium before introducing air or carbon dioxide may be helpful, especially if the foreign body absorbs the contrast agent.

DIAGNOSIS (p. 569)

Gastric foreign bodies are diagnosed by radiographic findings.

SURGICAL METHODS (pp. 569–571)

Rounded foreign bodies with a smooth surface can be removed by inducing vomiting 30 minutes after the animal has been fed a regular meal. In dogs, apomorphine can be used at a dose of 1 to 5 mg SC, but in cats, xylazine (1 mg/kg) is more effective.

Small foreign bodies can be retrieved by endoscopy. Large foreign bodies or foreign bodies with a rough surface that might injure the esophagus when retrieved by mouth are removed by gastrotomy. Stay sutures or Babcock tissue forceps are placed in the cranial surface of the stomach at each end of the incision and are used to rotate and lift the stomach and bring the site of incision into the abdominal wound. The incision is made in a relatively avascular area, approximately midway between and parallel to the greater and lesser curvature of the stomach and equidistant from the pylorus and cardia. The incision is large enough to allow the foreign body to pass without tearing.

A suction tube is used to remove fluid that spills from the stomach. Both one-layer and two-layer techniques may be used to close the incision. Gut is abjured because it may be absorbed too rapidly when exposed to gastric acid.

PROGNOSIS (p. 571)

Gastrotomy to remove foreign bodies has a favorable prognosis.

AFTERCARE (p. 571)

Electrolyte and acid-base imbalances are corrected by intravenous electrolyte solutions. Small amounts of drinking water are offered as soon as an animal has recovered from anesthesia. If drinking water is retained, feeding can be started 24 hours after surgery with small amounts of a bland diet.

COMPLICATIONS (p. 571)

Gastrotomy may be complicated by local or generalized peritonitis due to spillage of gastric contents into the abdominal cavity, but this is uncommon.

Gastroesophageal Reflux Disease
(pages 571–575)

Upper Gastrointestinal Bleeding
(pages 576–580)

INCIDENCE (p. 576)

Upper gastrointestinal bleeding may originate in the esophagus, stomach, or duodenum. It is a relatively rare sign that may occur in dogs and cats of all breeds and ages and is associated with other diseases such as chronic renal or hepatic disease, mast cell neoplasia, gastrin-producing neoplasia of the pancreas (Zollinger-Ellison syndrome), and gastric neoplasia. It may also be secondary to trauma, shock or sepsis, and disseminated intravascular coagulation or other clotting disorders and has been associated with the use of aspirin, dexamethasone, indomethacin, naproxen, and piroxicam.

PATHOPHYSIOLOGY (p. 576)

Upper gastrointestinal bleeding indicates mucosal damage in the esophagus, stomach, or duodenum. Esophageal lesions may be caused by gastroesophageal reflux or gastric acid hypersecretion. Lesions in the stomach and duodenum range from mild inflammation to severe ulceration. The latter can cause serious signs that may require surgical intervention.

This chapter discusses the pathogenesis of gastric and duodenal ulcers. Factors contributing to their development include reduced mucosal blood flow, reflux of bile salts from the duodenum into the stomach, and hypersecretion of gastric hydrochloric acid. The gastric and duodenal mucosa normally are covered with a layer of mucus that offers protection against the corrosive and digestive effects of gastric acid and pepsin. When the mucus layer is lost, the mucosa comes in direct contact with hydrochloric acid and pepsin, which may result in autodigestion and ulcer development.

Another important factor is reflux of duodenal contents into the stomach. Bile salts are more destructive than pancreatic juices because they act as detergents that solubilize lipid cell membranes and can inhibit ion transport systems. Gastric acid alone may produce gastrointestinal ulcers if it is secreted in excessive quantities.

Gastric ulcers may also be caused by aspirin, dexamethasone, indomethacin, naproxen, and piroxicam. These drugs decrease the secretion of gastric mucus and alter its biochemical composition, making it less resistant to digestion by proteolytic enzymes.

CLINICAL SIGNS (p. 576)

The most characteristic signs are hematemesis and melena. Chronic cases may show acute exacerbations due to hemorrhage or ulcer perforation.

LABORATORY FINDINGS (pp. 576–577)

In chronically affected patients, the most significant finding is microcytic, hypochromic anemia. Acute cases may show moderate normochromic anemia or no evidence of anemia if the loss of plasma equals the loss of erythrocytes. Chronic vomiting can cause electrolyte and acid-base imbalances. The most commonly found abnormality is metabolic acidosis, but metabolic alkalosis and respiratory acidosis and alkalosis may also occur.

RADIOGRAPHIC FINDINGS (p. 577)

Plain abdominal films may aid in the diagnosis of complications such as peritonitis or perforation. Esophageal, gastric, or duodenal ulcers may be diagnosed using positive-contrast or double-contrast radiography. Abrupt transition of the tissue surrounding the ulcer with normal gastric wall may be the most specific radiographic criterion of a malignant ulcer. Gastrointestinal ulcers may not be detected radiographically for various reasons.

DIAGNOSIS (p. 577)

The diagnostic process in patients with (upper) gastrointestinal bleeding includes determining and locating gastrointestinal bleeding and the underlying cause. Endoscopy, radiography, and scintigraphy have been used in small animals to localize the site of bleeding.

SURGICAL METHODS (pp. 577–579)

Surgical treatment of gastrointestinal bleeding is indicated in life-threatening hemorrhage and ulcer perforation. It should also be considered if gastrinomas are suspected or conservative management is unsuccessful.

The stomach and duodenum are exposed and inspected in a systematic way. The presence of ulcers may be suggested by adhesions, serosal scarring, and irregular, thickened areas in the gastric wall. The pancreas should be thoroughly inspected for nodules that might be gastrinomas, but it must be handled with great care to prevent postoperative pancreatitis.

Small ulcers are removed by elliptical excision. The incision is closed in one or two layers. Large ulcers in the pyloric part of the stomach are removed by a Billroth I gastrectomy. As an alternative procedure, the ulcer region may be oversewn with an omental or serosal flap.

Gastrinomas that are confined to one lobe of the pancreas are best removed by *en bloc* resection of the affected lobe and its regional lymph nodes. The cranial part of the right lobe is left intact to preserve the pancreatic ducts.

PROGNOSIS (p. 579)

Upper gastrointestinal bleeding due to stress ulcers has a favorable prognosis if the initiating condition can be treated successfully. The prognosis of bleeding due to chronic renal disease, chronic hepatic disease, or blood coagulation disorders depends on the prognosis of the underlying disease but is generally poor. The same applies to ulcers secondary to mastocytomas or gastric neoplasia, which are most commonly diagnosed in an advanced state. Little is known of the prognosis of gastrinomas in small animals.

AFTERCARE (pp. 579–580)

During the first 24 hours after surgery, the animal is carefully monitored for postoperative hemorrhage. Blood transfusions are given to compensate for preoperative and operative losses. Fluid and electrolyte balance is maintained by intravenous administration of electrolyte solutions until oral fluid intake is adequate.

Gastric Dilation-Volvulus Syndrome
(pages 580–591)

Gastric dilation-volvulus syndrome is an acute medical and surgical condition related to several pathophysiological effects occurring secondary to gastric distension and malpositioning. It occurs most commonly in large, deep-chested dogs. The disease can occur at any age but is most prevalent in older dogs.

PATHOPHYSIOLOGY (pp. 580–582)

Gastric dilation-volvulus syndrome is usually initiated by gastric accumulation of gas, fluid, or both, with some degree of functional or mechanical gastric outflow obstruction. Aerophagia is the most likely source of gas accumulation. The fluid component of gastric contents is a combination of ingesta, gastric secretions, and transudate from venous obstruction. The mechanism of gastric outflow obstruction is unknown.

Gastric dilation usually precedes volvulus of the stomach. Anatomically, a clockwise or counterclockwise rotation of the stomach occurs.

The most common rotation is clockwise (as viewed with the dog in dorsal recumbency). Displacement of the pyloric antrum and pylorus occurs from the right abdominal wall toward ventral midline, and passing over the gastric fundus and body to an area along the dog's left abdominal wall adjacent to the esophagus. The fundus displaces in a ventral direction toward the right abdominal wall, passing under the pylorus to a position along the right ventrolateral abdominal wall. The position of the spleen may vary depending on the degree of volvulus. It is often markedly congested and can undergo torsion on its own vascular pedicle.

Gastric dilation causes compression of the posterior vena cava and portal vein, resulting in secondary sequestration of blood in the splanchnic, renal, and posterior muscular capillary beds. Venous return to the heart is decreased, resulting in reduced cardiac output and arterial blood pressure. Hypotension and vascular stasis result in cellular hypoxia and a shift to anaerobic metabolism.

Portal vein occlusion can cause a decreased ability of the hepatic reticuloendothelial system to clear gram-negative endotoxins that are absorbed from a devitalized gastric mucosa. Endotoxemia produces further hypotension, decreased cardiac output, and increased venous sequestration.

Poor tissue perfusion and organ hypoxia have serious systemic effects. In the heart, focal myocardial ischemia and hypoxia can cause myocardial degeneration, inflammation, and necrosis. Decreased contractility and arrhythmias occurring secondary to myocardial ischemia, acidosis, and reperfusion injury contribute to cardiac dysfunction, causing reduced systemic blood flow. Vascular stasis, hypoxia, and acidosis can also predispose to the development of disseminated intravascular coagulopathy.

Respiratory dysfunction results from decreased pulmonary compliance and mechanical restriction of diaphragmatic movement by a dilated stomach. The clinical result of respiratory impairment, decreased cardiac output, and ventilation/perfusion mismatching is decreased blood oxygen tension and tissue hypoxia.

Increased gastric intraluminal pressure, portal hypertension, and venous thrombosis result in mucosal and mural venous stasis. Mucosal and submucosal gastric edema results. Vascular wall disruption occurs secondary to tissue hypoxia, resulting in mucosal and submucosal hemorrhage.

CLINICAL SIGNS (p. 582)

The typical dog with gastric dilation-volvulus syndrome has a progressively distended and tympanic cranial abdomen, nonproductive retching, hypersalivation, restlessness, and depression. Clinical signs associated with hypovolemic shock are generally present. Abdominal palpation reveals various degrees of gastric distension and splenomegaly.

DIAGNOSIS (p. 582)

Diagnosis of gastric dilation-volvulus syndrome is based on clinical signs and radiographic evaluation. Clinical signs alone do not differentiate simple dilation from gastric volvulus with dilation. Ability to pass a stomach tube is not a reliable criterion for differentiating simple dilation from volvulus. Plain abdominal radiographs with the dog in right lateral recumbency are generally diagnostic and are less stressful than ventrodorsal or multipositional views. The pylorus is normally gas filled and located dorsally; the fundus is located caudoventrally.

Pyloric displacement deep to the cardia signals counterclockwise torsion, whereas pyloric position superficial to the cardia suggests simple dilation.

PREOPERATIVE TREATMENT (pp. 582–583)

Initial medical management of gastric dilation-volvulus syndrome is appropriate therapy for hypovolemic shock and gastric decompression.

Gastric decompression via passage of an orogastric tube is performed after initiation of fluid therapy. If tube passage is unsuccessful, percutaneous gastrocentesis using an 18-gauge needle placed into the stomach can reduce the gaseous component of gastric dilation-volvulus syndrome.

If a dog is relatively stable based on cardiovascular clinical parameters, immediate surgery to decompress and reposition the stomach can be performed. Alternatively, decompression can be achieved by gastrotomy performed under local anesthesia.

Prolonged stabilization allows time for complete cardiovascular and metabolic stabilization, preoperative work-up, and transportation to a referral center if required. Failure to inspect and reposition the stomach immediately is a potential disadvantage of prolonged temporary stabilization. Perfusion to localized segments of malpositioned stomach may be decreased despite decompression. Another potential disadvantage of prolonged temporary stabilization is the increased frequency of cardiac arrhythmias that normally occur 12 to 36 hours after presentation.

SURGICAL TREATMENT (pp. 583–589)

Surgical treatment has three main goals: correction of gastric malpositioning, assessment and treatment of gastric and splenic ischemic injury, and prevention of recurrence by permanent fixation of the stomach to the abdominal wall.

The dog is positioned in dorsal recumbency. If gastric distension is present, an orogastric tube can be passed to decompress the stomach. After decompression, the stomach and spleen are repositioned. Splenectomy is indicated only if splenic necrosis occurring secondary to vessel avulsion or infarction is present.

Approximately 10 per cent of dogs have a devitalized gastric wall requiring surgical treatment. Determination of the presence and extent of gastric ischemic injury and secondary necrosis can be difficult. Thrombosis or avulsion of the short gastric and epiploic branches of the left gastroepiploic vessels along the greater curvature may not necessarily lead to gastric necrosis. No consistent objective parameters are available for the operative evaluation of gastric ischemic injury. Determination of gastric viability is based partially on serosal coloration, perfusion, patency of serosal vessels, and palpation of the gastric wall.

Pale greenish to grayish serosal areas are attributed to arterial or arteriovenous injury. This type of discoloration generally suggests ischemic or necrotic areas of gastric wall that require additional evaluation and possible resection. Black or blue-black serosal discoloration is mainly due to venous occlusion resulting in subserosal and intramural hemorrhage. Dark red hemorrhagic serosal areas are generally reversible lesions not requiring resection. Areas of questionable viability are re-evaluated 10 to 15 minutes after repositioning, because vascular supply and color can improve subsequently.

Palpation of the gastric wall can reveal thinning or stretching of the gastric wall, indicating possible devitalized tissue. Lack of active bleeding after incision into the gastric wall is useful in demonstrating the extent of gastric resection. Intraluminal assessment of the gastric mucosa as an indication of gastric mural viability is not recommended. The presence and extent of mucosal necrosis often determine the frequency and severity of postoperative gastritis, fluid, blood, and protein loss secondary to gastric ulceration. Mucosal anoxia results in subepithelial hemorrhage, necrosis, and ulceration.

Once the presence and extent of gastric ischemic injury and necrosis are determined, two surgical options are available. Partial gastrectomy or a partial gastric invagination technique can be used.

Partial Gastrectomy

Necrotic gastric wall is excised using a scalpel blade or Metzenbaum scissors to the level of viable gastric wall based on clinical parameters (e.g., serosal coloration and perfusion, gastric wall texture) and active arterial bleeding from the incisional edges. The gastrectomy incision is closed using a two-layer longitudinal closure.

After necrotic gastric areas are resected, a prophylactic gastropexy technique and thorough copious abdominal lavage are performed. In dogs with gastric rupture, open peritoneal drainage is recommended for the treatment of severe peritonitis. The prognosis is generally grave.

A partial gastric invagination technique is recommended in dogs with questionable gastric viability and is useful for avoiding the time delay and risk of abdominal contamination associated with a resection technique. The technique involves placing an inverting suture pattern into viable stomach wall. A double-layer closure using nonabsorbable suture material is placed in the seromuscular layer, resulting in invagination of nonviable stomach into the lumen. All dogs with this syndrome should have a prophylactic gastropexy to permanently prevent recurrence.

Tube Gastrostomy

Tube gastrostomy is relatively quick and technically simple. Problems with the technique include premature dislodgment of the tube secondary to balloon rupture, removal of the tube by the patient, local or generalized peritonitis or cellulitis associated with leakage of gastric contents around the tube, and persistent stoma drainage.

Surgical Technique

An 18 to 30 French Foley catheter is placed through a stab incision in the abdominal wall. A stab incision is made into the gastric wall, and the Foley catheter tip is placed into the gastric lumen. Absorbable sutures are preplaced between the pyloric antrum and abdominal wall. The tube is left in place for 7 to 10 days.

Circumcostal Gastropexy

Circumcostal gastropexy has a lower recurrence rate than tube gastrostomy and a stronger gastropexy site than with tube or permanent gastropexy.

Surgical Technique (pp. 586–587)

Modifications of the basic technique require a 5-cm by 1.5- to 3-cm flap of seromuscularis to be made from the ventral pyloric antrum, midway between the greater and lesser curvatures. A 5-cm incision is made over the most complete caudal rib (11th or 12th), through the parietal peritoneum and transverse abdominal muscle.

The gastric antral flap is passed from a craniodorsal to caudoventral direction around the rib. The flap is sutured back to its original seromuscular gastric margins using 2-0 or 3-0 absorbable suture material.

Belt-Loop Gastropexy

The technique is a modification of the circumcostal gastropexy; a seromuscular gastric flap is passed around a loop of transverse abdominal muscle instead of a rib.

Surgical Technique (pp. 587–588)

Permanent Incisional Gastropexy

Permanent incisional gastropexy is also a simple, quick method, avoiding the complications associated with tube gastropexy and the technical difficulties or complications associated with circumcostal or belt-loop gastropexy.

Surgical Technique

A longitudinal incision is made into the seromuscularis, located over the ventral surface of the pyloric antrum equidistant from the lesser and greater curvatures. An incision is also made into the peritoneum and internal fascia of the rectus abdominal or transverse abdominal muscles, located in the right ventrolateral abdominal wall. The edges of the gastric incision are sutured to the abdominal wall incision using a simple continuous suture pattern with 2–0 monofilament nonabsorbable material. The deeper (dorsal-cranial) incisional margins are sutured first, followed by the more superficial margin, creating an imperforate circular stoma. With disruption of mesothelial surfaces, deep infiltration of fibrous tissue into the abdominal and gastric muscles occurs at the gastropexy site. Long-term follow-up confirms formation of a strong, permanent gastropexy site.

POSTOPERATIVE COMPLICATIONS (pp. 589–591)

Many of the complications are secondary to the initial pathophysiological effects of the syndrome and gastric mural-mucosal ischemic injury.

Shock after surgery can result from inappropriate treatment of hypovolemic shock preoperatively, hypotensive effect of various anesthetic drugs, blood loss, gastrointestinal fluid sequestration, absorption of bacterial and tissue toxins, and secondary peritonitis.

Ventricular arrhythmias (e.g., ventricular and paroxysmal tachycardia, univocal and multivocal premature ventricular beats) are common after surgery, occurring in 40 to 50 per cent of dogs. The cause of ventricular arrhythmias is unknown. Treatment is instituted in dogs with ventricular arrhythmias greater than 15 to 20 per minute with signs of altered cardiovascular hemodynamics.

Treatment includes maintenance of normal hydration and correction of acid-base or electrolyte imbalances. Intramuscular antiarrhythmic therapy (procainamide, 6 to 15 mg/kg IM every 4 to 6 hours; or quinidine sulfate, 6 to 15 mg/kg IM every 4 to 6 hours) can be administered if arrhythmias are relatively infrequent and cause minimal clinical signs. Ventricular arrhythmias are usually treated with intravenous antiarrhythmic drug therapy. Lidocaine, 2 to 4 mg/kg as a slow intravenous bolus, is given until normal sinus rhythm occurs or a total dose of 8 mg/kg is administered. Maintenance administration of lidocaine as a continuous infusion (0.04 to 0.08 mg/kg/min) is necessary to maintain therapeutic levels. Signs of lidocaine toxicity include vomiting, muscle tremors, and convulsions. Lidocaine is temporarily discontinued if toxicity signs occur, and a lower dose is used. Refractory arrhythmias may respond to intravenous procainamide (0.5 to 1 mg/kg) or quinidine sulfate (0.04 to 0.08 mg/min).

Hypokalemia (serum K^+ <3.5 mEq/L) is the most common electrolyte imbalance. Empirical potassium supplementation in maintenance fluids (20 mEq/L) may be indicated.

Hypoproteinemia (total serum protein <5.2 g/100 ml) results from protein loss. Dogs with protein levels less than 3 g/100 ml may require plasma transfusions. Prolonged fluid therapy may also lower the hematocrit. In severe anemia, blood transfusions may be indicated.

Gastric ischemic injury and necrosis resulting in gastric perforation are infrequent. A positive cytological diagnosis of peritonitis secondary to gastrointestinal leakage indicates an exploratory laparotomy. Gastritis secondary to mucosal ischemic injury is common. Histamine H_2 receptor antagonists such as cimetidine (10 mg/kg IM TID) are recommended to increase pH of gastric contents.

CHAPTER 44

Small Intestine (pages 593–612)

SURGICAL DISORDERS (pp. 593–599)

Trauma

Trauma to the small intestine is uncommon. Intestinal and mesenteric injury may occur with bite wounds of the abdomen, when sharp objects or projectiles penetrate the abdominal wall, with self-inflicted injury after evisceration following dehiscence of an abdominal incision, and with blunt trauma due to motor vehicle accidents.

Clinical Findings

The cardinal signs of intestinal injury are vomiting, abdominal tenderness, bloody stools, or passage of bloody fluid from the rectum. Other signs include depression, anorexia, reluctance to move, and shock.

Radiographic Findings

Accurate diagnosis depends on the recognition of peritonitis. A small amount of free gas or none at all may be demonstrable in the abdomen, or gas escaping from ruptured intestines may be trapped, forming gas pockets between adhered loops of intestines.

Diagnosis

Suspected intestinal injuries are best evaluated by physical examination to detect penetration of the peritoneal cavity, abdominal tenderness, and proctorrhagia. Peritoneal lavage is invaluable; recovered lavage fluid containing bacteria, vegetable fibers, and toxic neutrophils indicates exploratory celiotomy. Patients with gunshot injury of the abdomen require prompt celiotomy.

Treatment

Treatment of shock and cardiovascular and pulmonary injury precedes or accompanies exploratory celiotomy and treatment of intestinal injury. Broad-spectrum antibiotics are administered preoperatively. After celiotomy, the abdominal cavity is thoroughly examined to locate all lesions. Adhesions between omentum and intestines or between adjacent intestinal loops are freed to permit inspection of the entire intestinal tract.

Small lacerations or holes in the intestines are débrided and closed with 3-0 synthetic absorbable material placed in simple interrupted or Lembert suture patterns. More extensive injuries are managed by intestinal resection and anastomosis. Contamination of the peritoneal cavity with intestinal contents is the principal cause of serious complications in intestinal injury. Postoperative support includes fluid, electrolyte, and nutritional therapy while closely monitoring for signs of peritonitis.

Mechanical Obstruction

Mechanical obstruction is the most common indication for intestinal surgery. Obstruction of the intestinal lumen may occur with foreign bodies, intussusception, neoplasia, and less commonly adhesions. Intramural intestinal hematoma causing intestinal obstruction has been reported in three dogs.

The nature and site of the obstruction influence the clinical signs. An object lodged in the proximal small intestine stimulates vomiting. Obstruction of the distal jejunum or ileum may not stimulate vomiting but result in distension of the intestinal lumen with fluid and gas. Strangulation of the intestine is an infrequent but dangerous and sometimes unsuspected complication of intestinal obstruction. Strangulation is considered in every animal with sudden and severe abdominal pain, a severe systemic reaction, often including shock that is out of proportion to that with intestinal obstruction, and a poor response to supportive treatment. Pressure produced by a foreign body or intussusception may cause venous stasis and edema followed by disruption of arterial flow and necrosis of the intestinal wall.

Foreign Body

Once an object has passed through the pylorus, the next smallest lumen is the distal duodenum and proximal jejunum, a common site of obstruction.

Clinical Findings

The signs of intestinal foreign body obstruction are variable, depending on the location of the foreign body and its propensity to cause vascular disruption and necrosis of the intestinal wall.

Radiographic Findings

The classic sign of mechanical obstruction is the presence of multiple loops of gas-dilated small intestine of various diameters.

Contrast examination of the small intestine permits confirmation of the diagnosis. Intraluminal obstruction often appears as a radiolucent area surrounded by contrast material outlining the foreign body.

Diagnosis

The diagnosis of foreign body obstruction is based on history, careful abdominal palpation, and abdominal radiographs.

Treatment

The treatment for foreign body obstruction is exploratory celiotomy. The abdomen is exposed by ventral midline abdominal incision of sufficient length to permit adequate inspection of the entire gastrointestinal tract.

If the foreign body has not caused vascular obstruction of the intestinal wall, it is removed through an enterotomy distal to the foreign body and slightly over it. If the foreign body has caused necrosis of the intestinal wall or if viability is in question, resection with end-to-end anastomosis is indicated. Small, sharp foreign bodies, such as a sewing needle, may be treated conservatively. Transit of the foreign object through the alimentary canal is monitored by periodic abdominal radiographs, and the animal is monitored for signs of peritonitis.

Linear Foreign Body

Linear foreign bodies (thread, nylon stocking, string) produce a unique form of intestinal obstruction more common in cats. String may extend through much of the intestinal tract and may be visible wrapped around the base of the tongue. The intestine progressively gathers itself in accordion-like pleats along the linear foreign body. As peristaltic waves continue to attempt to move the irritant along, the linear foreign body saws through the mesenteric side of the intestine. If the intestine is perforated, peritonitis develops. The inflammation and infection at the sites of laceration occasionally are walled off. In these cases, removal of the string is difficult and the intestines may not resume normal function postoperatively.

Clinical Findings

Linear foreign bodies cause signs of intestinal obstruction, with various degrees of vomiting, dehydration, anorexia, depression, and pyrexia.

Radiographic Findings

Radiographic findings include pleating of intestine loops, increased trapped intestinal gas bubbles, obstruction, and peritonitis.

Treatment

The string caught around the tongue is cut and the abdomen is explored. An enterotomy incision is made midway along the site of the string obstruction. As much string as possible is delivered by pulling gently and gradually; then the ends are cut. Additional enterotomies are spaced along the intestine to ensure removal of all string while minimizing the risk of lacerating the intestine. Even if it can be successfully extracted, the intestine may not resume normal function postoperatively.

Intussusception

Intussusception is produced by a vigorous contraction that forces the intestine into the lumen of the adjacent relaxed segment. The components of an intussusception include the invaginated section, called the *intussusceptum,* and the enveloping segment, called the *intussuscipiens.* The mesentery and blood supply to the intussusceptum are included in the invagination; venous obstruction can progress to arterial occlusion and necrosis. An intussusception can progress so that small intestine protrudes from the anus. Intussusception occurs most frequently in young animals, at the ileocecal junction.

Clinical Findings

The cardinal signs of intussusception are vomiting, abdominal pain, passage of bloody mucoid stools, and palpation of a sausage-shaped, minimally painful abdominal mass.

Radiographic Findings

The radiographic findings in intussusception are usually similar to those of mechanical obstruction of the intestine. Contrast radiography is usually necessary to differentiate an intussusception from other causes of intestinal obstruction.

Treatment

The treatment is exploratory celiotomy. The entire small and large intestine is carefully examined. An attempt is made to reduce the intussusception manually. One of the following will occur:

1. The intussusception can be successfully reduced.
2. The intussusception can be reduced, and the serosal surface and possibly a portion of the muscular layer of the intestine are split. These lacerations can be closed with simple interrupted 3-0 synthetic absorbable sutures.
3. The intussusception cannot be manually reduced, or after reduction, the involved segments of intestine are not viable.

If the intussusception cannot be reduced or the intestines are not viable, resection and anastomosis are necessary.

Many cases recur, some during surgery, and techniques should be used to prevent subsequent recurrence. The site of the intussusception can be sutured to the abdominal wall (enteropexy). A method we use successfully is intestinal plication—suturing the small intestine into accordion-like folds by simple interrupted sutures placed to unite adjacent serosal surfaces.

Adhesions

Adhesions rarely cause intestinal obstruction in small animals, although they frequently develop after traumatic and surgical wounds of the peritoneal cavity.

Neoplasia (see Chapter 154)

Mesenteric Torsion (p. 599)

PRINCIPLES OF SMALL-INTESTINAL SURGERY
(pp. 599–611)

Fluid Therapy

Animals with small-intestinal disease frequently require parenteral fluid replacement. Unless the fluid deficit is partially corrected before surgery, an animal may not survive an operation.

Antibiotic Prophylaxis

The decision to use antibiotics for prophylaxis in intestinal surgery is based on an estimation of the bacterial contamination that may occur during the surgical procedure. Prophylactic antibiotics are administered intravenously at induction of anesthesia and continued for a maximum of 24 hours after surgery.

Timing of Surgery

Surgery for mechanical obstruction of the intestines is performed as soon as possible after the diagnosis is made.

Assessment of Intestinal Viability (pp. 600–601)

Asepsis

Every effort is made to minimize bacterial contamination of the peritoneal cavity that occurs with intestinal surgery. The segment of intestine prepared for resection and anastomosis or enterotomy is "packed off" from the peritoneal cavity by layers of moist sponges or laparotomy pads. Intestinal contents are displaced from the resection site before the atraumatic forceps are clamped across the intestinal lumen.

Surgical drapes should be impervious to water. Instruments and equipment used during the intestinal resection and anastomosis or enterotomy are discarded after that procedure is completed, surgical gloves and gowns are changed, the peritoneal cavity is thoroughly lavaged, and closure of the incision in the mesentery and closure of the abdominal wall are performed with clean instruments and suture material.

Principles of Small-Intestinal Anastomosis

Modern surgical techniques for closure of intestinal wounds include various suturing patterns, mechanical stapling devices, and tissue adhesives.

Reconstruction of the intestinal tract after resection can be by end-to-end, end-to-side, or side-to-side technique. Although used in other alimentary tract procedures, a side-to-side or end-to-side technique has no advantages over an end-to-end anastomosis for the small intestine.

Types of End-to-End Anastomoses

The four main types of sutured end-to-end intestinal anastomoses in dogs and cats are the inverting, everting, invaginating, and approximating suture patterns.

The classic technique for human intestinal anastomosis is the two-layer inverting technique. This technique is usually performed with a first layer using a Connell suture pattern and a second layer of interrupted sutures in a Lembert pattern inserted to the level of the submucosa.

The everting intestinal anastomosis technique was developed in an attempt to increase the luminal diameter over inverting patterns. A horizontal mattress pattern has been described to evert all layers of the intestinal wall.

An end-to-end approximating suture technique has been popular with small animal surgeons. This technique was developed to improve intestinal healing by accurate realignment of cut layers of the intestinal wall and to minimize the possibility of luminal reduction, which may occur with an inverting suture pattern. The Gambee pattern is a simple interrupted suture that penetrates the lumen and passes through a small segment of mucosa and submucosa on the same side. The Poth and Gold pattern is a simple interrupted suture that is tied with sufficient tension to cut through the mucosa from beneath and the serosa and muscularis from above and hold just the submucosa in apposition. The appositional technique is a simple interrupted noncrushing suture. Mechanical stapling instruments have been used to create a functional end-to-end enteroanastomosis in man.

Intestinal Healing

Tensile Strength

Stapling Techniques

Stapled anastomosis lines show good anatomical layer alignment but more inflammation than suture techniques.

Luminal Diameter

The greatest decrease in luminal diameter occurred with the everting pattern, and the least occurred with the crushing pattern.

Conclusions

Approximating patterns offer several advantages over single- or two-layer inverting patterns: ease of application, increased luminal diameter at the anastomotic site, and more rapid mucosal regeneration. Approximating patterns also offer some advantages over the everting suture pattern: minimal adhesion formation, more rapid early healing, and better protection against leakage. Postoperative peritoneal adhesions at the anastomotic site are formed at a rate directly proportional to the amount of mucosa everted.

The simple interrupted and simple continuous approximating patterns cause less tissue ischemia at the anastomosis during the first 7 days after surgery than the simple interrupted crushing technique. The continuous approximating pattern causes less mucosal eversion and less postoperative peritoneal adhesion formation than the interrupted patterns.

If a leak occurs at the anastomotic site, the site is resected and the same suture pattern is used to create a new anastomosis. In most instances, a leak from an anastomosis results not from the choice of suture pattern but rather from some undetermined biological factor of wound healing or faulty surgical technique.

Role of the Omentum

Omentum wrapped around an anastomosis provides significant protection and greatly decreases the incidence of postoperative leakage from the anastomosis. Omentum can plug hernial defects, seal off infections and perforations, and impart new blood supply to viscera.

Techniques for Intestinal Anastomosis

Exposure and Examination of Intestines

The entire length of the intestines is thoroughly and gently examined before making a decision about a surgical procedure.

Intestinal Resection and Anastomosis (see also p. 604)

The procedure of choice is end-to-end appositional anastomosis. With disparity between the luminal diameter of the segments to be anastomosed, one of three techniques can be used: With minor luminal disparity, the spacing between simple interrupted sutures or the spacing between needle passes in a simple continuous pattern is greater on the larger lumen side than on the smaller lumen side, resulting in an end-to-end anastomosis without gap or pucker. With moderate luminal disparity, the intestine with the smaller lumen is transected at an angle rather than perpendicularly across the axis, creating a lumen of larger diameter. With marked luminal disparity, the intestinal wall opposite the mesenteric border is cut with scissors to create a spatulated end the same diameter as the larger intestinal segment.

The segment of intestine to be removed is selected after the vascularity of the intestine is assessed. The jejunal branches of the cranial mesenteric artery that supply the segment of intestine are doubly ligated with 3-0 chromic gut with a swaged-on taper needle. A space between the ligatures is left for transection.

Crushing clamps are placed across the intestine at the terminal arcade ligature adjacent to the diseased segment. The clamps are placed perpendicular to the axis of the intestine or angled slightly toward the normal segment to ensure adequate blood supply to the antimesenteric border. Noncrushing intestinal forceps are placed approximately 4 to 6 cm from the crushing clamps. Before these clamps are placed, intestinal contents are milked away from the resection site. The intestine is transected with a scalpel blade, using the crushing clamps as guides. The mesentery is transected with scissors, between each pair of ligatures on the jejunal artery branches.

A simple continuous suture pattern is started adjacent to the mesenteric border, the mesenteric border is sutured, and the pattern is continued around the circumference of the intestines. Using simple interrupted sutures, the first two sutures are placed at the mesenteric and antimesenteric borders. Mild traction is applied to these two sutures, the edges are aligned, and additional sutures are placed. Noncrushing intestinal forceps are used to position and rotate the intestines to facilitate suturing.

Sutures are placed approximately 2 to 3 mm from the cut surface and 3 to 4 mm apart. The sutures are passed through the wall to penetrate the submucosa, avoiding the mucosa, with appositional tension only. The anastomosis is inspected, and gaps or excess mucosal eversion is corrected by placement of additional sutures.

The defect in the mesentery is sutured with 3-0 or 4-0 absorbable suture material, avoiding the jejunal vessels. The anastomosis is washed with warm sterile saline and wrapped with omentum.

Enterotomy

Intestinal contents are expressed from the region of the enterotomy, and noncrushing intestinal forceps are placed across the intestine to minimize spillage. A full-thickness incision is made at the antimesenteric border with a scalpel. The incision may be enlarged as necessary with scissors.

Any everted mucosa is trimmed with scissors before closure is begun. The incision is closed using sutures of 4-0 or 3-0 synthetic absorbable material on a swaged-on cutting needle placed in a simple interrupted or continuous pattern.

Intestinal Biopsy

A full-thickness longitudinal specimen is removed from the antimesenteric border using a scalpel and fine atraumatic forceps. To prevent obstruction of the lumen, the defect is closed in a transverse manner using a single layer of simple interrupted sutures.

Abdominal Lavage and Drainage

After intestinal surgery is completed, the peritoneal cavity is lavaged with sterile saline solution at body temperature to minimize heat loss.

Lavage is effective because bacterial numbers are greatly reduced and debris that may reduce phagocytosis of bacteria is removed. All lavage fluid must be aspirated. Adding povidone-iodine solution to lavage fluid to prevent or treat peritonitis cannot be recommended. Experimental studies have shown that adding antibiotics to lavage fluid does not improve the survival rate of animals with experimental peritonitis when systemic antibiotics are given concurrently. The peritoneal cavity cannot be effectively drained by rubber drains or tubes.

Postoperative Care

Early resumption of oral intake of food and water encourages peristalsis and provides the most convenient route for assimilation of water, electrolytes, calories, and protein. The animal is offered a small amount of water the day after surgery. Once initial thirst has been satisfied and no vomiting has occurred, small amounts of bland food are given.

Three potential problems are abnormal fluid and electrolyte balance and impaired nutrition, complications of the abdominal incision, and adverse consequences of intestinal surgery such as peritonitis, adhesions, short-bowel syndrome, and adynamic ileus.

Peritonitis

After intestinal surgery, animals must be closely monitored for signs of peritonitis. Persistent vomiting is a prominent sign of peritonitis. Fever and leukocytosis are nonspecific indicators of inflammation and may be present with peritonitis. Abdominal radiographs show a lack of intestinal detail and a ground glass appearance.

The most valuable parameter for diagnosis of peritonitis is cytological study of abdominal fluid. Abdominocentesis to collect a sample of peritoneal fluid is performed, with syringe and needle, in the caudal right or left quadrant of the abdomen. If fluid is not obtained, diagnostic peritoneal lavage is performed. In animals with peritonitis, the predominant leukocytes are degenerating neutrophils showing karyolysis; bacteria are free in the fluid and possibly within neutrophils.

The tenets of treatment of peritonitis are (1) stop the source of bacterial contamination, (2) lavage the peritoneal cavity thoroughly with sterile warm fluids to flush out bacteria and debris, and (3) administer broad-spectrum antibiotics effective against enteric organisms.

Adhesions

Ischemic tissue within the peritoneal cavity is the strongest stimulus to formation of permanent adhesions. Irritating contaminants that enter the peritoneal cavity at laparotomy may cause granulomatous inflammation and fibrous peritoneal adhesions.

Short-Bowel Syndrome

Short-bowel syndrome is characterized by intractable diarrhea with impaired absorption of fats, vitamins, and other nutrients. Many factors may be responsible for short-bowel syndrome after intestinal surgery, including (1) extent and site of resection, (2) presence or absence of a functioning ileocecal valve, (3) function of the remaining digestive organs, and (4) time allowed for adaptation of remaining small intestine.

Malabsorption probably results from the rapid transit time and reduced small-intestinal mucosal surface area present in short-bowel syndrome.

The small intestine remaining after extensive resection undergoes compensatory changes. It increases in diameter, microvilli enlarge, and the number of mucosal cells increases, resulting in increased absorption per unit length. This adaptation of the remaining small intestine takes several weeks. During this period, parenteral supplementation of fluids, electrolytes, and nutrition may be necessary for survival.

Long-term medical treatments that may be of value in controlling diarrhea and providing adequate nutrition for dogs with short-bowel syndrome include frequent small low-fat meals, elemental diet supplements, and medium-chain triglyceride oil; vitamin, mineral, and pancreatic enzyme supplements; and medications including antidiarrheals, oral antibiotics, antacids, and bile salt-binding agents.

Vagotomy and pyloroplasty, reversal of single and multiple small and large intestinal segments, production of artificial sphincters, and construction of intestinal loops have been reported to treat short-bowel syndrome. These procedures have not been evaluated clinically.

Ileus

Ileus is a form of intestinal obstruction characterized by inadequate peristaltic activity usually involving the entire gastrointestinal tract. Loss of normal gastrointestinal motility may follow any abdominal operation and may also occur with diseases unrelated to the peritoneal cavity. The intestines rapidly distend with fluid and gas, resulting in impaired absorption. If left untreated, further distension causes greater impairment of absorption.

Clinical signs of ileus include vomiting, anorexia, and fluid and gas distension of the entire gastrointestinal tract. Treatment of ileus is difficult. Every effort is made to prevent this condition by attention to proper surgical techniques.

Metoclopramide, an effective antiemetic drug that enhances gastrointestinal motility, is used to treat ileus. It stimulates gastric contractions, accelerates gastric emptying, and stimulates smooth-muscle contraction in the small intestine. Metoclopramide is administered intravenously, intramuscularly, or orally at 0.2 to 0.4 mg/kg every 4 hours, or is added to intravenous fluid at 1 to 2 mg/kg/24 hr.

CHAPTER 45

Large Intestine (pages 613–627)

SURGICAL DISEASES (pp. 613–620)

Congenital Stenosis and Atresia

These abnormalities occasionally are hereditary, but there is usually no genetic basis for their development. The large intestine is less frequently involved than other areas of the intestinal tract.

The most common congenital anomalies of the large intestine in domestic animals are incomplete (stenosis) and complete (atresia) occlusion of the lumen.

The cause of congenital stenosis and atresia has now been postulated from clinical information. It has been shown experimentally that vascular insufficiency during embryological development is important in the occurrence of intestinal stenosis and atresia of the small intestine and colon.

Colonic Duplication

Enteric duplication is rare in humans and domestic animals. Colonic duplication has been categorized into three separate types:

1. Mesenteric cysts within the mesentery.
2. Diverticula of various lengths lined by epithelium and having a wall composed of smooth muscle.
3. Long colon duplication, characterized by duplication of the entire colon and rectum.

Megacolon

Megacolon is a term applied to a gross dilation of the large intestine. It is a functional disorder in which accumulated fecal material cannot be evacuated from the colon.

Obstipation

Intractable constipation, or obstipation, is an acquired condition that affects both dogs and cats. Primary obstipation is due to colonic impaction with foreign material. Secondary obstipation is caused by any other condition that obstructs the normal passage of feces or causes pain on defecation. If the distension becomes chronic, the colon dramatically increases in diameter, leading to irreversible degenerative changes.

Clinical Findings

Obstipation is more common in older animals. Anorexia, vomiting, tenesmus with passage of little or no stool or small amounts of liquid feces containing blood or mucus, and weight loss all are consistent with obstipation. Plain radiographs are indicated in all suspected cases of obstipation.

Chronic obstipation may be associated with anemia, as well as fluid, electrolyte, and acid-base abnormalities. Proctoscopy or exploratory celiotomy may be necessary for a definitive diagnosis.

Treatment

Fluid, electrolyte, and acid-base disturbances are corrected, obstruction is relieved, and the underlying cause is treated. Enemas and manual decompression are often necessary to relieve a chronic colonic impaction. It may be necessary to repeat the enemas and manual procedures for a few days to evacuate the colon completely. It is extremely important that these procedures be carried out gently to avoid trauma to the colon. Colotomy may be indicated in extreme cases when other efforts fail or trauma to the colon is likely. Once the impaction is removed, measures to prevent recurrence are initiated.

Idiopathic Megacolon

Idiopathic megacolon is an acquired disease in which no organic lesion can be found. It is a well-recognized entity in both man and cats.

Clinical Findings

The disease is characterized by recurrent and progressive episodes of constipation. Anorexia, vomiting, dehydration, depression, and weight loss have been associated with this condition. Abdominal palpation reveals a distended colon. Diagnosis can usually be made from history and physical examination alone; however, a complete evaluation including abdominal radiographs is performed to determine a definitive cause of the problem.

Treatment

Medical therapy for idiopathic megacolon is unrewarding in man and cats.

Good results have been reported in cats with the surgical technique of subtotal colectomy using either an enterocolostomy or a colocolostomy.

Traumatic Perforation

Injuries to the colon result from sharp or blunt trauma to the abdominal wall or from intraluminal trauma.

Clinical Findings

Perforation of the colon causes rapidly progressive peritonitis and septic shock. An inconsistent sign but a strong indicator of colonic trauma is passage of bloody feces or mucus.

Abdominal radiographs may show lack of abdominal organ detail and pneumoperitoneum.

The diagnosis of intestinal perforation can be confirmed by microscopic evaluation of fluid recovered by abdominal paracentesis or peritoneal lavage.

Treatment

An exploratory celiotomy is performed as soon as possible when perforation of the colon is suspected. Fluid replacement and treatment of shock with balanced electrolyte solutions are indicated. Broad-spectrum antibiotics are given as soon as possible.

A complete exploration is carried out in all cases, because multiple abdominal injuries may be present. Perforations of the large intestine are treated by débridement and primary closure or by resection and anastomosis, depending on the surgical findings. The abdomen is lavaged with warm saline, and culture and sensitivity testing are performed. Closure is usually routine except in cases of chronic or severe peritonitis, when the technique of open peritoneal drainage may be indicated.

Nontraumatic Perforation

A nontraumatic form of colonic perforation has been encountered in dogs after parenteral administration of dexamethasone following neurosurgical procedures. All dogs died within 10 days after surgery.

Dogs receiving dexamethasone occasionally develop bloody, mucoid diarrhea. It is advisable to discontinue the medication.

Clinical Findings

Anorexia, vomiting, depression, pyrexia, and abdominal pain were observed in reported dogs. Patients may be presented in shock, with death ensuing quickly.

Treatment

As with traumatic colonic perforation, supportive treatment for shock, administration of broad-spectrum antibiotics, and exploratory celiotomy are essential.

DIAGNOSTIC TECHNIQUES (pp. 620–621)
Endoscopy of the Colon

Endoscopic examination of the colon is a relatively safe, noninvasive procedure that is easy to perform and yields valuable information. Indications include evaluation of patients with chronic obstruction and diagnosis and monitoring, through biopsy, of such conditions as colonic polyp, neoplasia, irritable bowel syndrome, and inflammatory intestinal disease.

Proper preparation is essential to ensure good results. A 24-hour fast and a mild enema the evening before endoscopy may be effective. The use of isosmotic oral electrolyte lavage solutions containing polypropylene glycol has been advocated in dogs.

Patients are placed in right lateral recumbency so that the cecum and colon are less restricted in position and more easily examined. The top of the endoscope is lubricated and inserted into the anus. Air is insufflated, and the instrument is advanced slowly. The lumen is kept in focus during advancement to prevent entering a diverticulum or perforating the colon.

The entire colon is examined before biopsy specimens are taken.

Radiographic Examination of the Colon

Examination of the colon by plain radiographs is often inconclusive; however, if the colon is free of fecal material, films may be easier to interpret.

Endoscopy has generally supplanted the barium enema as a diagnostic method; however, barium enemas may be useful in cecal inversion and when endoscopic equipment is not available.

PRINCIPLES OF COLONIC SURGERY (pp. 621–623)
Preparation

To reduce the possibility of contaminating the abdomen with bacteria during open colonic surgery, mechanical emptying and cleaning are indicated. Most microbiological studies report that cleaning the colon does not significantly alter the concentration of cecal bacteria.

Antimicrobial Prophylaxis

Although there is controversy about how antibiotics should be used in large intestinal surgery, antimicrobial agents reduce the risk of infection. Metronidazole, which is absorbed from the intestinal tract, has been advocated in combination with neomycin or kanamycin. The number of anaerobes is significantly reduced if the preparation is started at least 48 hours before surgery. Another oral combination that has gained wide popularity is neomycin and erythromycin.

Healing and Suture Methods

A normal colonic wound is at its weakest until the third day after an anastomosis. The wound then rapidly gains strength so that by 7 to 11 days after surgery it resists bursting as well as nonoperated intestine. The goal of primary healing in the gastrointestinal tract can be attained and complications avoided if some important surgical principles are considered. Excessive tension at the surgical site can result in dehiscence and leakage.

Successful use of a mechanical stapling instrument for colocolostomy and ileocolostomy has been described in man. In an experimental study of normal dogs comparing hand-sutured with stapled colonic anastomoses, the anastomoses closed by staples were superior because they had the least tissue reaction, most mature fibrous connective tissue, lowest number of mucoceles and necrotic areas, least reduction in luminal diameter, and highest tensile strength.

Surgical Considerations

A complete abdominal exploration is carried out to define the full extent of the disease process and to put in perspective any other related or unrelated abdominal conditions.

The colon is gently isolated and "packed off" with moistened laparotomy pads to prevent contamination of the abdominal cavity and kept moist with warm saline. Meticulous hemostasis is used to prevent excess blood loss, to improve visibility, and to prevent free or clotted blood from acting as a medium for bacterial growth. Any gross leakage of intestinal contents is removed to maintain a minimally contaminated field.

The exteriorized colon is mechanically cleaned with saline-soaked sponges before relocation within the abdomen. The abdominal cavity is flushed with warm saline to remove any debris or blood clots. Drains may be effective to maintain drainage from a localized site in the abdomen; however, they are not effective for generalized abdominal drainage.

Open peritoneal drainage is only performed in advanced septic peritonitis and when proper nursing care is available.

Postoperative Considerations

The most significant postoperative complication is infection due to either contamination during the surgical procedure or leakage at the surgical site. Small amounts of water and a low-residue diet are offered on the day after surgery. Patients are usually discharged on the third postoperative day.

SURGICAL TECHNIQUES (pp. 623–626)
Colotomy

A simple longitudinal incision is made on the antimesenteric border to relieve an intraluminal obstruction or remove a foreign body. The incision is closed, without tension, in one or two layers. If there is any concern about tension at the suture line or lumen diameter, a resection and anastomosis are considered.

Resection and Anastomosis

The surgical anatomy of the area, especially the blood supply, is an important consideration. Carmalt forceps are placed across the colon at the transection sites. The colonic contents are milked away from the forceps for 3 to 5 cm, and noncrushing intestinal forceps, such as Doyen forceps, are applied. The colon is transected with a scalpel between the crushing and noncrushing forceps along the edge of the crushing forceps. Suturing is started at the mesenteric border. Simple interrupted penetrating sutures are placed until the antimesenteric border is reached. The intestine is turned 180°, and suturing is commenced at the mesenteric border until the antimesenteric border is again reached and the anastomosis is complete.

Typhlectomy (pp. 624–625)

Pull-Through Colonic Resection (pp. 625–626)

A pull-through resection of the colon is indicated when an anastomosis has to be made in the pelvic canal. There are few indications for this procedure in veterinary surgery, and complications, including anastomotic leakage and pelvic abscess, are common.

CHAPTER 46
Diseases of the Anus and Rectum (pages 627–645)

ANORECTAL STRICTURES (pp. 627–628)

Anorectal strictures usually occur secondary to proctitis, chronic anal sacculitis, penetrating foreign bodies, trauma, or perianal fistulas or as an iatrogenic complication of anorectal surgery. Carcinomas involving the rectal wall can cause secondary stricture formation.

Clinical Signs and Diagnosis

The majority of animals have dyschezia, constipation, and tenesmus. Secondary megacolon can occur in chronic cases. Digital rectal examination reveals the extent and location of the stricture. Deep biopsy of the stricture should be performed to allow differentiation of primary strictures from neoplasia.

Treatment

Superficial strictures involving the mucosa and submucosa can occasionally be successfully treated by bougienage. More extensive strictures require surgical treatment involving resection of the stricture using a partial or complete anoplasty procedure (e.g., rectal pull-through). Fecal incontinence, stricture formation, and wound dehiscence are potential complications of surgery.

ANAL AND RECTAL PROLAPSE (pp. 628–629)

Prolapse usually occurs secondary to tenesmus resulting from urogenital or anorectal disease.

Clinical Signs

With anal (partial) prolapse, only the mucosa protrudes from the anal opening. In rectal (complete) prolapse, a double-layer invagination of the rectum protrudes through the anal canal.

Small- or large-intestinal intussusceptions should be differentiated from rectal prolapse.

Treatment

Using general anesthesia or an epidural, the prolapse is reduced and a purse-string retention suture is placed at the anocutaneous line using nonabsorbable material. The purse-string suture is loosely tied, allowing insertion of a lubricated finger in large dogs or a thermometer in toy breeds or cats. A narcotic epidural injection can be given prior to anesthetic recovery to reduce rectal straining. A low-residue diet and stool softener are given after surgery. The purse-string is left in place for 3 to 5 days.

Colopexy

A routine caudal midline celiotomy is performed, and the prolapse manually reduced by applying traction on the colon. Once the prolapse is reduced, several sutures 1 to 2 cm apart in a single or double row are placed into the seromuscular wall of the descending colon and the transverse abdominal muscle. When the prolapsed segment is devitalized, necrotic, or severely self-traumatized, amputation and rectal anastomosis are performed.

Rectal Amputation

PERIANAL FISTULATION (pp. 629–633)

Perianal fistula or anal furunculosis is characterized by multiple chronic, ulcerating sinuses or fistulous tracts involving the perianal region.

Pathophysiology

The exact cause of perianal fistulation is unknown. In affected breeds, low tail carriage and a broad tail base may be predisposing defects causing poor ventilation, accumulation of fecal material, moisture, and glandular secretions.

Clinical Signs

Dogs with perianal fistula have a history of dyschezia, hematochezia, constipation, a malodorous mucopurulent discharge, pain associated with elevation of the tail, excessive licking of the perianal region, and personality changes.

Dogs may require heavy sedation or general anesthesia for elevation of the tail and examination of the perineum. Cleaning the purulent discharge from the area reveals multiple draining ulcers, sinuses, or fistulas with formation of secondary granulation tissue. The severity of lesions can vary from one or two localized draining tracts to 360° involvement. Rectal examination is performed to determine anal sphincter tone and to search for stenosis or inflammation directly involving the rectal wall or anal sphincter. The anal sacs are palpated and expressed if possible. Although the anal sacs are not usually the primary source of fistulas, they can be secondarily involved. With a dog sedated or anesthetized, all sinus and fistulous tracts are bluntly probed using a grooved director to determine the extent and depth of each tract and degree of communication.

The differential diagnosis of mild cases includes chronic anal sac abscesses. Fistulous tracts from anal sac disease are usually few and communicate directly with the anal sac. Perianal adenocarcinomas can be ulcerated, with multiple draining tracts, and can be confused with severe chronic perianal fistulas. Histological examination may be necessary to differentiate severe perianal fistulation from neoplasia.

Treatment

Medical treatment of perianal fistulas is usually unsuccessful.

Surgical treatment currently provides the most acceptable result. The various methods of surgical treatment include electrosurgery, cryosurgery, surgical débridement with fulguration of diseased tissue using chemical cautery, exteriorization and fulguration with electrocautery and open healing, and surgical resection of sinuses and fistulous tracts with primary closure or open healing of the wound. The main objective of surgical treatment is preservation of surrounding normal perianal tissues with complete removal or destruction of all diseased tissue. Each surgical technique has inherent advantages and disadvantages.

Surgical excision of perianal fistulas is one of the more favorable methods for treating the disease. The main objective of this technique is to excise all diseased tissue while preserving as much of the external anal sphincter as possible. The anal or rectal mucosa just cranial to the line of resection is sutured to the adjacent skin. Because secondary involvement of the anal sacs is common, bilateral anal sacculectomy is performed. After excision of all diseased tissue, the wound is thoroughly lavaged with isotonic fluid. The wound can be either left open to heal by second intention or closed primarily. In severe cases with multiple sinuses and fistulas involving the anus and external anal sphincter, partial or complete excision of the anus and sphincter may be required (e.g., partial or complete anoplasty).

Postoperative complications associated with surgical excision include fecal incontinence, flatulence, tenesmus, diarrhea, incisional dehiscence, constipation, anal stenosis, and recurrence of disease. Incisional dehiscence is encountered with excision and primary suturing techniques. Factors predisposing to dehiscence include excessive tension or motion across the incision, poorly placed sutures, and infection or ischemic injury to the incisional edges.

High tail amputation (caudectomy) can be used for treating severe perianal fistulas. The main rationale for this procedure is to decrease fecal contamination of the perineum and increase ventilation. The most common complication is recurrence.

Postoperative Complications

Complications can occur after any of the different surgical techniques used for treating perianal fistulas. The type of surgery and severity of the disease process determine the frequency of each complication. The more common and serious complications are anal incontinence, anal stricture, and recurrence of fistulas. All owners should be warned of the risk of recurrence.

BENIGN AND MALIGNANT TUMORS OF THE ANUS AND RECTUM (See Chapter 154) (pp. 633–638)

Rectoanal Polyps

The most common benign tumors involving the anorectal area are adenomatous polyps. Polyps can be sessile, raised, or pedunculated, and single or multiple. Gross and histological differentiation of polyps from rectal carcinomas can occasionally be difficult.

Clinical Signs

Blood and mucus may be present in the feces. Tenesmus can occur and if severe can cause secondary rectal prolapse. A dog is often seen after prolapse of the polyp from the anus.

Diagnosis

The majority of polyps involving the anal canal and distal rectum can be palpated. Histological examination is performed in all cases.

Treatment

Pedunculated and small sessile polyps can be removed from the anus and distal rectum using electrocoagulation, surgical excision with suture placement, or simple ligation. Larger sessile polyps involving a large area or circumference of rectal mucosa may require surgical techniques (e.g., intestinal resection) used for the removal of anorectal carcinomas.

Malignant Anorectal Neoplasia

Rectal or anal adenocarcinoma is the most common malignant tumor in dogs.

Clinical Signs and Diagnosis

Clinical signs associated with neoplasia of the anorectal region include diarrhea, dyschezia, tenesmus, passage of blood and mucus with feces, and painful defecation. The diagnosis of anorectal neoplasia requires physical examination, including digital rectal examination. Endoscopy or proctoscopy is useful in assessing the size and extent of the tumor and in obtaining biopsy specimens.

Preoperative Preparation for Anorectal Surgery

To decrease postoperative complications associated with wound infection and anastomotic dehiscence, effective preoperative intestinal preparation may be beneficial in dogs and cats. The main goal of large-intestinal preparation is to decrease fecal flow during surgery and reduce fecal bacterial numbers.

Surgical Treatment

The surgical approach and method of resection used to remove anorectal malignant tumors or invasive benign tumors depend on the location of the tumor. Tumor location can be divided into three regions as determined by physical examination and proctoscopic or endoscopic findings: (1) the colorectal junction and cranial third of the rectum, (2) the middle third of the rectum, and (3) the caudal third of the rectum and the anal canal. For tumors involving the colorectal junction and cranial rectal region, an abdominal colorectal resection and anastomosis are recommended. An ischial-pubic flap osteotomy is often required for additional surgical exposure. For tumors in the midrectal region, a dorsal perineal approach to the rectum has been described. For tumors involving the caudal third of the rectum and anal region, a rectal pull-through procedure or 360° anoplasty can be performed.

Abdominal Colorectal Resection and Anastomosis (pp. 635–636). Additional exposure of the cranial rectum is often necessary and can be achieved using a pelvic (ischial-pubic) flap osteotomy.

Dorsal Perineal Approach for Midrectal Resection. A purse-string suture is placed around the anus. An inverted U-shaped incision is made from the midpoint of one ischial tuberosity, extending dorsomedially over the top of the anus and ventrolaterally to the opposite ischial tuberosity. To expose the dorsal pelvic canal and rectum, the rectococcygeal muscle is undermined and transected near its attachment at the ventral surface of the coccygeal vertebrae. The nerves are closely associated with the peritoneal attachment to the rectum. Care should be taken to prevent damage to the caudal rectal nerve and autonomic nerve fibers located within the peritoneal reflection. Resections that include the peritoneal reflection may result in fecal incontinence due to nerve damage to the internal anal sphincter, even if innervation to the external sphincter is undamaged.

After the anastomosis is completed, the area is lavaged with warm sterile fluid. Two small Penrose drains are placed into the ischiorectal fossa.

Rectal Pull-Through Procedure (pp. 637–638). This procedure is indicated for tumors located in the caudal aspect of the rectum and anal canal. Location of the tumor and involvement of the external anal sphincter determine the location of the skin or mucous membrane incision.

Postoperative Complications

Anastomotic dehiscence with leakage and stricture formation are the most significant complications.

CONGENITAL ANAL AND RECTAL ABNORMALITIES
(pp. 638–640)

ANAL SAC DISEASES (pp. 640–643)

Diseases of the anal sac occur frequently in dogs and infrequently in cats. Disorders of the anal sac include impaction, sacculitis, abscesses, and neoplasia.

Pathophysiology

The secretory potential of the anal sac varies. Animals that produce large amounts of thick secretions and have an unusually small duct system or anal irritation have an increased risk of developing anal sac disease.

Diagnosis

Non-neoplasic anal sac disease consists of three types: impaction, sacculitis, and abscesses. All probably represent variations of the same process rather than separate diseases.

Clinical Signs

The characteristic signs of anal sac impaction or infection include frequent dragging or rubbing of the anus on the ground or carpet. The affected animal often persistently licks or bites at the anus, tail base, or skin on the side of the perineum, resulting in acute moist dermatitis.

Nonsurgical Treatment

The treatment for anal sac disease depends on the type of disease. Anal sac impaction and acute anal sacculitis are often treated conservatively. Recurrent episodes of severe impaction, anal sacculitis, abscesses, and anal sac adenocarcinoma are indications for anal sacculectomy.

Anal Sacculectomy (pp. 641–642)

Before surgical excision of an infected anal sac, the infection is treated medically. If surgery is performed during the acute inflammatory state, excessive friability of the anal sac may be encountered, resulting in incomplete removal of the anal sac and bacterial contamination of surrounding tissues. Surgical techniques for anal sac excision are closed or open.

The closed technique is performed by making a vertical incision over the anal sac and bluntly dissecting through the sphincter muscle until the sac is reached.

The open technique for anal sacculectomy is easy and quick to perform. This technique permits exposure of the secretory lining of the anal sac and helps ensure complete anal sac and duct removal.

Postoperative Complications

Careful surgical technique is necessary to prevent complications, including fecal incontinence, chronic draining tracts, tenesmus, and dyschezia. Fecal incontinence is a serious postoperative complication and may be associated with surgical trauma to the external anal sphincter and caudal rectal nerve during resection. Chronic draining tracts following anal sacculectomies result from incomplete excision of the mucosal lining of the anal sac or its duct.

RECTOCUTANEOUS FISTULAS (pp. 643–644)

Rectocutaneous fistulas are tracts located between the rectum and skin surrounding the anus, usually in the distal rectum.

Pathogenesis

Rectocutaneous fistulas can be caused by external trauma such as a bite wound or a penetrating object, internal trauma secondary to a fractured pelvis, or a rectal foreign body. Pararectal abscesses or ruptured anal sacs can evolve to rectocutaneous fistulas. Iatrogenic rectocutaneous fistulas can be a complication of anal sacculectomy or perineal herniorrhaphy.

Clinical Signs and Diagnosis

The primary sign of rectocutaneous fistulas is the presence of fecal material passing through the anus and pararectal wound.

Treatment

Surgical treatment involves placing Allis tissue forceps into the rectum via the anus and grasping the rectal wall at the cranial edge of the wound. The rectal wall at the cranial edge of the wound is gently undermined sufficiently to retract it to the mucocutaneous junction without tension. The mucous membrane between the mucocutaneous junction of the anus and the caudal border of the fistula is excised to provide a vascular base for the transposed rectal wall, and the cranial edge of the fistula is sutured to the mucocutaneous junction of the anus with nonabsorbable sutures. The fistula resolves spontaneously once the rectal defect is eliminated.

CHAPTER 47

Liver and Biliary System
(pages 645–677)

Surgical Diseases and Procedures
(pages 645–660)

DISEASES OF THE LIVER AND EXTRAHEPATIC BILIARY TRACT (pp. 645–648)

Trauma

Isolated liver injuries are uncommon, and the possibility of injuries to other organs must be considered. Blunt or penetrating abdominal trauma may injure the hepatobiliary system. Severe hemorrhage can result from large parenchymal fissures that cannot be managed by fluid replacement therapy, and exploratory celiotomy may be necessary to arrest bleeding.

Biliary tract rupture may also occur secondary to both blunt and sharp trauma. Recognition of biliary tract trauma most often is delayed from several days to 2 or 3 weeks. Clinical signs result from bile peritonitis.

Abdominal paracentesis using a multifenestrated catheter (dialysis catheter) with or without diagnostic peritoneal lavage increases the accuracy of assessment of hepatobiliary injury. With penetrating abdominal injuries such as gunshot wounds, immediate exploration of the abdominal cavity is indicated and careful, systematic examination of the liver lobes and extrahepatic biliary tree is performed.

The principles of hemorrhage control, débridement of devitalized tissue with precise biliary and vascular control, and extensive drainage of the perihepatic spaces are well accepted. Bleeding within the depths of the liver parenchyma can be managed by specific vascular ligation when a vessel can be identified. Electrocoagulation can be used selectively. Lobectomy is indicated when total or extensive disruption of a segment of a lobe has occurred or when it is the only technique that will control life-threatening hemorrhage.

Hepatic Abscess

Liver abscesses are rare in dogs and cats.

Cholelithiasis (p. 647)

Naturally occurring cholelithiasis in dogs and cats is rare.

Cholecystitis (pp. 647–648)

Like gallstones, cholecystitis is infrequently reported in dogs and cats. Terms used to describe cholecystitis include *acute, necrotizing, chronic,* and *emphysematous.*

Extrahepatic Biliary Obstruction

Extrahepatic biliary obstruction occurs when disease processes interfere with the normal flow of bile from the liver and gallbladder into the intestine. Neoplastic, lithogenic, inflammatory, parasitic, and congenital causes are known. Bile duct stricture due to chronic pancreatitis is the most common cause of extrahepatic obstruction in dogs. Icterus is the hallmark of physical findings but is not restricted to extrahepatic cholestasis. Diagnostic ultrasonography has become the single most useful noninvasive tool for demonstrating extrahepatic cholestasis.

SURGICAL PROCEDURES (pp. 648–659)

General Considerations

Regenerative Capacity

Removal of 70 to 80 per cent of the canine liver is tolerated, and the capacity for regeneration is well documented. A patient's general condition and the relative health of the remaining hepatic tissue have a more profound effect on survival than the amount of liver removed.

Metabolic Alterations

Hypoglycemia may occur within 48 hours of partial hepatectomy in humans and dogs. Glucagon levels in portal blood increase within hours after partial hepatectomy. AP and ALT levels are increased within 1 to 3 days of removal of 70 per cent or more of the liver in dogs. Plasma ammonia levels were significantly increased in anesthetized dogs that had 60 per cent hepatectomies.

Vascular Alterations

Ligation of the hepatic artery or disruption of portal blood flow to the liver results in increased blood flow in the remaining hepatic vasculature. Although ligation of the portal vein results in increased hepatic arterial flow, it is incompatible with life. Depending on the integrity of the portal system, the arterial blood supply to the liver can be interrupted without severely affecting hepatic function.

Antibiotic Therapy

Antibiotics are administered when hepatobiliary surgery is performed. The drug should be in a form suitable for intravenous administration and active against enteric organisms commonly encountered.

Approach and Exposure

The standard approach to the liver is through a ventral midline abdominal incision.

Other Considerations
Surgical Drainage

In dogs and cats, drains are infrequently used after hepatobiliary surgery.

Biopsy
Percutaneous Biopsy

Percutaneous biopsies are minimally invasive and are reserved for generalized diseases. Laparoscopic biopsy provides visual control of percutaneous biopsy and selectivity in site of biopsy.

Surgical Biopsy

A marginal biopsy sample is most easily taken by looping a ligature over a protruding portion of a liver lobe margin and crushing parenchyma as the ligature is tightened. A Keyes skin biopsy punch may also be used for sampling liver tissue either near the margin or from more central areas. A pledget of absorbable gelatin foam (Gelfoam) may be used to plug the biopsy defect and control hemorrhage.

Partial Hepatectomy

Indications for partial liver removal include localized masses such as abscesses or neoplasia, trauma, vascular alterations (arteriovenous fistula), and research. Various techniques can be used, such as parenchymal crushing, anatomical dissection, mass ligation, and surgical stapling.

Partial Lobectomy

Partial lobectomy implies separation of hepatic parenchyma through a portion of a lobe other than at the hilus. Sharp capsular incision improves the technical objective of leaving a smooth margin of exposed parenchyma on completion of the resection. The blunt end of a Bard scalpel handle is used to separate the hepatic parenchyma. Small vessels are encountered and are best occluded by electrocoagulation. Larger vessels (> 2 mm in diameter) are ligated or clipped with vascular occluding staples (Hemoclips) before transecting distally.

Complete Lobectomy (pp. 651–652)

In small dogs and cats, either of the left liver lobes can be removed after placing a single encircling ligature in an area that has been bluntly crushed with instruments or fingers. Mass ligation should not be used either in large dogs or for central or right division lobes.

General Considerations of Extrahepatic Biliary Tract Surgery (pp. 652–659)
Indications

Extrahepatic biliary tract obstruction and trauma are the two most common indications for biliary tract surgery.

Primary Repair

Primary repair of the extrahepatic biliary tree has been reported, but morbidity associated with surgical complications is frequent. Avulsion of the bile duct at its junction with the duodenum is most often not amenable to primary repair and requires bile flow diversion.

Stents

In traumatic injuries in which dilation of the duct has not occurred as in obstructive diseases, the small diameter of the bile duct limits primary choledochal repair and use of a stent in dogs and cats.

Bile Flow Diversion

Obstructive and traumatic diseases often irreversibly damage the functional integrity of the bile duct. In most cases, the gallbladder is only secondarily involved and can function as a conduit in the flow of bile to the intestine. When the bile duct is damaged distal to the entry of hepatic ducts from the right and left divisions of the liver, bile flow diversion can be easily achieved.

Surgery of the Gallbladder and Bile Duct

Cholecystectomy

Cholecystectomy is performed when a disease process of the gallbladder is primary in etiology or when the gallbladder is secondarily involved but has severe structural changes or is likely to be implicated in recurrent disease.

Cholecystectomy may be performed either by starting the dissection at the attachment of the fundus to the hepatic fossa and dissecting toward the cystic duct or by identifying the cystic duct and cystic artery and dissecting toward the fundus.

Bile is diluted and removed with abdominal lavage before abdominal closure. Cannulation of the bile duct is more important to ensure its patency. After cannulation, the stump of the cystic duct is ligated circumferentially. A sufficient stump is left to prevent encroachment of the ligature on the two hepatic ducts entering the bile duct near the entrance of the cystic duct.

Tube Cholecystotomy

Tube cholecystostomy is used for biliary decompression when the bile duct is temporarily obstructed, as in acute pancreatitis, but is expected to remain functional after the primary inflammatory process is resolved. An advantage of tube cholecystostomy is that positive-contrast cholangiography can be easily performed to determine bile duct patency before tube removal.

Choledochotomy

Direct incision into the bile duct is limited to chronic obstruction causing marked dilation of the duct. In such cases, direct duct exploration can be performed with a reasonable expectation of a secure ductal repair without leakage if the obstruction can be removed. Closure of the incision is achieved with 4-0 absorbable suture in a simple continuous or interrupted pattern.

Bile Flow Diversion

Cholecystoduodenostomy

Cholecystoduodenostomy is the procedure of choice for bile flow diversion in dogs and cats when the gallbladder is not directly involved in the disease process causing the bile duct obstruction.

Stoma contraction can be expected to decrease the original stoma size by 50 per cent. Because gallbladders vary in size in normal small cats and obstructed large dogs, an anastomosis that corresponds to the length of an incision from the gallbladder fundus to the infundibulum or up to 4 cm in length, whichever is shorter, is recommended.

The gallbladder is mobilized as described for cholecystectomy. Once mobilized, it is brought into apposition with the antimesenteric surface of the descending duodenum at the most tension-free site. The gallbladder is drained, and an appropriate cholecystostomy is made. A corresponding duodenotomy is made in the antimesenteric surface of the duodenum. Absorbable 3-0 suture material is used to create the anastomosis, using either a simple interrupted pattern or a continuous pattern.

Cholecystojejunostomy

Diversion of bile directly into the jejunum is a nonphysiological technique that should be considered only when diversion of bile into the duodenum cannot be accomplished. A physiological increase in gastric acid secretion occurs. An impairment of duodenal mechanisms responsible for inhibition of gastric secretion is postulated. Duodenal ulceration may develop.

Sphincter-Altering Procedures (pp. 658–659)

Tube Drainage

The biliary tract may be temporarily drained by inserting a polyethylene, Silastic, or rubber tube drain through the gallbladder or major duodenal papilla and into the bile duct. A cholecystotomy or duodenotomy over the major duodenal papilla is required to insert the drain.

Portosystemic Shunts (pages 660–667)

NORMAL VASCULAR ANATOMY

Blood is supplied to a fully developed liver by two afferent vessels: the hepatic artery, with well-oxygenated blood, and the portal vein, which drains blood from the splanchnic organs and spleen. All afferent blood must flow through the hepatic sinusoids before reaching the efferent vessels and the right heart. The hepatic veins represent the confluence of multiple tributaries draining the various liver lobes.

ABNORMAL VASCULAR ANATOMY

Portosystemic shunts in dogs and cats are recognized as a single anomalous vessel (76 per cent) or multiple extrahepatic shunts (24 per cent). Single shunts are congenital and may be located extrahepatically (53 per cent) or intrahepatically (23 per cent). Multiple extrahepatic shunts are secondary to portal hypertension, which may result from primary liver disease, manipulation of the portal circulation, or congenital arteriovenous fistula. Single extrahepatic shunts occur when any major splanchnic vessel bypasses or leaves the portal vein before the hepatic portal and communicates directly with the vena cava or other systemic vessel. Intrahepatic shunts occur when the fetal ductus venosus remains patent or other intraparenchymal portal-to-hepatic vein or inferior vena caval communications exist.

LIVER HEMODYNAMICS

The liver receives one-quarter of the total cardiac output, three-quarters of which is transported in the portal vein and the remainder in the hepatic artery. Portal venous pressures are 6 to 12 mm Hg, and hepatic arterial pressures are 80 to 120 mm Hg.

PATHOPHYSIOLOGY

The developmental pathophysiology associated with single shunts may differ significantly from multiple shunts, but the presenting clinical signs, biochemical profiles, and diagnostic tests may yield indistinguishable parameters.

Hematological values indicate mild anemia, microcytosis, hypoproteinemia (predominantly hypoalbuminemia), leukocytosis, and coagulation abnormalities. Serum biochemical abnormalities include decreased blood urea nitrogen, cholesterol, albumin, potassium, and glucose levels and ratios of branched-chain to aromatic amino acids, as well as increased retention of serum AP, serum ALT, serum aspartate transaminase, total bilirubin, blood ammonia, bile acids, and sulfobromophthalein. Bile acids are a sensitive indicator of hepatic dysfunction.

NEUROLOGICAL ABNORMALITIES AND HEPATIC ENCEPHALOPATHY

Most animals with portosystemic abnormalities have neurological dysfunction associated with hepatic encephalopathy The animals are often depressed and stuporous, appear blind, and press their head against walls or furniture. The predominant hypothesis describes coma-producing toxins that when combined with other metabolites produce effects disproportionate to their individual effects. Ammonia is the primary factor in this theory; it is produced primarily in the colon and small intestine from metabolism of dietary protein. The concentration of blood ammonia does not correlate well with the severity of clinical signs, but the presence of abnormally elevated blood ammonia levels in both the resting and the postprandial or post-tolerance states is a consistent diagnostic finding.

The possible causes of hepatic encephalopathy are numerous, and synergism between causative agents exists. Although the treatment of dogs with portosystemic shunts is surgical, recognition of the causes of encephalopathy is essential when the response to surgery is poor.

PATHOLOGY

Histopathological descriptions of liver morphology in dogs with portosystemic shunts are remarkably similar regardless of the presence of single or multiple shunts. The description is predominantly one of diffuse parenchymal atrophy with lobular collapse, compressed hepatic cords, close proximity of portal triads, inconspicuous portal veins, and proliferation of the small vessels, arterioles, and lymphatics.

DIAGNOSIS

Tentative diagnosis of portosystemic shunt can be made on the basis of history, clinical signs, and biochemical abnormalities. Abdominal radiographs may demonstrate a small liver, enlarged kidneys, cystic or renal calculi, and ascites. A definitive diagnosis of portosystemic shunt can be made with cranial mesenteric angiography, jejunal venography, transabdominal splenoportography, or nuclear scintigraphy.

These techniques are the diagnostic methods currently available to determine the location of the shunt before surgery. Although contrast radiography outlines the location of the shunts, it cannot be used as a prognostic indication of portal vascularization of the liver. Although blood flow to the liver is reduced in the presence of portosystemic shunts, the capacity of the liver to receive increased portal flow after shunt attenuation may be only moderately depressed and reversible with time.

MEDICAL THERAPY

Medical therapy of portosystemic anomalies is instituted before surgery. If surgical intervention is unsuccessful, medical management may alleviate clinical signs.

Prevention of signs of hepatic encephalopathy is a primary goal of treatment. Ureolytic and proteolytic bacteria may initially be reduced by administering oral aminoglycoside antibiotics (neomycin sulfate), but the long-term efficacy of these antibiotics is equivocal. Lactulose also alters the metabolism of amino acids by enteric bacteria and acts as a cathartic. When severe signs of hepatic encephalopathy are present, enemas with warm water, neomycin, lactulose, or other carbohydrates may reduce morbidity.

Poor ability to handle water loads and maintain adequate blood glucose levels has been observed both before surgery and in the immediate postoperative period. Antibiotics are administered to animals with septicemia or if liver enzyme elevations indicate active hepatic necrosis or damage. Penicillins are the antibiotics of choice for hepatic anaerobes (clostridia).

ANESTHESIA AND DRUG RESPONSE

Anesthetic protocols should reflect the impaired liver function in portosystemic shunts. Premedication with meperidine hydrochloride (2 to 4 mg/kg IM) and atropine (0.04 mg/kg IM) is recommended. Anesthetic induction may be produced by oxymorphone (0.1 to 0.2 mg/kg IV), ketamine (2 to 4 mg/kg IV) with diazepam (0.2 to 0.4 mg/kg IV), or gas. Anesthesia is usually maintained with isoflurane and supplemented with oxymorphone or diazepam if necessary. Cautious administration of dopamine hydrochloride (2.5 to 5.0 µg/kg/min; 80 to 200 µg in 500 ml 5 per cent dextrose in water to effect) may be necessary in severely hypotensive patients.

Sudden constriction of hepatic vein sphincters has been suggested to explain acute hepatic congestion. Glucocorticoids (Solu Delta Cortef, 20 mg/kg) are immediately administered, and manipulation of the liver and splanchnic vasculature is temporarily halted; all constricting ligatures are released if present.

SURGERY OF SINGLE EXTRAHEPATIC PORTOSYSTEMIC SHUNTS (pp. 670–672)

SURGERY OF INTRAHEPATIC PORTOSYSTEMIC SHUNTS (pp. 672–674)

SURGERY OF MULTIPLE EXTRAHEPATIC PORTOSYSTEMIC SHUNTS (pp. 674–675)

RESULTS AND COMPLICATIONS

Of patients with single extrahepatic portosystemic shunts, 90 to 95 per cent become functionally normal after surgical attenuation or obstruction of their anomalous vessel. Of single intrahepatic portosystemic shunts, 70 to 75 per cent improve clinically after surgical intervention. The majority of multiple extrahepatic portosystemic shunts (60 per cent) also improve after surgery.

Postoperative morbidity is most commonly caused by hypoglycemia. Potentially fatal portal hypertension occurs occasionally and is characterized by sudden hypotension and shock. Immediate surgical intervention to release the shunt ligature is necessary if severe splanchnic congestion develops.

Most dogs with intrahepatic shunt continue to have biochemical abnormalities postoperatively even if they have improved clinically. Postoperative nuclear scintigraphic studies indicate quantitative improvement of portal blood flow with time.

Postoperative morbidity is greatest with multiple extrahepatic portosystemic shunts. Caudal vena cava banding often produces ascites and pelvic limb edema. Ascites and limb edema usually improve over 4 to 6 weeks but if severe may be treated with diuretics. Biochemical abnormalities persist, although clinical improvement often occurs.

Less than 5 per cent of animals with portosystemic shunts are cats. Although the numbers are smaller, postoperative improvement seems less predictable.

CHAPTER 48

Surgery of the Exocrine Pancreas (pages 678–691)

SURGICAL DISEASES (pp. 678–686)
Pancreatitis

Inflammation of the pancreas is classified into acute, recurrent, and chronic forms.

In dogs, an acute, self-limiting pancreatitis characterized by mild interstitial edema of the gland is most common. Middle-aged, obese, sedentary female dogs are at risk for pancreatitis. Breeds with an incidence of pancreatitis higher than expected include miniature schnauzers and dachshunds. Pancreatitis is rarely detected in healthy, active dogs.

In cats, pancreatitis is characterized by chronic low-grade interstitial inflammation. Characterization of feline patients at risk for pancreatitis has not been made, although one investigator reported the condition in older cats (8 to 14 years).

Acute Pancreatitis
Etiology

The etiology of naturally occurring pancreatitis in dogs and cats remains obscure. Several factors have been associated with the condition. In dogs, high-fat diets, hyperlipidemia, hypercalcemia, drugs, thoracolumbar neurosurgery, infectious agents, and ischemia are considered precipitating factors in acute pancreatitis.

Pathophysiology

Acute pancreatitis is characterized by premature activation and release of proteolytic and lipolytic enzymes, which cause autodigestion of the gland. For pancreatitis to occur, the gland must be actively secreting digestive juices and enzymes, the excretory duct must be obstructed, and pancreatic acinar cells must undergo cytolysis and release of degradative enzymes. Intracellular breakdown of zymogen granules causes release of enzymes and conversion of trypsinogen into trypsin. Activation of trypsin is the key factor in initiation of the degradative biological cascades.

In addition to enzyme activation and direct tissue injury, trypsin is responsible for activation of the complement, coagulation, and fibrinolytic systems. The result is local and disseminated derangements of homeostasis, including hypotension, hemorrhage, and inflammation.

The culmination of a progressive hemorrhagic pancreatitis is irreversible shock associated with multisystemic organ failure. Hypotension, endotoxemia, septicemia, disseminated intravascular coagulation, and acute respiratory failure contribute to death.

Diagnosis

The anamnesis may include ingestion of a fatty meal, abdominal trauma, or long-term administration of corticosteroids. Vomiting, due to afferent stimulation from gastrointestinal and peritoneal irritation, is a common clinical sign. Abdominal pain and distension are present, and diarrhea secondary to paralytic ileus can also occur. The animal may have an elevated temperature due to pain, peritonitis, and pyrogen release. Transient diabetes mellitus may be present if pancreatic islet cells are being destroyed by the inflammatory process. In cats, icterus may be present because of the common duodenal opening of the bile and pancreatic ducts.

In patients with acute pancreatitis, the hematocrit and total serum proteins increase owing to hemoconcentration and fluid loss. With pancreatic necrosis and abscessation, neutrophilia with a regenerative left shift may occur. With disseminated intravascular coagulation and secondary fibrinolysis, coagulation profiles are abnormal and fibrin degradation products are present. Hyperlipemia and hypercholesterolemia in fasted serum samples suggest pancreatitis.

Serum amylase and lipase enzymes may parallel the inflammatory condition of the gland and are of value when assayed simultaneously. Experimental evidence suggests that increased serum lipase activity may be the most important indication of acute pancreatitis in cats.

Radiographic changes caused by acute pancreatitis include soft-tissue opacity in the region of the pancreas, a displaced duodenum, widening of the gastroduodenal angle, and segmental gas retention in the proximal duodenum or transverse colon.

Pancreatic biopsy via laparoscopy or during an abdominal exploration can be performed when other diagnostic procedures have failed to provide a definitive diagnosis.

Treatment

Medical Therapy. The goals of medical therapy are to reduce pancreatic secretions and normalize a patient's fluid, electrolyte, and acid-base imbalances. The pancreas is put to rest by ceasing all oral intake of foods, liquids, and medication for 2 to 5 days.

Intravenous fluid administration is necessary to correct fluid, electrolyte, and acid-base deficits; to replace losses due to vomiting, diarrhea, and abdominal sequestration; and to maintain homeostasis. Fluids are given at a rate of 60 ml/kg/24 hr, and urine output, packed cell volume, and total solids are evaluated to monitor the effects of fluid therapy. Central venous pressure should be checked in compromised patients to prevent fluid overload.

For relief of abdominal pain, meperidine hydrochloride (2 to 10 mg/kg SC) is given every 6 to 8 hours. Recommended protocols include penicillin (10,000 units/kg IV every 8 hours) used against anaerobes and an aminoglycoside (kanamycin, 5 mg/kg IV every 12 hours; or gentamicin, 1.8 mg/kg IV every 8 hours) used against gram-negative bacteria.

Surgical Therapy. Surgical intervention is not performed routinely for treatment of acute pancreatitis.

Surgical débridement, lavage, and drainage should be considered in severe pancreatitis with necrosis of the gland. Principles of surgery include careful débridement and resection of necrotic tissue; preservation of major vessels, nerves, and ducts unaffected by the disease; extensive lavage of the abdominal cavity with warm saline; and pancreatic drainage with sump drains or open peritoneal drainage.

Recovery and Aftercare

Care after surgery consists of no oral feedings for 2 to 5 days, continued intravenous fluid and electrolyte therapy, and broad-spectrum antibiotic therapy. Intravenous fluid and electrolyte replacement must be maintained until oral feedings can be used. Feedings can gradually begin with water as serum amylase and lipase values return to normal and vomiting does not occur.

In patients with abdominal drains, a warm sterile balanced electrolyte solution (500 ml for animals less than 15 kg and 1 L for those weighing more than 15 kg) is flushed into the abdomen two or three times a day.

Prognosis

Pancreatitis is an unpredictable disease characterized by varying degrees of severity.

Chronic Pancreatitis

In dogs, chronic pancreatitis results from repeated bouts of acute inflammatory disease causing progressive parenchymal destruction. In cats, the condition may be similar or associated with a persistent, smoldering, inflammatory process.

A celiotomy and biopsy of the pancreas may be required to establish a diagnosis of chronic pancreatitis in animals with vague abdominal signs of illness. Treatment for chronic pancreatitis is the same as for each episode of acute pancreatitis.

Exocrine Pancreas Neoplasia (see also Oncology Section)

In veterinary medicine, adenocarcinoma of the exocrine pancreas has a frequency ranging from 0.5 to 1.8 per cent of all tumors in dogs and 2.8 per cent in cats.

SURGICAL PROCEDURES (pp. 686–690)

Principles of Pancreatic Surgery

The success of pancreatic surgery is based on sound knowledge of regional anatomy, meticulous surgical technique, and the underlying disease process. Proper division of the shared blood supply of the right lobe of the pancreas with the proximal part of the duodenum is one of the most difficult aspects of pancreatic surgery. Pancreatitis infrequently can be caused by rough tissue handling and excessive surgical trauma to the gland.

Monofilament nylon, polypropylene, or synthetic absorbable material such as polydioxanone can be used in septic or neoplastic conditions. Gut suture is avoided because digestion of the suture due to enzyme leakage or sepsis is possible.

The duplicity of ductal openings and intrapancreatic communications should limit untoward effects of obstructive disease or surgical resection of pancreatic tissue. Leakage of enzymes into the abdominal cavity may not produce peritonitis because enzyme activation has not occurred.

The left lobe of the pancreas is seen in the deep leaf of the greater omentum. The right lobe is seen in the mesoduodenum, and the head and body are located along the duodenal-pyloric junction. With suspected malignancy of the pancreas, evaluation of adjacent abdominal viscera and regional lymph nodes is necessary to establish a prognosis and avoid unnecessary treatment.

Pancreatic Biopsy

Pancreatic biopsy can be performed with direct exposure during laparotomy. Either a shave biopsy or wedge excisional biopsy can be performed. Shave and wedge excision biopsies may cause transection of ducts or vessels, resulting in leakage or hemorrhage.

Partial Pancreatectomy

Partial pancreatectomy can be performed by dissection and ligation of the pancreatic ductule and blood vessels or by suture fracture technique. In the dissection ligation technique, the lobules are gently separated from the adjoining tissue by blunt dissection with a Halsted mosquito hemostat.

In the suture fracture technique, an incision is made through the mesoduodenum or omentum on each side of the tissue to be removed. Nonabsorbable suture material is passed from one incision to the other and around the tissue just proximal to the area being excised. This suture is drawn up into a ligature and tied, crushing its way through the parenchyma and ligating vessels, ductules, or ducts.

No impairment of carbohydrate or fat metabolism, maldigestion, or malabsorption was detected after removal of 80 to 90 per cent of the pancreas if the duct to the remaining portion was left intact.

Total Pancreatectomy (pp. 688–689)

Pancreaticoduodenectomy (p. 690)

Recovery and Convalescence

Adequate lavage and drainage after pancreatic surgery are essential if sepsis and necrotic tissue are present. Antibiotics are maintained at adequate levels during surgery and continued afterward for animals with sepsis or peritoneal drainage. Dehydration and electrolyte and acid-base disorders are treated with intravenous fluids during the first 24 hours after surgery. Water is offered in small amounts, and a small bland meal given 24 hours after surgery. Patients are monitored for pancreatitis and peritonitis. After total pancreatectomy, supplemental therapies for exocrine and endocrine pancreatic insufficiencies are necessary. Treatment of dogs with exocrine pancreatic insufficiency includes supplementation of meals with commercial pancreatic extract, feeding highly digestible diets, vitamin supplementation, and in rare cases antibiotic or glucocorticoid therapy. Animals with endocrine insufficiency require insulin therapy.

Respiratory System

CHAPTER 49

Functional Anatomy (pages 692–707)

UPPER RESPIRATORY TRACT (pp. 692–701)

The upper part includes the nose, nostrils, nasal chambers and their contents, paranasal sinuses, pharynx, and larynx.

Nose and Nasal Chambers
Nasal Plate

The hairless part of the nose of dogs and cats, the *nasal plate,* or planum nasale, is covered with thick keratinized epidermis. Noseprints are used for identification.

Nostrils and Nasal Vestibule

The *nostrils* (nares) and associated structures immediately inside the nasal vestibule impede the flow of air into the nasal chambers. Minor variations in form can be physiologically or clinically significant. The nostrils are bordered medially by a vertical pillar (the *columella*), which forms the rostral end of the nasal septum. The *nasal vestibule* is not empty (as in a human's nose) but is occupied by the swollen end of the ventral nasal concha, called the *alar fold* or *swell body.* It is this fold or its attachment to the wing of the nose that is typically excised in the treatment of stenotic nares.

Nasal Cavity

The nasal cavity is probably a dog's most variable feature, yet it is remarkably uniform in cats. The *nasal septum,* which divides the cavity in two, is mostly cartilaginous but does have an osseous periphery.

The caudal limit to the muzzle is ill defined. The ''stop'' that marks the limit of the forehead overlies the ethmoidal labyrinth so that the nasal chambers continue to extend caudally between and beneath the orbits.

The bulk of the muzzle is made up of two nasal fossae, irregular passageways between the nostrils and the openings into the nasopharynx (*choanae*). The fossae are almost filled with conchae, scrolls of bone or cartilage that project medially from the sides and roof and are covered with a vascular and glandular mucous membrane.

The air passages are restricted to narrow meatuses that are even narrower than in other domestic species. A thin, vertical common meatus is found on either side of the septum; it unites and is coextensive with the dorsal, middle, and ventral meatuses, which occupy the spaces between the conchae.

Paranasal Sinuses

Cats and dogs possess frontal sinuses and maxillary recesses. The maxillary recess is not a true sinus because it does not lie between two plates of a cranial bone but is instead bound laterally by the maxilla and medially by the ethmoid.

The *frontal sinus* is the largest and occupies the brow ridge and supraorbital process of the frontal bone. Right and left frontal sinuses are separated by a median septum. In dogs but not cats, each is composed of three separate cavities—lateral, medial, and rostral—which communicate separately via nasofrontal openings with the nasal fossa.

The *maxillary recess* is found at a level of the carnassial tooth between the orbit and infraorbital canal. It communicates with the middle meatus by a roomy nasomaxillary opening, which is flanked by the nasal conchae.

Nasopharynx

The respiratory tract develops mostly from the floor of the digestive tube, where it is in constant danger of being flooded with ingesta. The pharyngeal chiasma is an ingenious crossroads that has evolved to cope with this design flaw. The two roads are the nasopharynx and larynx in one direction and the oropharynx and esophagus in the other.

The nasopharyngeal conduit is a relatively large tubular space extending from the choanae to the intrapharyngeal ostium. Only its floor is extensively mobile.

Soft Palate

The soft palate forms the floor of the nasopharynx and the roof of the oropharynx. It is a mobile, valvelike partition that can be elevated to close off the proximal airway during swallowing or depressed to close off the oral cavity during nose breathing.

The soft palate is usually conspicuous on lateral radiographs because of the contrast afforded by air above and below it.

Larynx

The larynx supports two sets of ingenious valvular mechanisms, the epiglottis and the glottis. The epiglottis acts passively as a hinged lid that can be pushed over the entrance to the larynx and protects the lower airway against aspiration of liquids and solids during swallowing.

The glottis is a more refined, active valve made up of a pair of vocal folds and associated cartilages that encroach on the airway. It normally widens slightly during inspiration and narrows during expiration. As seals, they can close off the lower airway. As elastic membranes, they vibrate for phonation.

Cartilages

The larynx is a fibroelastic membranous tube in which stiff hyaline cartilages are embedded to maintain a patent airway and to provide support for the moving parts. The cricoid and thyroid mineralize early in life, especially in giant dogs, making them even stiffer and more conspicuous on radiographs. The ring-shaped cricoid, the most rigid, forms a chassis supporting the thyroid and paired arytenoid cartilages, which articulate with it.

Right and left arytenoid cartilages covered with mucous membrane intrude into the lumen of the larynx, with the gap between them forming the dorsal part of the glottal cleft (rima glottidis). A vocal ligament arises from the most ventral portion of both arytenoids (the vocal process). They stretch side by side and meet at the internal ventral midline of the thyroid, forming the core of the vocal folds and the ventral part of the glottal cleft. Rotating the arytenoids in a ventro-medial direction adducts the vocal folds.

Similar but smaller and less intrusive vestibular folds lie parallel to the vocal folds and rostral to them. The thyroid cartilage swings like a visor from the cricoid to assist in lengthening or shortening the vocal and vestibular folds.

The remaining cartilages are wholly or partly elastic. The principal element, the epiglottis, is pointed and V shaped in dogs and cats. The cuneiform process is elongated, and its ventral part gives rise to the vestibular fold (or false vocal cord).

The aditus laryngis is the irregularly shaped entrance to the larynx that lies between the aryepiglottic folds and their enclosed cartilages. Its widest part is found ventrally, abutting onto the rim of the epiglottis and the cuneiform processes. Its caudodorsal part is narrower, almost cleftlike, and lies between the cuneiform and corniculate tubercles.

Laryngeal Lumen

The larynx projects into the pharynx, and its entrance is held away from the pharyngeal wall. Fluids are unable to flow directly into the laryngeal lumen but are directed into the surrounding gutter-like recesses made up of the paired valleculae beneath the epiglottis and the piriform recesses on each side.

Dogs possess large laryngeal ventricles. Each is composed of two parts, a depression lying lateral to the vocal fold and a saccule situated lateral to the vestibular fold.

Cats do not have laryngeal ventricles.

Muscles

Extrinsic muscles of the larynx work with the muscles of the hyoid to elevate, depress, protract, or retract. Intrinsic muscles are striated and mostly concerned with movement of the vocal folds, especially their adduction.

Nerves and Vessels

The recurrent laryngeal branch of the vagus supplies all the intrinsic muscles of the larynx except the cricothyroid. The internal branch of the cranial laryngeal nerve is a sensory nerve to the laryngeal mucosa.

The cranial laryngeal artery provides the principal blood supply.

LOWER RESPIRATORY TRACT (pp. 701–707)

Trachea

C-shaped cartilages stiffen the elastic tubular trachea and keep it patent. They alternate with elastic annular ligaments that unite the cartilages and allow the trachea to stretch and bend without buckling.

The dorsal part of the trachea is free of cartilage and is composed of a wide band of mucosa, connective tissue, and tracheal muscle. In carnivores, this smooth muscle inserts on the external surface of the tracheal cartilages some distance lateral to their tips. Its contraction draws the ends of the cartilages together and even past one another so that they overlap like a key ring. This contraction narrows the airway and reduces the dead space, increasing the velocity of the ventilated air and perhaps assisting in expulsion of mucus during coughing.

The terminal trachea, carina, and pulmonary bronchi are supplied with blood via the bronchoesophageal arteries. The proximal vessels anastomose with the branches of the caudal thyroid arteries on the distal tracheal wall, and the distal vessels follow the bronchi into the lung parenchyma. Bronchial arteries supply the tissue of the lung (they are the *vasa privata,* in contrast to the pulmonary vessels, the *vasa publica*).

Transection of a bronchus near its origin interrupts its bronchial vessels and results in poor blood supply to the distal segment of the bronchus that is extrapulmonary.

Bronchial Tree

At its termination, the trachea divides into two short principal bronchi, which subdivide successively into lobar, segmental, and several smaller generations of bronchi.

The two principal bronchi continue without interruption into the caudal lobes of the lungs. The combination of principal bronchus and caudal lobar bronchus forms a single tapering conduit known unofficially as the *stem bronchus.* Six lobar bronchi are given off the principal bronchi, and each is recognizable on a lateral radiograph.

The two lungs can be subdivided into 20 to 30 bronchopulmonary segments, each a territory of lung supplied by a segmental bronchus. Despite this variability, it is possible to isolate one bronchopulmonary segment from its neighbors for partial lobectomy for metastatic disease. Elastic tissue is in abundance throughout the bronchial tree and contributes about one-third of the force tending to collapse the lungs (surface tension within the alveoli generating a further two-thirds).

Bronchioles are usually less than 1 mm in diameter and have no cartilaginous support.

Lungs

The lungs of dogs and cats are deeply fissured into distinct lobes. Fissuring allows the lungs to change shape with movements of the diaphragm or bending of the spine. Fissures are obliquely disposed and stand out on radiographs only when the pleura is thickened, fluid resides within them, or the adjacent parenchyma is consolidated.

Air within the lower respiratory tract is a superb natural radiographic contrast agent for the pulmonary vessels, bronchial tree, and other structures within the lungs and chest. During inspiration, the larger volume of air makes lung markings even clearer and other thoracic features more conspicuous.

Pulmonary Vessels

The differences between pulmonary arteries and pulmonary veins are less striking than between their systemic counterparts because of the lower pressure of the pulmonary circuit. The pulmonary veins are situated medial to the lobar bronchi. Their terminal portions may be seen subpleurally on the mediastinal surface of some lobes before they empty into the left atrium. Some deoxygenated bronchial venous blood drains into and dilutes the oxygenated pulmonary venous blood, but the larger bronchial veins drain into the azygos vein. Pulmonary lymphatics mostly drain into the three groups of tracheobronchial lymph nodes located around the tracheal bifurcation.

Pleura

The mesothelium of carnivores is supported on an unusually thin connective tissue layer. The caudal mediastinal pleura is so thin that it is transparent and ruptures easily. It is not normally fenestrated.

The lungs, covered with their own pulmonary pleura, are vacuum packed in large sacs of parietal pleura that are collapsed around them. Consequently, folds exist where parietal pleura is in contact with more parietal pleura. The potential spaces between the two layers are known as *pleural recesses;* they can open to receive the expanding lungs during inspiration or fill with air or fluid in pathological states.

Elsewhere, the parietal pleura is in contact with visceral (pulmonary) pleura except for the thin film of lubricating fluid. The parietal pleura is supplied by spinal nerves and is sensitive to tactile or thermal stimuli. The visceral pleura conveys afferents via autonomic nerves that only mediate pain.

CHAPTER 50

Pathophysiology of the Respiratory System (pages 709–724)

PHYSIOLOGY OF THE NORMAL LUNGS (pp. 709–720)

The primary function of mammalian lungs is to exchange gas between atmospheric air and venous blood returning from metabolizing tissues. Secondary functions include warming and humidifying inspired air, vocalization, and temperature regulation. The lung circulation has other nonrespiratory functions, such as filtration of emboli from blood and activation and metabolism of vasoactive substances. To ensure adequate gas exchange, the following processes must be maintained: (1) alveolar ventilation, (2) even distribution of inspired gas, (3) even perfusion of pulmonary capillaries, (4) diffusion of gases across the alveolar-capillary membrane, (5) matching of ventilation and perfusion, and (6) gas transport in blood.

Ventilation—Mechanics of Respiration

Normal resting ventilation is accomplished primarily by contraction of the diaphragm. The external intercostals, sternocleidomastoids, ventral serrati, and scalenes aid inspiration by moving the ribs in a rostral direction, pulling the lung surfaces outward.

Respiratory Pressures

Air enters and exits the lungs by moving along pressure gradients generated by changes in volume of the chest cavity. Pressure within the alveoli becomes subatmospheric during inspiration, returning to atmospheric at the end of inspiration. A positive alveolar pressure is produced during expiration as the lungs recoil, producing a pressure gradient that pushes air out of the lungs.

The magnitude of the alveolar pressure change depends on the movement of the diaphragm and chest wall and on the change in intrapleural pressure that develops.

Forces to Be Overcome During Ventilation

These forces include elastic structures that have to be stretched, airways that offer resistance to airflow, tissue that offers resistance to distortion, and surface tension in the alveoli that limits alveolar expansion.

Compliance

A pressure-volume curve describes the relationship between lung volume changes ($\triangle V$) produced by changes in pressure ($\triangle P$) throughout the range of lung volumes. The slope of the pressure-volume curve ($\triangle V/\triangle P$) is the pulmonary compliance at that lung volume; the steeper the slope, the greater the compliance.

Airway Resistance

This airway branching pattern results in an exponential increase in the cross-sectional area of the airways. Because resistance to airflow depends on the total number of airways, airway resistance decreases as the air moves more distally into the lungs. Total airway resistance has been partitioned for a dog's lungs. During quiet respiration, inspiratory resistance was 79 per cent nasal, 6 per cent laryngeal, and 15 per cent small airway. Expiratory resistance was 74 per cent nasal, 3 per cent laryngeal, and 23 per cent small airway. Measurements of total airway resistance (pressure gradient along the airways/airflow) reflect airway resistance of the upper airways and are not greatly affected by changes in small-airway diameter. Small-airway disease is difficult to diagnose until the disease has progressed to the stage at which small-airway resistance is markedly increased.

When airway resistance is increased, more energy must be generated to move air through the narrowed airways.

Surface Tension

Energy is used to overcome the tension at the surface of the alveoli. An air-liquid interface generates a high surface tension that resists deformation. However, measurements of surface tension indicate that the liquid lining the alveoli has a low surface tension because of the surface-active phospholipid surfactant synthesized by alveolar type 2 cells and secreted onto the alveolar surfaces.

Alveolar Ventilation (p. 743)

Expired ventilation can be measured by determining respiratory frequency and the tidal volume of each breath. Expired ventilation can be subdivided into alveolar ventilation and dead space ventilation.

$$\dot{V}_A = f(V_E - V_D) \text{ or } \dot{V}_A = \dot{V}_E - \dot{V}_D$$

Alveolar ventilation is indirectly related to arterial levels of CO_2. Small changes in $\dot{V}_A$ can markedly affect CO_2 levels and, subsequently, acid-base balance. In addition, intermittent positive-pressure ventilation can have significant cardiovascular effects. When air is forced into the lungs under positive pressure, blood flow into the chest from the peripheral veins is impeded. Thus, venous return decreases and cardiac output is reduced during periods of increased pressure. Exposure of the lungs to airway pressures greater than 20 mm Hg may cause overinflation of lung units and in diseased lungs may cause alveolar rupture and pneumothorax. Positive end-expiratory pressure reduces cardiac output and impairs gas exchange.

Blood Flow—Perfusion of Pulmonary Capillaries

An important component of gas exchange is maintenance of even perfusion of pulmonary capillaries with mixed venous blood. This function is performed by the pulmonary circulation.

Increases in pulmonary arterial pressure or pulmonary blood flow (cardiac output) result in reductions in pulmonary vascular resistance. This paradoxical effect is caused by the recruitment of previously closed capillaries and the distension of previously open capillaries. The increased cross-sectional surface area of the capillary bed decreases vascular resistance. Changes in lung volume also influence the caliber of vessels within the lungs. Pulmonary vascular resistance increases at high lung volumes.

None of the neurohumoral agents is as important in regulating pulmonary vascular tone as is a reduction in partial pressure of alveolar oxygen (P_{AO_2}). Local alveolar hypoxia causes smooth-muscle contraction in vessels supplying the hypoxic region of the lungs. This "hypoxic pulmonary vasoconstriction" is effective in directing blood flow away from hypoxic (poorly ventilated) areas of the lungs to better-ventilated areas of the lungs. This mechanism functions remarkably well in local regulation of vascular tone and in balancing ventilation and blood flow in the lungs.

Diffusion

Once ventilation brings air into the alveoli and perfusion brings blood into the pulmonary capillaries, O_2 and CO_2 are transferred across the tissue barrier separating air and blood. The gases move across the alveolar-capillary membrane by simple diffusion.

Ventilation/Perfusion Relationships

The result of nonuniform distribution of ventilation and perfusion is the development of gas exchange abnormalities.

The distribution of ventilation may be markedly affected by gravity. In a standing animal, gravitational forces acting on the lungs pull the lungs toward the sternum. The intrapleural space is compressed at the ventral surfaces and expanded along the dorsal aspects of the lungs. Intrapleural pressure is higher at the bottom of the lungs and lower at the top. Because intrapleural pressure is an expanding force, dorsal alveoli are exposed to a greater expanding pressure and therefore have a greater volume.

The distribution of blood flow is markedly affected by gravity. In a standing animal, dorsal portions of the lung are above heart level, whereas the ventral portions are below the heart, indicating that dorsal vessels should be poorly perfused and ventral vessels well perfused.

A description of potential maldistributions of ventilation or perfusion is actually not sufficient to predict gas exchange disorders; the balance between ventilation and blood flow in each individual alveolus or gas exchange unit is required. This parameter is the ventilation/perfusion ratio ($\dot{V}/\dot{Q}$). A perfect match of ventilation and perfusion is a $\dot{V}/\dot{Q}$ of 1.0. Little of the lungs has a $\dot{V}/\dot{Q}$ of 1.0. The dorsal portions of the lungs have a $\dot{V}/\dot{Q}$ in excess of 2.0, whereas the ventral portions have a $\dot{V}/\dot{Q}$ of approximately 0.8. This indicates that dorsal alveoli are relatively overventilated (or underperfused) and ventral alveoli are relatively underventilated (or overperfused). In diseased lungs, this normal nonlinear distribution can be altered even more, resulting in further mismatching of ventilation and blood flow.

Gas Transport in Blood

O_2 can be dissolved in plasma; the amount dissolved depends on the solubility and partial pressure of O_2 (PO_2). Despite a PO_2 of almost 100 mm Hg, the low solubility of O_2 results in only about 3 per cent of the O_2 being carried in the dissolved state. The second method of transport is in combination with hemoglobin.

The interactions between O_2 and hemoglobin are described by the O_2-hemoglobin dissociation curve. In the PO_2 range corresponding to the steep portion of the O_2-hemoglobin dissociation curve, O_2 unloading is facilitated at the tissue level. At a PO_2 of 80 mm Hg or more, only a small increase in O_2 saturation is observed. This relationship increases O_2 uptake into blood in the pulmonary capillaries. Dissolved CO_2 accounts for about 7 per cent of transported CO_2. CO_2 is primarily transported in the form of bicarbonate (HCO_3^-).

Control of Ventilation

Alveolar ventilation is precisely matched to metabolic needs so that arterial PO_2 and PCO_2 vary little with physical activity. From the extremes of sleep to intense running, ventilation is adjusted to maintain adequate O_2 uptake and CO_2 elimination. This precise control ventilation is accomplished by the integration of three different components. A central controller, or "respiratory center," generates the breathing rhythm and adjusts the tidal volume of each breath, and chemical and neural reflexes adjust ventilation to the needs of the animal.

Chemoreceptor reflexes are the most important regulators of ventilation. Changes in arterial PCO_2, PO_2, and pH alter ventilation by stimulating central and peripheral chemoreceptors. Of these chemical factors, the respiratory system is most sensitive to CO_2. The action of CO_2 is due to the diffusion of free CO_2 through the barrier. Once CO_2 is dissolved in the medullary extracellular fluid, it is hydrated to HCO_3^- and H^+. These H^+ ions stimulate chemoreceptors to elicit the "hypercapnic ventilatory response."

CO_2 can also stimulate the peripheral chemoreceptors located in the carotid and aortic bodies. Because H^+ ions cannot easily permeate the blood-brain barrier, ventilatory responses to acute changes in arterial pH are due to stimulation of peripheral chemoreceptors. If PaO_2 declines below 60 to 70 mm Hg, a vigorous ventilatory response is initiated. This "hypoxic ventilatory drive" may be essential for maintaining ventilation under a number of circumstances, particularly if CO_2 responsiveness has been altered by lung disease and acid-base disturbance.

The neural respiratory reflexes are less important in the control of normal ventilation but may be important when lung function is altered. The inflation stretch reflex (Hering-Breuer reflex) causes termination of inspiration as the lungs are inflated. Chest wall reflexes, such as the muscle spindle reflex, also seem to stabilize ventilation in the presence of changes in lung mechanics.

Lung Defense Mechanisms

Particles that settle on the mucus lining the airways are removed by the mucociliary cells. These particles may also be phagocytized by alveolar macrophages.

Initiation of the irritant reflex induces sneezing, coughing, and bronchoconstriction, causing forceful expulsion of noxious agents.

RESPIRATORY DYSFUNCTION (pp. 720–723)

Maintenance of normal arterial levels of O_2 and CO_2 and normal pH requires proper functioning of all of the processes of gas exchange. Even a slight structural or functional dysfunction can cause respiratory failure, with arterial hypoxemia, hypercapnia, and acidosis, which are caused by (1) alveolar hypoventilation, (2) impairment of diffusion, (3) pulmonary shunting, (4) ventilation/perfusion imbalance, (5) decreased inspired Po_2, or (6) altered blood gas transport.

Causes and Effects of Respiratory Dysfunction

Obstructive Conditions

Nasopharyngeal obstruction or compression is usually caused by stenotic nares, granulation tissue, polyps and tumors, palate deformations, foreign bodies, scarring secondary to trauma, or inflammatory disorders. The primary pathophysiological changes with nasal obstruction are increased airway resistance and decreased pulmonary compliance. The greatly increased nasal resistance necessitates a change to mouth breathing to avoid greatly increased work of breathing.

Obstruction of airflow in the large airways produces pathophysiological changes similar to those observed in nasopharyngeal obstruction. Increased inspiratory efforts result in markedly subatmospheric intrapleural and airway pressures distal to the site of obstruction. Active expiration may be caused by airway obstruction, and additional complications, such as distal airway closure, may occur. The dyspnea resulting from laryngeal or tracheal obstruction may be either inspiratory or expiratory. Chronic laryngeal or tracheal obstruction can also cause secondary pulmonary hypertension and right heart failure.

Restrictive Disorders

Interstitial and alveolar lung complications are less amenable to surgical correction but produce various pathophysiological changes. Lung fibrosis, lung compression due to space-occupying lesions, pneumonia, pulmonary edema, pulmonary contusion and ''shock lung,'' and constrictive pleuritis can cause interstitial-alveolar respiratory dysfunction.

A decrease in lung compliance is the primary defect in restrictive lung disorders; more energy is required to expand the lungs to the same extent, and the work of breathing is markedly increased. Restrictive conditions impair full expansion of the lungs most during exertion. Another important consequence of restrictive lung disorders may be diffusion impairment.

Chest wall pain and trauma, pneumothorax, diaphragm deformation and paralysis, diaphragmatic herniation, neoplasms, pleural effusion, and pleuritis can restrict movement of the chest wall or diaphragm, causing impaired ventilation.

Vascular Conditions (p. 723)

CHAPTER 51

Evaluation of the Surgical Respiratory Patient (pages 724–733)

PHYSICAL EXAMINATION (pp. 724–725)

In evaluating an animal with a suspected respiratory disorder, particular attention is paid to *inspection* of the breathing pattern, *auscultation* of the lungs, and *percussion* of the thorax.

Inspection

Animals that are not thermoregulating or are in pain generally adopt a pattern of breathing that minimizes the work of respiration. Elastic forces in the lungs are minimized by a *rapid and shallow* breathing pattern, whereas viscous forces in the lungs are minimized by a *slow and deep* breathing pattern. A normal animal balances the elastic and viscous forces in the lungs by adopting a normal breathing pattern. Patients with restrictive lung diseases (e.g., pulmonary edema, interstitial pneumonia, pulmonary fibrosis) adopt a rapid, shallow breathing pattern to reduce the high elastic forces present. Patients with obstructive lung disease (e.g., laryngeal paralysis, small-airway disease, bronchospasm) adopt a slow, deep breathing pattern to reduce airway resistance in the lungs. Patients with upper airway obstruction have an exaggerated effort predominantly during inspiration (usually with inspiratory stridor), whereas patients with lower airway obstruction have forced expiration. Careful inspection of the pattern of breathing can provide important information on the type of lung disease.

Auscultation

Normal breath sounds are generated in the large airways and are heard best when the stethoscope is placed over the cervical region or thoracic inlet. Changes in timing, loudness, and pitch of normal breath sounds at the thoracic wall result either from factors influencing the generation of breath sounds or from factors influencing the conduction of breath sounds to the thoracic wall. Several pathological and nonpathological factors can influence both the generation and conduction of normal breath sounds. Unfortunately, the multitude of factors influencing normal breath sounds and the uncooperative nature of animals can sometimes make interpretation of normal breath sounds difficult. Under conditions of normal quiet breathing, breath sounds auscultated at the thoracic wall are more pronounced during inspiration. Panting or inflammation of the large airways (i.e., tracheobronchitis) influences the quality and intensity of sound generated in the large airways, causing breath sounds to be increased under these conditions. Conduction of breath sounds to the chest wall is increased in underweight animals and by increased lung water (i.e., pulmonary edema). Under these conditions, breath sounds become more pronounced, especially during expiration. Conduction of breath sounds to the thoracic wall is diminished by obesity, fluid, or air in the pleural space (i.e., pleural effusion or pneumothorax).

Adventitious sounds are produced by pathological processes and are classified as discontinuous (crackles) or continuous (wheezes). The intensity, timing, pitch, and point of maximal intensity of adventitious sounds are characterized by the examining veterinarian. *Crackles* (rales) are discrete, nonmusical, explosive sounds that have no recognizable tone. More than one mechanism is responsible for the generation of crackles. Fine crackles are the result of sudden re-expansion of collapsed small airways and alveoli and are usually loudest during late inspiration. Fine crackles suggest small-airway or parenchymal lung disease. Interstitial pulmonary edema, interstitial pneumonia, and chronic pulmonary fibrosis are commonly associated with fine crackles. Coarse crackles are louder, longer in duration, and lower pitched than fine crackles. Coarse crackles are early or paninspiratory in timing and are generated by secretions in larger airways. Bronchopneumonia and severe pulmonary edema are often associated with coarse crackles. *Wheezes* (rhonchi) are continuous musical or whistling sounds that are generated by air passing through a narrowed airway. Wheezes occur primarily during expiration. Wheezing-like sounds heard during inspiration are most likely the result of referral of upper airway obstructive sounds (i.e., inspiratory stridor) to the lungs. High-pitched sounds are most frequently associated with small airways, and low-pitched wheezes are often associated with larger airways. A change in the pitch of wheezes following coughing suggests that they are due to secretions in larger airways. Small-airway disease, bronchospasm, mucosal edema or secretions, and bronchopneumonia are conditions that can be associated with wheezing.

Percussion

Percussion is an underused diagnostic skill that can quickly provide information about the pleural space. For percussion to be reliable, it must be performed regularly on animals with and without conditions involving the pleural space. Percussion is performed by placing one or two fingers firmly on a rib and then gently striking the fingers with the index and middle fingers of the opposite hand. Air in the pleural space produces a resonant sound on percussion compared with the normal thorax. Percussion is a highly reliable method of diagnosing pneumothorax and saves valuable time wasted taking thoracic radiographs in an emergency. Thoracic masses or pleural fluid produces dullness on percussion. A pleural fluid line can often be demonstrated during percussion if a patient is standing or sternally recumbent.

RADIOGRAPHY (pp. 725–729)

Plain Film Studies

Most respiratory patients can be radiographed with few precautionary measures; however, extra precautions must be taken with dyspneic patients. Dyspneic patients are radiographed only after proper stabilization and with minimal stress. Oxygen and equipment for ventilation should be readily available, and animals are continuously observed for signs of respiratory difficulty. A complete radiographic examination is performed if possible, but a minimal examination, lateral view(s) only, may be performed if an animal is extremely debilitated or dyspneic. The immediate safety of dyspneic animals is at all times given priority over obtaining additional radiographic views.

Nasal Cavity and Paranasal Sinuses

Accurate radiographic examination of the nasal cavity and paranasal sinuses requires general anesthesia. The open-mouth ventrodorsal view and the dorsoventral view of the nasal cavity with the film positioned in the mouth are the most valuable views.

Pharynx and Larynx

Inspiratory lateral views of the pharynx and larynx usually provide the most information.

Trachea

Lateral radiographs of the trachea are most informative. A ventrodorsal radiograph is made if tracheal deviation is suspected because of mass lesions within the mediastinum. If fluoroscopy is available, dynamic tracheal movements with inspiration and expiration can be observed.

Lungs

Routine radiographs of the thorax are made on inspiration, with exposure times of 1/20 of a second or less. The entire thorax is included on the film from the thoracic inlet to the most caudal extent of the lungs. The diaphragm and a large portion of the liver are included because the caudal portions of the lungs are superimposed over these structures. Lateral and dorsoventral or ventrodorsal radiographs constitute a complete study in most cases.

Contrast Studies

Bronchography

Bronchography outlines the mucosal surfaces of the trachea and bronchi with radiopaque contrast material.

Pulmonary Angiography

Pulmonary angiography is a technique of injecting iodinated contrast material intravascularly to opacify pulmonary arteries and veins. Pulmonary angiography is useful for detecting congenital pulmonary vascular abnormalities, pulmonary thromboembolism[2], and changes associated with pulmonary hypertension.

BLOOD GAS ANALYSIS (pp. 729–732)

Besides physical examination and thoracic radiography, arterial blood gas analysis is the single most effective means of evaluating pulmonary disease in veterinary patients. It is the only readily available test that provides quantitative information about pulmonary function.

Ventilation

By definition, *hypoventilation* is present when the Pa_{CO_2} in a patient is elevated (i.e., > 40 mm Hg). Conversely, *hyperventilation* is present when the Pa_{CO_2} is decreased.

Gas Exchange

The three basic mechanisms of impaired gas exchange are *diffusion impairment, shunt,* and *ventilation/perfusion* (V̇/Q̇) *mismatch.* Shunt occurs when unoxygenated venous blood bypasses the pulmonary gas exchange areas of the lung and directly mixes with the oxygenated arterial blood. The result is hypoxemia. Shunts can be either intracardiac (e.g., tetralogy of Fallot) or intrapulmonary (e.g., collapsed lung lobe). V̇/Q̇ mismatch is the most common cause of hypoxemia in patients with pulmonary disease. $\dot{V}/\dot{Q}$ mismatch occurs when ventilation and blood flow are not closely matched in various regions of the lungs.

Interpretation

Normal arterial blood gases for patients breathing room air at sea level are approximately 40 mm Hg and 98 mm Hg for the $PaCO_2$ and PaO_2, respectively. When hypoxemia is the result of impaired gas exchange, then the PaO_2 is low but the $PaCO_2$ is normal.

If the hypoxemia is the result of diffusion impairment, breathing O_2 immediately corrects the hypoxemia. If there is no response to breathing O_2, the most likely mechanism of impaired gas exchange is shunt.

ENDOSCOPY (pp. 732–733)

General anesthesia is required for most endoscopy in animals to prevent damage to the animal and equipment. Deep general anesthesia is needed to examine the upper respiratory system, especially the nasal passages. A lighter plane of anesthesia can often be used if it is augmented by a topical anesthetic. Atropine sulfate is avoided because it decreases secretions of the mucous membranes, allowing the surfaces to become dry.

Rhinoscopy

Rhinoscopy is indicated primarily when nasal foreign bodies are suspected on the basis of the history, physical examination, and nasal radiographs.

Laryngoscopy

The larynx may be examined with a rigid laryngoscope used for endotracheal intubation or with a flexible endoscope as part of a tracheobronchoscopic examination.

Tracheobronchoscopy

Tracheobronchoscopy is performed using a flexible endoscope and an adapter that allows passage of the endoscope through the endotracheal tube while gas anesthesia is maintained.

CHAPTER 52

Upper Respiratory System
(pages 733–776)

CONGENITAL ANOMALIES (pp. 733–745)

Stenotic Nares

Stenotic nares are frequently found in brachycephalic dogs and occur with other conditions causing resistance to airflow. Interference with inspiration by the obstructed nares can lead to secondary airway changes (i.e., everted saccules, laryngeal collapse, tracheal collapse), but the reverse does not occur.

Clinical Signs

The principal sign of stenotic nares is inspiratory dyspnea, which is relieved by open-mouth breathing.

Surgical Approach

The wing of the nostril is examined to determine the amount of tissue to be removed for optimal airflow. The wing of the nostril is continuous with the alar fold as it tapers caudally to the alar cartilage. Part of this fold may need to be excised to open the airway. This tissue is highly vascular and bleeds profusely when incised. Pressure against the first incision of the wedge with a suction tip controls the hemorrhage and removes most of the blood as a second incision is made. Electrosurgery should not be used, because too much tissue is destroyed. Epinephrine-soaked cotton-tipped swabs are helpful in reducing the hemorrhage as the edges are sutured together.

Vertical Wedge. The technique of removing a vertical wedge from the wing of a nostril and extending the incision caudally to include part of the alar cartilage has been useful in eliminating stenosis.

Horizontal Wedge. A second method removes a wedge of the nostril in a medial to lateral direction.

Lateral Wedge Resection. A third method for enlarging stenotic nares is resection of a portion of the caudolateral border of the wing of the nostril and a triangle of skin adjacent to it.

Postoperative Care. The surgical site is kept clean and protected from rubbing (self-mutilation) with an Elizabethan collar. Additional medical care is usually not needed.

Cleft Palate

Congenital diseases of the primary and secondary palate have been reported in both dogs and cats and can be associated with other skeletal defects. The primary palate consists of the lip and premaxilla, whereas the secondary palate comprises the hard and soft palates. The incomplete closure of these structures is attributed to inherited, nutritional, hormonal, mechanical, and toxic factors.

Nutritional, hormonal, and mechanical factors enhance the formation of clefts in genetically predisposed fetuses. Growth of the palatine plates must compete successfully with growth of the skull width to achieve midline closure of the palatine plates.

Toxic agents and intrauterine viral infections can produce animals with clefts if the insult occurs at a very specific time in fetal development (25th to 28th day in dogs).

Clinical Diagnosis

Primary cleft palate is obvious at birth as an abnormal fissure in the upper lip (harelip). Clefts of the secondary palate are more common and frequently go unnoticed until a neonate demonstrates signs of poor growth; drainage of milk from the external nares during or after nursing; coughing, gagging, and sneezing while eating; and respiratory tract infection (rhinitis, laryngotracheitis, and inhalation pneumonia).

Clefts of the primary and secondary palate cause conditions similar to those described for secondary palate cleft, plus inability to nurse.

Tube feeding is easy, puppies adapt to it quickly, and it allows surgical treatment to be delayed until an animal is 6 to 8 weeks old. At this time, the tissues are more mature and have better holding strength, and there is more working room in the small oral cavity.

Surgical Technique

Meticulous care of tissue is needed at all stages of the cleft reconstruction. Crushing or drying of tissue cannot be tolerated. The injection of epinephrine solution or the use of electrosurgical equipment is avoided. Retraction is done with traction sutures and fine skin hooks. All sutures (4-0 to 6-0) have swaged-on needles.

Patients are placed in ventral recumbency during repair of clefts of the primary palate and in dorsal recumbency for those of the secondary palate. The oral and nasal cavities are flushed clear of debris with saline and then four to six times with a tissue-compatible antiseptic.

Cleft of the Primary Palate

The main objective in repairing the primary palate cleft is closure of the nasal floor. Without adequate closure of the nasal mucosa over the cleft, realignment of the remaining tissue is meaningless, because dehiscence with secondary repair requires taking down the lip closure.

Cleft Lip (Harelip)

The objective of cleft lip closure is to align the natural adjoining edges of the cleft so that the distance from the ventral nostril to the free ventral edge of the lip is the same on the cleft and unaffected sides. The ventral rim of the nostril and the floor of the rostral nasal passage must make a smooth, sealed junction. The alveolabial sulcus is established to provide mucosal continuity of the oral side of the cleft.

The normal side of the nose and muzzle is measured for width of the normal lip in the same area as for the cleft. This dimension is compared with the two edges of the cleft. If it is different, one edge of the cleft is shortened by resecting a wedge of tissue or is lengthened by making an incision perpendicular to the cleft edge, which is stretched open, aligned, and sutured to the opposing edge.

Complete Primary Cleft Palate

Complete cleft of the lip is repaired as described whether it occurs alone or in conjunction with a cleft of the premaxilla. The mucosal defect in the premaxilla cleft is closed first with two mucoperiosteal flaps raised from the nasal floor. The incisions at the junction of nasal and gingival mucosa are continued caudally along the edge of the cleft in the premaxilla to the caudal extent of the cleft. These mucosal edges are undermined to create two long narrow flaps (nasal and oral) along each side of the cleft premaxilla. The two nasal flaps are sutured together, closing the nasal floor over the cleft. Simple interrupted absorbable sutures (4-0 to 6-0) are preplaced and tied sequentially caudal to rostral, with knots buried in the submucosa.

The defect in the premaxilla may be slow to heal, and a free periosteal graft has been used to improve this. The rostral edge of the mucosal flaps is used to close the rostral nasal floor by suturing it to the ventral rim of the nostril. The remaining hard palate and gingival cleft are closed by similar flaps raised along the ventral edge of the cleft in the premaxilla. These flaps are sutured on the oral midline.

Growth of the premaxillae and palate may be abnormal (shortened, deviated), with simultaneous closure of the lip and palate defects, as a result of aggressive undermining of the graft tissue over the bones involved and increased lip pressure after closure. Closure of the palate defect followed later by the lip defect closure reduces this abnormal bone growth.

Complete Bilateral Clefts of the Primary Palate
(p. 739)

Clefts of the Secondary Palate (pp. 739–740)

Cleft Hard and Soft Palate (pp. 740–745)

Surgical Repair (pp. 740–743)

Hard Palate. Elevating two mucoperiosteal flaps of the hard palate mucosa and subsequently suturing them together at the midline produce a more anatomically correct closure that has the potential for bony union of the palate. The double-layer mucosal closure described later is technically more difficult but provides a strong, reliable repair with the potential for achieving nearly normal tissue architecture after healing is complete. This latter procedure is advantageous because bone production in the palate does not occur until it is covered by soft tissue. Bone is laid down next to the bone covered by the mucoperiosteal flap.

Bilateral flaps of mucoperiosteum, based on the nasal sides of the cleft, are raised along the length of the hard-palate cleft and are used to close the nasal cleft in the mucosa.

Excessive tension on the oral mucosa suture line (usually related to a wide bony cleft) requires a second mucoperiosteal flap from the opposite side of the hard palate. The second flap allows adequate tension release and cleft coverage without superimposition of the oral and nasal suture lines.

Soft Palate. Repair of a soft-palate cleft, with or without a coexisting hard-palate cleft, is performed with either overlapping flap technique or midline appositional two- or three-layer closure.

The *overlapping flap* technique produces two flaps, one based on the nasal side and the other on the oral side of the palate. A second flap of comparable size is developed with a nasal base on the opposite side of the soft-palate cleft. The nasally based mucosal flap is sutured into the nasal mucosal defect left by elevating the orally based flap. The orally based mucosal flap is stretched into the oral defect left by raising the nasal flap.

The *appositional repair* of a soft-palate cleft uses two- or three-layer closure and bilateral relaxing incisions.

Postoperative Care

Most of the postoperative care is related to maintenance of adequate alimentation without placing tension on the suture lines. A wide cleft with a tenuous closure should be bypassed with a pharyngostomy (but *not* nasogastric) tube so that a patient can be fed without disturbing the incisions. Patients with a supple palate after a two- or three-layer closure can be fed gruel for 24 to 48 hours and soft food in 72 hours. Dry food is not introduced into the diet for 6 weeks.

Edema or infection is rarely a problem. Dehiscence is the result of motion, tight sutures, or tension. Nonabsorbable oral sutures are not removed.

Long-term Dehiscence. The reconstructed palate of a neonate grows rapidly, stretching and thinning some of the hard-palate closures. This process results in various sizes of oronasal fistulas, which are repaired after a patient is 8 to 10 months old (see the later section on oronasal fistula).

Overlong Soft Palate

Incidence. Approximately 80 per cent of cases of overlong soft palate are found in brachycephalic dogs.

Signs. The severity of inspiratory dyspnea depends on the length and congestion of the soft palate and other restrictive or obstructive conditions present. Gagging and coughing are frequently accompanied by rattling or snoring during ventilation, especially inspiration.

Surgical Procedures. The intention of palate resection is to shorten the soft palate so that its free border lies slightly rostral to the tip of the epiglottis or just covers it with the tongue in a normal position.

Postoperative Care. Steroids are useful in decreasing edema. Antibiotics are not needed.

TRAUMA TO THE UPPER RESPIRATORY TRACT
(pp. 745–751)

External Nares (Nostrils)

Lacerations. Patients with lacerations of the nose, nostrils, and proximal nasal passage are evaluated as soon as possible to prevent additional tissue loss as a result of drying or infection. Adequate but not unnecessary débridement to remove foreign material and nonviable tissue is followed by copious flushing of the remaining tissue with saline and tissue-compatible antiseptic. This area has an abundant blood supply, and relatively long narrow flaps of tissue are viable and are retained.

Soft Stents for Nostrils

These are used to hold the flaps and grafts of the mucosa against the nasal walls and to provide gentle counterpressure against a denuded surface to retard granulation tissue growth while the mucosa regenerates.

The stent must slide easily against the mucosa, conform to the shape of the nostril and passageway, and fill but not distend the nostril to obtain mucosal growth without pressure points.

Traumatic Split Palate (see Chapter 142)

Cats are prone to a midline fracture of the maxilla with laceration of the soft tissue of the hard palate in falls from heights (high-rise syndrome) and occasionally in vehicle accidents. The majority of these injuries heal without surgical repair of the palate.

Oronasal Fistula (pp. 746–747)

Oronasal fistula occurs secondary to tooth extraction, resection or irradiation of nasal and maxillary neoplasia, and penetrating injury of the palate or maxilla. The presence of infection, necrotic tissue, or food in the nasal passage leads to chronic rhinitis and nasal discharge.

Basic Considerations. Surgical closure of an oronasal fistula depends on a mucosal advancement or rotation flap(s) well supported with submucosa and fascia that when sutured in place provide an airtight seal. A two-layer (mucosal and submucosal) suture closure is more secure.

Oronasal fistulas are either *healed* (mucosal continuity between oral and nasal cavities) or *nonhealed*. Healed fistulas provide surgical alternatives, because one or more of the oral flaps can be based at the edge of the fistula, obtaining their blood supply from the nasal vessels.

Postoperative Care. Patients are allowed to eat and drink 24 hours after surgery. Only soft food is allowed for 6 weeks, and bones are permanently eliminated from the diet.

A pharyngostomy tube may be used in patients with a tenuous closure of a large defect. Gruel feedings are given through this tube until the tissues are healed and have reasonable strength after 3 to 4 weeks.

Surgical Approaches to Nasal Passages

Dorsal Nasal Approach (pp. 748–751)

The standard approach to the nasal passage is via a dorsal midline incision, caudal to the *nasal plane*, to the medial canthi.

Ventral Approach to Rostral Nasal Passages (pp. 750–751)

The ventral rostral approach provides a more cosmetic and adequate approach to the turbinates, nasal passages rostral to the cribriform plate, and frontal sinus. Two approaches can be made to the nasal passage via incision of the hard palate, rostral to the foramina of the major palatine neurovascular bundle.

Ventral Approach to Caudal Nasal Passages (p. 751)

The caudal nasal passages are approached via midline incisions in the hard and soft palates. The palatine bone is removed and discarded. The palatine vascular pedicle is kept intact to maintain adequate blood supply to the soft tissues of the palate.

Ventral Approach to the Nasal Pharynx (p. 751)

A midline incision in the soft palate is used to approach the nasal pharynx. The incision can extend through the caudal edge of the soft palate, but if this extension can be avoided, closure is technically simpler. A mandibular symphysiotomy may be necessary to expose the nasopharynx through the soft-palate incision.

NASAL FOREIGN BODIES (pp. 751–752)

Most small foreign bodies that gain access to the external nares and nasal passages are filtered from the air by the rostral turbinate system and expelled by sneezing. They occasionally become embedded in the mucosa and cause severe inflammation.

Signs

Epistaxis and *excessive sneezing* occur in both acute and chronic stages of inflammation and infection. A unilateral mucopurulent discharge accompanies the foreign body and can conceal the location of the foreign body.

Diagnosis

An otoscope can be used to examine the rostral nasal passage, and the foreign body is occasionally seen and removed with small alligator forceps. A small, flexible fiber-optic bronchoscope or ridged arthroscope allows a better view. Radiographic examination is useful in determining the presence of radiopaque foreign bodies. A rostrally located foreign body can be removed with forceps.

Surgical Approach

Inaccessible foreign bodies should be surgically removed through a dorsal or ventral approach to the nasal passage.

CHRONIC SINUSITIS (pp. 752–753)

Chronic sinusitis occurs in cats as the result of mucosal damage secondary to feline viral rhinotracheitis or calicivirus.

Sinus Flushing

The location of the trephine hole varies with the age of the cat. Curette biopsy and swab cultures are obtained as soon as the sinuses are opened. Small-diameter tubing (intravenous tubing) is placed through the hole and into the sinus. The sinuses are flushed two to three times a day with a trypsin solution (one part trypsin powder to two parts water), 0.5 to 1.5 ml per sinus, to aid in dissolving the heavy mucus.

Sinus Drainage

A more radical approach to *frontal* sinusitis is needed if the sinonasal opening remains occluded after flushing. The nasosinus ostium on the affected side is enlarged and the turbinate resected to allow exudate to drain into the nasal passages.

Sinus Obliteration

Bilateral sinus involvement unresponsive to medical therapy has been treated in cats by obliterating the sinuses. The sinuses heal and become occluded with fibrous tissue and bone during the ensuing 6 to 12 months. Recurrent mucocele can be a problem unless all mucosa is removed.

Reconstruction of Apertures into the Frontal Sinuses

The apertures are enlarged to 1.0 to 1.5 cm with a bone bur, and a piece of 0.125-mm silicone rubber sheet rolled into three or four thicknesses is laid loosely in each opening so that it extends into the nasal cavity. The openings left after the removal of the rubber sheeting close rapidly with granulation tissue if they have not re-epithelialized.

LARYNGEAL DISORDERS (pp. 753–762)
Laryngeal Collapse

Laryngeal collapse occurs as a result of either cartilage fracture (trauma) or loss of the supporting function of the cartilages. The latter condition is common in brachycephalic breeds and is considered part of the brachycephalic airway syndrome. The sequence of changes that occur in the larynx develops as a secondary effect from other forms of upper airway stenosis pre-existing in these patients. Collectively, these obstructive conditions predispose dogs to abnormal stresses within the larynx that lead to progressive distortion and ultimate collapse of the arytenoid cartilages (stages 1 to 3).

Pathophysiology

The first stage in the pathogenesis of laryngeal collapse involves eversion of the laryngeal saccules into the cavity of the glottis. This is caused by an abnormal negative pressure created at the glottis during inspiration. During stage 2, the cuneiform process of each arytenoid cartilage, which normally extends to the caudolateral region of the pharynx during inspiration, loses its rigidity and gradually collapses into the laryngeal lumen. In stage 3, the corniculate process of each arytenoid cartilage, which normally maintains the dorsal arch of the glottis, collapses toward the midline, resulting in complete collapse of the larynx.

Surgical Treatment

A temporary tracheostomy is necessary to ensure an adequate airway during surgery and during postoperative recovery. Dogs with stenotic nares, an elongated soft palate, or everted laryngeal saccules are treated for these conditions first. Dogs with persistent stage 2 disease, even after resection of the soft palate and nares, may require partial arytenochordectomy to enlarge the laryngeal opening (see the later section on partial laryngectomy). Dogs with stage 3 laryngeal collapse may not show significant improvement when treated with partial laryngectomy. An alternative treatment for dogs with severe laryngeal collapse that does not improve after resection of the elongated soft palate, stenotic nares, or laryngeal saccules is a permanent tracheostomy (see Chapter 53).

Laryngeal Paralysis

Laryngeal paralysis in dogs and cats usually occurs from an interruption of the innervation to the intrinsic muscles of the larynx. Disruption of the normal nerve transmission of the vagus or recurrent laryngeal nerves may be either congenital or acquired (idiopathic, traumatic, polyneuropathic, or iatrogenic). The congenital form may be an early manifestation of a polyneuropathy frequently found in older dogs and cats. The result is a failure of the arytenoid cartilages and vocal folds to abduct, leading to mechanical airway obstruction. Idiopathic acquired laryngeal paralysis, the most common form, usually afflicts large dogs older than 9 years.

Diagnosis

A high-pitched noise in the laryngeal region on auscultation suggests laryngeal stenosis. The diagnosis is based on laryngoscopy under light anesthesia.

Animals with laryngeal paralysis are unable to abduct the arytenoid cartilages and vocal folds during inspiration. The majority of animals with laryngeal obstruction have bilateral dysfunction of the dorsal cricothyroid muscles.

Medical Treatment

Most animals in a cyanotic crisis precipitated by upper airway obstruction recover initially with medical therapy. Oxygen is administered by mask. Hyperthermic animals (temperature $> 105°F$ [$40.5°C$]) must be cooled with an alcohol or ice-water bath. Corticosteroids (intravenous dexamethasone, 0.2 to 1.0 mg/kg BID) reduces laryngeal inflammation and edema.

Surgical Treatment

Laryngeal surgery is directed at removing or repositioning laryngeal cartilages that obstruct the rima glottidis.

Arytenoid Cartilage Lateralization. This procedure has been used successfully to treat laryngeal paralysis in cats and dogs. It can be performed unilaterally or bilaterally, depending on the relative increase in glottic diameter desired to produce an airway of adequate size yet prevent aspiration.

Either of two techniques can be used: (1) Suture the arytenoid to the caudodorsal part of the thyroid cartilage or (2) suture the arytenoid cartilage to the dorsocaudal part of the cricoid cartilage. The latter provides an adequate laryngeal airway with only a unilateral tieback.

Partial Laryngectomy Per Os. Partial laryngectomy for the treatment of laryngeal paralysis involves removal of one or both vocal folds and unilateral resection of the corniculate, cuneiform, and vocal processes of the arytenoid cartilage. Difficulty in swallowing or aspiration has not been a problem. The size of the airway created may be equivalent to abduction of the vocal folds and arytenoid cartilages in normal dogs under light anesthesia.

Partial Laryngectomy—Ventral Laryngotomy Approach. The indications for this approach are similar to those for oral laryngectomy. It is particularly useful in small patients weighing less than 7 kg. The size of the functional airway created is more difficult to appreciate unless the airway is observed *per os.*

Postoperative Treatment

A broad-spectrum antibiotic is administered at the time of surgery and continued for 3 to 5 days after surgery. Corticosteroids (prednisolone, 0.5 to 1.0 mg/kg; dexamethasone, 0.2 to 0.5 mg/kg) are used to minimize laryngeal edema and inflammation during the first 1 to 3 days. Patients fed canned dog food swallow discrete boluses of food, reducing the chances of aspiration. Strenuous exercise and barking are discouraged for at least 6 weeks.

Complications of Partial Laryngectomy

Coughing, gagging, and periodic retching caused by edema and inflammation are common after surgery. Fatal aspiration pneumonia may occur. Laryngeal stenosis can develop after partial laryngectomy. Persistent airway aspiration secondary to dysphagia can be prevented by total laryngectomy or laryngeal diversion in conjunction with a permanent tracheostomy.

Reinnervation of Laryngeal Muscles

The major problem in reinnervation of the recurrent laryngeal nerve is the reinnervation of both abductor and adductor muscles by the same nerve bundles, causing stimulation of both muscle groups simultaneously during inspiration and expiration (laryngeal synkinesis). The result is quivering uncoordinated movement of the arytenoid cartilage during respiration.

Surgical Technique. Most dogs and cats with clinical signs of laryngeal paralysis have involvement of both recurrent laryngeal nerves and may need a tracheostomy to provide an adequate airway until reinnervation occurs. The nerve selection for reinnervation of the abductor muscle is based on the length of the distal segment of the recurrent laryngeal nerve available to reach the phrenic nerve or the motor branch of C1.

Everted Laryngeal Saccules

The saccules (ventricles) evert in response to a decrease in pressure that is created within the larynx during inspiration. Everted tissue rapidly becomes edematous and partially occludes the ventral rima glottidis. The saccule is grasped with long hemostats or Allis forceps, and rostral traction applied. The saccule is amputated at its base.

Reverse Sneeze

An intermittent problem in many toy breeds is frequently manifested as an upper respiratory spasm. It is associated with retention of the epiglottis over the rima glottidis with entrapment by the soft palate.

Inflammation of the Larynx

Inflammation of the laryngeal tissue causing dyspnea must be differentiated from surgically correctable laryngeal obstruction.

DEVOCALIZATION (pp. 762–764)

The aim of devocalization is to remove laryngeal tissue that can emit sound. Devocalization, whether partial or complete, does not cause obvious adverse psychological effects. Dogs appear to enjoy the act of barking as much as the sound produced, and devocalization does not suppress their enthusiasm.

Vocal Cordectomy—Per Os

Excision of the vocal folds is accomplished by securing the cord with long-handled (bayonet type) biopsy forceps while long-handled Metzenbaum scissors are used to make controlled cuts in the vocal fold and vocal muscle. Care should be taken to avoid disrupting the ventral commissure of the vocal fold by leaving 1 to 2 mm of ventral cord and muscle. Eventually, 60 per cent of these dogs develop scar tissue at the surgical site, allowing them a muted bark.

A more extensive resection for debarking *per os* involves bilateral removal of the true vocal fold, vocal muscle, vocal process, and the ventral cuneiform cartilage and false vocal fold. The key to the success of this method is to remove the entire vocal process or most of it. If the vocal process remains, it holds any unresected tissue toward the midline, increasing the chance for transverse webbing (between the vocal apparatus). Resection of the false vocal fold and ventral cuneiform cartilage removes this apparatus from use in phonation. The ventral commissure is spared, as noted.

Vocal Cordectomy—Ventral Laryngotomy (Laryngofissure)

This is the recommended approach when devocalization is essential.

The false and true vocal folds (including the vocal muscle) and ventral arytenoid projections (vocal and cuneiform processes) are removed with scissors and rongeur forceps. Mucosal defects are sutured. A similar laryngotomy procedure can be used in cats. Dogs have been successfully muted by excising only the mucosa of the laryngeal ventricles. It implicates the ventricle in the vocalization process or supports the need to eliminate the mobility of both the true and false vocal folds to effectively reduce the bark.

Postoperative Care

It is essential that dogs be allowed limited exercise and be discouraged from barking for 4 to 6 weeks after surgery. Corticosteroids can be used for 2 to 3 days after surgery to reduce edema and inflammation of the surgical site.

LARYNGEAL TRAUMA (pp. 764–766)

Stents for Laryngeal and Tracheal Repair

After resection or realignment of obstructing tissue, it is difficult to prevent transverse adhesion of the dorsal (arytenoid) or ventral (vocal fold) commissures, collapse of damaged cartilage, and excessive granulation tissue production during healing of large defects in the mucosa. Stents are generally used to maintain normal tissue contour, separate adjacent healing surfaces, retard the proliferation of granulation tissue toward the airway lumen, and hold a mucosal graft adjacent to the airway wall while it heals into its new bed.

Most materials are not suited for use as stents because they are not soft enough or are of improper size. Pressure points, sharp edges, and inflexibility are not tolerated by the delicate tissues of either larynx or trachea.

LARYNGEAL STENOSIS (pp. 766–771)

Obstruction of the larynx by granulation tissue and cartilage degeneration and collapse results in progressive reduction in airway diameter. These lesions vary from partial diaphragm or web stenoses to broad-based scar tissue covered by mucosa. Focal and circumferential involvement can occur. Laryngeal stenosis is a complication of laryngeal surgery and other trauma.

Glottic Stenosis

Etiology

Various types of trauma lead to primary or secondary glottic stenosis (see laryngeal trauma). Transluminal webs of mucosa-covered granulation tissue occur after injury to both arytenoids or both vocal folds (i.e., arytenoidectomy, vocal cordectomy). Prolonged intubation is a major cause of laryngotracheal injury, leading to long segmental stenoses in man. Similar stenoses have been noted in dogs.

Diagnosis

Laryngeal stenosis secondary to granulation tissue manifests as progressive dyspnea after a traumatic incident or prolonged intubation. A patient with early signs of dyspnea can have as much as a 60 per cent reduction in lumen size and remain clinically unchanged for weeks. Direct examination of the entire system from the nasopharynx to the trachea by endoscopy is the best method to assess lesions. Tomography may assist in the evaluation of the lesion, especially if the area is too small to allow passage of a bronchoscope.

Treatment

In surgical patients, the best treatment is to prevent stenosis by accurate tissue apposition, and in acutely injured patients, by surgical exploration and reconstruction within 24 hours of injury.

Mechanical Dilation. Dilation is best suited for lesions that are less than 4 weeks old, in conjunction with intralesional corticosteroids and excessive granulation tissue removal with biopsy forceps.

Surgical Repair. Many narrow-based (rostrocaudal) adhesions heal with an adequate glottic opening after simple sharp excision of the web via the oral or ventral thyrotomy routes. Recurrence may be a problem if the mucosa is not sutured to close the defect or a keel stent is not placed.

Broad-based adhesions approached via ventral thyrotomy must be sharply resected to normal tissue to re-establish the airway. High recurrence rates are reduced by mucosa flap coverage of the tissue exposed by scar removal or by stenting. Recurrence can be prevented by placing a piece of silicone rubber sheeting or keel in the airway between the granulating surfaces and keeping it in place with sutures.

A tracheotomy is made three or four rings below the larynx, and a tracheostomy tube placed. It is maintained during and after surgery until the stent is removed.

Subglottic Stenosis (pp. 768–771)

Laryngorrhaphy (pp. 768–769)

Cricolaryngotomy with Splintage (p. 769)

Caudal Segmental Laryngeal Resection

Patients with glottic stenosis involving the cricoid cartilage or neoplasia of the ventral airway respond well to partial cricoid resection and reconstruction using the proximal trachea. The procedure replaces the resected ventral aspect of the cricoid cartilage with the ventral one-half to two-thirds of the first one to three tracheal rings. This procedure can be performed in puppies and kittens without interference in adequate growth of the larynx or trachea.

Pedicled Periosteal Patch

A simpler but less anatomically correct method is to use the periosteal covered end of the sternomastoid muscle to close the defect in the cricoid cartilage.

Postoperative Care. Patients are given antibiotics before surgery, maintained on them for 3 days, and monitored for airway obstruction. Tracheostomy is generally not needed.

Laser Excision

Vaporization of glottic and subglottic stenoses with carbon dioxide (CO_2) laser has met with varied success in dogs and man.

PROLIFERATIVE DISORDERS OF THE LARYNX
(pp. 771–774)

Granulomatous Laryngitis

The proliferating lesions are found around the arytenoid processes and cause laryngeal stenosis. Regression of the lesion usually occurs with debulking of the mass and steroid therapy.

Neoplasia of the Larynx (see Chapter 162)

Primary neoplasia of the larynx is rare in dogs and cats.

Voice alteration is an early sign of masses in the larynx (particularly the vocal cords). Progressive encroachment on the airway results in partial obstruction and respiratory noise or distress.

Segmental Hemilaryngectomy

Small tumors involving mucosa of the vocal cord and adjacent superficial tissues can be excised via cordectomy or hemilaryngectomy. If the tumor is limited to the vocal cord, a standard vocal cordectomy is performed (see devocalization). If the tumor involves mucosa outside the vocal cord, the mucosal incisions are deepened into the thyroid cartilage, and the full-thickness laryngeal segment is removed. The mucosal and cartilage defects are repaired by replacing large tissue defects with free tissue implants or by suturing cartilage and soft tissue to re-establish normal tissue continuity.

Free tissue implants (i.e., costal cartilage, buccal mucosa, thyroid muscle, or combinations of these) are used only when most or all of the thyroid and arytenoid cartilages and covering mucosa are resected.

Suturing the remaining tissue is the more common method of repair of smaller defects. The thyroid cartilage resection is continued dorsally to include its full thickness and height to allow the cranial segment of the thyroid cartilage to be moved caudally and sutured to the caudal segment.

"Rotary Door" Myocutaneous Flap. A method has been developed to bring vascularized epidermis into the laryngeal defect using a myocutaneous flap from the ventral cervical region. Myocutaneous flap repair of the larynx and trachea provides a stable, reliable reconstruction of large, full-thickness defects. A permanent tracheostomy is constructed in the distal cervical trachea. The tracheostomy is left in place until the patency and stability of the airway are adequate, as estimated by obstructing the tracheostomy.

Postoperative Care. The tracheostomy is maintained through the postoperative period (2 to 10 days) or until the wound or graft site is stable. Antibiotics are given and continued postoperatively for 5 days. Pharyngostomy tube feeding is used for 10 to 14 days to reduce tissue motion.

Total Laryngectomy (pp. 773–774)

Tumors involving both sides of the larynx are treated by total laryngectomy.

CHAPTER 53

Lower Respiratory System
(pages 777–804)

DISEASES OF THE TRACHEA AND BRONCHI (pp. 777–791)

Collapsing Trachea

Incidence

Collapsing trachea is most common in miniature or toy breeds.

History

The condition is reported in dogs of all ages, with an average age of 7 years. Signs of respiratory distress have usually been evident for 2 years. Dyspnea is noted during inhalation (cervical trachea) or exhalation (thoracic trachea) or both.

Pathophysiology

If the tracheal rings are reasonably normal and the dorsal membrane is redundant or weak (grades 1 and 2), the membrane is drawn into the cervical tracheal lumen during inspiration and forced into the intrathoracic trachea during expiration, resulting in a functional stenosis. When the cartilaginous rings are hypoplastic or fibrodystrophic, they are weak and lack the ability to maintain their C configuration. These rings are shorter and collapse dorsoventrally to form either a flattened oval or a slitlike lumen (grade 3 or 4). Abnormal rings in the cervical region collapse on inspiration, whereas those in the thoracic portion collapse on expiration. The weak thoracic and bronchial cartilage allows intrathoracic airway collapse during expiration, resulting in higher expiratory pressure and increased pulmonary vascular resistance.

Diagnosis

Digital palpation of the trachea incites severe coughing spasms and hypoxia. Palpation of the cervical trachea reveals a dorsoventral flattened trachea with narrow borders. Hyperextension of the occipitoatlantal joint may increase the severity of the dyspnea owing to dorsoventral tracheal flattening. Radiographs and fluoroscopy of the lateral cervical and thoracic trachea taken in an unanesthetized patient during inspiration and expiration can be diagnostic. Endoscopy is the best technique to evaluate the trachea and bronchi before surgery.

Surgical correction of a collapsing trachea should not be undertaken unless the remainder of the upper respiratory system is free of obstruction. If bronchial collapse is present, surgical support of the trachea may not significantly alter a dog's clinical condition.

Methods of Repair

Dorsal Tracheal Membrane Plication. This technique is used with reasonable success in patients that have a lax tracheal membrane (grades 1 and 2).

Preoperative Preparation. Antibiotics are given before surgery and continued for 24 hours. Viscous tracheal secretions, caused by atropine, are difficult to remove and can lead to tracheal narrowing.

Surgical Approach. A right lateral dissection is made to expose the dorsal aspect of the trachea. The width of the lax tracheal membrane is reduced by plication with interrupted horizontal mattress sutures of 3-0 or 4-0 monofilament nonabsorbable suture.

Internal Stents. Long-term internal support of a weak trachea in a dog using a straight tubular stent has not been successful because it dislodges, becomes obstructive, or is coughed out. Internal tracheal support as an emergency method for maintaining an airway can be achieved with an endotracheal tube placed through a tracheotomy site.

Tracheal Ring Transection. Satisfactory improvement in the cross-sectional area of the trachea has been obtained with transecting alternate tracheal rings at the ventral midline.

Postoperative Care. Patients are confined to a cage for 5 to 10 days. Dogs may have to remain on oxygen for 2 to 4 days.

External Support. Plastic split rings have been made to partially encircle the trachea. When they are sutured to the ring, the airway wall is held in an expanded form. The split rings are placed two or three tracheal rings apart to provide the flexibility needed for tracheal movement. These rings are implanted without interfering with the vascular and nerve supply of the larynx or trachea.

Postoperative Care. Antibiotics are given for 5 to 10 days and corticosteroids for at least 3 days after surgery. Patients frequently have a persistent cough during the healing phase. The persistent cough may be related to a collapsing mainstem bronchus or myocardial disease. Bronchoscopy is used to evaluate the internal structure of the trachea and bronchi 30 to 45 days after surgery.

Internal Injury to the Trachea

Injury During Intubation

Injury of the tracheal mucosa by prolonged use of high-pressure, low-volume cuffed endotracheal or tracheostomy tubes is directly related to the pressure exerted by the inflated cuff and the tip of the tube on the tracheal wall. Pressures one to three times systemic blood pressure are attained at initial contact points as the cuff is expanded to occlude the trachea.

Endotracheal tubes sterilized with ethylene oxide cause mucosal irritation or necrosis unless they are properly degassed.

Tracheal Stenosis (pp. 781–782)

Foreign Body of Trachea and Bronchi

History. The history of an acute onset of coughing and possibly dyspnea is common.

Diagnosis. Radiopaque foreign bodies are confirmed with flat film radiographs. Radiolucent foreign bodies can be demonstrated by positive-contrast bronchography and bronchoscopy.

Therapy for Retrievable Foreign Body. Foreign bodies in the trachea or mainstem bronchus are removed from most patients with a rigid hollow bronchoscope or flexible fiber-optic endoscope and appropriate grasping equipment.

Postoperative Care. Patients with purulent exudate and bronchiole wall damage are treated with antibiotics and bronchodilators for 3 to 5 days.

Therapy for Nonretrievable Foreign Body. Broad-spectrum antibiotic therapy is initiated before surgery. A lateral thoracotomy at the appropriate interspace is used to approach the affected lung, and tissue is inspected for consolidation and palpated for location of the foreign body. A decision must be made whether to perform bronchotomy or lobectomy to remove the foreign body.

Lobectomy is considered when most of the visible bronchus is severely damaged or the lung lobe consolidated. Mucosal loss with submucosal damage exceeding one-third the circumference of the bronchus usually leads to airway stenosis.

External Injury to the Trachea and Bronchi

Persistent peritracheal, subcutaneous, or mediastinal emphysema indicates the need for a careful examination for tracheal or bronchial damage.

Cervical Trachea

Small lesions are commonly self-limiting and undiagnosed. Lacerations of the trachea may be severe enough to produce significant subcutaneous and mediastinal emphysema.

Extensive tissue damage frequently accompanies penetrating bite and gunshot wounds.

Emergency Care. Intubation *per os* or through the laceration is carried out quickly to gain control of the airway. The extent of damage is determined, and appropriate care is given to damaged nonairway structures.

Surgical Approach. Cartilage and mucosa of the trachea are débrided, aligned, and sutured in position with fine monofilament nonabsorbable material. General alignment of cartilage and mucosa can be aided by an intraluminal stent placed through a tracheotomy incision (i.e., Montgomery T tube or tracheostomy tube).

Postoperative Care. Drainage of the peritracheal area is required until the infection is controlled. Broad-spectrum bactericidal antibiotic therapy is started before exploration and continued for 10 days after surgery.

Intrathoracic Trachea and Bronchus

Penetrating injury or inward collapse of the chest wall during impact causes significant damage to the trachea and mainstem bronchi. Minor punctures or lacerations supported by healthy peritracheal tissue are self-limiting. Unsupported lacerations, especially involving the distal trachea and bronchi, may cause extensive pneumomediastinum and 109tension pneumothorax.

Surgical Approach. Preferably, a sternotomy is initially performed to give access to the entire thorax. Flooding the pleural space with saline aids in locating the leak.

Tracheal Transection (p. 784)

Tracheal and Bronchial Resection and Reconstruction

Preoperative Evaluation and Preparation

Resection of the trachea is not undertaken until the lesion and the proposed segment for resection are evaluated in relation to the procedure. Preparations must be made for maintenance of ventilation during all phases of the procedure. Preoperative radiographs should be available at the time of surgery. These should have adequately localized the lesion for resection and identified any other possible lesions in the respiratory system.

Endoscopic evaluation of the mass and biopsy of the lesion should have been carried out before initiating definitive procedures. Endotracheal tube length is selected so that the cuffed portion of the tube reaches into the distal portion of the trachea beyond the anastomosis. A sterile endotracheal tube and Y extension should be available for distal segment intubation. This setup allows greater flexibility for distal dissections by being able to move the intubated segment independently from the upper trachea.

Limitations on Tracheal Resection

Dehiscence and stenosis occur in adult dogs when 50 per cent of the trachea is resected. A similar lesion develops in puppies (6 to 8 weeks old) after approximately 25 per cent of the tracheal length (eight to ten rings) has been resected and in older puppies (12 to 18 weeks old) after 35 to 38 per cent (14 rings) has been resected.

The lateral walls of the anastomosis are the first to dehisce, and dehiscence progresses to the ventral wall as more tension is applied.

These stress points can be reduced by applying tension sutures in the tracheal wall and maintaining cervical flexion during a 1- to 2-week period of healing.

Suturing Techniques

In all but small or older animals, the simple interrupted suture pattern penetrating the cartilaginous rings adjacent to the incision is the best method to obtain tissue alignment. Tracheal rings of young or very small animals and older animals may fracture. Accurate mucosal alignment is desirable for at the anastomosis because defects in mucosal continuity may lead to granulation tissue growth, scarring, and possibly stenosis. The addition of tension sutures significantly reduces incisional separation and granulation tissue production in anastomoses with excessive tension on the primary suture line.

Cervical Trachea (p. 787)

Intrathoracic Trachea (pp. 787–788)

Distal Thoracic Trachea and Carina (pp. 788–789)

Bronchial Resection and Anastomosis

Disruption of the mainstem bronchus requires anastomosis of the bronchus, or the remaining lung lobes supplied by the distal segment are lost. Anastomosis of bronchi is difficult because of their small size and incomplete cartilage rings. A primary suture line of simple interrupted absorbable sutures is placed with mucosal alignment as the goal. Cartilage plates may be incorporated in the sutures only if they allow mucosal alignment. The anastomosis is wrapped with peritracheal adipose tissue or omentum brought through the diaphragm with its blood supply intact.

Replacement of Tracheal Wall (pp. 790–791)

Partial Replacement
Segmental Replacement
Tracheal Allografts

TRACHEOTOMY/TRACHEOSTOMY (pp. 791–794)

Indications

Tracheotomy is indicated for either life-threatening upper respiratory obstruction or the anticipation of its development. It is the best if not the only method to maintain prolonged ventilatory support for a critically ill but conscious surgical patient during the postoperative recovery period. Stenosis occurs more frequently when the tracheal rings are transected or partially resected.

Temporary Tracheotomy (Emergency)

Emergency tracheostomy in most cases of neck swelling is made difficult by distortion of tissue. A needle on a syringe containing saline is used to locate the trachea. Intraluminal position of the needle is verified by the appearance of free air bubbles on aspiration. The needle is used as a guide for the scalpel. An incision is made along the lateral side of the needle on the ventral midline and is deepened until the scalpel enters the trachea. A closed curved hemostat is placed through the incision and into the lumen. The incision is spread with the hemostat while the tube is placed into the tracheotomy.

Transverse Tracheotomy

Transverse tracheotomy is used for intubation of less than 6 hours. No tissue is removed from the tracheal wall because the incision is made between the tracheal rings, through the annular ligament and mucosa.

A roll of towels or cotton may be placed under the neck to cause dorsiflexion in the cervical region, assisting in keeping the trachea near the skin surface and the site open. The interspace between the fourth and fifth tracheal rings is incised through the annular ligament and mucosa. A suture is left in the fifth ring so that the ring can be manipulated during intubation or reintubation at a later time if the tube should become dislodged.

Tube Removal. As soon as the upper airway has been re-established and the tracheotomy is no longer needed, the tube may be removed and the trachea suctioned clear of fluid and debris. The surgical site is allowed to granulate or is sutured with four or five interrupted absorbable sutures placed around the tracheal rings. Accurate tissue approximation decreases granulation tissue formation at the surgical site.

Tracheal Flap. A U-shaped incision, based at the second tracheal ring and extending two or three rings distally, is made in the ventral aspect of the trachea. The flap is raised as a door so that the endotracheal tube or tracheostomy tube may be placed. The flap technique is best suited for long-term intubation (weeks to months). After extubation, the tracheostomy site is débrided free of granulation tissue and the flap mobilized and sutured into its original bed.

A vertical incision made through the ventral midline of tracheal rings is *not* advisable for a tracheostomy.

Tube Placement. Proper sizing and tube alignment within the trachea allow prolonged use without damage to the mucosa and cartilage.

Permanent Tracheostomy

The surgical site is centered over the fourth to sixth tracheal rings, and a midline approach to the trachea is made. The dissection is carried along the lateral walls of the trachea so that it can be elevated to the skin. Approximately 3 cm of the dorsal aspect of the trachea is freed from surrounding soft tissue. Nonabsorbable monofilament suture (3-0) is used to suture the medial edges of the sternohyoid muscle bellies together dorsal to the trachea.

In the first technique, the ventral aspect of four tracheal rings is removed, leaving the mucosa intact. The section of tracheal wall removed in this manner should be approximately 50 per cent larger than the final desired size of the tracheostomy. Redundant skin or subcutaneous fat must be excised to leave a smooth conformation and an even transition between the skin surface and the tracheal mucosa at the anastomosis. The skin is anastomosed directly to the tracheal mucosa using simple interrupted sutures of 4-0 absorbable material.

A second type of permanent tracheostomy uses skin flaps and full-thickness tracheal wall flaps made at 90° angles to each other. The incision in the trachea is an H shape but is placed so that two flaps are formed at the cranial and caudal ends of the incision. These flaps are raised to suture to the skin. At the same time, a pair of skin flaps equal in width to the length of the tracheal incision are raised from the midline incision. These are depressed toward the tracheal lumen to be anastomosed to the incision in the mucosa along the lateral edge of the tracheostomy. This produces a rectangle tracheostomy, eliminates the high-tension points, and provides complete mucocutaneous anastomosis around the entire tracheostomy.

Postoperative Care

Long-term care of a permanent tracheostomy site entails cleaning the opening, removing hair or foreign debris, and applying ointments such as boric acid or petroleum jelly to the mucocutaneous junction.

ACQUIRED LUNG DISEASE (pp. 795–798)
Abscess

Lung abscess and associated pyothorax are more common in cats than dogs, although they are relatively uncommon in both. Abscess formation is secondary to many problems—foreign body, chronic lung infection (i.e., bacterial bronchopneumonia, bronchiectasis), penetrating wounds, or vascular obstruction and neoplastic tissue.

History

This condition is a chronic debilitating disease with various degrees of respiratory distress, persistent low-grade fever, and severe leukocytosis with a degenerative left shift. The pleural space may have to be lavaged and drained before a definite radiographic diagnosis can be made.

Surgical Approach

The incision into the thorax is made with great care, because adhesions of lung lobes to the lateral wall are common. The involved lung lobe is located, and a partial or complete lobectomy is performed. Two lobes are occasionally involved. The remaining interlobar fissures are explored, and adhesions between lung lobes freed until all lobes are movable and loculated areas of exudate are cleared.

Bronchiectasis

Chronic respiratory disease can result in or be caused by saccular or cylindrical dilations of bronchi, bronchioles, or both. Lobectomy of the affected lobes is the definitive treatment in patients with one or two involved lobes. Patients with more than two lobes involved are treated medically.

Foreign Body

Barbed seeds or hulls (grass awns) and other small bodies inhaled into the bronchi resist dislodgment by coughing and work their way along the small air passages. A plant awn frequently breaks into parenchymal tissue and causes a septic focus that develops into an abscess.

History

Vague and intermittent signs of respiratory disease may be noted. A temporary response to antibiotic therapy is common.

Diagnosis

Radiographic examination may show an area of increased lung density compatible with local atelectasis, bronchopneumonia, abscess, or granuloma.

Surgical Approach

Partial or complete lobectomy is the method of choice for removing deep-seated lung foreign bodies.

Lung Laceration

Lung lacerations are usually small and resolve on their own or with the aid of chest drainage to control the accumulation of air and blood in the chest. Before surgical intervention, a serious effort is made to locate the laceration. Thoracoscopy has been used to locate lacerations and cauterize bleeding points with good success. All penetrating wounds of the chest are explored as soon as a patient is stabilized. Hemorrhage into the chest greater than 2 ml/kg/hr, and unresolving or uncontrollable pneumothorax with chest drainage are reasons for exploratory thoracotomy.

Surgical Approach

Superficial unsealed lacerations are closed with a simple continuous inverting mattress suture (Lembert type) of absorbable suture (4-0 or 5-0). Deep lacerations into the lung parenchyma may involve vessels and airways that leak profusely.

The base of the involved lobe is gently cross-clamped (noncrushing vascular forceps or finger hold) to reduce or stop air and blood flow. The wound is explored for lacerated bronchioles and vessels, and these are individually ligated with fixation ligatures. The edges of the laceration are apposed by a loose Lembert or simple continuous suture technique to realign the pleural surface.

The lobe is evaluated for ventilation and perfusion after the leaks are controlled. If either appears to be compromised, a partial or complete lobectomy is performed.

NEOPLASTIC DISEASE OF THE LUNG (see Chapter 162)
(pp. 798–802)

Lobectomy

Partial Lobectomy

Lesions involving the distal two-thirds or less of a lung lobe can be excised using partial lobectomy.

The area of the lung lobe to be removed is identified, and a pair of crushing forceps are placed across the lobe at the resection level. A continuous overlapping hemostatic/pneumostatic suture (3-0 or 4-0 absorbable suture) is placed 4 to 5 mm proximal to the forceps. The suture is tied at its beginning and at its end so that adequate tissue compression is achieved, and a piece (8 to 10 cm long) is left at each side of the lobe to control the lung. The lung lobe is incised on the proximal side of the forceps, leaving a narrow strip of uninjured lung distal to the compressing suture. The edge of the lung incision is oversewn with a very closely spaced simple continuous pattern of absorbable suture (4-0 or 5-0).

Partial lobectomy in the proximal third of the lobe encounters relatively large bronchi and blood vessels. These are ligated individually with suture ligatures (fixation ligatures) to reduce hemorrhage or air leak, and the lung edge is sutured as previously described. If no fluid or air accumulates in the chest cavity within the first 24 hours, the chest drain is removed.

Complete Lobectomy

The arterial supply to the lobe is approached first to control blood flow to the lobe, preventing congestion and reducing the chance of severe arterial hemorrhage as the hilar dissection is made.

A simple ligature of 2-0 or 3-0 suture material (nonabsorbable) is tied at the proximal end of the artery near its branch point. A similar suture is placed distal to the point at which the artery is transected. A transfixing suture is tied 1 mm distal to the proximal suture to prevent its migration. The artery is transected between the two distal sutures.

The lobe is retracted dorsally, and the pulmonary vein is approached on the ventral side of the bronchus. The vein is ligated as for the artery. Care should be used to ensure that the venous drainage from other lung lobes in the area is not interfered with by incorporating an adjacent vein in the ligatures.

The bronchus is cross-clamped with two pairs of crushing-type forceps proximal and distal to a convenient point for transection close to the lung lobe. The bronchus is transected between the forceps, and the lung is removed. The bronchus, near its origin and proximal to the remaining clamp, is sutured with preplaced interrupted horizontal mattress sutures (2-0 to 3-0 nonabsorbable monofilament suture). The bronchus is transected just distal to these sutures, leaving minimal noncrushed bronchus remaining distal to the mattress sutures. A simple continuous suture pattern is used to oversew the mucosa and cartilage on the distal end of the bronchus (3-0 or 4-0 absorbable suture). Complete coverage of the raw tissues exposed during surgery aids in decreasing adhesions, reduces postoperative air leaks, and speeds healing of the exposed stumps.

Necrotic Lobes

Resection of a torsive lung lobe occasionally requires handling friable tissue and vessels containing large loose clots and autolyzed blood. Such lobes are retracted gently and not untwisted until the pedicle is clamped.

Pneumonectomy (pp. 800–802)

Acute restriction of more than 60 per cent of the pulmonary artery outflow is fatal in dogs. Because the right lung is larger than the left, a right pneumonectomy removes more than 50 per cent of the lung and is likely to be fatal. Excision of an entire left lung is tolerated if the right lung is healthy.

Pneumonectomy is accompanied by secondary changes in the contralateral lung and the myocardium. The lung remaining after pneumonectomy is more sensitive to positive end-expiratory pressure, as manifested by a greater increase in the pulmonary vascular resistance with a given level of positive end-expiratory pressure. This is correlated with a lower cardiac output.

The main bronchus has trachea-type cartilage rings, which resist collapse, and the sutures or staples tend to cut through the bronchus. Closure can be reinforced by suturing a piece of dermis, pericardium, or fascia over the closure.

Care of Respiratory Patients
(pages 804–819)

Surgical intervention frequently results in reduced respiratory function. These changes occur secondary to diminished diaphragmatic and chest wall muscle activity, causing decreased inspiratory effort. Decreases in ventilatory muscle function and diminished sighs lead to atelectasis, retained secretions, and pneumonia. Respiratory status must be evaluated carefully, and therapeutic measures implemented so that morbidity and mortality can be minimized.

BRONCHIAL HYGIENE (pp. 804–808)

Bronchial hygiene is the maintenance of clear airways and removal of secretions from the tracheobronchial tree. Retained secretions lead to pulmonary malfunction: (1) Retained secretions in the airway lead to an inflammatory response in the underlying mucosa, narrowing the airway lumen, and increased airway resistance. Consequences of increased airway resistance include an increase in the work of breathing. (2) Retained secretions that obstruct bronchioles lead to atelectasis of the involved lung segment. The consequences of atelectasis are reduced gas exchange and an additional increase in the work of breathing secondary to decreased lung compliance. (3) Retained secretions and atelectasis predispose to bacterial pneumonia.

Cough

Coughing is the most important defense against retained secretions when the mucociliary escalator is dysfunctional. This high-velocity airflow mobilizes excess mucus from the small airways toward the pharynx.

Airway Hydration

Although the nasopharynx is the principal site of heat and fluid transfer, the mucous blanket of the tracheobronchial tree supplies water and heat to inspired air. The mucous layer is the primary source of water and heat for inspired air if an animal is mouth breathing or if the nasopharynx is bypassed by an endotracheal or tracheostomy tube. Hyperventilation, dry inspired air (e.g., dry medical gases), and fever cause increased water loss from the respiratory tract and dehydration of the tracheobronchial mucous blanket. Inadequate hydration leads to impaired ciliary activity, impaired mucus movement, retention of viscous secretions, and inflammation and necrosis of the ciliated epithelial cells, predisposing to atelectasis and pneumonia.

Fluids are administered systemically or locally to maintain hydration of the mucous layer. It is difficult to maintain hydration with local fluid therapy alone if a patient is dehydrated.

Local Fluid Therapy

Humidifiers and nebulizers are used to administer fluids directly to the tracheobronchial tree. Humidifiers saturate gas with water vapor without producing particulate water, whereas nebulizers produce an aerosol (a suspension of very fine particles of liquid in a gas). The risk of transmitting bacteria from a contaminated humidifier reservoir fluid is very low, because humidifiers do not produce particulate water. Conversely, the potential for bacterial transmission with nebulizers is high because they produce small-droplet aerosols that contain the particulate matter present in the reservoir. Only sterile solutions are nebulized.

In general, humidifiers are helpful in preventing dehydration of airways but are unable to deliver fluids, whereas nebulizers are able to deliver fluid even to the point of systemic overhydration. Chest physiotherapy should be performed after nebulization to facilitate removal of these hydrated secretions from the respiratory tract.

Nebulized Medications

Nebulizers may be used to deliver medications directly to the respiratory system. Nebulization of 1 to 2 per cent sodium bicarbonate solutions is beneficial in decreasing the viscosity of mucus. Acetylcysteine therapy can be accomplished by nebulizing 3 to 10 ml of a 10 per cent solution three or four times daily or instilling 0.25 to 2.0 ml directly into the airway hourly. Delivery of a bronchodilator concurrently with acetylcysteine is recommended to reduce bronchospasm.

Nebulization of antibiotic solutions is controversial. Higher concentrations in respiratory secretions may be achieved with nebulization than with systemic therapy because many antibiotics penetrate the blood-bronchus barrier poorly. Nebulization of the steroid beclomethasone dipropionate (Beclovent) results in minimal systemic absorption.

Complications of Aerosol Therapy

Complications of aerosol therapy include swelling of retained secretions, bronchospasm, fluid overload, and nosocomial infections.

Chest Physiotherapy

Postural Drainage

Postural drainage uses different body positions to allow gravity to remove secretions from diseased areas. Recumbent animals are repositioned so that they are in a different body position every 2 hours to prevent retention of secretion and atelectasis in dependent lung segments.

Encouraging Deep Ventilations

Deep ventilations should be encouraged in all postoperative patients to prevent atelectasis and improve coughing. Early ambulation is recommended to encourage deep breathing. The intensity of activity should be the maximum that is tolerated and not stressful to a patient.

Chest Percussion

Chest percussion is performed by forcefully striking the chest wall with cupped hands over the diseased lung segment. The sudden compression of air over the chest wall produces a mechanical energy wave that is transmitted through the chest wall to the lung tissue to mobilize retained secretions.

The sequence of care for respiratory patients is first to deliver airway nebulization, then perform chest percussion (usually in conjunction with postural drainage), and finally encourage deep ventilations with mild to moderate exercise.

ARTIFICIAL AIRWAYS (pp. 808–811)

Endotracheal tubes or tracheostomy tubes are the primary artificial airways used in small animal patients. The indications for establishing an artificial airway in animals are to provide prolonged ventilation support, bypass upper airway obstructions, and facilitate airway clearing. If a patient requires an artificial airway for more than a few hours, a tracheostomy tube is inserted.

Tracheostomy Tubes

If a tracheostomy tube is being placed for prolonged ventilatory support, a cuffed tube is required. It is desirable to select a tube that has an interchangeable inner cannula so that it is easier to clean the tube and occlusion of the tube is less likely.

Tracheostomy Care

Within 24 hours of tracheostomy tube placement, the trachea becomes colonized with bacteria from the oropharyngeal flora. It is recommended that ventilator circuits be changed every 24 to 48 hours to prevent contamination. If the tracheostomy tube is to be handled or suctioned, sterile surgical gloves are worn.

Airway Clearing by Suction

Airway clearing is required to prevent occlusion of the tube with secretions and to remove retained secretions, because tracheostomy tubes prevent patients from coughing. Tracheostomy tubes bypass the heat and humidification normally provided by the upper airway. The inspired air should be humidified to prevent dehydration of the mucous blanket. If humidification is not possible, 0.1 ml/kg of sterile saline, with a minimum of 1 ml and maximum of 5 ml regardless of an animal's weight, is directly instilled into the trachea every 1 to 2 hours to help maintain airway hydration. Aseptic technique and sterile equipment are always used when suctioning.

Before suctioning, patients are preoxygenated for a few minutes using 100 per cent oxygen to minimize hypoxemia. The suction catheter is inserted without a vacuum until an obstruction is detected. The catheter is then retracted slightly to prevent occlusion of a bronchus, and intermittent suction is applied while rotating the catheter between the thumb and forefinger as the catheter is removed. The total time that the catheter is placed into the airway should not exceed 10 to 15 seconds to prevent severe hypoxemia.

Tracheostomy Wound Care

Wound care is performed two or three times daily. The tracheostomy site is cleaned with cotton-tipped applicators soaked in 3 per cent hydrogen peroxide and then rinsed with sterile saline. After cleaning, an antiseptic or antibacterial ointment and new sterile dressing are applied.

Cuff Inflation

The cuff is inflated so that a slight leak is detected when airway (tracheal) pressures are maximal. To detect air leaks, the diaphragm of the stethoscope is placed over the trachea adjacent to the tube cuff.

Tracheostomy Tube Removal

The tracheostomy tube is removed and replaced with a smaller one if possible. Patients are then observed for the next 10 minutes to evaluate ventilation through the upper airway and around the tube. If respiration is not labored, the orifice of the tube is occluded. When ventilation is adequate with the small tube occluded, the tube is removed and the tracheostomy site is occluded. If ventilation is still adequate, the tracheostomy is surgically repaired or allowed to heal by granulation.

MANAGEMENT OF ACUTE RESPIRATORY FAILURE
(pp. 811–816)

Oxygen Therapy

Increasing fractional inspired oxygen concentration (FIO_2) can be beneficial to respiratory patients by increasing alveolar oxygen concentrations to improve oxygen exchange and prevent hypoxemia.

Indications for Oxygen Therapy

Increasing FIO_2 is an effective therapy for hypoxemic patients with diffusion impairment (e.g., emphysema), high ventilation/perfusion ($\dot{V}/\dot{Q}$) mismatch (e.g., pulmonary thromboemboli), or hypoventilation (e.g., general anesthesia). Low $\dot{V}/\dot{Q}$ mismatch or right-to-left shunts secondary to alveolar collapse and lung consolidation cause hypoxemia that is generally unresponsive to oxygen therapy and usually requires airway pressure therapy (continuous positive airway pressure [CPAP] or positive end-expiratory pressure [PEEP]) to restore normoxemia.

Oxygen Masks

Oxygen masks are an excellent short-term method for administering oxygen. Relatively high gas flows ($\geq$ 10 L/min) should be used to prevent carbon dioxide from building up inside the mask. The mask should fit closely to minimize dead space but should not be airtight, or hypercapnia will occur.

Nasal Oxygen Therapy

Nasal cannulation is an excellent method for delivering long-term oxygen therapy. This procedure can be performed with local anesthesia, by placing the animal's head in a nose-up position and instilling 0.5 to 1 ml of proparacaine ophthalmic solution into a nostril. The nose is held up for 30 to 60 seconds to allow the local anesthetic to act. After waiting for an additional minute, the instillation is repeated so that good local anesthesia is obtained. Polyurethane nasogastric feeding tubes or rubber urethral catheters are commonly used for nasal cannulation. A number 6 French tube is used for cats and small dogs, and a 10 French tube is appropriate for large dogs.

The distance from the nares to the carnassial tooth is measured, and the catheter tip is lubricated with 2 per cent lidocaine jelly. The tube is directed in a ventromedial direction into the ventral meatus for the premeasured distance. After the tube is in place, it is sutured to the perinasal skin. An anesthetic machine or other regulated source of oxygen is used. It is imperative that the administered oxygen be humidified to prevent dehydration of the airways. Oxygen flow rates of 50 to 125 ml/kg/min are required to obtain an FIO_2 of 0.4. The only disadvantage is poor tolerance of the tube by some patients. Elizabethan collars may be required to prevent catheter removal.

Tracheal Oxygen Therapy

Transtracheal catheters can also be used to administer oxygen. A "through-the-needle" 16-gauge intravenous catheter with side holes placed near the tip can be passed through the cricothyroid membrane or between tracheal rings to deliver oxygen.

Oxygen Cages

Oxygen cages can also be used to administer oxygen. It is necessary that temperature and humidity be regulated and carbon dioxide be eliminated from the system. Simply placing an animal in an enclosure with a high oxygen flow is not appropriate.

Complications of Oxygen Therapy

Complications of oxygen therapy include pulmonary oxygen toxicity, retrolental fibroplasia, absorption atelectasis, and hypoventilation. Pulmonary oxygen toxicity results from the production of oxygen free radicals, which damage cells of the respiratory system. Exposing dogs to 100 per cent oxygen produced compromised lung function within 24 hours and resulted in death within 50 to 60 hours. An F_{IO_2} of 0.5 is safe for chronic oxygen therapy in dogs and cats.

Airway Pressure Therapy

Positive airway pressure may be delivered during inspiration, expiration, or both inspiration and expiration.

Inspiratory Airway Pressure Therapy

Positive-pressure ventilatory support is indicated when Pa_{CO_2} is greater than 50. The primary benefit is that the ventilator is able to perform the work required to maintain alveolar ventilation. There are three disadvantages of positive-pressure ventilation: (1) Increases in inspiratory airway pressure result in increased mean airway pressure and cause increased intrathoracic pressure. Increased intrathoracic airway pressure can inhibit venous return to the heart and reduce cardiac output. (2) Increases in alveolar pressure can reduce blood flow to the dorsal lung and increase blood flow to the gravity-dependent ventral regions of the lungs. (3) Excessive airway and alveolar pressures can traumatize the lungs, causing pneumomediastinum, subcutaneous emphysema, and pneumothorax.

Guidelines for Positive-Pressure Ventilation

Although general guidelines can be used when placing an animal on positive-pressure ventilation, patients must be closely monitored and the ventilator adjusted to provide optimal therapy.

The rate of ventilation should be between 8 and 15 breaths per minute, with slower rates used for larger dogs and higher rates used for small dogs and cats. The ratio of inspiration to expiration is 1:2 to 1:3. Minute ventilation (tidal volume × ventilation per minute) is 150 to 250 ml/kg/minute. If a patient fights the ventilator, blood gas is monitored to rule out inadequate ventilation (elevated Pa_{CO_2}), nonrespiratory acidosis, and hypoxia. If inadequate ventilation, metabolic acidosis, and hypoxia are not present, pain and anxiety are the most likely causes of fighting the ventilator.

Expiratory Airway Pressure Therapy

Expiratory airway pressure therapy is indicated if gas exchange failure is present. The primary benefit of expiratory pressure therapy is that it prevents and reverses both small-airway closure and alveolar collapse. With airway pressure therapy, it is possible to maintain PaO_2 above 70 mm Hg at a FIO_2 less than 0.6. PEEP is defined as an expiratory airway pressure in which the airway pressure is maintained above atmospheric at the end of expiration. CPAP is similar to PEEP except that positive airway pressures are maintained throughout the entire breathing cycle. In a clinical setting, PEEP is most commonly delivered in conjunction with positive-pressure ventilation in patients with combined ventilatory and gas exchange failure. CPAP is most commonly used to provide expiratory pressure therapy to patients with gas exchange failure alone.

In most patients, 5 to 10 cm H_2O of PEEP or CPAP may be administered safely. If cardiac output can be monitored, up to 15 cm H_2O may be delivered.

Patient Monitoring

Intensive monitoring is required for airway pressure therapy, including mucous membrane color, hydration, thoracic auscultation, pulse rate and character, and body weight.

Discontinuing Airway Pressure Therapy

When removing an animal from positive-pressure ventilation, it is helpful to switch to intermittent mandatory ventilation. In patients receiving PEEP/CPAP, gradually decrease the FIO_2 to less than 0.5, and then decrease PEEP/CPAP to 3 cm H_2O. If blood gases and clinical assessment indicate that gas exchange is adequate, it is usually safe to discontinue therapy and use oxygen alone.

ANTIBIOTIC THERAPY (pp. 816–818)

Definitive antibiotic therapy is based on sensitivity test results, because gram-negative bacteria possess unpredictable antibiotic resistance.

Culturing Techniques for the Lower Respiratory Tract

Appropriate techniques for obtaining samples from the lower respiratory tract include transtracheal aspiration, bronchial wash, bronchoscopy, transthoracic lung aspiration, and lung biopsy.

Transtracheal Aspiration

Transtracheal aspiration is an extremely valuable technique for obtaining samples from the lower respiratory tract for culture and cytological study.

The technique involves insertion of a 16- or 18-gauge needle through the needle catheter, through either the cricothyroid membrane or between tracheal rings in the lower cervical trachea, with the animal in sternal recumbency with its head extended. Local anesthesia is preferable. When the catheter has been inserted, a three-way valve is placed on the hub of the catheter and two syringes are attached. One syringe is filled with either 0.9 per cent sodium chloride or lactated Ringer's solution, and the other is used to aspirate the sample. Immediately after instilling 2 to 10 ml of fluid, the three-way valve is turned and suction is applied. A total of 0.5 to 2 ml/kg is instilled, but only 1 to 3 ml is recovered.

Bronchial Washing

The animal is anesthetized with a short-acting anesthetic and intubated with a sterile tracheal tube. A sterile catheter is passed down the endotracheal tube, and sterile saline or lactated Ringer's solution is instilled and aspirated as described for transtracheal aspiration.

Transthoracic Lung Aspiration (p. 817)

SUPPORTIVE THERAPY (p. 818)

Cardiovascular System

CHAPTER 55
Surgical Anatomy (pages 820–826)

The ribs displace cranially more readily than caudally when a rib space is opened, so structures located in the caudal third of the rib space may be exposed more completely if the incision is made one rib space more caudally.

VESSELS (pp. 820–821)

Venous return to the heart is supplied by the cranial and caudal venae cavae. Both vessels lie to the right of the mediastinal tissue and enter the right atrium. The azygos vein is the last branch to enter the cranial vena cava.

The pulmonary trunk and its branches carry unoxygenated blood to the lungs. The trunk arises from the pulmonary fibrous ring and divides into the right and left pulmonary arteries. The pulmonary trunk contacts the aorta along its medial surface as the vessels spiral and cross each other. The ligamentum arteriosum arises before the bifurcation of the pulmonary trunk and passes to the aorta.

The ascending aorta arises from the fibrous base of the heart and turns dorsocaudally and to the left as the aortic arch and descending aorta. The first large branch to leave the aortic arch is the brachiocephalic trunk, which terminates in the common carotid arteries and the right subclavian artery.

NERVES AND INNERVATION (pp. 821–823)

The autonomic nervous system, sympathetic and parasympathetic branches, provides the innervation to the heart. The autonomic nervous system controls heart rate, rate of impulse transmission, and force of contraction. Parasympathetic innervation is provided by the vagus nerve. Sympathetic fibers are distributed to both the atria and ventricles. These fibers originate in the thoracic spinal cord.

PERICARDIUM (p. 823)

The pericardium is divided into an outer fibrous part and an inner serous part. The apex is continued to the ventral part of the diaphragm, where it becomes the sternopericardiac ligament. The serous pericardium has parietal and visceral layers. The parietal layer is fused to the fibrous pericardium. The visceral layer is firmly attached to the heart muscle.

HEART (p. 823)

The heart lies obliquely in the thorax with the base directed craniodorsally and the apex directed caudoventrally. A small area on the caudodorsal surface adjacent to the apex is closely associated with the diaphragm. The remainder of the heart predominantly faces the sternum and ribs. The heart usually extends from the third rib to the sixth rib, but variation is seen in different breeds.

Internally, the heart is divided into four chambers, which can be identified by superficial external landmarks. The coronary groove, which contains the major coronary vessels, demarcates the atria and ventricles. The interventricular grooves separate the right and left ventricles.

CORONARY VESSELS (p. 824)

Blood supply to the myocardium is provided by the right and left coronary arteries, arising from the aortic bulb beyond the aortic valve. The left coronary artery is a short trunk that divides into the circumflex, paraconal interventricular, and occasionally septal branches. The circumflex branch lies in the coronary groove and passes to the left and across the caudodorsal surface of the heart and turns toward the apex of the heart. Here it becomes the subsinosal interventricular branch (caudal descending coronary artery). Branches of the circumflex artery supply both the atria and ventricles.

Venous return to the heart is primarily through the coronary sinus to the right atrium. The coronary sinus is the termination of the great coronary vein, which lies in the dorsodextral part of the coronary groove.

The right cardiac veins return blood from the right ventricle and enter the small cardiac veins or right atrium directly. The small cardiac veins are microscopic channels that enter all heart chambers but predominate in the right ventricle and right atrium.

ATRIA (p. 824)

The right atrium receives venous blood from the systemic circulation and venous return from the coronary vessels. The right auricle is a blind appendage that leaves the cranial surface of the right atrium and extends ventrally. The left atrium consists of a main chamber and a left auricle. The left auricle lies caudal to the pulmonary trunk and overlies the proximal portion of the paraconal interventricular groove.

VENTRICLES (pp. 824–825)

The right ventricle, which is crescent shaped in cross section, lies cranial and ventral to the left ventricle in the thoracic cavity. Because it functions in a lower-pressure system, the right ventricular wall is thinner than the left. The entrance to the right ventricle is controlled by the right atrioventricular valve. Blood leaving the right ventricle passes through the pulmonic valve.

The left ventricle is conical and, because it functions as the systemic pump, has a thicker, more muscular wall than the right ventricle. The interventricular septum is composed of a small dorsal membranous portion and a more extensive ventral muscular portion. The membranous portion lies under the septal cusp of the right atrioventricular valve.

VALVES OF THE HEART (pp. 825–826)

The atria and ventricles are separated on either side by the right and left atrioventricular valves. They attach peripherally to the fibrous skeleton and are stabilized by multiple chordae tendineae. Innervation to the valve leaflets arises from the atrial subendocardium. The right atrioventricular valve (tricuspid valve) has two cusps, the septal cusp and the parietal cusp. These cusps merge at their extremities and may form subsidiary cusps. The left atrioventricular valve, the mitral valve, is also a bicuspid valve. The semilunar valves normally consist of three leaflets attached peripherally to the aortic or pulmonic fibrous ring. The free border of each cusp has a nodule in the middle that helps to complete the valve closure during diastole. The pulmonic valve consists of right, left, and intermediate cusps. The aortic valve consists of right, left, and septal cusps.

CONDUCTION SYSTEM (p. 826)

Cardiac impulses normally originate at the sinoatrial node, which is located at the junction of the cranial vena cava and right atrium. Conduction across the atrium from the sinoatrial node to the atrioventricular node occurs via the three internodal pathways (anterior, middle, and posterior). The major conducting load is carried by the anterior internodal pathway.

The atrioventricular node begins in the septal wall of the right atrium. The atrioventricular bundle (of His) emerges from the atrioventricular node and continues ventrally through the fibrous base of the heart. The bundle divides into the right and left bundle branches. The right bundle branch traverses the septum as a single structure that branches near the right ventricular apex. The left bundle branch is broader and fans over a more diffuse area. The bundle branches terminate in the endocardium as Purkinje fibers.

CHAPTER 56
Pathophysiology of Cardiac Failure (pages 826–841)

Heart failure is *circulatory failure* caused by cardiac dysfunction. Circulatory failure is an inability to provide adequate cardiac output at an acceptable venous pressure.

CLASSIFICATION OF HEART FAILURE (p. 827)

Heart failure can be categorized according to anatomical description, severity and nature of clinical signs, and etiology.

Anatomical descriptions refer to the locus of primary malfunction, often referenced to a valve or cardiac chamber. The nature of clinical signs refers to whether physical disabilities are due primarily to a reduction in cardiac output (sometimes referred to as *forward* failure) or due to fluid retention and congestion/edema (i.e., *backward* failure). An important implication is that heart failure is not necessarily associated with any one particular physiological abnormality.

ETIOLOGY OF HEART FAILURE (pp. 827–830)

Several congenital conditions can impair cardiac function and induce heart failure. Congenital volume overload can develop in response to developmental alterations in the structure and function of cardiac valves (causing regurgitation) or arise from left-to-right shunts.

Volume Overloads

Acquired valvular regurgitation is common in older small dogs and usually involves a process known as *endocardiosis*. Valvular regurgitation is a common manifestation of dilative cardiomyopathies in cats and large dogs. Traumatic damage to valves or their support structures and inflammatory disease (endocarditis) are encountered less commonly.

Rhythm Disturbances

Disturbances in cardiac rate and rhythm have deleterious effects on cardiac output and cardiac filling pressures, but the impact is mild and alone is insufficient to induce heart failure. Exceptions are occasionally encountered when the ventricular rate becomes either very slow (< 30 to 40 beats per minute [bpm] or very fast (> 250 bpm for dogs, > 300 bpm for cats).

Diastolic Dysfunction

Diastolic dysfunction involves abnormalities in the rate, extent, and pressure associated with ventricular relaxation and filling. The heart cannot sustain a higher volumetric output than what is supplied by venous return. This "return" is the degree of diastolic ventricular filling. If the compliance of the ventricles is reduced or if the duration of diastole is reduced, diastolic filling and stroke volume decrease.

When compliance *is* reduced or when the diastolic duration is too short (extreme tachycardia), ventricular filling can be less.

Pressure Overloads

The most common causes of an increased pressure load are the presumed heritable obstructive deformities of the semilunar valves or surrounding tissue.

Systolic Dysfunction

Systolic myocardial dysfunction is a primary problem in idiopathic cardiomyopathy and a common secondary sequel to other forms of heart disease. Theoretically, systolic impairment can develop because of interference with myocardial function at a cardiac *chamber* level as well as a *cellular* level.

Cellular mechanisms are probably more important than chamber mechanisms in most forms of myocardial failure. These can include changes in the quantity of myocardial cells or functional changes within the cell.

Cell Excitation

Cell excitation requires cell depolarization and intracellular calcium influx, which is subject to modification by various autonomic and endocrine factors.

The amount of calcium entering the cell during depolarization must be extruded during the repolarization and resting parts of the cardiac cycle. Calcium extrusion is largely accomplished by a membrane-bound sodium-calcium countertransport mechanism.

Excessive influx of excitation calcium may be a cause of myocardial failure in some experimental models. Altered intracellular calcium concentration can be detrimental to myocyte function beyond its role as a trigger for contractile protein interactions.

Intracellular Calcium Activation (pp. 829–830)

Contractile Filament Interactions (p. 830)

Energy Transduction (p. 830)

PRIMARY CHANGES INDUCED BY HEART DISEASE
(pp. 830–834)

Heart failure is a complex state that includes various alterations in hemodynamic, neurological, endocrine, and biochemical parameters. Three features are universal and exist to some degree in all forms of heart failure: reduced cardiac output, decreased arterial pressure, and increased venous pressures in the systemic or pulmonary circulations.

The primary reduction in cardiac output initiates either a decline in mean arterial pressure, a rise in venous pressure, or more commonly both. A rise in venous pressure increases the hydrostatic force for filtration. The effect of a major reduction in arterial pressure is an impairment in perfusion of the vital organs (brain and heart).

With the exception of rhythm failure resulting from severe brady-cardia, the primary decrease in cardiac output is due to a reduction in *effective* ventricular stroke volume.

A decline in cardiac output initiates an obligatory reduction in global or regional perfusion and delivery of oxygen to tissues and a decrease in systemic arterial blood pressure.

The primary effects on preload, afterload, and contractility differ depending on the principal abnormality. These loads and contractility are particularly important hemodynamic factors because they are major determinants of stroke volume and myocardial oxygen requirements.

Cardiac Loads

Preload and *afterload* refer to forces acting on (within) the ventricles during the diastolic and systolic phases of the cardiac mechanical cycle, respectively.

Preload is the stretching force applied to a muscle or cardiac chamber during diastole and is usually referenced to the last or end-diastolic moment of diastole.

The stretch of a muscle strip or cardiac chamber is determined by the prevailing stretching force (preload) and the passive compliance (or stiffness) of that chamber. If compliance remains the same, an increase in preload promotes an increase in sarcomere stretch (muscle strip length or cardiac chamber volume) and consequently an increase in systolic performance and stroke volume.

Afterload, like preload, is a force acting on or within the myocardium. It represents the composite force *opposing* myocardial shortening during systole. Stated another way, afterload is the force that must be overcome before myocardial shortening and ejection can occur. The greater the force of opposition (afterload), the less the extent of myocardial shortening and ejection.

Contractility

Contractility is a parameter that originally referred to the vigor or strength of contraction of the myocardium independent of any modification by the prevailing preload and afterload. It had been previously thought that contractility was largely embodied in the amount of calcium that bathed the contractile proteins in systole and possibly also the affinity of the troponin-tropomyosin complex to calcium. Newer evidence shows that both the magnitude of calcium release and the sensitivity of the contractile proteins can be modulated by changes in preload.

Changes in Loads and Contractility: Volume Overloads

Volume overloads are typically associated with moderate to severe increases in diastolic ventricular volumes (hence radius) and pressure, with little change in wall thickness. The result is a moderate to severe increase in diastolic stress or preload. The effect on afterload is not as consistent. Most volume overloads, at least during systole, have an abnormal patency between two or more cardiac chambers or major vessels. One chamber usually represents a low-pressure ''relief'' region during the contraction of the remaining high-pressure chamber. The change in afterload in volume overload disorders varies, generally being greatest for pulmonic or aortic regurgitation and patent ductus arteriosus and least for atrioventricular valve regurgitation and intracardiac left-to-right shunts. Contractility disorders are not a *primary* feature of volume loads nor even inevitable secondary changes.

Pressure Overloads

The primary effects of pressure overloads are qualitatively similar to volume overloads, with some important quantitative differences. Because of a primary fall in stroke volume, end-diastolic volume and pressure increase. The initial response is an increase in preload volume and pressure, and hence preload is usually much smaller than with volume overloads. In contrast, afterload is markedly increased in pressure overloads, at least initially because of the high systolic pressures needed for effective ejection. Contractility increases transiently after imposing an increased afterload—the Anrep effect.

Systolic Dysfunction

By definition, contractility is depressed as the primary event in heart failure caused by systolic myocardial failure.

Diastolic Dysfunction

Diastolic myocardial disorders differ from the preceding forms of heart failure in that an increase in preload is not a predominant feature. The primary effects on contractility have not been resolved and probably depend on the underlying condition.

Rhythm Disorders

The effects of severe rhythm abnormalities on loads and contractility depend on whether tachycardia or bradycardia exists. With tachycardia sufficient to cause heart failure, preload is often decreased. Bradycardias sufficient to induce heart failure are often characterized by changes exactly opposite to those with tachycardias. Preload is increased owing to the increase in diastolic ventricular volume afforded by longer filling time. Afterload is variable.

SECONDARY EFFECTS OF HEART DISEASE (pp. 834–837)

Physiological responses to primary effects of heart disease develop quickly, often within seconds. Some can persist indefinitely, whereas others can be sustained only for brief periods. Many of these secondary effects have clear origins, being manifestations of neural, endocrine, renal, and morphological changes. Other responses, including some of the peripheral vascular responses, are mediated by mechanisms that are not fully understood. All can be significant contributors to the complex state known as heart failure.

Cardiovascular Priorities

The available physiological "resources" are activated to maintain three important hemodynamic variables: arterial blood pressure, tissue perfusion (flow), and venous pressures. Physiological "priorities" must be established. These priorities are designed to (1) sustain blood flow to the critical organs (brain and heart), (2) provide blood flow to the remaining noncritical organs, and (3) prevent venous pressures from exceeding the threshold for edema, in that order.

Initial Responses

A reduction in renal blood flow elicits a decline in urine volume and an increase in blood volume, venous return, and cardiac filling. Stretch receptors in the aortic arch and carotid sinuses perceive pressure by the degree of vessel wall stretch. The effects of reduced renal perfusion and baroreceptor unloading are concerted. They act together to increase effective circulating blood volume, improve cardiac output, and maintain blood pressure. Multiple physiological control systems are competing for overall control of the circulation, with the autoregulatory and cardiopulmonary receptor systems opposing the renal blood flow and arterial baroreflex systems. The effects of the latter two usually predominate. These initial responses develop quickly and are powerful but cannot be sustained.

Intermediate (Endocrine) Responses

One of the most important hormonal changes is activation of the renin-angiotensin-aldosterone system. A decrease in blood flow to the kidneys is sensed by intrarenal baroreceptors in the afferent artery, stimulating the local release of renin. Renin release also is stimulated by increased renal sympathetic nerve activity of the arterial baroreflex response.

Antidiuretic hormone (ADH) levels are elevated in congestive heart failure. In quadrupeds, the major stimulus is probably mediated through unloading of the arterial baroreceptors, although angiotensin II can serve as a direct stimulant. Inhibition of ADH release is provided by excitation of the low-pressure cardiac baroreceptors. ADH has well-known effects on the collecting ducts of the kidneys, promoting water retention and expansion of blood volume.

Chronic (Structural) Responses

One of the most important and universal responses of the heart to disease and abnormal loads is hypertrophy of the myocardium. Neural, endocrine, and renal responses are probably adequate to sustain a stressed cardiovascular system for days to weeks, but hypertrophy is probably essential for long-term survival.

Myocardial protein may increase by up to 50 per cent in as little as 48 hours after the imposition of increased loads. The benefits of hypertrophy are at least twofold. First, hypertrophy increases the number of contractile filaments and presumably the composite force that can be generated during systole. Second, hypertrophy can act to normalize the preload and afterload abnormalities that accompany heart disease.

The cost of hypertrophy is the increase in vascularity required to supply the increased mass. Companion animals generally have a high capacity for collateral vascular development, but even this can be exceeded by hypertrophy.

EFFECTS OF HEART FAILURE ON VASCULAR FUNCTION (pp. 837–839)

The task of sustaining an effective circulation is shared equally by the heart and blood vessels. The contribution of blood vessels to circulatory control is manifested by changes in regional and total vascular resistance. These changes are manifested by neural and endocrine stimuli, local metabolic modifiers, and the passive properties described by the structural compliance of the vessel wall.

In *severe* heart failure, vascular responsiveness may decline. Because impairment to so many stimuli is observed, the explanation may be at least partially mechanical, probably due to an increase in the passive stiffness of the vessel wall.

SUMMARY (pp. 839)

Heart disease can result from five physiological abnormalities. Regardless of etiology, the primary effects of heart disease include decreased cardiac output and mean arterial pressure and increased venous pressure. A series of responses are available to restore these primary abnormalities, including neural changes, endocrine activation, and myocardial hypertrophy. The overall compensatory response does not proceed as a simple transference of responsibility from one control system to another. The total response involves extensive interactions characterized by amplification of some factors and attenuation of others. Some patients develop a new compensated state of heart failure in which cardiac output and arterial pressure can be maintained at rest despite advanced cardiac disease. In some animals, compensatory reserve is eventually exhausted, culminating in noticeable clinical signs at rest.

CHAPTER 57

Diagnostic Methods (pages 842–855)

ANAMNESIS (p. 842)

Despite the development of new diagnostic techniques and equipment, a complete history and physical examination are important. The breed may offer a clue to the diagnosis because certain cardiac diseases have breed predispositions. The history includes identification of the complaint, a history of the current problem, and past and environmental and vaccination history. Data concerning growth and activity of littermates are helpful. An animal's diet is also important, because weight control and limited sodium intake may be part of therapy. An owner's desired use for the pet is considered in selecting therapy and evaluating prognosis. It is important to assess whether clinical signs are referable to the cardiovascular system.

PHYSICAL EXAMINATION (p. 842)

A complete physical examination is directed at evaluating the entire animal and identifying all abnormalities. A history of cardiovascular problems may focus additional attention on the cardiac and pulmonary systems. The neck is examined for jugular distension or a jugular pulse.

AUSCULTATION (pp. 843–844)

Auscultation is best performed with an animal standing to allow the heart and lungs to assume normal positions. All areas of the heart and lung field are auscultated. The heart is evaluated over the pulmonic, aortic, mitral, and tricuspid valve areas. The remainder of the chest, thoracic inlet, neck, and head is examined for radiation of murmurs. Both the diaphragm and bell of the stethoscope are used to identify high- and low-frequency murmurs. The lung fields are examined over multiple sites on both sides.

A first heart sound (S_1) associated with atrioventricular valve closure and a second heart sound (S_2) at the time of semilunar valve closure are normally heard. The third heart sound (S_3) occurs during diastole and rapid ventricular filling. The fourth heart sound (S_4) is heard just before S_1 and is associated with atrial contraction.

Cardiac Murmurs

Turbulent flow can produce auscultable murmurs. These murmurs may be innocent flow murmurs heard most frequently in young animals, murmurs arising from physiological changes such as anemia with a packed cell volume less than 15 per cent, or murmurs due to cardiac disease. Evaluation of a murmur includes identification of time of occurrence, duration, type, intensity, location on the thoracic cavity, and radiation.

PHONOCARDIOGRAPHY (p. 844)

ELECTROCARDIOGRAPHY (pp. 844–846)

Changes in the ECG may be associated with cardiac enlargement, myocardial disease, conduction disorders, and dysrhythmias.

Cardiac Enlargement

Changes in duration and amplitude of the P wave may occur with atrial enlargement. The right atrium depolarizes first and provides the initial part of the P wave. Left atrial depolarization occurs later, producing the remainder of the P wave. When the right atrium enlarges, portions of the right and left atrial depolarization overlap, and this superimposition results in increased P-wave amplitude. In left atrial enlargement, the second half of the P wave is prolonged, resulting in an increased P-wave duration.

Left ventricular enlargement is often associated with increased amplitude of the R waves in leads facing the left ventricle. Other changes with enlarged left ventricles include prolongation of the QRS complex, ST segment slurring, and increased T-wave amplitude. A mean electrical axis of greater than $+100°$ in a dog is a useful indicator of right ventricular enlargement.

Myocardial Damage

An ECG can be used to recognize some types and degrees of myocardial damage. Alterations that might be expected include the development of deep Q waves, particularly in cases of transmural myocardial damage. Elevation or depression of the ST segment is a rapidly developing response to myocardial hypoxia or injury. Finally, changes in repolarization of injured myocardial tissue may produce T-wave alterations.

Conduction Disorders

Conduction disorders may involve any level of the conduction pathway. The abnormalities may range from alterations in impulse generation to delayed conduction or complete obstruction of conduction.

Dysrhythmias

Atrial enlargement predisposes to myocardial changes that may alter automaticity and also favors re-entry pathways that can perpetuate abnormal rhythms.

Premature atrial depolarizations are identified by the early appearance of P waves with abnormal conformation. These P waves are usually followed by normal QRS complexes. Atrioventricular nodal or junctional premature depolarizations are also usually followed by normal QRS complexes. The P wave, if visible, is inverted because of retrograde conduction through the atria.

Atrial fibrillation may occur with congenital or acquired disorders. The ECG is characterized by the absence of discernible P waves, an irregular ventricular rate, variable second-degree atrioventricular block, and a rapid ventricular rate.

Ventricular dysrhythmias may range from periodic ventricular premature depolarizations to ventricular tachycardia with only occasional capture or fusion beats. The QRS complexes usually appear bizarre and are prolonged.

RADIOLOGY (pp. 846–849)

A radiograph rarely gives direct evidence of the kind of cardiac disease present but rather demonstrates changes in the thoracic structures that occur in response to cardiac disease.

Contrast Radiography

Although general assessments can be made from plain radiographs, contrast radiography allows evaluation of wall thickness, chamber and vessel size, and flow patterns.

Intravascular angiography may be accomplished in a nonselective manner through percutaneous catheterization of the jugular or cephalic vein or selectively after direct catheterization of right- or left-sided structures through the jugular vein, carotid artery, or femoral vessels.

Nonselective venous angiography is less precise but more easily and rapidly accomplished. Chemical restraint is usually required, but the depth and duration are shorter than for selective catheterization. The technique can be adapted to private practice, and although a rapid film changer is helpful, manual techniques are adequate.

Iothalamate meglumine, approximately 1 ml/kg, is injected rapidly. The first film is taken just before completion of the injection and at intervals of 0.5 to 1.0 second, thereafter depending on the tentative diagnosis. Adjustments in timing must be made in animals with prolonged circulation times.

CARDIAC CATHETERIZATION AND SELECTIVE ANGIOGRAPHY (pp. 849–851)

Cardiac catheterization is used to confirm a tentative diagnosis, identify additional abnormalities, and evaluate the nature and severity of a lesion.

Cardiac catheterization provides assessment of pressures, oxygen tensions, cardiac output, and shunt quantitation. All of this information may not be necessary in every case, and a protocol for the most complete and efficient evaluation should be prepared for each patient.

Surgical Approach

The surgical approach for cardiac catheterization may use the carotid artery and external jugular vein or the femoral vessels.

Catheter Selection and Technique (pp. 849–850)
Pressure Recordings

Pressure tracings are recorded from all chambers and vessels entered. A slight (< 5 mm Hg) pressure gradient may exist between the right ventricle and pulmonary artery in normal dogs. Left atrial pressure is usually evaluated indirectly via the pulmonary artery wedge pressure because the left atrium is difficult to catheterize. Both aortic and pulmonic stenosis produce pressure gradients between the ventricular chamber and related great vessel. This information is obtained by recording pressures as the catheter is pulled from the pulmonary artery to right ventricle or left ventricle to aorta.

Cardiac Output Measurement

Cardiac output determinations are accomplished by indicator dilution techniques.

Oximetry

Oximetry is useful in diagnosis and quantitation of shunts. Left-to-right shunts are recognized by increased right-sided oxygen saturation.

Selective Angiography

Selective angiography is accomplished by direct catheterization of the desired vessel or chamber. Because the catheter can be placed at the desired injection site, less contrast medium is required and better demonstration of the lesion obtained. If all data obtained by catheterization are integrated, a clinician can determine systolic and diastolic chamber size, valve orifice area, vascular resistance, and regurgitant flow.

ECHOCARDIOGRAPHY (pp. 851–854)

Echocardiography uses the imaging capabilities of ultrasound to identify and evaluate various cardiac structures. The ultrasound transducer acts as a transmitter and receiver. It generates high-frequency sound waves that reflect or echo from cardiac structures and then collects these reflected waves so they can be integrated and displayed on an oscilloscope.

Several different modes of echocardiogram can be obtained, each with particular advantages and disadvantages. An M-mode, or motion, echocardiogram does not allow viewing of most structural lesions but is the preferred method for obtaining cardiac measurements. A two-dimensional echocardiogram is obtained by using mechanical or electronic scanning transducers to obtain multiple images that are continuously updated to give a two-dimensional picture with real-time motion. Many abnormalities of cardiac structure and function can be seen directly. Spectral Doppler echocardiography applies the Doppler principle to the evaluation of blood flow velocity. This information can then be used to identify areas of turbulent flow. Color flow Doppler echocardiography allows viewing of blood flow toward and away from the transducer, plus observation of turbulent flow.

M-mode echocardiography is used primarily for obtaining measurements of chamber size as well as indices of ventricular function. An M-mode echocardiogram produces an "ice pick" view of the heart; however, if combined with two-dimensional echocardiography, the location of the ice pick can be carefully selected. This combination improves accuracy and validity of M-mode measurements.

Two-dimensional echocardiography permits viewing the heart in both long-axis and short-axis views with real-time motion. Anatomical structures and relationships in two-dimensional echocardiograms of normal dogs are established. Cardiac measurements can also be obtained from the two-dimensional echocardiogram as well as the M-mode recording. Structural abnormalities that are not apparent with M-mode recordings can be seen on a two-dimensional echocardiogram.

An echocardiogram is able to provide both qualitative and quantitative information about the significance of various congenital heart defects. Nevertheless, the available information may be insufficient to confirm a diagnosis or adequately assess the severity of a defect.

The Doppler principle is used to determine blood flow velocity and direction at specific sites in the heart and great vessels. Doppler studies are highly dependent on a patient's anatomy, the experience of the ultrasonographer, and the patient's cooperation. Acceptable studies cannot always be obtained.

Cardiac catheterization may be necessary to obtain peak-to-peak pressure gradient, which is still the basis for many surgical decisions in pulmonic and aortic stenosis.

Our criteria for making surgical decisions may have to change, because pressure gradients obtained with Doppler are maximum instantaneous pressure gradients in awake or sedated animals rather than peak-to-peak gradients in anesthetized patients.

MISCELLANEOUS DIAGNOSTIC PROCEDURES (p. 854)

CHAPTER 58

Cardiac Disorders (pages 856–889)

CONGENITAL CARDIAC DISORDERS (pp. 856–877)

Development

In a developing fetus, the heart forms from a single tube and through a series of bends and separations eventually becomes a four-chambered structure.

During fetal development, connections between the two parallel circuits—the developing right side of the heart and the developing left side—allow shunting from right to left because of the high resistance to pulmonary flow. In the late stages of fetal development or shortly after birth, the shunts (atrial, ventricular, and ductal) close. If any of the fetal openings persist, the high pressure in the left side directs the shunt from left to right.

Malpositioning

Ectopia cordis, an uncommon anomaly, is a malpositioning of the heart, usually in the neck. *Dextrocardia*, or positioning of the heart apex to the right of the thorax rather than the left, is an occasional radiographic finding. The concept of *situs* relates the heart to body organ positioning. *Situs solitus* is the normal relationship. *Situs inversus* is a congenital anomaly, rarely reported in animals but probably much more common than is recognized, in which the body organs are positioned in mirror image.

Venous Anomalies

Major systemic venous anomalies are described in Chapter 47. The remaining significant venous anomaly associated with cardiovascular disease is persistence of the left anterior cardinal vein or left anterior vena cava. This anomaly causes no physiological problems.

Physiology of Left-to-Right Shunts

The most common disorder of the right atrium is atrial septal defect. This defect and combination defects involving the atrial septum are more common in cats.

Other left-to-right shunts are ventricular septal defect and patent ductus arteriosus. The pathophysiology of left-to-right shunts is related to the pressure or flow developed in the corresponding right chambers and lungs and the volume overload and failure of the left side of the heart. The fetal connections (foramen ovale, interventricular foramen, and ductus arteriosus) allow shunting of blood from the fetal high-pressure right side of the heart to the low-pressure left side, therefore bypassing the developing lungs. If persistence of the opening between the two parallel circuits continues, the flow or shunt is from the postnatal high-pressure left side to the low-pressure right, a left-to-right shunt. The left side of the heart continues to meet the body's needs, so output is increased by the shunt volume. Because of shunting from the left side to the right, the volume of blood in all chambers of the shunt circuit is increased. This shunt includes the pulmonary arteries, pulmonary capillaries, and pulmonary veins and may be diagnosed by the characteristic radiographic appearance of overcirculated lungs. Pulmonary edema may occur, producing the pulmonary signs of left-to-right shunts. In ventricular septal defect and patent ductus arteriosus, the additional volume of blood that the left ventricle must pump may cause the left ventricle to fail.

Atrial Septal Defects

The physical findings with atrial septal defect are related to the shunt from left atrium to right atrium, to right ventricle, to pulmonary vasculature. Clinical findings with atrial septal defect include a flow murmur associated with the increased blood flow across the pulmonary valve. The second heart sound is frequently split owing to the delay in closure of the pulmonary valve that results from the increased volume.

Electrocardiographic (ECG) findings with atrial septal defect reflect the amount of additional work load of the right side of the heart.

The diagnosis of atrial septal defect is established by radiography, echocardiography, and cardiac catheterization. Oxygen saturation measurements taken from the anterior vena cava and right atrium show an oxygen increase from the veins to the atrium.

Surgical correction of atrial septal defect has been reported. The prognosis in animals with isolated atrial septal defect is favorable. Careful management of salt level and reduction of activity are adequate for maintenance.

Endocardial Cushion Defect

In cats, endocardial cushion defect or atrioventricular canal defect is the second most common congenital lesion. The embryonic endocardial cushions form the ventral portion of the atrial septum, the dorsal portion of the ventricular septum, and portions of the mitral and tricuspid valves. Total endocardial cushion defects, therefore, can produce a butterfly-shaped opening at the center of the heart, including a low atrial defect, a high ventricular defect, and lesions in the atrioventricular valves. The signs of endocardial cushion defect are associated with mitral valve regurgitation and the large left-to-right shunt at the atrial or ventricular level, producing extreme pulmonary flows, pulmonary edema, and usually death due to respiratory failure. The diagnosis of endocardial cushion defect is made by echocardiography, in which the defects or valve lesions can be seen. Successful treatment of the lesion in cats has not been reported, but pulmonary artery banding (see Chapter 60) might be effective in reducing the increased pulmonary blood flow.

Tricuspid Valve Disorders (p. 861)

Ventricular Septal Defect

The lesion occurs in approximately 1:2,000 live births in dogs. It may be more common in cats, in which it is the most common congenital heart defect.

Ventricular septal defects can occasionally be found in the ventricular muscle toward the apex but are much more commonly located high in the ventricular septum. Animals with ventricular septal defect exhibit pulmonary edema due to increased pulmonary pressure and flow because of the shunt from the left to the right ventricle. A pulmonary-to-systemic flow ratio of more than 2.5:1 is necessary to produce symptoms and therefore require treatment.

Ventricular septal defect murmur radiates to the right chest wall, as with a lesion at the tricuspid valve. The murmur is pansystolic and has a slight crescendo-decrescendo quality. The murmur frequently radiates to the thoracic inlet via the aortic arch and brachiocephalic vessels. If the ventricular defect is severe enough to produce extreme flows to the right side, a crescendo-decrescendo murmur may be heard at the pulmonary valve. The presence of a second murmur at the pulmonary area usually suggests flow severe enough to warrant treatment. The ECG findings associated with ventricular septal defect include mild left ventricular enlargement and perhaps right ventricular enlargement. Right-axis deviation and right ventricular hypertrophy suggest developing pulmonary hypertension and more severe disease. Radiographically, the heart is enlarged on both sides. The pulmonary vasculature is increased.

The diagnosis of ventricular septal defect is established through the physical findings, the ECG and radiographic findings, the echocardiographic findings, plus venous angiography. Cardiac catheterization can also be used to demonstrate the severity of the pressure changes.

Indications for surgical or medical treatment of ventricular septal defect are (1) an audible flow murmur in the pulmonary area, (2) enlargement of the pulmonary artery on a dorsoventral radiograph, (3) a diagnostic echo or angiogram, or (4) a shunt ratio of 3:1 or more.

Open heart surgical repair has been reported. It carries a moderate mortality, but repair is total and the animal can be expected to live a normal life. The palliative procedure, pulmonary artery banding, is effective and safe in both dogs and cats.

The prognosis in ventricular septal defect is favorable. A small percentage of defects close spontaneously. Approximately 75 per cent of dogs and probably a similar percentage of cats with the defect do not have pulmonary-to-systemic flow ratios of greater than 2.5:1 and do not need treatment.

Pulmonic Stenosis

Pulmonic stenosis is one of the most common congenital cardiac disorders. The lesion can be supravalvular (in the pulmonary artery), valvular (affecting the valve, usually by fusion of the valve cusps), subvalvular (a very common fibrous lesion just beneath the valve in the right ventricle), or muscular infundibular. The term *pulmonary valve dysplasia* has been used to describe a frequent form of the disease in animals in which the obstruction includes the valve and the immediate subvalve tissue.

Valvular pulmonic stenosis, subvalvular pulmonic stenosis, and valve dysplasia are the most common types of pulmonic stenosis in small animals. Muscular infundibular pulmonary stenosis is the normal response to obstruction but can occur independently. Physical findings of pulmonic stenosis include a crescendo-decrescendo systolic murmur, heard best at the base of the heart on the left side, which is characteristic and tends not to radiate.

The laboratory findings of pulmonic stenosis include right ventricular hypertrophy and right-axis deviation on ECG and the right-sided cardiac enlargement seen on all radiographic views. A poststenotic dilation of the main pulmonary artery is a usual finding.

A venous angiogram differentiates pulmonic stenosis from the two lesions that appear similar. On the angiogram, the approximate location of the obstruction and the severity of the right ventricular hypertrophy can be seen.

ECG can also be used to indicate severity. Right-axis deviation generally correlates well with the severity of right ventricular hypertrophy. Right-axis shifts to 180° have consistently been found in animals that prove by catheterization to be surgical candidates. Animals with demonstrated pulmonic stenosis and right-axis deviation of greater than 180° or wall thickness more than three times normal are invariably surgical candidates; however, the severity should be confirmed by cardiac catheterization.

Supravalvular pulmonic stenosis is most easily repaired by a conduit circumventing the obstruction. Valvular or discrete subvalvular pulmonic stenosis or valve dysplasia can be treated in several ways. Our preferred procedure for mature animals is a modification of the inflow occlusion–pulmonary arteriotomy procedure popularized by Swan. Immature animals needing surgical repair for pulmonic stenosis at the valve level are most successfully treated with the patch graft technique. The simplest surgical techniques are the bistoury and modified Brock procedures for incising or removing the obstruction. Muscular pulmonic stenosis is the most difficult to manage surgically, but the patch graph technique is the most effective surgical treatment. Open heart surgical repair has been successful for the muscular type; other techniques have limited success.

Surgery for pulmonic stenosis is recommended if evidence of severe hypertrophy, failure, syncope, or increasing wall thickness is found. In adults, systemic pressure of 120 mm Hg in the right ventricle or a gradient of 100 mm Hg across the valve indicates a need for surgical repair. In immature animals, right ventricular pressure of greater than 70 mm Hg indicates the need for surgery.

Severely affected animals with pulmonic stenosis may live to adulthood but usually die of right-sided heart failure or arrhythmia by 1 to 2 years of age. Mildly affected animals with right ventricular pressures less than 70 mm Hg can be expected to live a normal life. Dogs with severe muscular pulmonic stenosis, either primary disease or secondary to other pulmonic stenosis, have a grave prognosis.

Tetralogy of Fallot

Tetralogy of Fallot is the most common cyanotic congenital cardiac disorder in dogs and cats. The disorder includes (1) ventricular septal defect; (2) muscular pulmonic stenosis; (3) over-riding or rightward positioning of the aorta; and (4) right ventricular hypertrophy secondary to pulmonic stenosis. Cyanosis results from the obstruction of pulmonic stenosis that produces increased right ventricular pressure, causing venous blood to flow through the ventricular defect and mix with oxygenated blood in the aorta.

Animals with tetralogy of Fallot show weakness, failure to thrive and grow, exercise intolerance, and generalized cyanosis. A systolic murmur is present at the base of the heart. The murmur may not always be present if the abnormal flow is not turbulent. The presence of severe polycythemia implicates a right-to-left central shunt. The diagnosis is suggested by finding severe right ventricular enlargement on ECG and radiography. Confirmation of the diagnosis is made by a venous angiogram.

Treatment for tetralogy is either palliative or curative. Palliative procedures may be medical or surgical. Medical palliation currently used with success in dogs, cats, and humans depends on reduction of the muscular obstruction associated with the pulmonic stenosis. Many surgical techniques are used for tetralogy of Fallot, the most commonly used in animals being the Blalock or Potts anastomosis. Total corrective procedures require open heart surgery and resection of the muscular obstruction with closure of the ventricular defect. Results of treatment of tetralogy are fair. Without treatment, few animals survive to 1 year of age.

Eisenmenger's Complex (p. 869)

A condition similar to tetralogy of Fallot but much less common is Eisenmenger's disease, which consists of ventricular septal defect and severe pulmonary hypertension producing right-to-left ventricular shunt. Signs are identical with tetralogy of Fallot.

Because of permanent pulmonary vascular damage, no treatment is available for Eisenmenger's disease. *Eisenmenger's syndrome* is a term defining any left-to-right shunt producing pulmonary hypertension and resultant right-to-left shunt.

Mitral Valve Abnormalities

Congenital abnormalities of the mitral valve have signs referable to heart failure with mitral regurgitation, as noted with cardiomyopathy.

Aortic Stenosis

Left ventricular outflow tract lesions, aortic stenosis, and similar aortic disorders are extremely common in dogs but rare in cats. Valvular aortic stenosis is rare, but subvalvular fibrous aortic stenosis is hereditary (autosomal dominant).

Animals affected with subvalvular aortic stenosis have a history of syncope or a family history of sudden death. On examination, affected dogs have a crescendo-decrescendo systolic murmur that is heard best at the base of the heart on the left side or in the right anterior thorax near the sternum and radiates into the thoracic inlet and up the neck. Arterial pulses are weakened. ECG findings include left ventricular hypertrophy in approximately half the cases, left-axis deviation, and occasional dysrhythmias or ST segment alteration. Echocardiography may reveal the subvalvular lesion, the left ventricular wall thickening, and echo densities apparently due to fibrosis of myocardium in severe cases.

Diagnosis of aortic stenosis is established by a venous angiogram with the radiograph taken in the levo phase approximately 6 to 8 seconds after the injection. If aortic stenosis is mild, animals live a normal life. If the disease is severe, syncopal episodes, probably related to severe ventricular dysrhythmia, or sudden death occurs. The indications for therapy are syncope, ST segment change on the ECG, or catheterization findings of left ventricular outflow tract gradient of greater than 70 mm Hg. Animals with left ventricular pressures of greater than 220 mm Hg (left ventricular-aortic gradients of 100 mm Hg or more) are usually symptomatic and die early.

Several medical treatments suggested for aortic stenosis use beta-adrenergic blockers to lessen the obstruction. Surgical resection of the obstruction has been successful in dogs. Left ventricular-aortic conduits have now been used to bypass the obstruction but have a high mortality.

Transposition of the Great Arteries

Transposition complex is an unusual cardiac abnormality rarely encountered in animals.

Aortic-Pulmonary Window

The defect is an opening between the aorta and the pulmonary artery at the ascending portion of the aorta. It resembles a severe patent ductus arteriosus. Because in appearance and physical findings it resembles patent ductus arteriosus, aortic-pulmonary window is an important differential diagnostic consideration in animals suspected of having patent ductus arteriosus.

Patent Ductus Arteriosus

The most common congenital cardiac disorder is patent ductus arteriosus, which results from failure of closure of the ductus arteriosus, the normal fetal connection between the aorta and pulmonary artery. Patent ductus arteriosus occurs in approximately 1:750 live births in dogs but is much less common in cats. In dogs, this disorder is hereditary and is assumed to be polygenic. There is approximately a 4:1 female/male distribution.

The diagnosis of patent ductus arteriosus in dogs or cats is usually made by auscultation of the characteristic continuous or "machinery" murmur in asymptomatic animals presented for vaccination. If the disease is untreated, signs of pulmonary edema and left-sided heart failure follow. The left ventricle, because of the large volume it must pump, dilates and hypertrophies, causing dilation of the mitral annulus and mitral regurgitation in approximately half the animals. If mitral regurgitation occurs, development of pulmonary edema is increased, and signs of unthriftiness, exercise intolerance, and occasionally cough and poor growth are exacerbated.

ECG evidence of left ventricular hypertrophy and, rarely, late right ventricular hypertrophy can be found. The nearly pathognomonic murmur, in addition to radiographic findings of pulmonary overcirculation, dilation of the descending aorta due to the ductus diverticulum, and left ventricular enlargement, confirms the diagnosis.

Patent ductus arteriosus is treated surgically. Animals allowed to continue untreated risk development of mitral regurgitation, left ventricular enlargement, permanent pulmonary vascular damage, atrial fibrillation, and death. Small animals seldom live to 1 year, but large animals may live to 5 years.

A small number (1 to 2 per cent) of animals with patent ductus develop right-to-left shunt. Regardless of the cause of right-to-left shunting patent ductus, affected animals have differential cyanosis and weakness in the rear legs. Owing to the severely desaturated arterial blood supply to the kidneys, erythropoietin is released, and severe polycythemia is found.

The prognosis for animals with patent ductus arteriosus, if treated early, is excellent. Approximately 1.5 per cent of dogs with ligation of the ductus develop recanalization, and a second operation with division of the ductus is needed.

Aortic Arch Obstructions

Obstructions to the aortic arch are rare.

Persistent Right Aortic Arch

Included in this group of diseases are anomalous subclavian arteries, double aortic arch, and most commonly persistence of the right aortic arch. The right arch becomes the permanent aortic arch, but blood flow is physiologically normal. No cardiovascular problems develop. Still, the esophagus and trachea are trapped in a vascular ring. Persistent right aortic arch is almost certainly hereditary.

Animals with persistent right aortic arch have characteristic clinical signs. The animals regurgitate after eating, usually starting at the time of weaning. When the animal begins to eat semisolid or solid food, the obstruction to the esophagus is manifested by regurgitation. The diagnosis of persistent right aortic arch or other vascular ring anomaly is made by barium swallow study. Treatment for vascular ring anomalies and persistent right aortic arch is surgical. Treatment must be started before distension of the esophagus becomes severe.

Preoperative management of animals suspected of having persistent right aortic arch includes liquid diet, feeding on an incline to aid in flow of the liquid food into the stomach, and frequent small feedings. The surgical treatment is division of the ligamentum arteriosum. Postoperative management is identical to the preoperative care and should be continued for 1 to 4 weeks, depending on the amount of distension of the esophagus at the time of surgery. Patients are slowly returned to a normal diet, frequency of feeding, and consistency and height of the food.

ACQUIRED CARDIAC DISORDERS (pp. 877–888)

Mitral Regurgitation

The vast majority of acquired disorders are associated with mitral valve regurgitation, which affects 1:12 dogs older than 5 years, with a slight preference for males. The condition is associated with degenerative changes on the mitral valve leaflets, poor coaptation, and eventual dilation of the mitral annulus. Mitral regurgitation develops slowly and often produces no clinical signs for up to 5 years after the first development of the disease.

The pathophysiology of left heart failure and mitral valve disease described in Chapter 56 should be reviewed. Measurements in spontaneous mitral regurgitation in dogs have demonstrated that a regurgitant fraction (the portion of left ventricular blood ejected to the left atrium) of approximately 60 to 70 per cent is necessary before pulmonary signs and failure develop.

The clinical signs of mitral regurgitation are generally attributed to problems with the lungs; the usual presenting complaint is a dry, hacking cough. The animal is elderly, and abnormal respiratory sounds may be heard. A pansystolic plateau murmur heard best on the left thorax at the fourth or fifth rib space is audible. The murmur radiates dorsally. Atrial arrhythmias and left ventricular hypertrophy may be noted on ECG. The lateral thoracic radiograph shows a loss of posterior waist and elevation of the trachea. On the dorsoventral radiograph, pulmonary densities and enlargement of the left atrial appendage are helpful for the diagnosis. Pulmonary venous patterns, interstitial patterns, and in very severe cases alveolar patterns may be present in the lungs.

In animals, surgical treatment of significant mitral regurgitation has been successful on few occasions. The mitral valve has been successfully replaced in the dogs, and new valved conduits show promise.

Animals with mitral regurgitation seldom have significant problems for several years after the onset of the disease. Rarely is myocardial failure a problem. When needed, medical treatment with diuretics and perhaps vasodilators or angiotensin-converting enzyme inhibitors is used.

Atrial fibrillation may be a sequel to mitral regurgitation because of the enlargement of the left atrium in large animals. This severe consequence can be fatal and is aggressively treated. Because of the continuing degeneration of the mitral valve tissues, the chordae tendineae supporting the mitral valve occasionally tear. At this time, acute increase in left atrial pressure occurs, and subsequent dilation of the left atrium is not sufficient to buffer the pressure, causing acute pulmonary signs.

Tricuspid Regurgitation

A valvular lesion of the right side of the heart that is analogous to mitral regurgitation is tricuspid regurgitation. Signs associated with this lesion arise from the systemic veins, particularly the veins of the liver. It is invariably present with mitral regurgitation but develops at a slower rate and usually has a later onset. The murmur of tricuspid regurgitation is pansystolic, is heard best on the right side at the fourth intercostal space, and tends not to radiate. Signs of the disease are ascites and previous mitral valve disease. Treatment for tricuspid regurgitation is similar to treatment for mitral regurgitation.

Dirofilariasis

In some geographic areas, the most commonly acquired heart disease affecting dogs is dirofilariasis (heartworm infestation), which is caused by the parasite *Dirofilaria immitis*. Dogs have various responses to the presence of heartworm, from almost no apparent effect to severe pulmonary hypertension, right-sided heart failure, and death.

The diagnosis of dirofilariasis is easily established. Physical examination revealing a split second heart sound (due to right ventricular emptying delay) and harsh respiratory lung sounds with laboratory findings of leukocytosis (particularly eosinophilia) and the presence of microfilariae in the blood (detected by one of the microfilaria detection laboratory tests) establish the diagnosis. The prognosis for recovery from dirofilariasis is favorable. Severely affected dogs have excellent recovery after heartworms have been removed.

An unfortunate sequel to heartworm heart disease is the postcaval syndrome. Postcaval heartworm disease, by definition, is fatal within 72 hours. Signs of postcaval syndrome are acute onset of weakness, collapse, and rapid onset of hemolysis with resultant anemia and hemoglobinuria. Treatment for postcaval syndrome is emergency surgical removal of the offending worms. The postcaval removal (Jackson) technique is a remarkable emergency lifesaving procedure.

Endocarditis

Infections of cardiac structures produce serious consequences in dogs. Bacterial infections of the heart tend to embolize to other organ systems, most frequently those tissues with the greatest blood supply. Septic emboli from the heart should be considered as a possible cause whenever multiple organ infection is suspected or multiple organ pain is detected. Treatment for bacterial endocarditis is aggressive antibiotic therapy, preferably with the appropriate antibiotic established by culture and sensitivity testing.

Complete Heart Block

The major cardiac arrhythmia of surgical significance in dogs is complete heart block. The condition develops because of damage to the atrioventricular node or bundle of His, completely interrupting the conduction from the atrium. A ventricular rhythm is established, with a heart rate of approximately 40 beats per minute. The prognosis for patients with complete heart block is grave unless a pacemaker is implanted.

Cardiomyopathy

Feline Cardiomyopathy

Feline cardiomyopathy is one of the most common major feline diseases and is the major cause of heart disease in cats. The disease may be either congestive or hypertrophic.

The etiology of feline cardiomyopathy is not completely known, but usually the congestive form is due to taurine-deficient diets.

The feline cardiomyopathy syndrome presents clinically as one of two basic disease processes: a disease of systolic malfunction (congestive cardiomyopathy) or diastolic malfunction (hypertrophic cardiomyopathy). Cats with either type of disease have similar signs. An animal is usually presented with mild to severe respiratory dysfunction, open mouth breathing and weakness, and an occasional cough or sneeze.

Congestive Cardiomyopathy. Diagnosis of congestive cardiomyopathy is based on the history, the physical findings, and the presence of dysrhythmia on ECG. The diagnosis is confirmed by echocardiography. Without an echocardiogram, confirmation of type of cardiomyopathy is most easily accomplished by venous angiogram.

Treatment for congestive cardiomyopathy is preventive by using well-developed feline diets supplemented with taurine. The use of diuretics and digitalization may be effective, but the long-term prognosis is grave.

Hypertrophic Cardiomyopathy. The cause of hypertrophic cardiomyopathy is unknown. The diagnosis is made by the ECG findings, venous angiogram, and, most important, the echocardiogram. The thick-walled, small-lumen left ventricle seen on echocardiography is pathognomonic.

Hypertrophic cardiomyopathy may be helped by beta-adrenergic blockade. Supportive therapy with diuretics can be recommended. Prognosis for cats with non–taurine-deficient feline cardiomyopathy syndrome is poor, the average life expectancy (after signs appear), regardless of therapy, being approximately 1 year. When pulmonary edema and pleural effusion are present, diuretics are important in prolonging life.

Embolization is a sequel in one-third of cats with feline cardiomyopathy. The most common location is at the bifurcation of the aorta, producing a ''saddle thrombus.'' Cats surviving aortic embolus average one recurrence within 6 months.

Canine Cardiomyopathy

The disease most often affects males of the large and giant breeds, particularly Dobermans. It can be caused by a virus. The diagnosis of congestive cardiomyopathy in a dog is established by the following criteria: (1) a large male with a history consistent with heart failure; (2) physical findings of tachycardia, respiratory distress, abnormal lung sounds, and ascites or edema; (3) ECG evidence of atrial or ventricular arrhythmias; (4) echocardiographic evidence of large, dilated, thin-walled ventricular chambers; and (5) radiographic evidence of tremendous enlargement of the heart, particularly the atria. Findings of poor ventricular wall motion, a thin ventricular wall, and poor contractility on two-dimensional echocardiography have become diagnostic.

Dogs with congestive cardiomyopathy usually have mitral regurgitation because of dilation of the left ventricle and the mitral annulus. The treatment for congestive cardiomyopathy in dogs is medical, and the prognosis is poor.

Hypertropic Cardiomyopathy. A condition manifested by sudden death and a hypertrophied left ventricle has been described in dogs. Hypertrophic cardiomyopathy in dogs is more common than previously anticipated and should be considered in sudden death of an otherwise healthy dog.

ECG findings may include left ventricular hypertrophy, conduction disturbances, and ST segment alterations. Echocardiographic evidence of abnormal thickening of the septum and free wall or asymmetrical septal hypertrophy with a septum-free wall ratio of greater than 1.3:1 is strong evidence of the disease. Effective treatment for hypertrophic cardiomyopathy in dogs has not been confirmed.

Pericarditis

Pericarditis, or reactive pericardial disease, is occasionally reported. Animals with pericarditis usually have signs associated with pericardial tamponade. The diagnosis is established by low-amplitude recording on all leads of the ECG, the radiographic appearance of a circular heart on all views, and the classic echocardiographic signs of effusion.

The treatment for pericarditis and pericardial disease is pericardiocentesis (see Chapter 60).

Tumors of the Heart

Discussion of tumors of the cardiovascular system can be found in Chapter 155.

CHAPTER 5.9

Principles of Vascular Surgery (pages 890–893)

INSTRUMENTS

Vascular cutting instruments must be sharp and free of imperfections. Rough edges on vessel walls invite deposition of proteins and cells, which can lead to thrombosis. Forceps are available in many sizes and shapes. Only atraumatic instruments are used to grasp vascular tissues.

The variety of vascular clamping instruments is tremendous. Clamps such as DeBakey ring-handle bulldog clamps are especially useful. Full-size vascular clamps may be required to reach deep vessels.

A fine pair of Olsen-Hegar or Mayo-Hegar needle holders suffices for most vascular procedures. In procedures involving use of 5-0 or 6-0 suture, a Castroviejo-style needle holder is helpful; the locking mechanism eliminates the ratchet catch and resulting gross movements necessary with more conventional needle holders.

All of these instruments are available in pediatric sizes and weights, but these are unnecessary, because vessels as small as 3 mm can be successfully sutured with the instruments described.

SUTURES

Only sutures with swaged-on needles are appropriate for vascular anastomoses. The diameter of suture used for particular applications depends on a surgeon's preference and the material. Generally, 5-0, 6-0, and 7-0 sutures are sufficiently strong for most peripheral arteries and all feline vascular anastomoses. Aortic grafts in large dogs may require 4-0 sutures.

For most applications in small animal practice, a three-eighths circle or one-half circle taper-point needle is appropriate. These fine needles must be used with care because they bend easily unless passed through the tissues with a rotational motion.

VASCULAR PROSTHESES (pp. 891–892)

Vascular prostheses consist of textile or nontextile synthetic and fresh or preserved biological types. All currently available grafts function adequately when placed in high-flow, low-resistance vessels such as the aorta.

Synthetic Grafts

All synthetic grafts are fabricated from polymers. Depending on the particular polymer and method of fabrication, a graft can be called a textile or a nonwoven graft. Dacron grafts are textiles, while polytetrafluoroethylene and polyurethane grafts are nonwoven. Dacron prostheses use knitted, woven, or velour construction. Ultrathin grafts are applicable to all vessels in canine and feline practice. Teflon and polyurethane are the two polymers most commonly used in nonwoven synthetic grafts.

Polyurethane grafts are a recent development. These grafts apparently preferentially absorb albumin, an activity that renders them nonthrombogenic. Despite porosity, they do not require preclotting. These are the most compliant grafts available, a characteristic that increases patency.

Biological Grafts

Biological grafts include both preserved and fresh conduits. The most commonly available prosthesis is glutaraldehyde-tanned human umbilical vein. A second type of preserved vascular graft is the dialdehyde starch-tanned bovine heterograft.

The most widely used and successful vascular prosthesis is fresh autogenous vein. Heparinized cold (39.2°F [4°C]) whole blood is the preferred storage medium. Mechanical hyperdistension of venous grafts causes degenerative changes throughout the wall, with increased early thrombosis.

Fresh veins elongate when pressurized in the arterial system. This property must be taken into account when the graft is trimmed. When veins are considered for use as vascular grafts, more centrally located vessels are frequently thin and prone to pseudoaneurysm formation. Venous branches are ligated rather than cauterized.

ANTICOAGULANT DRUGS (pp. 892–893)

Most vascular procedures involve agents to prevent blood clotting. These drugs may be used before, during, or after surgery. They may also be used in combination and can cause serious complications if misused. Heparin is the most widely used anticoagulant. It can be given subcutaneously but is usually administered intravenously. Heparin is sold in various concentrations. One milligram of heparin is equal to 100 units. Intravenously, the dose of heparin is 1 to 2 mg/kg of body weight. Heparin activity is monitored by measuring the activated clotting time. In most animals, 2 mg/kg produces an activated clotting time of more than 600 seconds (normal is 80 to 100 seconds), which is considered total anticoagulation. Heparin can be neutralized with protamine sulfate.

Dicumarol and warfarin act as anticoagulants by competitive antagonism with vitamin K. Prothrombin time is the best test to monitor warfarin therapy. Whole blood transfusions combined with vitamin K can be used if hemorrhage is severe or prothrombin time is greatly prolonged.

Aspirin acts as an anticoagulant by inhibiting the release of prostaglandins E_2 and F_2 from platelets, thus inhibiting platelet aggregation. In cats, aspirin is administered orally at 25 mg/kg/day. To maintain adequate blood levels in dogs, aspirin is administered every 8 hours at 25 mg/kg. Dipyridamole prevents platelet aggregation and adherence and release of platelet factors and enhanced graft patency when used with aspirin.

CHAPTER 60

Basic Cardiac Surgical Procedures (pages 893–918)

Anesthesia for cardiac surgery is discussed in Chapter 66. Excellent anesthesia is the single most important factor in successful completion of a cardiac surgical procedure. Fortunately, the surgeon can monitor two major cardiovascular and anesthesia variables during most procedures—depth of anesthesia (by blood pressure determination) and ventilation (by observing the color of the left atrium).

First, the animal is maintained in as light a plane of anesthesia as possible; second, drug administration or other nonphysiological manipulations are limited before, during, and after the surgery.

BIOPSY TECHNIQUES (pp. 894–895)

Biopsy is rarely performed on the cardiovascular system. Biopsy techniques are used primarily to evaluate myocardial muscle or to assess cardiac tissue with the diagnosis of cardiomyopathy.

Pericardiocentesis

The one cardiac biopsy technique that is routinely used clinically is pericardiocentesis for assessment of pericardial fluid.

Pericardiocentesis is accomplished at the "cardiac notch," which is the area on the right side where lung does not cover the heart. The cardiac notch area is safe for pericardiocentesis because no coronary arteries (high-pressure vessels) are located on that area of the heart and the heart chamber below the costochondral junction is the moderately thick-walled, relatively low-pressure right ventricle.

CARDIAC CATHETERIZATION (pp. 895–897)

The purposes of cardiac catheterization are to measure intracardiac pressures and oxygen saturations and to position the catheter for selective angiograms (see Chapter 57). Cardiac catheterization can be done without the use of fluoroscopy, but fluoroscopy with image intensification should be used.

Femoral artery catheterization allows easier retrograde entry into the left ventricle and left atrium. The femoral vein can be used for entry to the right atrium and ventricle, but catheter manipulation into the pulmonary artery is difficult in small animals. The carotid artery and jugular vein are always approached from the right side. The carotid, jugular, and femoral vessels can be sacrificed without interfering with normal function in dogs.

THORACOTOMY (p. 897)

Left lateral thoracotomy in the fourth intercostal space can be used for nearly all common clinical cardiac surgical procedures (see Chapter 31).

COMMON CARDIAC SURGICAL CONDITIONS
(pp. 897–915)

Patent Ductus Arteriosus

The most common cardiovascular surgical procedure is ligation of a patent ductus arteriosus (see Chapter 58). Animals with the anomaly die unless it is corrected. The younger the animal, the better the success rate.

The ductus arteriosus is ventral to the aorta, dorsal to the pulmonary artery at the point where the vagus nerve crosses between the two vessels, and beneath or medial to the vagus nerve. The thrill produced by the continuous turbulence at the ductus can be palpated ventral and anterior to the ductus, at the point where the blood flow from the shunt is reflected off the pulmonary artery near the pulmonary valve. This point corresponds to the position where the murmur is best heard during physical examination, which in large dogs may be 5 cm from the ductus itself. Palpation posterior and dorsal to the heart may reveal a second thrill as a result of mitral regurgitation if left ventricular dilation has occurred.

Results of patent ductus arteriosus correction are excellent. The only additional recommendation is that the animal be neutered because the condition is hereditary. Approximately 1.5 per cent of animals with patent ductus ligation have recanalization of the ductus. With recanalization, the murmur returns, usually within 2 months of operation. A recanalized patent ductus is divided and sutured. Division and suturing of the patent ductus are difficult. The structure is very short, and placement of two clamps with division between allows little tissue for the suture line. This technique is used only by individuals with previous experience in vascular surgery.

Aortic Arch Anomalies

Anomalies of the aortic arch—persistent right aortic arch, double aortic arch, and anomalous arch arteries—obstruct the respiratory and gastrointestinal tracts. These diseases constitute the vascular ring anomalies, in which the esophagus is constricted because of the anomalous vessel (see Chapter 58).

Persistent Right Aortic Arch

The most common of the aortic arch anomalies is persistent right aortic arch. The trachea and esophagus are encircled by the base of the heart ventrally, the right aortic arch to the right, the dorsal aorta dorsally, and the ligamentum arteriosum and pulmonary artery to the left. Blood flow is normal, but tight constriction on the esophagus produces obstruction when solids or large pieces of food are eaten.

Surgical correction of persistent right aortic arch is palliative because the ligamentum is cut, freeing obstruction to the esophagus. If the esophagus has dilated to more than twice its normal diameter, surgical results are not ideal.

Pulmonic Stenosis

Pulmonic stenosis is one of the most common cardiac diseases amenable to surgery. There are several types (see Chapter 58), and each has a preferred surgical correction.

Diagnosis

Diagnosis of correctable pulmonic stenosis is based on clinical signs, increasing right ventricular hypertrophy, or elevated right ventricular pressure. With severe right ventricular hypertrophy, results of surgery are poor.

Modified Brock Technique

The Brock or modified Brock procedure is effective in muscular and some subvalvular stenoses. The technique consists of excising fibromuscular obstruction in the right ventricle with a rongeur. The advantage of the Brock procedure is its simplicity. It requires a few additional instruments and is safe. The major disadvantage is the inability to directly observe the tissue being excised.

Bistoury Technique

The bistoury technique for incision of valvular or fibrous subvalvular pulmonic stenosis is performed just like the Brock procedure. Instead of an infundibular rongeur, a teat bistoury is inserted through a pursestring suture into the right ventricle and passed through the obstruction. Cuts are then made in the valvular or fibrous subvalvular ring.

Valve Dilator Technique

If available, valve dilators can be introduced as in the Brock or bistoury technique. Valve dilators are effective for fibrous valvular, subvalvular, and valve dysplasia types of pulmonic stenosis.

Pulmonary Arteriotomy

We prefer an inflow occlusion pulmonary arteriotomy for valvular, immediate fibrous subvalvular, or dysplastic pulmonic valve stenosis. The procedure was originally performed using hypothermia, but even though hypothermia allows additional time for observation of the lesion, the time needed for this operation is so short that it can be safely accomplished without hypothermia.

At normal temperatures, inflow can be safely occluded for as long as 4 minutes. However, the time should be kept to less than 3, preferably 2, minutes.

The major advantage of this procedure is the ability to directly observe the valvular or subvalvular lesion. Pulmonary arteriotomy inflow occlusion is more difficult than the Brock and bistoury techniques, and the results are poorer in young animals. As a result of scarring, the pulmonary valve annulus diameter is fixed at the completion of the pulmonary arteriotomy and does not grow. In a very young animal, this remaining diameter, though normal at the time, becomes stenotic as the animal grows.

Patch Grafting

A modified patch graft for repair of pulmonary outflow tract disease can be large, extending from the pulmonary artery to well down onto the right ventricle. As a result, it can be effective in valvular pulmonic stenosis, pulmonary valve dysplasia, subvalvular pulmonic stenosis, and some muscular pulmonic stenosis. The technique is the most effective and the preferred technique for young animals that are expected to grow to more than double their size at the time of operation. The patch can be placed so that there is redundant tissue at surgery and the growing animal will not have stenosis when it matures.

The graft is cut as a double ellipse to fit from the pulmonary artery across the obstructive lesion to the right ventricle.

The technique is effective in valvular, subvalvular, and muscular stenosis and valve dysplasia. The disadvantages of the technique include (1) the presence of foreign material on the heart; (2) the occasional aberrant coronary artery that crosses the right ventricular outflow tract, negating use of the procedure; (3) difficult identification of the lumen in severely hypertrophied ventricles; and (4) placement of the cutting wire without direct observation.

Conduits

A Dacron vascular conduit from pulmonary artery to pulmonary artery is the most effective method of repair of supravalvular pulmonic stenosis. The circulation is re-established around the obstruction, and the pulmonary valve is retained to function normally. There are no complicating factors.

We have had poor results with placement of conduits from the right atrium to the pulmonary artery (the Fontan procedure). This technique is used for animals with severe obstructive right ventricular disease due to severe muscular hypertrophy or with major obstruction at the tricuspid valve in addition to abnormalities of the right ventricle.

Open Heart Techniques

Open heart surgical techniques have been used in animals to repair pulmonic stenosis. The techniques of cardiopulmonary bypass are described in Chapter 61.

Ventricular Septal Defect

The currently recommended surgical treatment for adult ventricular septal defect in dogs and cats is the palliative procedure of pulmonary artery banding. Banding the pulmonary artery creates a supravalvular pulmonary stenosis to increase right ventricular pressure. In large ventricular defects, the left-to-right shunt flow depends on the pressure gradient between the left and right ventricles. For a given defect, the higher the gradient, the more blood is shunted from the left to the right ventricle and consequently to the lungs, producing pulmonary disease. Surgery for ventricular septal defect is not necessary unless pulmonary symptoms develop (see Chapter 58). These symptoms occur when pulmonary-to-systemic flow ratio is greater than 2.5:1. With pressure elevation in the right ventricle, the gradient between the left and right ventricles is decreased, and consequently the left-to-right ventricular shunt is decreased. If pulmonary artery banding is used, the right ventricular pressure elevation must be sufficient to reduce the left-to-right shunt but not so much to produce right ventricular failure or, even more seriously, right-to-left shunt.

Tetralogy of Fallot

Medical therapy is currently the most efficacious treatment for tetralogy in dogs (see Chapter 58). In at least 25 per cent of affected animals, the disease does not respond to beta-adrenergic blockage, and surgery is considered.

The palliative procedures, Blalock and Potts anastomoses, have been successfully used and should be considered for tetralogy not responsive to medical management. The Blalock anastomosis returns partially oxygenated arterial blood to the lungs to be fully oxygenated through an end-to-side anastomosis from the left subclavian to the pulmonary artery. A similar result is accomplished by the Potts anastomosis, but the pulmonary artery is directly anastomosed side to side to the aorta. The increased systemic oxygenation can alleviate signs of the disease.

Animals undergoing these palliative procedures still have tetralogy, but the clinical response to hypoxemia and the cyanosis is frequently relieved.

Heartworm Removal

Surgical removal occasionally is the preferred therapy for severe dirofilariasis. The procedures for heartworm removal are varied, depending on the position of most of the worms and the physical condition of the animal.

Jugular Venotomy

The simplest surgical treatment for dirofilariasis is removal via the jugular vein in the vena cava syndrome (see Chapter 58). The presence of the worms in the vena cava and right atrium makes them readily accessible. The disease is fatal without surgery, but long-term survival after surgery is approximately 85 per cent.

Pulmonary Arteriotomy

The procedure of choice is an inflow occlusion pulmonary arteriotomy, as described earlier for pulmonic stenosis. At least 90 per cent of adult heartworms in the heart and pulmonary arteries can be removed by this technique.

Right Ventricular Removal

A second approach for heartworm removal is through a purse-string-sutured incision in the right ventricle, similar to that used in Brock technique for pulmonary stenosis, described earlier. The advantages are limited blood loss and simplicity, but the disadvantage—inability to observe and therefore remove worms in the area—makes this technique a poor choice.

Inflow Occlusion and Right Ventriculotomy

An alternative approach for heartworm removal is by median sternotomy, inflow occlusion, and opening of the right ventricle. The advantage of this technique is direct observation of the right ventricle. Disadvantages are related to tearing of the stay sutures in the right ventricle and possible major blood loss before a reinforcement suture line can be completed.

Surgical Disorders of the Pericardium

Pericardial Effusion

Surgical diseases of the pericardium include pericarditis and the effusion and granulomatous response to pericarditis (see Chapter 58). Most cases of surgical pericarditis can be treated by pericardiocentesis. When this fails, the pericardium can be removed. Pericardial effusion associated with pericarditis must have been treated unsuccessfully by pericardiocentesis at least twice and usually three times before pericardiectomy.

In pericardiectomy, it is important to remove as much pericardium as possible. Removal of a small portion of the pericardium (pericardial window) alleviates signs for a short time, but adhesions to the heart usually form, and pericardial effusion returns.

Pericardial Diaphragmatic Hernia

Pericardial diaphragmatic hernia, an uncommon condition that may be either congenital or acquired, can be easily treated surgically. The condition is frequently associated with defects of the sternum or umbilical hernias if congenital and is usually associated with trauma if acquired. The surgical approach is transabdominal median sternotomy, from midsternum to umbilicus. The pericardium is incised so that a pericardial sac can be reformed around the heart. The remaining portion of the pericardium-diaphragm is closed to form the new diaphragm. The heart and pericardium must be separated from the diaphragm so that adhesions, which may cause erosion of the heart at the diaphragm or sternum, do not develop.

Feline Aortic Embolism

The major arterial disease in small animals is embolization, encountered in feline cardiomyopathy (see Chapter 58). Aortic embolectomy is performed to remove the embolus from the distal division of the aorta (see Chapter 62). If surgery is delayed for 6 to 8 hours, there is little advantage over medical management of the disease. Cats must be carefully anesthetized because they are critically ill with the underlying cardiomyopathy. Even with successful surgery, most cats die within 1 year as a result of the cardiomyopathy.

Complete Heart Block

Consistently successful pacemaker implantation has been accomplished only recently, primarily because of the increased availability of pacemakers. Animals with complete heart block are critically ill, and surgical therapy is an emergency procedure.

In a dog in otherwise good health, the pacemaker is implanted after a transvenous temporary pacemaker is inserted into the right ventricle. After a normal heart rate has been established by temporary pacemaker, the animal can be anesthetized in the usual manner. Anesthesia of animals in complete heart block is a high-risk procedure.

The postoperative complications associated with pacemakers include infections associated with foreign bodies, serum pockets near the battery pack, poor pacemaker control of the heart, pleural effusions, and battery failure.

COMPLICATED CARDIAC SURGICAL CONDITIONS
(pp. 915–917)

Subvalvular Aortic Stenosis

Subvalvular aortic stenosis, hereditary in dogs, can be corrected by a closed technique using a valve dilator, open heart surgical resection, or a left ventricle-to-aorta conduit. Aortic stenosis is corrected only if the gradient from the left ventricle to the aorta is severe.

The criteria for surgery for aortic stenosis are (1) the animal must be less than 6 months of age; (2) the left ventricular-to-aortic gradient must be 100 mm Hg or greater; and (3) the animal must be large enough for the surgical technique to be accomplished effectively.

All severely affected dogs with aortic stenosis are at risk of a late (5 to 7 years) postoperative complication of congestive cardiomyopathy. It is unlikely that these dogs would live to develop this complication if they had not had their aortic stenosis corrected. The problem may be associated with preoperative fibrosis and calcification due to severe aortic stenosis.

CHAPTER 61

Extracorporeal Circulatory Support (pages 918–922)

The purpose of a cardiopulmonary bypass unit is to take over the function of a patient's heart and lungs while surgical correction of defects in these organs takes place in a bloodless and motionless field.

COMPONENTS OF THE CARDIAC BYPASS UNIT
(pp. 918–920)
Cannulas

A single venous cannula can be positioned in the right atrium or the venae cavae may be cannulated individually. The arterial return cannula can be placed in the femoral artery, carotid artery, or aortic arch.

Priming Solution

The cardiopulmonary bypass "prime" is the minimum volume of fluid required to fill the tubing and reservoir of the bypass unit before onset of circulatory support. Whole blood prime has the advantage of its oxygen-carrying ability, but it increases the blood's viscosity and the amount of hemolysis occurring during the bypass. The use of a non-hemic prime leads to hemodilution but has the advantages of reduced need for donated blood, decreased blood viscosity, lessened damage to blood elements, and increased perfusion of the microcirculation.

Oxygenator

The oxygenator mixes the venous blood with the fresh gases. The two types of oxygenators that are available commercially are the bubble type, in which there is a direct gas-blood interface, and the membrane type, which has a semipermeable barrier between the gas and blood.

Reservoir and Heat Exchanger

Regulation of blood flow during the bypass procedure requires a reservoir in the cardiopulmonary bypass unit. Control of the patient's body temperature is important during the bypass procedure.

Pumps

Variable-speed roller pumps are used in the bypass unit to pump the volume of blood needed for physiological homeostatis.

CARDIAC ASSIST PUMPS (p. 920)

Intra-aortic balloon pumps synchronized with the electrocardiogram provide counterpulsation during diastole to help force arterial blood to the peripheral tissues. Assist devices can also bypass the ventricles completely; a pumping chamber accepts blood from the left atrium and forces it into the aorta via cannulas.

PHYSIOLOGICAL CHANGES SECONDARY TO CARDIAC BYPASS AND ASSIST (pp. 920–921)

Blood

Shear forces and surface tension can cause hemolysis of red blood cells or may damage the cell membranes so that they are removed by the patient's reticuloendothelial system. White blood cells are damaged by forming adhesions with abnormal surfaces. Platelet function decreases after cardiac bypass. Denaturation of plasma proteins and alteration of blood lipids may lead to coating of red blood cells and agglutination. Alterations in serum electrolyte concentrations are common during cardiac bypass. Epinephrine is released from a patient's adrenal medulla during cardiac bypass. Likewise, sympathetic nerve endings release norepinephrine.

Heart

Blood, gas bubbles, or particulate matter may form microemboli in the arterial supply from the cardiopulmonary bypass unit and cause infarction of the myocardium. The lactic acidosis that normally occurs with cardiac bypass, when coupled with the sodium and water retention, can result in acute congestive failure. Ventricular fibrillation during cardiac bypass either may be induced or may occur spontaneously.

Lungs

Pulmonary damage is one of the major causes of postoperative death in patients after bypass. *Perfusion lung* is a syndrome characterized by atelectasis, pulmonary edema, and perivascular and alveolar hemorrhage. This condition is usually fatal in dogs.

Brain

The most severe bypass complication affecting the brain and central nervous system is an embolic crisis.

Kidneys

Although the kidneys can be affected by embolic infarction, the most common problem is postoperative anuria.

PHARMACOLOGY OF CARDIAC BYPASS (p. 921)

Heparin is usually given intravenously at an initial loading dose of 200 to 400 units/kg of body weight (2 to 4 mg/kg) just before inserting the bypass cannulas. Other drugs that are considered in the management of patients undergoing cardiac bypass include alpha-blockers, such as acepromazine (1 mg/kg), which improve the blood flow to peripheral tissues and decrease the effects of a patient's own catecholamines. Shock doses of corticosteroids are used to help stabilize capillary membranes and reduce lysosomal disruption.

HYPOTHERMIA (pp. 921–922)

Body core temperatures of around 82.4°F (28°C) decrease the normal metabolic demands for oxygen by about 50 per cent. Such temperatures should be maintained during procedures in which a patient's circulation is reduced. Body temperatures of 73.4° to 77°F (23°C to 25°C) can be used in combination with coronary infusion of a 41°F (5°C) cardioplegic solution to permit the complete cessation of blood flow for prolonged periods.

Surface hypothermia can be used when short to moderate (30 minutes) duration circulatory arrest is needed and bypass equipment is not available. Although surface hypothermia requires less specialized equipment, the technique is labor intensive and lacks the control afforded by a cardiopulmonary bypass unit. Rewarming a patient after surface hypothermia is much more difficult than the cooling process, and patients must be monitored for development of systemic metabolic acidosis.

CHAPTER 62

Peripheral Vascular Procedures and Disorders
(pages 922–929)

ARTERIOTOMY (pp. 922–923)

Arteriotomy is incision of an artery and is the basic procedure in vascular surgery. The care with which an arteriotomy is made can influence a procedure's ultimate outcome. Patients are heparinized when a vessel is to be totally occluded for an arteriotomy. Incisions are made perpendicular to the vessel wall to prevent necrotic edges that can result from a beveled incision. Loosely adherent adventitia is removed to avoid dragging it into the vessel lumen with the suture material. During handling of the vessel edges, care is taken not to pinch them in the forceps' jaws, because pinching can damage endothelium and precipitate thrombosis. Arteriotomies are closed with either simple continuous or interrupted sutures.

VENOTOMY (p. 923)

Venotomy is rarely indicated in veterinary surgery.

ANASTOMOTIC TECHNIQUES (pp. 923–925)

The most common anastomotic techniques are end to end and end to side. Most prosthetic grafts are sewn end to side. End-to-end direct reconnection of vessels is the procedure of choice only when the ends can be approximated without tension. End-to-side anastomosis is most often used to join grafts to vessels. It offers the advantages of not totally occluding flow, a longer anastomosis (lessening the possibility of thrombosis), and an enlarged lumen at the anastomotic site. To minimize turbulence, grafts are attached at an angle of about 30° to the vessel. Anastomotic length should be at least twice the diameter of the involved vessel.

PERIPHERAL DISORDERS (pp. 925–929)

Dogs and cats suffer very few primary vascular disorders. All injuries involve vascular trauma, which may be signified by hemorrhage or hematoma. Even the most severe hemorrhage from peripheral vessels can often be temporarily stopped with direct pressure. Most vascular injuries can be repaired by either direct suturing, end-to-end anastomosis, or implantation of a prosthetic conduit.

End-to-end direct reanastomosis of severed vessels is often very difficult. It must be accomplished with complete lack of suture line tension. If there is any doubt about the amount of tension required to hold the ends together, a prosthesis should be considered.

When major vessels are traumatized, repair should be considered. Repair of major vessels usually involves a prosthetic conduit.

Arteriovenous fistula is an abnormal communication between an artery and vein that does not involve a capillary bed. It can be congenital or traumatic in origin. All types of arteriovenous fistulas are uncommon in dogs and rare in cats. The majority involve extremities. In response to the greatly lowered total peripheral resistance, even moderate-sized fistulas can cause serious overloading of the heart, with only slight diminution of flow to the distal limb.

Diagnosis of arteriovenous fistula in the extremities is usually not difficult. A continuous murmur, similar to that of patent ductus arteriosus, can be heard at the fistula site. A thrill may be present. Pulsation of veins in the area is an inconsistent finding.

Treatment of arteriovenous fistulas is surgical separation of the arterial and venous systems and interruption of the arterial supply. The separation must be complete, or the fistula will gradually re-establish itself. If the exact fistula site cannot be located, the arterial supply and venous drainage must be ligated and divided both above and below the area. Incomplete closure or partial interruption of the arterial supply can result in a condition worse than the original.

Closure of large fistulas in main arteries may require prosthetic conduits to bypass the affected area and supply blood to distal tissues. Ideally, if the connection can be identified, the artery and vein are separated and repaired individually. Small fistulas and fistulas located distally on a limb are best treated by either ligation of the arterial supply or arterial embolization.

Concomitant with the increased use of prosthetic grafts is an increased incidence of complications. These can be disastrous, especially when infection is involved. Prophylactic antibiotics are indicated in all vascular procedures.

Despite the most careful precautions, a small proportion (approximately 1 per cent) of grafts become infected. Untreated graft infections have a very high mortality rate, perhaps 100 per cent if the aorta is involved. Once a diagnosis of graft infection is made, the patient should be prepared for surgical exploration of the area and probable graft removal.

The most common vascular disorder requiring surgical intervention is aortic embolism due to feline cardiomyopathy. Clinically, cats with aortic embolism are usually presented with a sudden onset of pain and posterior lameness or paralysis. One or both femoral pulses are diminished or absent. The affected hindlimb is cooler than normal and possibly swollen. The gastrocnemius muscles may be in spasm, and more general signs of shock (pale mucous membranes, dyspnea, weakness) are usually present. Cardiac auscultation frequently reveals abnormal heart sounds or murmurs.

Treatment of aortic embolism is surgical removal. When surgical treatment is not begun within 6 hours, there is little chance for improvement, and secondary complications usually develop. Even when successful treatment is given within several hours of onset, the chance of long-term (greater than 1 year) survival is only about 50 per cent owing to the underlying heart disease. Fluids are administered intravenously and should contain additional sodium bicarbonate (e.g., 1 mEq/10 ml).

Before the aorta is opened, the cat is heparinized (2 mg/kg). The aorta is opened longitudinally over the embolus, which can usually be removed easily with fine forceps. When all visible embolus has been removed, each occlusion is temporarily released to flush out remaining tiny emboli. Blood flow to the hindlegs is re-established slowly to dilute the amount of acidic, hyperkalemic blood suddenly entering the circulation.

Once an animal has recovered from embolectomy, a long-term treatment plan aimed at the underlying cardiac disease must be instituted. In all cases, anticoagulants must be continued for the life of the animal.

Hemolymphatic System

CHAPTER 63

The Hematopoietic System
(pages 930–941)

Physiology and Pathophysiology
(pages 930–937)

HEMATOPOIESIS (pp. 930–933)

In adult dogs and cats, nearly all blood cells, other than lymphocytes, are produced in the bone marrow, and multipotential stem cells of the bone marrow are probably responsible for all blood cell formation. During intrauterine development, before bone cavities are formed, blood cells are first formed in the yolk sac and later in the liver and spleen. During fetal life, the liver is usually more hematopoietically active than the spleen. At birth, all areas of bone marrow cavities are hematopoietically active.

A structured hierarchy of pluripotential, oligopotential, and unipotential stem cells participates in development of various formed blood elements (erythrocytes, granulocytes, monocytes, lymphocytes, and thrombocytes). They remain in a resting stage until acted on by appropriate environmental or humoral stimuli.

It is currently envisioned that erythrocytes, all leukocyte types, macrophages, and megakaryocytes originate from a single pluripotential stem cell of mesenchymal origin—the hematopoietic stem cell.

The proliferative capacity of stem cells decreases with age. Therefore, after severe bone marrow damage such as with irradiation or panleukopenia virus infection, stem cells repopulate the bone marrow and hematopoiesis resumes, but older animals recover more slowly than younger animals.

Erythropoiesis

Production of erythrocytes is controlled by both humoral and local microenvironmental factors. The major mechanism of erythropoiesis regulation is modulation of renal erythropoietin release in response to variation in renal tissue oxygenation. Erythropoietin production and release are influenced by hormonal and neural influences also. Activation of the beta-adrenergic nervous system increases erythropoietin production in both normal and hypoxic animals. Prostaglandins or prostacyclin mediates erythropoietin production via activation of adenylate cyclase, increasing renal cortical cyclic adenosine monophosphate concentrations.

The rate of erythrocyte production remains fairly constant in normal individuals but can increase tenfold during marked erythroid hyperplasia. This marked increase in erythrocyte production is controlled primarily by the rate at which progenitor cells (mainly erythroid–colony-forming unit cells) differentiate to rubriblasts and initiate a maturing erythropoietic unit.

Erythrocyte life span is about 80 to 90 days in cats and 110 to 120 days in dogs.

Granulopoiesis

Granulopoiesis is the production of neutrophils, eosinophils, and basophils. It is regulated by poorly understood interactions between numerous stimulatory and inhibitory factors, many of which are yet to be classified.

The developmental stages, immature to mature, of the granulocyte series are the myeloblast, progranulocyte (promyelocyte), myelocyte, metamyelocyte, band cell, and segmented granulocyte (mature neutrophil, eosinophil, and basophil). Maturation time from the myeloblast to mature, peripheral blood, segmented neutrophil is estimated to be from 3.5 days to 2 weeks.

The peripheral blood half-life of neutrophils is about 6 to 10 hours. It decreases during inflammation and increases during corticosteroid therapy and hyperadrenocorticism.

Monocytopoiesis

As with granulopoiesis, the production of monocytes is regulated by numerous factors and, at this time, is not completely understood. Monocytes are less differentiated than granulocytes when released from the bone marrow. As a result, monocyte bone marrow transit time is much less than that of granulocytes. Mature monocytes may be produced in as little as 10 hours.

Lymphopoiesis

Lymphopoiesis and lymphoid physiology and pathophysiology are discussed in greater detail in Chapters 66 and 159.

Thrombopoiesis

The production of thrombocytes (platelets) is regulated by variation in the concentration of thrombopoietin, which is controlled by total platelet membrane surface area. The productive unit is the megakaryocyte. The maturational stages of thrombopoiesis are megakaryoblast, promegakaryocyte, megakaryocyte, and thrombocyte or platelet.

PERIPHERAL BLOOD CHANGES ASSOCIATED WITH PHYSIOLOGICAL AND PATHOLOGICAL CONDITIONS
(pp. 933–937)

Erythrocyte Changes

Physiological Influences

Age. At birth, in both dogs and cats, the mean corpuscular volume (MCV) and mean corpuscular hemoglobin (MCH) are markedly greater than in adults; the hematocrit (Hct), hemoglobin (Hgb) concentration, and mean corpuscular hemoglobin concentration (MCHC) are about the same as in adults; and the erythrocyte count is markedly less than in adults.

Epinephrine Release. Epinephrine release sometimes causes redistribution of the erythrocyte mass into the larger veins that are used for collection of blood samples. As a result, the Hct, Hgb, and RBC values may be increased.

Gestation. Gestation causes a decrease in Hct, Hgb, and erythrocyte values.

Pathological Conditions

Polycythemia. Polycythemia is a relative or absolute increase in erythrocyte mass. It is denoted by increased Hct, Hgb, and erythrocyte values. Polycythemias are relative when Hct, Hgb, and erythrocyte values are increased but the total erythrocyte mass is not. Relative polycythemias are caused by dehydration and erythrocyte redistribution (splenic contraction).

Polycythemias are absolute if the increases in Hct, Hgb, and erythrocyte values reflect an actual increase in the total erythrocyte mass. Absolute polycythemias are uncommon in dogs and cats.

Anemia. Anemia is a relative or absolute decrease in erythrocyte mass. It is denoted by decreased Hct, Hgb, and erythrocyte values. An anemia is relative if the Hct, Hgb, and erythrocyte values are decreased but the actual erythrocyte mass is not. Most if not all relative anemias are caused by hemodilution produced by conditions such as pregnancy, administration of fluids, and sodium retention during heart disease.

An anemia is absolute when the actual erythrocyte mass is decreased. Absolute anemias are caused by conditions that result in blood loss (hemorrhage), increased erythrocyte attrition (hemolysis), or decreased erythrocyte production. Anemias caused by hemorrhage or hemolysis are regenerative, and evidence of erythroid hyperplasia (polychromasia, reticulocytosis, and anisocytosis) can be detected in peripheral blood smears if a patient has been anemic a sufficient length of time (usually 3 or 4 days). The regenerative response during hemolytic anemia is greater than during hemorrhagic anemia.

Total protein concentration can often help differentiate hemorrhagic anemia from hemolytic anemia. During hemorrhagic anemia, total protein concentration usually is decreased because of plasma protein loss, whereas during hemolytic anemia, total protein concentration usually is normal or increased owing to concurrent inflammation or free hemoglobinemia. Lowest values for total protein concentration are generally reached between 12 and 24 hours after hemorrhage. Hct, Hgb, and erythrocyte values may not decline below normal limits until 12 to 24 hours after hemorrhage and may not reach lowest values until 48 hours after hemorrhage.

Conditions that cause hemolysis include immune-mediated mechanisms, oxidative injury to hemoglobin and erythrocyte cell membranes (Heinz body anemias), erythroparasites (babesiosis, hemobartonellosis), vascular disease (microangiopathic anemia due to vasculitis or vascular neoplasms—hemangiomas and hemangiosarcomas), and erythrocyte plasma membrane alteration as in severe liver disease.

Nonregenerative anemia may be caused by bone marrow suppression alone or in conjunction with hemorrhage or hemolysis. When bone marrow suppression alone causes anemia, polychromasia and reticulocyte counts are markedly reduced.

Leukocyte Changes

Leukocyte changes include increases and decreases in the total leukocyte count, increases and decreases in the absolute and relative individual leukocyte counts, and changes in leukocyte morphology.

Physiological Conditions

Age. The total leukocyte count is highest in young animals and gradually decreases with age.

Epinephrine. Factors such as pain, fear, excitement, and exercise can cause demargination of previously marginated leukocytes and result in dramatic increases in leukocyte counts.

Glucocorticoid Release. Glucocorticoid administration and occasionally endogenous glucocorticoid release result in a delayed increase in neutrophil numbers of two to three times normal. Lymphopenia and eosinopenia develop concurrently in both dogs and cats, and monocytosis may develop in dogs.

Pathological Conditions

Inflammation. Inflammation may cause neutropenia or mild, moderate, or marked neutrophilic leukocytosis or may be associated with a normal leukocyte count. Inflammation may also cause an increase in immature neutrophils (i.e., a left shift) and toxic changes in neutrophils.

Bone Marrow Suppression. Conditions that cause bone marrow suppression are discussed in Chapter 64.

Neoplasia. Neoplasia of the hematopoietic system is covered in Chapter 158.

Surgical Patients with Hematopoietic Dysfunction (pages 937–941)

PREOPERATIVE EVALUATION

The primary purpose of preoperative hematological evaluation is to prevent hemostatic complications and to ensure erythrocyte numbers are adequate for tissue oxygenation in case of blood loss.

CLASSIFICATION OF ANEMIA IN SURGICAL PATIENT

Nonregenerative anemias show a decreased reticulocyte count and are classified on the basis of erythrocyte morphology. Cats are particularly susceptible to nonregenerative anemia secondary to infections. Examination of the bone marrow in a patient with a nonregenerative anemia is helpful in defining the cause of the anemia.

One specific cause of aplastic anemia that may be surgically correctable is hyperestrogenism associated with a Sertoli cell tumor in a dog.

Regenerative anemias fall into two categories: blood loss (hemorrhagic) and hemolytic.

Microcytic, hypochromic anemia is most commonly the result of iron deficiency. Any patient with unexplained iron deficiency should be evaluated for gastrointestinal blood loss. If medical causes such as parasites, chronic inflammatory bowel disease, or ulceration are eliminated, surgery may be indicated for diagnosis and therapy.

Autoimmune hemolytic anemia is associated with neoplasia, the use of certain drugs, recent vaccination, or primary immune-mediated disease. The antibody-coated erythrocytes are removed from the circulation by fixed macrophages, primarily in the spleen. Treatment includes immunosuppressive drugs or splenectomy.

TISSUE OXYGENATION IN ANEMIA

Reduced oxygen delivery to peripheral tissues is the most important adverse effect of anemia. The reduced oxygen-carrying capacity of the blood is compensated by increased cardiac output and a shift to the right of the oxyhemoglobin dissociation curve, which increases oxygen delivery to the tissues.

In deciding whether to proceed with surgery in an anemic patient, the surgeon should consider the urgency of the surgery, the cause of the anemia, and the patient's ability to compensate for the lowered hematocrit. Oxygen therapy preoperatively and administration of at least 30 per cent oxygen with inhalant anesthetics allows maximal oxygenation of the blood. In postoperative management of anemic patients, one should try to prevent shivering, which greatly increases oxygen consumption. Overhydration must be avoided during treatment of chronically anemic patients because cardiac enlargement, especially left ventricular hypertrophy, may occur as a component of the compensatory response.

TREATMENT OF PATIENTS WITH ACUTE BLOOD LOSS

Except for acute loss of more than one-third of the circulating blood volume, a blood transfusion normally is not needed.

Isotonic crystalloids are most commonly used as replacement for acute blood loss. Because normal saline and lactated Ringer's solution have no colloidal osmotic effects, plasma volume equilibrates with the extracellular space. Therefore, crystalloids must be infused at three to four times the intravascular volume. Hypertonic saline in a 7 per cent solution (300 to 600 mOsm) has been used as an alternative to isotonic crystalloid solutions in hypovolemic shock.

Fresh-frozen plasma should be reserved for replacement of coagulation factors because volume expansion can be accomplished with crystalloids or colloids without the risk of exposure to foreign antigens and citrate.

Dextrans are colloids of high-molecular-weight polysaccharides. Dextran 40 (10 per cent solution) expands blood volume at a rate of twice the volume infused. Dextran 70 (6 per cent solution) expands blood volume 1.25 times its volume or exerts oncotic pressure about twice that generated by albumin. Hydroxyethyl starch is a high-molecular-weight starch solution with oncotic properties similar to those of plasma.

In general, when a transfusion is required, packed erythrocytes may be used for all but the most acute life-threatening hemorrhages. Sluggish microcirculation may be avoided by diluting the erythrocytes with 0.9 per cent saline.

SURGICAL CONSIDERATIONS IN GRANULOCYTOPENIC OR IMMUNOSUPPRESSED PATIENTS

Granulocytopenia is defined as a neutrophil count of less than 1000/μl. Acute overwhelming sepsis is the most life-threatening postoperative complication in granulocytopenic patients. Any change in the normal postoperative course is an indication for immediate use of bactericidal antibiotics.

IMMUNOSUPPRESSIVE VIRUSES

Neutropenia in dogs and cats often has a viral origin. Feline leukemia virus (FeLV) or feline immunodeficiency virus (FIV) viremic cats are prone to the development of leukemia or lymphoma, bone marrow suppression, immune deficiency, and other disorders such as glomerulonephritis or reproductive disorders. Both viruses exert their immunosuppressive effects on T-lymphocytes, but this immunosuppression may coexist with neutropenia, making these cats susceptible to a broad range of infections. About one-third of FIV-infected cats in the immunosuppressed stage of disease are anemic. If surgery is necessary, the risks should be considered but necessary procedures performed.

HEMATOPOIETIC NEOPLASIA

Neoplasia causes many disturbances that are expressed as paraneoplastic syndromes. Cytopenias can result from decreased or ineffective production within the bone marrow, increased destruction of cells, or sequestration in the spleen. Decreased production of platelets is the most common cause of thrombocytopenia in patients with neoplasia. Hemangiosarcoma is one of the major causes of sudden or recurring internal hemorrhage in older dogs. Hypercalcemia is present at the time of diagnosis in approximately 25 per cent of dogs with lymphoma.

CHAPTER 64

Bone Marrow (pages 942–948)

FUNCTION AND ORGANIZATION OF THE BONE MARROW

The main function of the bone marrow in dogs and cats is hematopoiesis of nonlymphoid cells.

Hematopoiesis in growing animals occurs within the medullary areas of the long and flat bones. In mature animals, active marrow is present mainly in the flat bones, which include the ribs, sternum, pelvis, and vertebrae.

GROSS ANATOMY

The color of bone marrow in young animals is dark red because of the increased erythropoiesis. Decreased hematopoiesis occurs normally with age, causing the color to change to red with white mottling due to fat infiltration. Blood supply to the bone marrow primarily comes from the periosteal and muscle arterioles. Capillaries form sinuses at the osteomyeloid and paratrabecular junctions. Blood cells are released into these and connecting sinuses located within the hematopoietic tissue.

HISTOLOGY

The main supporting tissues consist of the outer cortex and projections of bony trabeculae, which compartmentalize the hematopoietic tissue. Lining these trabeculae are endosteal cells, which include osteoblasts and osteoclasts.

Hematopoietic elements have an organized arrangement with islands of erythroid precursors associated with iron-containing macrophages. Megakaryocytes also develop in clusters. Granulocytes are found both diffusely within the marrow parenchyma and focally at the osteomyeloid or paratrabecular junctions. Normal lymphoid cells may be found as small aggregates termed *follicles* or *nodules* within the bone marrow of dogs and cats.

INDICATIONS FOR BONE MARROW EVALUATION

Anemia

Bone marrow examination is not indicated for acute blood loss or for regenerative anemias, especially if responsive to therapy. Persistent, poorly regenerative or nonregenerative anemias require bone marrow examination.

Leukopenia

Reduced leukocyte numbers may reflect lymphopenia, which often indicates primary or secondary immunosuppression. Persistent neutropenia may require bone marrow evaluation to determine whether precursors exist.

Thrombocytopenia

Accurate assessment of the number and morphology of megakaryocytes is best determined by bone marrow core and aspirate biopsy.

Unexplained Elevations in Cell Numbers

Bone marrow examination is recommended to confirm the presence of absolute polycythemia, which can occur as a rare neoplastic disorder or can develop secondary to renal tumors.

Extreme leukocytosis in the absence of a major site of inflammation or tumor growth should indicate evaluation of the bone marrow.

Benign thrombocytosis must be distinguished from neoplastic conditions such as essential thrombocythemia. In the latter condition, the bone marrow contains increased numbers of abnormal megakaryocytes.

Abnormal Circulating Cells

The presence of abnormal or dysplastic circulating cells always requires bone marrow evaluation. Dysplasia may result from altered nuclear or cytoplasmic maturation with resulting asynchronous development.

Blast cells indicate improper release or production of bone marrow precursors and are seen with marrow injury or neoplasia.

Clinical Staging of Malignancies

Bone marrow evaluation is used to determine the presence of disease or the clinical stage of plasma cell myeloma, lymphoma, or mast cell tumor. Buffy coat examination may reveal circulating neoplastic cells, but this is often time consuming and frequently unrewarding. Their presence in blood may reflect their release from damaged, infiltrated tissues without actually originating from the bone marrow.

Evaluation of Iron Stores (p. 944)

EXAMINATION OF THE BONE MARROW

Aspiration Biopsy Versus Core Biopsy

Aspiration biopsy provides excellent morphological detail of bone marrow cells. Focal changes of the stroma best appreciated by core biopsy include inflammation, neoplasia, marrow necrosis, osteolysis, or myelofibrosis. For maximum information, the two techniques are performed together and interpreted along with a blood sample drawn the same day.

Sites of Biopsy

For dogs, the dorsal iliac crest is the most popular location because it is readily accessible. Because smaller dogs and cats have a thin dorsal ilial crest, one may obtain transilial core samples. For obese or very muscular dogs, the craniolateral part of the greater tubercle of the humerus is the site preferred because of lack of muscle, fat, or subcutaneous tissue in this region. In small dogs and cats, the proximal femur may also be used to obtain marrow samples, but this area is less accessible.

Preparation

Sedation or local anesthesia (e.g., lidocaine) is often sufficient for aspiration and core biopsies. The area is surgically scrubbed and draped, and sterile gloves are used. A stab incision is made in the skin with a number 11 scalpel blade.

Aspiration

The aspiration needle with stylet in place is rotated to penetrate the cortex several millimeters so that it becomes firmly embedded. The stylet is removed, and suction is produced to draw marrow into the syringe.

Core Biopsy

Core biopsy is performed similarly to aspiration except that the stylet is removed before the instrument penetrates the bone. To cut and retain the bone sample, the needle is sharply rotated both clockwise and counterclockwise several revolutions. The needle is withdrawn with a twisting motion.

Complications

Complications are rarely encountered during bone marrow aspiration or core biopsy.

INTERPRETATION OF THE PATHOLOGIST'S REPORT
(pp. 946–947)

Aplasia or Hypoplasia

The term *aplastic anemia* is used when numbers of erythrocytes, granulocytes, and platelets are reduced in circulation and the bone marrow lacks active marrow. Cytologically, hypoplasia can refer to a relative decrease in a cell line. Animals admitted for tumor resection and receiving antineoplastic agents should be evaluated for the presence of drug-related myelosuppression.

Hyperplasia

The bone marrow under conditions of strong regeneration is characteristically hyperplastic. This may be anticipated from examination of the peripheral blood. Hyperplasia may be present during the preregenerative period or under conditions of ineffective hematopoiesis.

Myelodysplasia

The term *dysplasia* refers to abnormal growth of cells. Dysplasia may affect one cell line (e.g., erythroid, as occurs in lead toxicity) or more commonly two or more cell lines along with peripheral cytopenia.

Neoplasia (see also Chapters 63 and 158)

New or uncontrolled cell growth within the bone marrow can arise primarily from hemolymphatic tissue or secondarily from metastasis of a nonhematopoietic tumor. Common malignancies that metastasize include lymphoma, mast cell tumor, and mammary adenocarcinoma. Primary malignancies include acute or chronic lymphoid or myeloid leukemias.

Necrosis, Myelofibrosis, Reactivity

The bone marrow may be damaged by infection, drugs, chemicals, neoplasia, radiation, or immune destruction. When the insult is severe enough, permanent and irreversible necrosis may occur. If marrow injury is moderate, attempts to repair the affected area may result in increased numbers of reticulin and collagen fibers. This condition, termed *myelofibrosis,* is considered a secondary response and may be reversible. When marrow injury is mild, with minimal cell destruction, a reactive response usually occurs.

BONE MARROW TRANSPLANTATION (p. 947)

CHAPTER 65

Spleen (pages 948–961)

GROSS ANATOMY (p. 948)

The spleen lies in the left anterior quadrant of the abdomen, in a dorsoventral orientation. The spleen is attached to the greater omentum along a ridge, called the *hilus,* that runs the length of its visceral surface. The parietal surface is convex.

Through the hilus, arterial vessels and sympathetic nerves enter the spleen and venous vessels and lymphatics leave the spleen. Venous blood from the spleen empties into the portal vein and subsequently flows through the liver. The spleen has efferent but no afferent lymphatic vessels. Smooth-muscle cells in the blood vessels, capsules, and trabeculae are innervated by sympathetic fibers from the celiac ganglion. The spleen has no parasympathetic nerve supply.

The abundance of smooth-muscle cells in the spleen of dogs and cats enables it to contract, a property not shared by the human spleen. Relaxation of smooth muscle is induced by anesthetics such as barbiturates or tranquilizers such as acetylpromazine, allowing congestion of the red pulp with blood and resulting in marked splenic enlargement.

MICROSCOPIC ANATOMY (pp. 948–949)

White Pulp

The lymphatic tissue of the spleen consists primarily of lymphocytes and macrophages supported by a scaffolding of branched connective tissue called *reticular cells.* The meshwork of supporting cells and extacellular fibers produced by them is called the *reticulum.* The white pulp is distributed along the course of arterial vessels. Within the white pulp are zones rich in T-lymphocytes and zones of B-lymphocytes.

The white pulp is separated from the surrounding red pulp by a region called the *marginal zone.*

Red Pulp

The red pulp consists mainly of arterial capillaries, small venous vessels, and a reticulum filled with macrophages and blood. Blood is delivered into the red pulp reticulum from the terminal segments of arterial capillaries, which are continuations of the central arteries of the white pulp. These arterial capillaries are surrounded by a sheath composed of reticular cells and highly intertwined macrophages. This structure is the *periarterial macrophage sheath,* or ellipsoid. The periarterial macrophage sheath is the primary particle filter in the spleen of dogs and cats.

In dogs and cats, the terminal portion of each arterial capillary leaves its periarterial macrophage sheath and opens into the red pulp reticulum. Blood cells and plasma discharged from arterial terminations flow through the reticulum to constitute vascular pathways of an intermediate circulation interposed between arterial and venous vessels. The major anatomical difference and the basis for the major functional difference between the spleen of dogs and cats is the structure of the venous vessels in the red pulp.

SPLENIC FUNCTIONS (pp. 949–951)

The Reservoir

Ninety per cent of the erythrocytes entering the spleen of a resting dog or cat pass through it as quickly as do erythrocytes flowing through a conventional capillary bed (about 30 seconds). At any time, the spleen contains 10 per cent or more of the total erythrocyte mass of a resting dog or cat. Contraction of the spleen ejects most of this reservoir of erythrocytes and raises the packed cell volume of blood in the circulation. The presence of a readily available splenic reservoir of erythrocytes has physiological importance. A pool of slowly moving platelets is also maintained in the red pulp. Approximately one-third of the total platelet mass is in the spleen at any time.

Reticulocyte Sequestration and Surface Remodeling

Reticulocytes released from the marrow are transiently sequestered in the red pulp. While there, they lose some of their surface membrane to acquire the shape and size of mature erythrocytes.

Erythrocyte Culling and Pitting

Among the most important functions of the red pulp are the recognition and removal or modification of aged or damaged erythrocytes. Complete removal of an erythrocyte from the circulation is called *culling; pitting* is the selective removal of intraerythrocytic inclusions.

In pitting, rigid intracellular inclusions such as nuclei, Howell-Jolly bodies (nuclear remnants), Heinz bodies (precipitated hemoglobin), and intracellular parasites are pinched from an erythrocyte as it squeezes between endothelial cells of the sinus wall. The erythrocyte, freed of its inclusion, may continue to circulate unless it is severely damaged during pitting.

Erythrocytes with reduced pliancy may be trapped in the red pulp until phagocytized or may fragment into smaller pieces that re-enter the circulation.

The reticulum of the red pulp is crowded with macrophages that have receptors for the Fc portion of immunoglobulin G (IgG) and for complement (C3b). Erythrocytes bearing even small amounts of IgG or complement are likely to become bound to macrophages. Normal erythrocytes at the end of their life span are culled from the circulation by macrophages in the spleen, liver, and bone marrow.

The only known difference in function between a dog's and cat's spleen is the inability of a cat's spleen to pit intracellular bodies from the erythrocyte. The lack of pitting ability accounts in part for the frequent finding of Heinz bodies in erythrocytes of nonanemic cats.

Although a cat's spleen inefficiently removes intraerythrocytic inclusions, it nevertheless can free erythrocytes of the epicellular parasite *Hemobartonella felis*. Removal of the spleen or concurrent diseases that suppress macrophage function permit *Hemobartonella* to rise to detectable levels, revealing the latent infection.

Immune Responses and Protection in Septicemia

The red pulp, marginal zone, and white pulp act in defense against blood-borne bacteria and in response to blood-borne antigens. Bacteria and particulate antigens that are deposited at arterial terminations in the red pulp and marginal zone are phagocytized by macrophages. The spleen is also the first site of production of specific immunoglobulin M (IgM) antibody in blood-borne bacterial infections.

Some of the blood-borne particulate antigens deposited in the marginal zone are transported into lymphatic nodules, resulting in stimulation of B-lymphocyte proliferation, formation of germinal centers, and antibody production.

Hematopoiesis

The splenic red pulp is a site of blood cell production during fetal development and to a limited extent postnatally. Splenic hematopoiesis in dogs and cats becomes more prominent in certain diseases (see Chapter 63).

MECHANISMS OF SPLENOMEGALY (pp. 951–952)

Symmetrical Splenomegaly

Purely congestive splenomegaly, the result of vascular disorders, is rarely encountered in small animals. Congestive splenomegaly due to splenic torsion often accompanies gastric dilation-volvulus, although it may occur in the absence of gastric involvement. Symmetrical splenomegaly with increased sequestration and destruction of blood cells may be secondary to macrophage recruitment and proliferation in infectious diseases, especially those caused by organisms that infect macrophages and stimulate mononuclear phagocytes.

Splenomegaly may be associated with hemolytic anemia in patients in whom the spleen is a major site of erythrocyte destruction. In myeloid neoplasia, the splenic red pulp is infiltrated with neoplastic

cells, the degree of symmetrical splenomegaly depending on the
and course of the disease. Neoplasia of lymphoid tissue affects
spleen in varied ways; splenic white pulp involvement may lead to
symmetrical or asymmetrical splenic enlargement.

Asymmetrical Splenomegaly

Primary tumors of vascular cells, connective tissue, or smooth muscle
produce single or multiple nodular growths on the spleen. Subcapsular
splenic hematoma due to trauma usually produces a single focal enlargement, whereas nodular hyperplasia frequently occurs as multiple
nodules of various sizes.

REGENERATION OF THE SPLEEN (p. 952)

After traumatic rupture of the spleen, multiple splenules may be found
throughout the abdomen, a condition called *splenosis.* Spleen regrowth
rarely occurs after surgical removal of an intact spleen.

SURGICAL DISEASES OF THE SPLEEN (pp. 952–956)

Primary splenic neoplasia, splenic torsion, and severe splenic trauma
are the most common indications for total splenectomy. Life-threatening destruction of peripheral blood cells by the spleen may be an
indication for total splenectomy.

Splenic Neoplasia

Splenic neoplasia is the most common reason for total removal of the
spleen in dogs, with hemangiosarcoma the most common primary
splenic neoplasm. Although total splenectomy has in the past been the
recommended treatment for primary splenic neoplasia, it apparently
has little influence in increasing survival time of animals with hemangiosarcoma.

Torsion of the Spleen

Splenic torsion occurs when the spleen twists or rotates on its vascular
pedicle, occluding vessels to the splenic hilus. The condition frequently accompanies gastric dilation-volvulus but may occur alone.
Splenic torsion typically occurs in large or giant-breed dogs.

Acute Isolated Splenic Torsion

Discomfort is an early sign of acute splenic torsion. Excessive salivation, drooling, gagging, or retching may occur. Signs of cardiovascular
collapse and shock develop within several hours.

   Treatment involves cardiovascular resuscitation and exploratory celiotomy. Intravenous fluids, shock doses of glucocorticoids, and perhaps whole blood should be administered. If possible, the patient is
stabilized physiologically before anesthesia and exploratory surgery.

   Torsion greater than 360° may occur. If the pedicle can be untwisted, the splenic artery and vein and their branches are examined
for thrombosis. If thrombosis is present, total splenectomy is necessary. In the absence of thrombosis, whether restoration of splenic
blood flow will relieve the organ of its entrapped blood can be determined after several minutes.

Chronic Isolated Splenic Torsion

Anatomical derangements and treatment of the less acute clinical form
of splenic torsion are similar to those described for the acute form,

...te type frequently occurs with a history of vague ...rt, usually of several days' duration. In some ...ormation, such as a recent whelping or the admin- ...lmintics, may cloud the clinical picture.

...dings include an increased heart rate and slightly in- ...ase... ...piratory rate. Body temperature is usually elevated. The abdomen may be distended, and a large intra-abdominal mass may be palpated.

Anemia and dehydration often develop after several days of splenic pedicle obstruction. The packed cell volume may reach 20 per cent, with a reduction in hemoglobin and erythrocyte count. White blood cell counts may range between 15,000 and 50,000 cells/μl, manifested primarily as a neutrophilia. Proteinuria, hemoglobinemia, hemoglobin-uria, and bilirubinuria are frequently detected in more chronic splenic torsion. These findings indicate extensive erythrocyte destruction within the spleen. Pancreatitis is a potential complication of splenic torsion.

Response to treatment is usually rapid in both acute and chronic splenic torsion once the spleen has been removed or the splenic vessels are untwisted.

Splenic Trauma—Hematoma (pp. 954–955)

TOTAL SPLENECTOMY (pp. 956–957)

The spleen is exposed via a ventral midline abdominal incision. Beginning at the free or distal end of the spleen and ending at its head or proximal end, the splenic hilar vessels and then the short gastric arteries all are double ligated and transected. Folds of the thin gastro-splenic ligament must also be severed. An alternative technique is to ligate the short gastric arteries and the splenic artery distal to the branches that supply the left limb of the pancreas. This procedure may be faster than ligation at the splenic hilus and does not lead to ischemia of the greater curvature of the stomach.

In splenic torsion, the twisted splenic pedicle is not permanently ligated *en masse* because the vessels within the large amount of ligated tissue may dislodge, leading to life-threatening hemorrhage.

PARTIAL SPLENECTOMY

Partial splenectomy is recommended whenever possible, especially in cases of splenic trauma in which only one portion of the spleen is involved. It is not recommended for splenic neoplasia, even though the obvious tumor mass may grossly involve one portion of the spleen.

The obvious advantage of partial splenectomy is the retention of splenic function, which is important in dogs and cats that may be latent carriers of *Hemobartonella* and *Babesia* organisms.

Several partial splenectomy techniques have been described; they differ primarily in the method by which the splenic parenchyma is transected and handled to prevent hemorrhage. Regardless of the method used, hilar vessels that supply the portion of spleen to be removed are double ligated and transected. A color difference is noted between ischemic and perfused splenic tissue. This line of demarcation is used as the guideline for splenic excision.

SPLENIC REIMPLANTATION (pp. 957–958)

PERCUTANEOUS BIOPSY

Histological evaluation of splenic tissue is necessary to establish a diagnosis in splenomegaly. Malignant lymphoma, myelogenous leukemia, and nonvascular tumors such as fibrosarcoma and leiomyosarcoma may be diagnosed by percutaneous splenic biopsy. Percutaneous procedures may be contraindicated if hemangiosarcoma is suspected because of the possibility of inducing life-threatening hemorrhage or peritoneal metastasis. In addition, percutaneous biopsies of splenic abscess may lead to leakage and peritonitis.

Techniques for performing percutaneous splenic biopsy include punch biopsy, needle aspiration, and fine-needle aspiration. Fine-needle aspiration is currently recommended because of its simplicity, the excellent tissue samples that it yields, and its low risk of complications.

SPLENIC BIOPSY AT CELIOTOMY

Needle or punch biopsy is indicated when gross examination suggests splenic metastasis from a neoplasm such as a hepatic or pancreatic carcinoma. Incisional splenic biopsy is indicated when diffuse splenomegaly is present. Primary splenic neoplasms are removed by total splenectomy; incisional biopsy is not recommended in such cases, particularly for tumors of vascular origin. Hemorrhage from the biopsy site may be difficult to control; it may occur after the abdomen has been closed.

COMPLICATIONS OF SPLENECTOMY

Hemorrhage is the major complication of partial and total splenectomy. All vessels occluded with ligatures or hemostatic clips must be examined for hemorrhage before the abdomen is closed.

Ischemic pancreatitis is a potential complication of partial or total splenectomy. Vascular supply to the left limb of the pancreas arising from branches of the splenic artery may be accidentally transected, resulting in disruption of pancreatic blood flow. Ligations at the splenic hilus prevent this.

HEMATOLOGICAL AND PHYSIOLOGICAL CHANGES AFTER SPLENECTOMY

Postsplenectomy hematological changes may differ from one species to another. In dogs, the number of Howell-Jolly bodies and nucleated erythrocytes is higher after splenectomy, reflecting loss of pitting. Increased numbers of target cells may be found in blood smears from splenectomized dogs. Platelet counts in dogs may rise and remain elevated for prolonged periods after splenectomy.

Although *Hemobartonella canis* usually does not produce clinically apparent hemolytic anemia, splenectomy of infected dogs promotes detectable parasitemia. Splenectomy of dogs infected with *Babesia canis* may also permit recrudescence of clinical anemia.

CHAPTER 66

Lymphatics, Lymph Nodes, and Tonsils (pages 962–977)

Lymphatics and Lymph Nodes
(pages 962–973)

The lymphatic system functions as an appendage of the cardiovascular system, collecting and transporting plasma proteins from the capillary filtrate back to the blood.

EMBRYOLOGY, HISTOLOGY, AND ANATOMY

Lymphatic Vessels

Lymphatics arise as epithelial buds from the mesonephric veins, anterior cardinal vein, and wolffian body. Two paired lymph sacs (jugular and iliac) and two unpaired lymph sacs (retroperitoneal and cisterna chyli) coalesce to form the thoracic duct, right lymphatic duct, and cisterna chyli.

Lymphatic capillaries possess a wider and more irregular lumen than blood capillaries. They have a discontinuous basement lamina, the endothelial cell junctions generally lack the tight junctions characteristic of blood capillaries, and anchoring filaments bind the lymphatic endothelium to the adjoining connective tissue.

The superficial lymphatic capillaries of the extremities drain into a valved group of vessels at the junction of the dermis and subcutaneous tissue. The fluid drains into afferent lymphatics, which collectively drain into regional lymph nodes. Efferent lymphatics from the lymph nodes drain into larger lymphatic ducts.

The thoracic duct is the common trunk of all lymph vessels, with the exception of the right lymphatic duct, which drains the right side of the head and neck, right forelimb, and possibly the heart, lungs, and diaphragm.

The entire lymphatic system, with the exception of the lymph capillaries and lymph nodes, has numerous valves. Valves at the junction of the thoracic duct and the venous system prevent back-flow of blood into the thoracic duct.

Lymph Nodes

Lymph node architecture is relatively uniform throughout the body and reflects its functional capacity as an accessory route for the return of interstitial fluid to the blood stream and as an important arm of the immune response. The cortex of the lymph node contains follicles that are composed of lymphocytes (primarily B cells) and phagocytes encircling small accumulations of larger lymphoid cells called *germinal centers*. The paracortical region consists of dense cords of small lymphocytes that are predominantly T cells.

PHYSIOLOGY OF LYMPH FORMATION AND FLOW
(pp. 963–964)

The primary function of the lymphatic system is to regulate the interstitial fluid by providing a route to return to the circulation those substances that have been leaked from the vascular bed but not reabsorbed. Sixty to 70 per cent of all ingested fats are conveyed to the blood stream via the thoracic duct. In animals, more than one-third of the protein that is lost into the interstitial space is cleared by lymphatics; the remainder is returned by venular capillaries.

Lymph is formed at the capillary level as a balance between hydrostatic and colloid osmotic pressures within the interstitial and intravascular spaces. Lymph propulsion along the larger lymphatic vessels is affected by both intrinsic and extrinsic forces. Intrinsic forces result from active contraction of smooth muscle in the lymphatic wall.

DIAGNOSTIC EVALUATION OF THE LYMPHATIC SYSTEM (pp. 964–965)

Lymphangiography

Direct or indirect lymphangiography is used to identify and define normal and abnormal lymphatic vessels. With the indirect technique, contrast agent is injected into a tissue, such as a lymph node, and allowed to be passively absorbed by lymphatics. Direct lymphangiography is injection of contrast agent directly into either peripheral or mesenteric lymphatics, depending on the area of interest.

An improved view of the central lymphatics, particularly the thoracic duct, can be obtained by injecting into a mesenteric rather than a peripheral lymphatic.

Lymphoscintigraphy

Lymphoscintigraphy is a safe, reproducible, and noninvasive technique using radionuclides to image regional lymph node drainage systems. It is based on the transport of a subcutaneously injected radioactive colloid through the lymphatic system. The two most commonly used radioactive colloids are ^{99m}Tc-labeled dextran and ^{99m}Tc-labeled antimony sulfide.

Pathological lymph nodes may fail to pick up the radioactive colloidal compounds and are poorly seen, whereas obstruction of the lymphatics may delay or halt the normal flow of activity.

CLINICAL APPROACH TO LYMPHADENOPATHY (pp. 965–968)

Physical Examination

The age and physical condition of the patient are important. It is important to note the distribution of the adenopathy. If one of a localized set of lymph nodes is involved, the sites drained by these lymphatics are carefully examined for infection, inflammation, or neoplasia. If several peripheral lymph nodes are involved, systemic antigenic stimulation or primary lymphoid neoplasia is considered. If lymphadenopathy is noted distal to a lesion, lymphatic obstruction is suspected because normal lymphatic flow is unidirectional. The presence of lymph nodes that are not normally palpable is also significant.

Radiography

Survey radiographs of the thorax, abdomen, and cervical region may help confirm internal lymphadenopathy. Ultrasonography and computed tomography scanning can detect lymph node enlargement and are particularly helpful in occult internal locations that are inaccessible to palpation.

Aspiration Cytology

The techniques most clinically useful in evaluating patients with lymphadenopathy are fine-needle aspiration cytology and lymph node biopsy. Lymph node cytology can be invaluable as a screening test. Proper slide preparation is extremely important with these aspirates. Accurate interpretation of a lymph node aspirate must be based on knowledge of the normal cellular population.

The term *reactive hyperplasia* indicates increased numbers of plasma cells, a moderate increase in the number of inflammatory cells, or an enlarged node that is cytologically normal. This is a nonspecific diagnosis but implies that the node is responding to the presence of antigen. The distribution of the adenopathy helps determine if the antigen is a local or systemic challenge.

Suppurative lymphadenopathy implies an infiltration of neutrophils and is most often associated with response to a local bacterial infection. This diagnosis suggests a need for culture and sensitivity testing and investigation of the area drained by this node. Increased numbers of macrophages are seen with granulomatous reactions and are most commonly associated with fungal infections. Allergic and parasitic skin diseases may lead to a dermatopathic lymphadenopathy that is often composed of increased numbers of eosinophils. An eosinophilic response can also be associated with phycomycosis and mast cell disease.

Tumor types that commonly metastasize via lymphatics include carcinomas, melanosarcomas, mast cell tumors, and transmissible venereal tumors.

Lymph Node Biopsy

Incisional (wedge) biopsy of lymph nodes is indicated primarily in areas where excisional biopsy may be difficult to perform because of a node's size or location, including nodes that are located close to major vascular or nervous structures. Alternatively, a *needle punch* biopsy can be performed using an instrument such as a Tru-Cut disposable biopsy needle.*

Excisional biopsy of superficial lymph nodes, such as the popliteal lymph nodes, can be performed under local anesthesia if a patient's condition dictates; however, short-duration general anesthesia facilitates extirpation of lymph nodes. The node must be handled gently to prevent damage and distortion of the architecture. At this point, the lymph node can be sectioned to provide samples for aerobic and anaerobic cultures, fungal cultures, and histopathological and cytological study. Impression smears can be made by lightly blotting the cut edge of the node with absorbent paper and touching the sample lightly to a glass slide before placing the tissue in formalin.

Complications associated with lymph node biopsy are rare, and there are no absolute contraindications.

SPECIFIC DISORDERS OF PERIPHERAL LYMPHATIC VESSELS (pp. 968–972)

Lymphangitis

The lymphatic system's role as a ''filter'' for antigens and particulate matter makes it particularly susceptible to secondary infection and inflammation. As a result of carrying organisms and their inflammatory products, affected lymphatic vessels may become inflamed and occluded.

---

*Travenol Laboratories, Inc., Deerfield, IL.

Physical abnormalities may include local swelling with pain and heat, lameness, and draining lesions with abscesses. Particularly with acute reactions, the lymph nodes may be enlarged and painful (lymphadenitis). If total lymphatic obstruction is caused by inflamed lymphatics and activated lymph nodes, then subcutaneous edema of the area may ensue.

Appropriate treatment of lymphangitis generally leads to complete recovery with restoration of normal lymphatic function. Symptomatic care includes moist hot compresses or hydrotherapy to manage swelling, encourage enhanced circulation, and promote drainage. Depending on the underlying etiology, systemic antimicrobial or antifungal therapy is initiated. Surgical exploration is indicated to provide drainage or to remove foreign material and indurated tissues.

Lymphedema

Lymphedema is an accumulation of fluid in the interstitial space, particularly in the subcutaneous fat, due to a failure of the lymphatic system. Failure of the lymphatic system results in accumulation of plasma proteins in the interstitial fluid, causing an increase in interstitial fluid colloid osmotic pressure. This in turn causes more water to move into the interstitial space, resulting in edema.

Primary lymphedema is due to an abnormality or disease of lymph conduction elements of the lymphatic vessels or lymph nodes. Secondary lymphedema is caused by disease in the nodes or vessels that did not begin in the lymphatic system or that follows surgical excision of lymphatics or lymph nodes.

Lymphedema typically presents as a spontaneous, painless swelling of the extremities, with pitting edema. In severely affected animals, all four limbs as well as the trunk may be edematous. Congenital lymphatic abnormalities may not result in lymphedema until the animal is several years of age.

In poodles, peripheral lymphedema is an autosomal dominant trait. The diagnosis of lymphedema is made after ruling out other causes of edema, such as congestive heart failure, hypoproteinemia, and hepatic or renal failure. Contrast radiography may help define the lymphatic abnormalities in dogs with lymphedema. Lymphangiographic patterns noted in affected limbs include an absence of vessels (aplasia), a reduction in vessel numbers (hypoplasia), and an increased number of dilated or ectatic vessels (hyperplasia). Lymphoscintigraphy may also help detect abnormalities in peripheral lymphatic vessels and lymph nodes.

Treatment of lymphedema may involve either conservative management (massage, pressure bandages) or surgery. However, because of inconvenience associated with long-term conservative management, such therapy is not feasible for most owners. Diuretics, such as chlorothiazide, may be beneficial in mild or moderate lymphedema in dogs. Benzopyrones reduce lymphedema in man.

Surgical therapy of lymphedema in dogs has not been well evaluated, and results of reported cases are difficult to assess owing to the lack of consistent classification techniques, comparable measurements of severity, and the paucity of long-term results; none of the techniques is uniformly successful.

Cellulitis is a common complication of lymphedema in man and dogs.

Intestinal Lymphangiectasia

Intestinal lymphangiectasia, the most common lesion associated with severe canine protein-losing enteropathy, may occur as a primary abnormality of the lymphatic system or may be secondary to other disease processes. It is characterized by pathological dilation of the intestinal lymphatic network in the mucosa, bowel wall, and mesentery; however, there is no correlation between the apparent severity of lymphatic dilation and protein loss. The protein loss is not selective, resulting in panhypoproteinemia.

Primary intestinal lymphangiectasia is generally associated with diffuse lymphatic abnormalities including lymphatic dysplasia of the extremities and thoracic duct obstruction. Affected individuals may have chylothorax, chylous ascites, or subcutaneous chyle instead of gastrointestinal disturbances or concurrently.

Secondary intestinal lymphangiectasia may occur subsequent to systemic venous hypertension, with resultant increased pressures in the intestinal lymphatic network. Abdominal lymphatic hypertension probably occurs secondary to increased flow through the thoracic duct.

The clinical signs associated with intestinal lymphangiectasia include diarrhea, lethargy, weight loss, ascites, edema, and respiratory difficulty due to pleural effusion. Because no simple test can confirm the gastrointestinal tract as the site of protein loss, it is generally implicated by ruling out other potential causes of hypoalbuminemia.

The treatment of intestinal lymphangiectasia has involved feeding a low-fat diet such as Prescription diet R/D* or W/D* or a home-made diet with most of the dietary fat being composed of medium-chain triglycerides. Short- and medium-chain triglycerides are primarily absorbed by the portal system, thereby bypassing the lymphatics. Secondary intestinal lymphangiectasia may respond to corticosteroids.

Neoplasia of the Peripheral Lymphatics (p. 972)

The Tonsils (pages 973–977)

ANATOMY

The paired palatine tonsils are masses of lymphoid tissue in the lateral walls of the oropharynx caudal to the palatoglossal arch and ventral to the soft palate. The base of the tonsil is in the dorsolateral aspect of the tonsillar crypt. In young dogs, much of the tonsil may protrude from the tonsillar crypt and be exposed to the pharynx. This is rare in cats.

PHYSIOLOGY AND PATHOPHYSIOLOGY

The tonsillar crypts of normal dogs and cats contain a diverse bacterial flora, including potential pathogens. The normal host immune mechanisms can effectively deal with a small number of these pathogens, but larger numbers may lead to clinical infection. Therefore, the tonsils may serve as a portal of entry for these or other bacterial or viral pathogens. The tonsils can also act as a reservoir for pathogens during an inapparent infection or convalescence or when the host is an asymptomatic carrier of infection.

DISEASES
Tonsillitis

Primary tonsillitis is usually a bilateral inflammation that can be either acute or chronic. This condition is more frequent in dogs than cats, often afflicts small dogs, and is uncommon in dogs over 1 year of age.

*Hill's Pet Products, Topeka, KS.

Tonsillectomy is contraindicated for treatment during an episode of acute tonsillitis, when it may result in further spread of the infection to adjacent or distant tissues.

Chronic Tonsillitis
Etiology of Tonsillitis

Primary causes of tonsillitis include bacteria, viruses, and foreign bodies. The most common pathogenic bacteria isolated from patients with tonsillitis are alpha- and beta-hemolytic streptococci, staphylococci, and coliforms in both dogs and cats.

Secondary tonsillitis can occur as a result of other disease processes. One category includes causes of pharyngeal irritation, such as recurring vomiting or regurgitation due to megaesophagus, pylorospasm, or gastric neoplasia. Periodontal disease and licking distant infected tissues, such as infected skin or anal sacs, can lead to chronic contamination of the mouth with pathogens.

Tumors of the tonsil, such as squamous cell carcinoma or tonsillar lymphosarcoma, are always part of a differential diagnosis when enlarged or otherwise abnormal tonsils are found. A foreign body such as a grass awn or a piece of wood lodged in a tonsil or crypt may cause inflammation and swelling.

Diagnosis and Case Selection

The three main indications for tonsillectomy are (1) chronic recurrent tonsillitis that is unresponsive to antibiotics, (2) acute tonsillar enlargement causing mechanical interference with swallowing or airflow, and (3) neoplasia.

TONSILLECTOMY TECHNIQUES (pp. 975–977)

The objectives are complete removal of the tonsillar tissue, minimal tissue trauma, and maximal hemostasis. The three most common techniques for tonsillectomy are described in the parent text. Once removed, the tonsil is divided and submitted for bacterial culture and antibiotic sensitivity testing, impression smears, and histopathological examination.

Histopathology (p. 976)

Prognosis (p. 976)

Aftercare

After tonsillectomy, aspiration of blood or saliva may lead to pneumonia or hypoxia. To help prevent these complications, the endotracheal tube is left in place until the animal is making voluntary attempts at swallowing. An animal's normal diet can be resumed on the fourth or fifth postoperative day. Complete healing of the area occurs by 10 days to 2 weeks after surgery.

Complications

Hemorrhage may occur during the first 24 hours after surgery. Localized pharyngitis present before surgery may persist. Regrowth of incompletely removed tonsillar tissue is possible, requiring subsequent removal if clinical signs persist.

CHAPTER 67

The Thymus (pages 977–983)

ANATOMY AND HISTOLOGY
THYMIC PHYSIOLOGY

The thymus has close ties to the endocrine system and is responsible for early postnatal lymphocytopoiesis. Thymic development peaks at approximately 4 to 5 months after birth (just before sexual maturity), and the gland begins to involute when deciduous teeth are lost. Involution is rapid early but is never complete and is characterized by a loss of cortical lymphoid structure. The thymus is important to immunological defense mechanisms, especially cell-mediated immunity. Thymic epithelial cells also release soluble factors (identified as thymic hormones) that seem to enhance immune function.

The magnitude of immunosuppressive effects of thymectomy are age and species dependent. In rodents, neonatal thymectomy causes severe immunodeficiency with consequent loss of T cells and cachexia due to chronic unopposed infection. In small animals, postnatal thymectomy has a less adverse effect on immune function because prenatal development of immunocompetence is more advanced. Nevertheless, if thymectomy is performed, each patient should be monitored for evidence of T-cell deficiency, such as development of autoimmune disease, certain malignancies, and chronic infection.

THYMIC INVOLUTION

Thymic involution in normal small animals occurs with the onset of sexual maturity and the loss of deciduous teeth. It may be influenced by increasing blood levels of adrenal corticosteroids and the decreasing influence of growth hormone.

THYMUS-RELATED DISEASE

Thymus-related disease is rare but may include thymic hypoplasia, hyperplasia, branchial cysts, myasthenia gravis, and thymic hematoma. Thymic hypoplasia in bull terriers is associated with decreased plasma zinc levels and is an autosomal recessive disorder known as *lethal acrodermatitis*.

The most common disease associated with thymic disease in dogs is acquired myasthenia gravis. Congenital myasthenia gravis is not associated with autoantibody or thymic disorders. Many reports have described myasthenia gravis associated with thymoma in dogs. Damage to antigen common to both skeletal muscles and thymic epithelium or myoid cells may explain the relationship resulting from this autoantibody disorder. The efficacy of thymectomy for treatment of acquired myasthenia gravis in dogs is unknown.

In dogs, lymphoma, lung adenocarcinoma, testicular tumors, mammary carcinoma, astrocytoma, and pheochromocytoma have been reported concurrently with thymoma. A failure of thymus-dependent immune surveillance may be responsible for this association. In cats, myositis, megaesophagus, reduced esophageal motility, acute moist dermatitis, and hypogammaglobulinemia have been reported to be associated with thymoma. Spontaneous fatal thymic hemorrhage has been reported in dogs. Affected dogs usually are younger than 2 years, and the hemorrhagic incident occurs during thymic involution.

THYMIC SURGERY

The most common indication for thymic surgery is neoplastic disease involving the thymus.

THYMOMA

Thymoma is the most common primary tumor of the thymus gland in dogs and cats. It is a neoplasm of thymic epithelium with variable numbers of non-neoplastic lymphocytes and can be classified as invasive or noninvasive. Thymoma usually occurs in very old animals, but invasive thymoma has been reported in a 3½-year-old dog.

Animals with noninvasive thymomas may have no clinical signs or nonspecific signs. Clinical signs include those expected for a large space-occupying thoracic mass (e.g., exercise intolerance, coughing, dyspnea, dysphagia, or weight loss) or those of a particular paraneoplastic syndrome. Invasive thymomas produce clinical signs similar to noninvasive forms but may also produce cranial vena cava syndrome (pitting edema of the submandibular area, neck, thoracic inlet, and forelimbs) and are usually associated with pleural effusion. Thoracic radiographs generally reveal a large mass in the left cranioventral thorax. Clinical laboratory data are usually normal in dogs and cats with thymoma. In dogs, a marked mature lymphocytosis ($\sim$ 20,000 cells/μl) may be seen.

Definitive diagnosis of thymoma may be made by transthoracic needle biopsy in some dogs and cats. In some animals, excisional biopsy is required. Exploratory thoracotomy is often necessary to determine the character of the tumor (invasive versus noninvasive) in the absence of clinical data suggestive of malignancy or invasiveness. Benign and malignant thymomas are difficult to differentiate histologically.

Surgical resection of a thymoma in dogs can be performed by lateral thoracotomy or median sternotomy. Because most thymomas are large by the time an animal is admitted to the hospital, a median sternotomy is usually necessary. In cats, resection of a thymoma can be accomplished by lateral thoracotomy, but rib transection may be required if the mass is large. Surgical excision of invasive thymomas is usually unrewarding because of the vital structures invaded by the tumor. Adjunctive treatment of thymoma has still not been well documented in small animals. In dogs, recurrence of thymoma after resection does occur, but the paucity of long-term reports makes it difficult to draw concrete conclusions.

Other tumors that involve the thymus and may require surgery include thymic lymphoma, carcinoid, germ cell tumors, thymic carcinoma, and thymolipoma. The thymus may also be invaded secondarily by neoplasia from another site.

THYMIC CYSTS (p. 982)

Thymic branchial cysts may occur as a mediastinal mass or in the subcutis of the neck.

Nervous System

CHAPTER 68
Neurological Examination and Localization (pages 984–1003)

The evaluation of animals suspected of having neurological disease includes the history, signalment, physical examination, and neurological examination. The objectives are to (1) determine if neurological dysfunction exists, (2) localize the lesion, (3) determine the extent (severity) of the lesion, and (4) determine the cause of the neurological dysfunction. A complete examination is important because very subtle changes may differentiate neurological diseases with similar presentations. Brief examinations may lead to erroneous or short-sighted conclusions.

SIGNALMENT AND HISTORY

Signalment considers an animal's breed, age, sex, and use. Certain physical and neurological disorders occur with increasing frequency in each of these categories. The history often helps characterize the disease process as acute, chronic, progressive, or static.

PHYSICAL EXAMINATION

Examination is thorough and conducted in a logical, organized manner. Techniques used in physical examination are observation, palpation, percussion, and auscultation. The order of the physical examination is less important than the consistency with which the order is followed.

NEUROLOGICAL EXAMINATION (pp. 987–991)

Mental Status

A normal animal is bright and alert and responsive to its environment and all external stimuli in an expected, appropriate manner. Altered levels of consciousness are depression, delirium, stupor (semicomatose), and coma.

Gait and Posture

A wide-based stance often indicates disequilibrium associated with cerebellar or vestibular dysfunction or occasionally high cervical or generalized peripheral nerve disease. Conscious proprioceptive deficits may be displayed by knuckling of the paws and can indicate loss of sensory function, motor function, or both. Nonweightbearing lameness is infrequently encountered with neurological disease and is more likely associated with orthopedic disease.

Cranial Nerve Examination

The cranial nerve examination evaluates specific areas of the brain stem and the peripheral nerve component of each cranial nerve.

Cranial nerve I (olfactory) is evaluated by observing the blindfolded animal after placing food or a nonirritating volatile substance, such as cloves, under the nose. Tests used to evaluate vision (cranial nerve II, optic) include the menace response (cranial nerve II, cranial nerve VII, facial; cerebellum), visual following (cranial nerve II), and pupillary light reflexes.

The pupillary light reflex tests function of cranial nerve II to the optic chiasm and the oculomotor (cranial nerve III) parasympathetic pathway. Position and movement of the globe involve cranial nerves III (motor portion), IV (trochlear), and VI (abducent). The ophthalmic branch of cranial nerve V is tested by the palpebral reflex and the corneal reflex. These tests also evaluate motor function of cranial nerves VII (palpebral) and VI (corneal).

Drooping of the muzzle is a sign of cranial nerve VII motor dysfunction. Sensory evaluation of the head and face assesses the maxillary and mandibular branches of cranial nerve V. Head tilt is associated with cranial nerve VIII (vestibular branch) dysfunction, and torticollis is associated with dysfunction of the neck muscles innervated by cranial nerve XI (accessory). Ear movement is controlled by cranial nerve VII. The cochlear branch of cranial nerve VIII is evaluated by hearing tests.

POSTURAL REACTIONS (pp. 991–994)

Postural reactions are most helpful in detecting the presence of subtle deficits in strength and coordination when the gait is normal.

Wheelbarrowing

The thoracic limbs are tested by picking up the pelvic limbs and moving the animal forward.

Hemistanding and Hemiwalking

The thoracic and pelvic limbs on one side are held off the floor or ground to evaluate the animal's ability to stand and move laterally on the contralateral limbs.

Hopping Response

Abnormalities include conscious proprioceptive deficits, deficits in motor function, and dysmetria.

Extensor Postural Reaction

The normal response is extension of the pelvic limbs and an orderly backward stepping.

Placing Reaction

The test is conducted in two parts: tactile placing and visual placing. Abnormal responses can indicate deficits in sensation, motor ability, or vision.

Conscious Proprioception

Each limb is tested by placing the dorsal aspect of the paw in contact with the floor. The normal response is a quick return of the paw to the normal position. A delayed or absent response is abnormal and can denote involvement of the afferent system (loss of position sense) or the efferent system (decreased motor control [paresis]) or both.

Righting Response

The normal response requires functional vestibular and proprioceptive abilities.

SPINAL (SEGMENTAL) REFLEXES (pp. 994–998)

Spinal reflexes are elicited through a reflex arc that includes the receptor, afferent peripheral nerve pathway, spinal cord synapse(s), efferent peripheral nerve pathway, and effector muscles. Spinal reflexes aid in localization and are recorded as normal, exaggerated (hyper-reflexic), depressed (hyporeflexic), or absent (areflexic).

Myotatic Reflexes

A synonym for myotatic reflexes is *stretch reflexes*. Tendons and muscles involved in the myotatic reflex test should be stretched (loaded) before percussion with a pleximeter to produce the proper response.

The triceps reflex is evaluated by placing the finger over the insertion of the triceps muscle, just proximal to the olecranon process of the elbow. The biceps reflex test is performed by placing the index finger over the distal end of the biceps and bicipital tendons at the elbow and tapping the finger with the pleximeter.

The patellar reflex is elicited by placing the stifle in a slightly flexed position, thereby stretching the patellar tendon, and percussing the tendon with the pleximeter.

The sciatic nerve and its branches can be evaluated using several different reflexes, including the cranial tibial and gastrocnemius reflexes. Another test is to tap between the greater trochanter and the ischiatic tuberosity with the pleximeter.

The cranial tibial reflex is elicited by tapping the limb directly below the lateral tibial tuberosity with the stifle and hock in extension. The gastrocnemius reflex test can be performed by flexing the hock and striking the index finger placed over the distal end of the gastrocnemius tendon with the pleximeter.

Flexor Reflexes

Presence of the flexor reflex response should never be confused with the ability to perceive pain. The flexor reflex can usually be elicited by pinching the web areas between the toes with the fingers. Hemostats are used only when additional stimulus is needed to elicit a response.

Other Segmental Reflexes

The crossed extensor reflex is assessed at the same time as the flexor reflex. With an animal in lateral recumbency, the reflex occurs when the limb (thoracic or pelvic) on the top side is withdrawn and at the same time the (contralateral) limb on the lower side extends.

The perineal or anal sphincter reflex and, in males, the bulbourethral reflex evaluate function of the pudendal nerve and the S1 through S3 spinal cord segments.

The cutaneous trunci reflex (formerly the *panniculus reflex*) is elicited by lightly stimulating the skin on both sides of the dorsal midline with a blunted hypodermic needle or small hemostats, beginning in the region of the fifth lumbar vertebra and continuing cranially to the cervicothoracic junction. The expected response is a contraction or "rippling" of the cutaneous trunci muscle on both sides of the dorsal midline at the point of stimulation and forward to the cervicothoracic junction.

OTHER TESTS OF SPINAL FUNCTION (pp. 998–999)
Hyperpathia

Hyperpathia is noted when an animal shows pain in response to pressure on the vertebral transverse processes or spinous processes or on the paraspinal musculature. In the thoracic and lumbar regions pain is often accompanied by a reflex tightening of the abdominal muscles.

Nociception (Deep Pain Perception)

A test for deep pain perception is often the most important prognosticator and is a reliable indicator of functional integrity of the spinal cord. It is performed on each limb and at the tail by applying painful stimuli to the digits or the end of the tail. Only conscious recognition of the stimulus denotes intact nociceptive pathways because mere withdrawal of the limb (flexor response) does *not* imply that the animal can feel the stimulus.

Superficial (Cutaneous) Nociception Testing

The skin is first grasped with hemostatic forceps and pinched with additional closing of the forceps. For the animal to perceive the sensation, not only the afferent peripheral nerve but also the pathways to the somatosensory cortex must be intact.

LESION LOCALIZATION (pp. 999–1000)
Assessment of Neurological Examination Findings

The initial step is to determine if the deficits can be attributed to a single lesion or if the problem is multifocal. Next, the location is categorized as either above or below the foramen magnum to allow the examiner to explore the components of the cranial vault or the spinal cord as possible locations of the lesion. Other categories considered are paroxysmal, episodic, and those associated with muscle or peripheral nerve diseases (neuropathic, myopathic). Each category is defined by the anatomical location and specific neurological deficits that result from disease within that anatomical space.

Anatomical Classification of Deficits

Familiarity with the categories described allows grouping of abnormal findings representing anatomical localization of the lesion. Multifocal disorders have signs that reflect two or more categories. Examples are animals with spinal trauma affecting two regions of the spinal cord.

NEUROLOGICAL DIAGNOSIS (p. 1000)
Differential Diagnosis
Diagnostic Plan

The diagnostic plan begins with the minimum data base. Additional laboratory data may be necessary (e.g., fasting blood glucose levels).

Spinal diseases warrant radiography. Potential diagnoses are listed according to the etiology classification (e.g., degenerative) and the usual disease history of an acute-onset progressive, acute-onset non-progressive, or chronic progressive illness.

SPECIAL NEUROLOGICAL EXAMINATIONS

Neurological Examination of Neonates

Neonates (puppies and kittens less than 4 weeks of age) often respond differently to the various neurological tests because their nervous system is still developing.

Small Animal Coma Scale

Animals presented for head trauma may exhibit various neurological signs, but most confusing is an animal presented in an altered state of consciousness. To evaluate these animals more accurately and to provide a more objective means of serial evaluation, the Small Animal Coma Scale was developed in 1985.

CHAPTER 69

Electrodiagnosis (pages 1003–1008)

ELECTROMYOGRAPHY

Electromyography is the recording and interpretation of striated muscle electrical activity. Diseases of the motor neuron cell body, ventral nerve root, nerve plexus, peripheral nerve, neuromuscular junction, and muscle fiber all may cause electromyographic abnormalities.

Electrical activity of striated muscle is characterized by the presence or absence of waveforms, the types of waveforms seen, and their configuration and time of occurrence (at rest or during voluntary activity).

Normal Electromyographic Activity

Normal electromyographic activity consists of insertional activity, motor unit potentials, and infrequent spontaneous waves. Normal muscle at rest is electrically silent, and persistent spontaneous activity should be considered abnormal. Motor unit potentials are noted during involuntary muscle contraction and when a motor nerve is stimulated (M response).

Abnormal Electromyographic Activity

Insertional Activity. Prolonged insertional activity is found 6 to 10 days after peripheral nerve injury.

Fibrillation Potentials. Spontaneous, repetitive action potentials increase for several weeks after denervation.

Positive Sharp Waves. Positive sharp waves are associated with denervation and sometimes primary muscle disease. They have an initial positive deflection with a slower negative component.

Myopathic Potentials. Myopathic waveforms are a continuous discharge of potentials with varying amplitude, duration, and frequency.

Reinnervation Potentials. As denervated muscle is reinnervated, motor unit potentials are initially low amplitude and polyphasic but soon become larger than normal. The presence of these potentials is a favorable prognostic sign, particularly if they appear early in the recovery period.

NERVE CONDUCTION STUDIES (pp. 1004–1005)

Motor Nerve Conduction

Motor nerve conduction velocity and M response can provide information to help determine the location of nerve lesions and the prognostics. Two different M responses are generated from a muscle by stimulating the nerve supplying that muscle at two separate sites along its course.

If a nerve has been severed or severely traumatized, stimuli supplied above the site of injury do not produce the M response. The success of surgical repair of peripheral nerve injuries can be evaluated by electromyography, motor nerve conduction velocity measurement, and evaluation of the quality of the M response.

Sensory Nerve Conduction

In sensory nerve conduction studies, action potentials are recorded directly from the nerve after stimulation of a cutaneous sensory nerve field.

H-Wave Reflex

In the H-wave reflex, different sensory impulses from a peripheral site of nerve stimulation are conducted to the spinal cord, where alpha motor neurons are activated to discharge different impulses resulting in generation of a compound muscle section potential, the H reflex.

F-Wave Reflex

The F wave is produced after a peripheral nerve is stimulated below the intensity necessary to cause H-wave production. Antidromic conduction in motor nerve fibers activates the motor neuron to generate an efferent nerve impulse.

SOMATOSENSORY EVOKED RESPONSES (pp. 1005–1006)

Somatosensory Evoked Potentials

This technique uses signal averaging to record responses in the cervical spinal cord and cerebral cortex after stimulation of a peripheral nerve. The presence or absence of this response seems to correspond clinically to the presence or absence of deep pain perception in dogs and therefore may be useful in evaluating spinal cord injury in stoic animals.

Spinal Evoked Potentials

In this procedure, the stimulus is applied to a peripheral nerve as with somatosensory evoked potentials, but the response is recorded from an electrode inserted near the intervertebral space or dorsal lamina of the vertebra. Because they can be used to discretely evaluate the sensory pathways of small sections of the spinal cord, spinal evoked potentials can provide valuable localizing information. Loss of response past a particular vertebra can accurately localize a lesion, and the conduction velocity of afferent pathways can be calculated. As with somatosensory evoked potentials, interpretation should be undertaken with the understanding that sensory function can be preserved with permanent motor loss.

MOTOR EVOKED POTENTIALS (pp. 1006–1007)

Sensory evoked potentials may persist despite permanent loss of motor function. The advantage of a test of spinal cord motor function is obvious. The generation of efferent spinal cord signals after cerebral stimulation has long been described, but only recently have techniques been developed for clinical use of motor evoked potentials. Stimulation can be direct cortical (requiring craniotomy), transcranial, or spinal; both electrical and magnetic stimulation pulses have been evaluated. Recording electrodes are placed as described for spinal evoked potentials at various levels of the spinal cord. Signal-averaging capabilities are needed. In dogs, a noninvasive technique for generating and recording motor evoked potentials has been described.

MISCELLANEOUS TECHNIQUES (p. 1007)

Electroencephalography

An electroencephalogram is a continuous graphic recording of the electrical activity of the cerebral cortex, obtained through scalp electrodes. The activity thus recorded varies considerably with techniques, restraint, a patient's age and state of consciousness, head size, and environment.

Auditory Evoked Responses

The auditory evoked response (also known as the brain-stem auditory evoked potential) is a complex brain-stem response to auditory stimuli. Signal-averaging equipment is necessary to record this potential.

CHAPTER 70
Neuroradiology

Conventional radiography remains the primary method of diagnostic imaging in veterinary neurology. Radiographic contrast procedures improve diagnostic accuracy but may be technically difficult or dangerous, especially when evaluating brain disease. Improvements in the quality and safety of myelographic contrast agents have broadened the application of myelography for diagnosis of spinal cord lesions in veterinary practice. Referral of patients for computed tomography (CT), magnetic resonance imaging (MRI), or scintigraphy is considered when there is clinical evidence of a brain lesion or a spinal lesion that cannot be accurately assessed by conventional radiographic techniques.

PRINCIPLES OF ADVANCED IMAGING TECHNIQUES
(pp. 1008–1009)

Scintigraphy

Scintigraphy, also known as *radionuclide imaging, nuclear imaging,* or *radioisotope scanning,* is the application of gamma-emitting radio-tracer techniques to view organs and systems in living organisms. Radionuclide images are obtained by administering a tracer dose of radiolabeled compound (radiopharmaceutical), which is selectively accumulated in or excluded from specific organs or tissues. A gamma camera (also known as a scintillation camera) is used to obtain a visual image of the pattern of radionuclide accumulation in a patient.

Anatomical detail is far superior on radiographs, but radionuclide images offer physiological or functional information because the pattern of radioactivity depends on physiological distribution of the radiopharmaceutical.

Computed Tomography

CT generates cross-sectional images with excellent anatomical detail. CT can resolve structures as small as 1 mm and can distinguish tissue density differences of 0.5 per cent or less.

A number of cross-sectional images, or "slices," are made at intervals of 1.5 to 10 mm to examine a particular area of the body. The ability of the computer-generated images to display small differences in tissue opacity allows viewing the ventricles without intrathecal injection of contrast material. Organic iodine contrast media can be injected intravenously to accentuate the opacity of vascular structures on CT images.

Animal patients must be heavily sedated or anesthetized for CT. A complete examination of the brain of a dog may require 1 hour or longer.

Magnetic Resonance Imaging

MRI creates diagnostic cross-sectional images using the physical principle of nuclear magnetic resonance. One advantage of MRI is that no ionizing radiation is used in the procedure, so there is no danger of radiation exposure to the patient. The phenomenon of nuclear magnetic resonance is created when certain atomic nuclei are placed in a strong magnetic field, are stimulated by radio waves, and subsequently re-emit some of the absorbed energy in the form of weak radio signals. Acquisition of an adequate signal usually requires a number of minutes; animals must be anesthetized or heavily sedated to remain motionless during the entire procedure.

Unlike CT or conventional radiography techniques, MRI signal intensity does not depend on tissue density but rather on the complex interaction of physical parameters, including proton density, T1 and T2 relaxation times, proton bulk motion, diffusion, magnetic susceptibility, and chemical shift. Therefore, the appearance of structures as light or dark on magnetic resonance images bears no relation to their appearance on CT or conventional radiographic images. On magnetic resonance images, bone produces almost no signal and appears as a black or void component of the image. The major advantage of MRI is its ability to provide detailed images of soft tissue.

IMAGING THE SKULL AND BRAIN (pp. 1009–1015)

Diagnostic imaging of the head is indicated to evaluate animals with clinical and neurological signs of a brain lesion, to locate fractures in animals that have suffered significant head trauma, and to assess for invasion of the calvarium when neoplasms are present in the nasal cavity, sinuses, or other adjacent tissues.

Routine examination of the skull always includes at least lateral and ventrodorsal or dorsoventral projections. True lateral positioning is accomplished by placing radiolucent wedge-shaped sponges under the mandible. The ventrodorsal projection of the skull is preferred over the dorsoventral projection because the calvarium is closer to the film, resulting in better radiographic detail and less distortion. Precise positioning accurately displays bilateral symmetry of the skull, which is useful in interpreting unilateral radiographic abnormalities.

Additional radiographic projections may be made, depending on the nature and location of the suspected abnormality. Frontal projections of the skull may be particularly useful in assessing fractures and evaluating the frontal sinuses. Open-mouth projections with the x-ray beam directed at the palate allow a view of the nasal cavity, cribriform region, and rostral calvarium without superimposition of the mandibles and tongue. When radiographs are used to assess deep involvement of masses adjacent to the calvarium, at least one projection is made with the beam tangential to the lesion so that the mass is profiled on the radiograph.

Interpretation of radiographs of the skull can be difficult because of the complex osseous structure, superimposition of the bony elements, and subtle nature of some abnormalities. A thorough knowledge of the radiographic anatomy of the skull is required.

Findings on survey radiographs may be normal in many animals with significant lesions of the central nervous system. Intracranial hemorrhage and brain contusion may occur with or without fracture of the skull. Intracranial masses usually are fluid opacity; they can be seen on survey radiographs only when there is mineralization, as in some meningiomas and chronic inflammatory masses. For these reasons, additional imaging procedures are necessary for accurate assessment of most diseases affecting the brain.

Radiographic Contrast Procedures

Cerebral arteriography can be used to identify masses and vascular abnormalities within the brain. The procedure is technically difficult because it requires selective catheterization of an artery supplying the brain, and it places patients at risk because of direct injection of contrast medium into the brain. Cavernous sinus venography requires injection of contrast medium into a vein that drains into the cavernous sinus. Ventriculography is performed by injecting either positive (organic iodine) or negative (air) contrast medium into the lateral ventricles. The procedure can be used for confirming a diagnosis of hydrocephalus and determining the extent of ventricular enlargement.

Scintigraphy

Radionuclide brain imaging is a safe, noninvasive technique that is sensitive in detecting lesions larger than 1 cm in diameter. Radionuclide brain imaging does not allow differentiation of tumors and inflammatory lesions. Abnormalities are detected as a result of deficit in normal physiologic function rather than unique metabolic properties of the lesion. Lesions appear as areas of increased activity or "hot spots" on scintigraphic images.

Computed Tomography

CT allows an excellent view of the skull and brain. CT images can be used to diagnose subtle skull fractures, intracranial hemorrhage, invasion of the calvarium by neoplasia, hydrocephalus, brain infarcts, and intracranial masses such as neoplasia and abscesses. Identification of abnormalities is based on changes in radiographic opacity, displacement of normal structures (particularly the ventricles), and contrast enhancement of structures.

Images can be acquired with both bone and soft-tissue window settings, allowing accentuation of bone structures on one series of images and soft-tissue structures on another. CT images allow identification and precise localization of most anatomical brain lesions. The images also allow some evaluation of the extent and biological behavior of the lesion but do not allow identification of the histological nature.

Unfortunately, brain neoplasms cannot be distinguished from non-neoplastic lesions by CT characteristics in all cases. Quantitative and dynamic studies may eventually allow more precise noninvasive determination of the nature of brain lesions.

Magnetic Resonance Imaging

Diagnostic-quality magnetic resonance images of the brain can be obtained from dogs and cats.

MRI is more sensitive than CT in detecting brain abnormalities. CT may be more sensitive with subtle bone involvement or mineralization in the lesion. MRI also offers the prospect of increased specificity in diagnosis of brain lesions. It was initially hoped that MRI would inherently distinguish neoplastic from non-neoplastic lesions. Although this has not happened, manipulation of imaging sequences may allow distinction between different tissues.

Contrast enhancement of magnetic resonance images can be accomplished by intravenous injection of the paramagnetic contrast medium gadolinium (Gd)-DTPA.

IMAGING THE SPINE (pp. 1015–1021)

Diagnostic imaging of the spine is indicated when vertebral or spinal cord abnormalities are identified by clinical signs, neurological examination, or electrodiagnostic evaluation. Vertebral fractures, luxations, congenital anomalies, tumors, and infections can usually be identified on conventional radiographs. Symmetrical positioning of the spine is essential for critical radiographic evaluation and usually requires general anesthesia. Spinal pain causes involuntary axial muscle contraction with distortion of vertebral alignment even in cooperative patients.

Both lateral and ventrodorsal projections of the spine are included in all complete radiographic examinations. The spine is radiographed in multiple short segments so that the vertebrae being evaluated are near the center of the x-ray beam. Geometrical distortion (which increases with distance from the central ray) interferes with critical evaluation of intervertebral disc space width and other subtle signs. Additional radiographs may be necessary to fully evaluate a suspected lesion in any region. Because most of the spine is covered by thick muscle mass, high-contrast radiographic techniques of less than 80 kVp are used.

Survey radiographs allow accurate determination of the location and nature of a lesion in cases of direct vertebral involvement but do not allow a direct view of the spinal cord. Spinal cord involvement may be diagnosed by inference when there is vertebral displacement, evidence of intervertebral disc herniation, or osseous destruction or proliferation. Contrast radiography or alternate imaging procedures are considered when survey radiographs do not allow accurate localization or adequate assessment of the extent of a spinal cord abnormality.

Myelography

Myelography is accomplished by intrathecal injection of radiographic contrast medium to allow a view of the spinal subarachnoid space and the outer margins of the spinal cord. Because intrathecal injection of contrast medium always poses some risk of complication, myelography is not used when survey radiographs allow adequate diagnosis and treatment planning or when additional diagnostic information does not alter the course of treatment.

Myelography is performed with patients anesthetized. Phenothiazine-derivative tranquilizers, including acepromazine, are avoided in patients undergoing myelography because they potentiate seizures, particularly when used with metrizamide.

Two sites are commonly recommended for subarachnoid puncture and injection of myelographic agent: the cerebellomedullary cistern at the atlanto-occipital joint and the lumbar subarachnoid space at L4–L5 or L5–L6. The cerebrospinal fluid is examined visually, and if it is cloudy or grossly hemorrhagic, the myelographic procedure is aborted. It is essential that both lateral and ventrodorsal projections be made because significant spinal cord compression can be missed in any single projection.

Extradural lesions are the most common and can be caused by intervertebral disc herniation, ligamentous hypertrophy, fractures, luxation, or tumors arising outside the meninges. Intramedullary lesions are those arising within the spinal cord, including cord tumors, cord edema due to trauma, and hematomyelia. Intradural/extramedullary lesions arising within the subarachnoid space are uncommon and are most often tumors of spinal nerves.

Epidurography and Sinus Venography (p. 1019)

Scintigraphy

No scintigraphic procedure affords a view of the spinal cord, but radionuclide bone imaging can be used as a screening procedure for vertebral lesions, and it is more sensitive than conventional radiography. Radionuclide bone imaging may be particularly useful in identifying early or multiple sites of vertebral metastasis or intradiscal osteomyelitis.

Computed Tomography and Magnetic Resonance Imaging

CT and MRI offer the possibility of directly viewing the spinal cord in addition to surrounding structures. CT is particularly applicable to evaluation of osseous lesions and myelography. MRI allows a better direct view of soft tissues. Accurate positioning of dogs and cats can be difficult because their spines are long and mobile. The small diameter of the cord also makes spinal MRI more challenging in animals than in man.

CHAPTER 71

Pathogenesis of Diseases of the Central Nervous System

(pages 1022–1037)

THE BRAIN

Anatomy

The brain, cerebrospinal fluid (CSF), and cerebral blood volume are virtually incompressible, and their total volume remains constant. An increase in any one of these three compartments is accompanied by a reciprocal decrease in another, or intracranial pressure increases.

Intracranial space-occupying lesions initially may be accommodated through transfer of CSF to the spinal subarachnoid space or reduction of cerebral blood volume. These compensatory mechanisms are eventually overcome if the lesion becomes too large or interferes with either CSF or venous outflow. Resultant increased intracranial pressure (> 200 mm H_2O or 15 mm Hg) may impede cerebral blood flow (see the later section on Cushing response) or lead to displacement (herniation) of portions of the brain through foramina or ventral to dural septa.

The speed of onset of the inciting lesion is important in determining whether brain herniation occurs and the severity of neurological dysfunction. Factors that may precipitate herniation in animals with brain disease include the administration of volatile anesthetic agents and aspiration of CSF.

Distinct barriers exist between the blood and brain (blood-brain barrier) and blood and CSF (blood-CSF barrier). The blood-brain barrier is formed by a complex cellular system consisting of endothelial cells, pericytes, perivascular microglia, astrocytes, and basal laminae. Specialized adaptations of brain endothelial cells form the barrier. The blood-CSF barrier is formed by tight junctions at the apical end of the choroid epithelium rather than at the capillary endothelium of the villus.

These barriers physically insulate the healthy brain from blood-borne injurious agents such as microorganisms and certain chemicals but also impede delivery of therapeutic agents.

Physiology

The brain largely depends on oxidative metabolism of glucose for its unusually high energy requirements. Factors causing either a reduction in mean arterial pressure or an increase in intracranial pressure may impede the brain's blood supply.

Pressure Autoregulation

Coupling of cerebral blood flow and mean arterial pressure is termed *pressure autoregulation*. This process maintains the brain's blood supply at a constant rate despite fluctuations in mean arterial pressure between 50 and 160 mm Hg. The myogenic theory attributes pressure autoregulation to pressure-sensitive smooth muscle in cerebral vessel walls. Other theories attribute pressure autoregulation to changes in local tissue pressure and sympathetic innervation of cerebral blood vessels. Pressure autoregulation is impaired by brain disease.

Cushing Response

Increased intracranial pressure evokes a corresponding increase in systemic arterial pressure (Cushing response) that maintains cerebral blood flow. The Cushing response is more resilient than pressure autoregulation, at least with regard to hypoxia.

Metabolic Autoregulation

Cerebral blood flow also varies according to the metabolic needs of brain tissue. Metabolic autoregulation is impaired by head injury.

Chemical Regulation

Cerebral vessels are also sensitive to the arterial partial pressures of oxygen (PaO_2) and carbon dioxide ($PaCO_2$). Systemic hypoxia induces cerebral vessel dilation, leading to increased cerebral blood flow. Brain tissue oxygenation is maintained until PaO_2 falls to 20 mm Hg. Further reduction in oxygen tension necessitates anaerobic glycolysis, and energy requirements are no longer met. Fluctuations in $PaCO_2$ have an even more potent effect on cerebral vessel tone. Systemic hypercapnia causes cerebral vessel dilation. Resultant enhancement of blood flow prevents cerebral acidosis.

Response to Disease

Most brain diseases cause gliosis, proliferation and congestion of vessels, and at least some edema. In addition, many result in necrosis (malacia), hemorrhage, and inflammation.

Necrosis

Brain necrosis is liquefactive and can be focal or diffuse. Softening of the brain subsequent to necrosis is termed *encephalomalacia*.

Ischemia, Hypoxia, Hypoglycemia. Reduction of either brain oxygen or glucose causes neuronal necrosis. Causes of cerebral hypoxia include diminution of PaO_2 (hypoxic hypoxia), depletion of blood hemoglobin (anemic hypoxia), impaired tissue use of oxygen (histotoxic hypoxia), and reduction of the brain's blood supply (cerebral ischemia) due to either selective impairment of cerebral blood flow (oligemic hypoxia) or reduced cardiac output (stagnant hypoxia). Reduction of brain glucose may occur because of either cerebral ischemia or systemic hypoglycemia.

Classic studies provide indisputable evidence of irreversible neuronal injury following 4 to 6 minutes of cerebral ischemia. However, some brain function may return after periods of complete ischemia lasting as long as 60 minutes. This finding suggests that variables other than the duration of ischemia contribute to the severity of injury. One such variable is the quality of cerebral blood flow after the initial ischemic insult.

Regardless of the exact pathogenesis, the metabolic effects of ischemia are manifested morphologically within 12 hours by neuronal shrinkage and eosinophilia (ischemic cell change). With diffuse cerebral ischemia, a patient may die before other lesions develop.

The occurrence of ischemic cell change in animals and man with nonischemic forms of cerebral hypoxia and systemic hypoglycemia suggests that these conditions have pathogenetic mechanisms similar to ischemia. Status epilepticus in man and dogs also causes diffuse cerebrocortical ischemic cell change. That neurons are involved in these conditions but glia and other non-neuronal cells are spared has been termed *selective neuronal necrosis.* All three of these processes involve energy depletion due to either inhibition of energy production (ischemia and hypoglycemia) or increased consumption (epilepsy).

Trauma. Many animals with traumatic neurological dysfunction have no demonstrable brain lesion (concussion) or only focal subpial hemorrhage with minimal malacia (contusion). Others have extensive malacia, intracranial hemorrhage, or both subsequent to the combined effects of brain laceration and vascular tears. These primary effects of trauma often cause physiological deregulation leading to brain herniation within 12 hours.

Inflammation. Release of lysosomal enzymes by degenerating neutrophils and macrophages causes necrosis. Lesions may occur focally, as with bacterial abscess formation, or diffusely owing to disseminated encephalitis. Diffuse inflammatory processes often have a perivascular distribution, especially with concomitant vasculitis. Selective involvement of either gray matter (polioencephalitis) or white matter (leukoencephalitis) may be noted.

Hemorrhage

Intracranial hemorrhage may be extradural, subdural, subarachnoid, intraventricular, or intracerebral.

Trauma. All cranial trauma probably causes at least minimal subclinical intracranial hemorrhage. Most epidural hematomas are associated with linear skull fractures that tear meningeal vessels, particularly the middle meningeal artery. Subdural hematomas usually form either subsequent to tearing of a surface vein or because of exteriorization of intracerebral hemorrhage. Most intracerebral hematomas are associated with focal application of force, as with missile injuries and depressed skull fractures.

Vascular Disease. Primary cerebrovascular disease is unusual in dogs and cats. Conditions that cause vasculitis may also lead to cerebral infarction or hemorrhage. Vasculitis has been recognized in several infectious diseases of dogs and cats, including feline infectious peritonitis, canine parvovirus infection, and Rocky Mountain spotted fever.

Edema

Brain edema occurs after most cerebral diseases. Diffuse involvement increases intracranial pressure, resulting in brain ischemia and herniation.

Cytotoxic Edema. The principal cause of cytotoxic edema is hypoxia-induced failure of the cellular sodium pump.

Vasogenic Edema. Vasogenic edema occurs when any factor increases cerebrovascular permeability, allowing escape of fluid into the extracellular space. Principal causes of vasogenic brain edema in dogs and cats include encephalitis, head injury, and brain tumors.

Interstitial Edema. Hydrocephalus is the lone cause of interstitial brain edema. Most cases of hydrocephalus in animals occur because of defective absorption of CSF, either because of intraventricular obstruction to flow (noncommunicating) or secondary to lesions at the arachnoid villi within the subarachnoid space (communicating).

Neoplasia

Most brain neoplasms develop as solitary masses that grow primarily by expansion and seldom metastasize to points either within or outside the central nervous system.

THE SPINAL CORD (pp. 1030–1035)

Anatomy

Movement of the spinal cord in response to compressive extramedullary lesions is restricted not only by the surrounding vertebrae and meninges but also by the nerve roots as they leave the spine. The spinal cord often becomes trapped between one of these structures and the offending lesion. Less frequently, extradural masses encircle the spinal cord, because their growth follows the route of least resistance.

The gradual onset of many compressive lesions allows time for spinal cord accommodation, so initial neurological dysfunction may be minimal. With continued compression, neural function is lost in a predictable sequence. Conscious proprioception is lost first, followed by voluntary motor activity, superficial (primary) pain sensation, and deep (secondary) pain sensation. The sequence of neurological deterioration may reflect greater sensitivity to pressure of large, heavily myelinated fibers that convey position sense and motor function, compared with the lightly or nonmyelinated polysynaptic pathways responsible for pain sensation. One study showed that histological changes occurring after 7 hours of slow, graded compression were consistent with ischemia. Other studies indicate that mechanical factors are more important than ischemia.

Physiology

Spinal Reflexes

Spinal reflex activity is mediated locally and occurs independently of thought. Nevertheless, spinal reflexes are influenced considerably by both descending and ascending pathways.

Spinal Shock. Areflexia caudal to a lesion following acute functional spinal cord transection is termed *spinal shock*. It occurs because of sudden interruption of facilitory brain stem and forebrain input to spinal neurons. Spinal shock is a transient condition that varies in depth and duration with the degree of cerebral dominance over the brain stem (encephalization). It lasts only hours in carnivores.

Hyperreflexia. Most dogs and cats with acute spinal cord injury have recovered from spinal shock when first examined and exhibit either normoreflexia or hyper-reflexia. Extensor reflexes are especially prone to hyper-reflexia. The most plausible explanation is a loss of supraspinal inhibition to extensor neurons concomitant with the loss of facilitation responsible for spinal shock.

Mass Reflex. Spinal reflex activity in dogs and cats may become markedly exaggerated several months after functional spinal transection.

Crossed Extensor Reflex (p. 1032)
Schiff-Sherrington Phenomenon (p. 1032)

Spinal Cord Blood Flow

Normal spinal cord blood flow to gray matter (50 to 60 ml/100 g/min) is approximately five times that of white matter (10 to 15 ml/100 g/min) in dogs and cats. This amount of spinal cord blood flow is maintained despite fluctuations in mean arterial pressure in a way analogous to cerebral blood flow pressure autoregulation. Spinal cord blood flow also varies directly with the $Paco_2$. Both chemical regulation and pressure autoregulation are impaired by spinal cord trauma.

Histopathological effects of spinal cord ischemia are similar to those induced by acute impact injury. Both are characterized by central hemorrhagic necrosis, suggesting that ischemia may contribute to the pathogenesis of acute spinal trauma.

Two principal mechanisms have been proposed to explain the reduction of spinal cord blood flow after acute injury: vascular and neurovascular. The vascular theory attributes ischemia to direct effects of trauma on vessel walls, resulting in vasospasm, vascular tears, endothelial cell swelling, and thrombi. However, some believe that the most important factor is vasospasm induced by vasoactive agents. Intervention directed at modulating deleterious effects of oxygen radicals, endorphins, calcium, and excitatory amino acids has been beneficial experimentally. Similarly, benefit has been attributed to the glucocorticoids and to agents such as thyrotropin-releasing hormone that may act independently to increase spinal cord blood flow.

Response to Disease

Responses to spinal cord and brain disease are similar.

Necrosis

Acute spinal cord injury often results in central hemorrhagic necrosis in dogs and cats. The most common cause is acute intervertebral disc herniation. The severity of histological changes varies directly with the force of impact. Measures directed at reversing this process may be beneficial in treating spinal cord injury in dogs and cats.

Myelomalacia also occurs subsequent to ischemia induced by vascular occlusion due to fibrocartilaginous emboli originating from the intervertebral disc.

Demyelination and Hypomyelination

Demyelination, a breakdown or loss of normal myelin, is a pathological hallmark of several human diseases, most notably multiple sclerosis.

The pathogenesis of demyelination in canine distemper encephalomyelitis is of particular interest to veterinarians. Considerable interest has been focused on cytopathic effects of the canine distemper virus on glial cells. Demyelination may occur because macrophages responding to virus infection secrete oxygen radicals that are toxic to oligodendrocytes.

The process of concomitant degeneration of the axon and its myelin sheath distal to the point of separation from the neuronal cell body, called *wallerian degeneration*, is the most common form of demyelination in dogs and cats. It is particularly marked after chronic spinal cord compression.

Dogs and cats have numerous congenital diseases in which myelination is either delayed or faulty or in which myelin, axons, or both degenerate later in life. Many of these conditions selectively involve the spinal cord, resulting in neurological signs *indistinguishable* from those caused by spinal cord compression. Veterinary surgeons are *obligated* to be familiar with these diseases. Unnecessary diagnostic procedures or surgery might otherwise be performed.

Edema

Vasogenic edema is an integral component of the process of central hemorrhagic necrosis. Edema increases intraluminal spinal cord pressure, causing further compression of its vascular and neural structures. Therapeutic measures directed at the removal of edema are important in the resolution of spinal injury.

Neoplasia (see also Chapter 157)

In dogs and cats, approximately 50 per cent of spinal tumors are extradural, 30 per cent are extramedullary, and 20 per cent are intradural-intramedullary.

CHAPTER 72

Surgical Approaches to the Spine (pages 1038–1047)

VENTRAL APPROACH TO THE CERVICAL VERTEBRAE

The ventral approach is indicated for ventral slot decompression (Chapter 75), disc fenestration (Chapter 75), atlantoaxial instability, and treatment of some classifications of spondylopathies (Chapter 74).

A ventral midline incision is made from the larynx to the sternum. Reflection of the trachea to the left side protects the esophagus and exposes the paired longus colli muscles. The disc spaces are located just caudal to the ventral processes of the vertebrae.

DORSAL APPROACH TO THE FIRST AND SECOND CERVICAL VERTEBRAE

A dorsal approach is indicated for repair of atlantoaxial instability (Chapter 73) and fractures of the first and second cervical vertebrae (Chapter 78) and for hemilaminectomy for tumors associated with spinal cord segments C1 and C2.

A dorsal midline incision is made from the external occipital protuberance to the dorsal process of the fourth cervical vertebra. The incision is continued on the midline between the paired bellies of the cervicoscutularis, cervicoauricularis superficialis, and platysma muscles.

DORSAL APPROACH TO THE MIDCERVICAL VERTEBRAE

The dorsal approach is indicated for repair of fractures and luxations of vertebrae C2 through C5 (Chapter 78) and for dorsal laminectomy or hemilaminectomy of vertebrae C2 through C5.

An incision is made along one side of the nuchal ligament and between the paired bellies of the rectus capitis dorsalis major (cranially) and the spinalis et semispinalis cervicis and multifidus cervicis (caudally).

DORSAL APPROACH TO THE CAUDAL CERVICAL VERTEBRAE

The dorsal approach is indicated for dorsal laminectomy or hemilaminectomy of C5 through T3 and open reduction of fractures or luxations of C5 through T3 (Chapter 78).

The dorsal spines of T1 through T3 can be removed for dorsal laminectomy because the nuchal ligament is continuous with the supraspinous ligament.

DORSAL APPROACH TO THE THORACOLUMBAR VERTEBRAE

The dorsal approach is indicated for dorsal laminectomy and hemilaminectomy, fenestration of thoracolumbar discs (Chapter 75), and reduction of thoracolumbar fractures and luxations (Chapter 78).

The skin incision is made slightly off the dorsal midline and extends three vertebrae cranial and caudal to the vertebrae to be exposed. The multifidus, interspinalis, and rotatores longi muscles are elevated from the spinous processes and vertebral arches one vertebra cranial and caudal to the affected vertebrae with a periosteal elevator.

DORSOLATERAL APPROACH TO THORACOLUMBAR DISCS

The dorsal approach is indicated for fenestration of intervertebral discs from T9 to L7 (Chapter 75).

A dorsal incision is made 1 cm off the midline, extending two vertebrae cranial and caudal to the segment of the spine to be fenestrated. The multifidus and longissimus muscles are separated by blunt dissection from caudal to cranial.

DORSAL APPROACH TO THE SACRUM

The dorsal approach is indicated for dorsal laminectomy for cauda equina syndrome (Chapter 77), intervertebral disc herniation, spinal cord tumors, and repair of fractures and luxations of the sacrum and seventh lumbar vertebra (Chapter 78).

CHAPTER 73

Atlantoaxial Instability
(pages 1048–1056)

ANATOMY

The atlantoaxial joint allows rotational movement of the head on the vertebral column. Rotation is centered around the odontoid process (dens) of the axis, which projects rostrally into the bony ring formed by the atlas.

The restricted rotational movement allowed by this joint is complemented by the dorsoventral movement of the occipital condyles on the atlas and the complex movements of the cervical vertebrae, to allow free motion of the head in all directions.

PATHOLOGY

Traumatic injuries can occur at any age or in any type of animal as a result of forceful flexion of the head.

If the dens is absent, is malformed, or has no ligamentous attachments, the dorsal atlantoaxial ligament must bear all the stress of head flexion. Any of these lesions compromises atlantoaxial stability or jeopardizes the spinal cord by encroachment into the spinal canal. The dorsal atlantoaxial ligament may be congenitally weakened, but even when normal it weakens and ruptures if it alone is expected to stabilize the atlantoaxial joint. The end result is atlantoaxial joint instability.

Instability alone is not associated with clinical signs; the instability leads to spinal cord trauma resulting in pain or upper motor neuron tetraparesis. The severity of clinical signs depends on the degree of injury to the spinal cord.

DIAGNOSIS

Trauma is part of the history in most cases of atlantoaxial instability.

The presenting and neurological signs usually include cervical pain and various degrees of proprioceptive or motor deficits in the rear legs only or in all four legs.

Confirmation of the clinical diagnosis is obtained by a well-positioned lateral radiograph that shows the fracture or abnormal separation of the dorsal arch of the atlas and the dorsal spine of the axis. A flexed lateral view may be necessary to demonstrate instability, but extreme care should be taken when flexing if the dens is intact or deviated dorsally. Further displacement of an intact dens into the spinal canal may precipitate respiratory paralysis and death.

PROGNOSIS

The prognosis depends on the degree of trauma inflicted on the spinal cord.

TREATMENT

Conservative management has been advocated in animals with minimal clinical signs. Movement of the head and neck is restricted by using a neck brace constructed of padded splint material. Recurrence is common after this treatment.

Surgical therapy may be performed to decompress the spinal cord or to stabilize the atlantoaxial joint. Because most surgeons agree that anatomical reduction and appropriate fixation will result in decompression, specific decompression techniques are rarely used.

Dorsal Approach

A doubled length of heavy (0 to 1) nonabsorbable suture (braided polyester) is threaded under the dorsal arch of the atlas.

Two widely separated small holes are drilled through the dorsal spine of the axis. The suture is cut, and the cut ends are passed through the holes in the spine of the axis. These two ends are tied to the corresponding free ends with the axis and atlas held in alignment. This double sling helps prevent rotational as well as rocking movement.

Ventral Approach

The ventral approach is used with the intention of fusing the atlas to the axis or for fracture repair. The more substantial bone available ventrally allows the choice of one of several orthopedic fixation techniques to achieve stability. Pins alone, pins and methacrylate, and plates all have been used successfully. All of these techniques benefit from a cancellous bone graft in the joint space or at the fracture site.

FRACTURES

The lack of bone and the critical structures in close proximity to the vertebrae make fixation difficult. Careful and accurate implant placement is essential to ensure a satisfactory outcome.

CHAPTER 74

Caudal Cervical Spondylomyelopathy

(pages 1056–1070)

Disorders of the caudal cervical vertebrae and intervertebral discs (spondylopathy) resulting in compression of the spinal cord (myelopathy) in large dogs, particularly Doberman pinschers and Great Danes, have been termed *caudal cervical spondylomyelopathy* or wobbler syndrome.

ANATOMY (p. 1056)

PATHOPHYSIOLOGY (pp. 1056–1060)

Regardless of the specific cause, compression of the spinal cord results in electrophysiological conduction abnormalities, demyelination, and myelomalacia.

Congenital Osseous Malformation

Congenital osseous malformation of the cervical spine principally affects Great Dane and Doberman pinscher puppies within the first or second year of life. Congenital osseous malformation most commonly affects C3 to C7 vertebral bodies.

Cervical Vertebral Instability/Chronic Degenerative Disc Disease

Cervical vertebral instability/chronic degenerative disc disease is principally a disorder of middle-aged to older Doberman pinschers, presumably caused by degenerative intervertebral disc disease and resultant vertebral instability of the C5–C6 or C6–C7 intervertebral disc or both. Hypertrophy or hyperplasia of the dorsal annulus fibrosus results in ventral compression of the spinal cord that varies with neck position.

Vertebral Tipping

Ligamentum Flavum Disease or Vertebral Arch Malformation

Instability may result in hypertrophy or hyperplasia of the ligamentum flavum, causing dorsal spinal cord compression. Patients with vertebral arch malformation may have either a genetic predisposition or nutritional imbalance or both. This form of spondylomyelopathy principally occurs in the caudal cervical spine C4–C7 of young Great Danes (5 months to 2 years of age).

Hourglass Compression

Compression of the dorsal, ventral, and lateral aspects of the spinal cord resulting in an hourglass configuration occurs mostly in young Great Danes.

PRESENTATION (pp. 1060–1061)

Historical, clinical, and neurological examination of patients with caudal cervical spondylomyelopathy generally suggests a lesion in the caudal cervical spinal cord. The presence and degree of ataxia, tetraparesis, and forelimb and hindlimb reflex changes are helpful in determining the neuroanatomical location as well as the severity of the lesion. Information concerning age and breed may assist specific classification of caudal cervical spondylomyelopathy.

DIAGNOSIS

Although plain radiography is helpful in diagnosing caudal cervical spondylomyelopathy, myelography is essential to evaluate the level (affected intervertebral space or spaces), location of the lesion in the spinal canal (dorsal, ventral, lateral), and degree of spinal cord compression. Stress myelography is mandatory to determine the dynamic component of a compressive lesion.

TREATMENT (pp. 1062–1067)

Medical management consists of strict rest and confinement, support with a neck brace, use of a body harness in place of a neck collar, and glucocorticoids or nonsteroidal anti-inflammatory medications.

Ventral Decompression

Ventral decompression (slot) alone has been used successfully in patients with lesions caused by chronic vertebral instability, chronic degenerative disc disease, and vertebral tipping. A ventral slot is created at the affected intervertebral disc space with a high-speed surgical burr.

The major disadvantage of ventral decompression alone is failure to remove the entire compressive lesion and possible instability caused by the slot.

Decompression and Stabilization Using Polyvinylidine Spinal Plates

Techniques that use decompression and stabilization for patients with dynamically compressive lesions allow the annulus fibrosus to stretch, relieving compression. With stabilization, atrophy of the annulus fibrosus occurs, further improving decompression.

The approach and slot are performed as described for ventral decompression, but the slot is carried only to the level of the inner cortical layer. The affected intervertebral space is pulled into linear traction with a modified Gelpi retractor. The configuration of the slot must be precisely created to accommodate a full cortical allograft. A polyvinylidine spinal plate is placed on the ventral surface of the adjacent vertebral bodies to secure the bone graft in the slot.

Postoperative care includes strict confinement and a neck brace for 4 to 6 weeks. Advantages of this technique over ventral decompression alone include adequate spinal cord decompression without entering the spinal canal, reduced risk of iatrogenic spinal cord trauma, and improvement in the rate and duration of recovery. The major disadvantage is the high incidence of implant failure in patients that do not tolerate a neck brace.

Decompression and Stabilization with Steinmann Pins and Bone Cement

From 2 to 3 mm of distraction is applied to the affected intervertebral space using the modified Gelpi retractor previously mentioned.

Autogenous cancellous bone is placed into the distracted space. Two 7/64- or 1/8-inch Steinmann pins are inserted into the vertebral body cranial and caudal to the affected intervertebral space. Sterile polymethyl methacrylate is molded around each pin. Advantages of this technique include adequate spinal cord decompression without entering the spinal canal; reduced risk of iatrogenic cord trauma; improvement in the percentage, rate, and duration of recovery; and no requirement for a neck brace.

Decompression and Stabilization with Harrington Rods

Harrington spinal distraction rods provide distraction and stabilization in patients with cervical vertebral instability without the need for a vertebral spreader. This technique is most useful in patients with two adjacent lesions (generally C5–C6 and C6–C7). The Harrington spinal distraction rod consists of a threaded 58-mm bolt, two nuts, and two distraction hooks. There is a high incidence of implant failure in patients that do not tolerate a neck brace.

Inverted Cone Decompression

Dorsal Laminectomy

The length of the laminectomy may be from three-fourths of the length of each vertebra up to a continuous laminectomy extending from C4 to C7. Transarticular hemicerclage wires or lag screws may be necessary for additional stability.

This technique does not alter the underlying causes of caudal cervical spondylomyelopathy, but relief of spinal cord compression is achieved. Owners are given a guarded prognosis for neurological recovery.

AFTERCARE (p. 1067)

SELECTION OF SURGICAL TECHNIQUE AND PROGNOSIS (pp. 1067–1069)

Congenital Osseous Malformation

Patients with congenital osseous malformation generally have an unfavorable prognosis.

Cervical Vertebral Instability/Chronic Degenerative Disc Disease, Vertebral Tipping, Hourglass Compression

Patients with cervical vertebral instability/chronic degenerative disc disease, vertebral tipping, or hourglass compression with pain, paraparesis, or ambulatory tetraparesis have a greater than 90 per cent chance of recovery to an acceptable neurological status.

Ligamentum Flavum Disease or Vertebral Arch Malformation

The prognosis is generally guarded to favorable depending on the degree of neurological deficit.

LONG-TERM COMPLICATIONS (p. 1069)

Fusion of one intervertebral space may lead to an increase in stress on the adjacent intervertebral discs. This increased stress may predispose those intervertebral discs to cervical vertebral instability/chronic degenerative disc disease or may accelerate subclinical degeneration.

CHAPTER 75
Intervertebral Disc Disease
(pages 1070–1087)

ANATOMY OF THE DISC AND RELATED STRUCTURES
(pp. 1070–1071)

An intervertebral disc is interposed in every intervertebral space except C1–C2. Intervertebral discs unite adjacent vertebral bodies to form amphiarthroidal joints. Each disc consists of two distinct regions: (1) an ovoid center of gelatinous material, the *nucleus pulposus,* which originates from the embryonic notochord; and (2) an outer annulus fibrosus composed of fibrocartilaginous material arranged in concentric layers. The ventral and lateral portions of the annulus are 1.5 to 3 times thicker than the dorsal annulus. The propensity of the nucleus to herniate dorsally into the vertebral canal is explained by its eccentric position within the annulus. The cranial and caudal borders of an intervertebral disc are formed by hyaline cartilaginous end-plates, which cover the epiphyses of the vertebral bodies.

Several ligamentous structures adjacent to the intervertebral discs provide support, which varies in different regions of the spine. These include the dorsal and ventral longitudinal ligaments and the intercapital ligaments. The presence of stabilizing intercapital ligaments from T1–T2 through T9–T10 and possibly T10–T11 accounts for the greatly reduced incidence of disc herniation in this area compared with the cervical, caudal thoracic, and lumbar regions of the spine.

The internal vertebral venous plexus (vertebral sinuses) consists of left and right thin-walled, flattened, valveless vessels that extend along the floor of the vertebral canal from the skull to the caudal vertebrae.

PHYSIOLOGY OF THE DISC AND PATHOPHYSIOLOGY OF DISC EXTRUSION (pp 1071–1073)

The intervertebral discs form cushions between adjacent bony vertebrae to allow movement, minimize and absorb shock, and unite segments of the vertebral column. When compression of the disc occurs, shock is absorbed by displacement of the incompressible nucleus in all directions and by distension of the annulus. Mechanical efficiency of a disc depends on the quality and quantity of its matrix components. Nutrition of the discs is by diffusion from the cartilaginous end-plates and is facilitated by normal vertebral movement.

In chondrodystrophoid dogs, chondroid metaplasia occurs between 8 months and 2 years of age, with 75 per cent or more of all intervertebral discs undergoing some degeneration by 1 year. The degenerate nucleus often undergoes dystrophic calcification, further compromising its function. Failure is often manifested by complete rupture of the dorsal annulus and an explosive upward extrusion of a large volume of nuclear material into the vertebral canal. This event, termed a Hansen type I disc protrusion generally occurs in dogs between 2 and 7 years of age, with a peak incidence at 4 to 5 years.

In nonchondrodystrophoid dogs, intervertebral disc degeneration occurs later in life, generally causes less severe signs, and involves a different metaplastic process. Partial rupture of annular bands and a domelike bulging of the dorsal annulus are typical.

PATHOGENESIS OF CANINE DISC DISEASE
(pp. 1073–1075)

The ability of the spinal cord to tolerate displacement depends on the dynamic force of compression. Compressive masses with equal velocity and volume produce more severe signs in the thoracolumbar region than in the cervical region because of a smaller ratio of cord diameter to vertebral canal diameter in the latter.

In chronic progressive compression, dynamic force is low and the spinal cord can compensate for a surprising degree of displacement before clinical signs occur. When the compensatory mechanisms of the spinal cord are exceeded, local hypoxia develops and demyelination, axonal degeneration, and malacia occur. With acute, complete Hansen type I extrusions, the dynamic force of compression is often very high. Spinal cord damage due to acute compression ranges from slight demyelination to total necrosis of gray and white matter.

With progressive degrees of spinal cord compression, increased ischemia and demyelination occur. Accordingly, different neurological functions are lost in a predictable order according to the degree of myelination and the diameter of the fibers that mediate a given type of function (Fig. 75–3). Large, heavily myelinated fibers mediating conscious proprioception are the first to be affected; intermediate-sized fibers mediating voluntary motor function and slightly smaller fibers mediating superficial pain appreciation are affected next; and small fibers mediating deep pain appreciation are the last affected. During recovery, functions return in reverse order, with deep pain appreciation returning first and conscious proprioception last.

Hansen type I extrusions generally cause a focal compressive myelopathy. A progressive ascending-descending hemorrhagic myelomalacia occasionally ensues.

Another mechanism by which intervertebral disc disease can cause paresis or paralysis is fibrocartilaginous embolism leading to spinal cord infarction. These emboli probably originate from a degenerative nucleus pulposus, but the exact anatomical routes by which they gain access to the spinal cord microvasculature remain controversial.

CERVICAL DISC DISEASE (pp. 1075–1080)

Incidence

Chondrodystrophoid and other small breeds are at greatest risk, with dachshunds, toy poodles, and beagles accounting for more than 80 per cent. Cervical disc lesions occur most commonly at C2–C3, with involvement progressively decreasing from C3–C4 to C7–T1.

Clinical Signs

Severe neck pain is the most common sign associated with cervical disc lesions. A stiff gait, lowered head, guarded neck, and spasms of cervical cutaneous and shoulder muscles are typical manifestations of the pain. Referred pain to a front leg ("root signature") and an associated orthopedic-like lameness occurs in up to 50 per cent.

Diagnosis

A presumptive diagnosis of cervical disc protrusion or extrusion is based on signalment, history, and physical examination. The diagnosis of cervical disc protrusion/extrusion is confirmed by radiographic procedures and surgery. Myelography is strongly recommended for nearly all patients that have cervical disc disease for which surgical decompression is planned (see Chapter 70).

Staging and Prognosis

Symptomatic patients can be subdivided into three basic groups: (1) first episode involving neck pain only; (2) repeated episodes of neck pain only; and (3) neck pain and concurrent neurological deficits. Medical therapy or prophylactic intervertebral disc fenestrations are often recommended for dogs in group 1; surgical decompression with removal of the compressive mass is often appropriate for dogs in group 2; and surgical decompression is almost always advisable for dogs in group 3.

Prognosis for complete recovery after cervical disc extrusion is generally favorable but depends on several factors; anatomical location, dynamic factors influencing severity of the lesion, and treatment. Although many dogs respond to conservative treatment, recurrence rates of 33 per cent or more occur. When cervical disc extrusion causes nonambulatory tetraparesis, important prognostic factors include location of the lesion, duration of nonambulatory status before and after surgery, and forelimb sensory status.

Treatment

Medical Therapy

Principles include attentive nursing care, restricted physical activity, and cautious use of anti-inflammatory drugs or muscle relaxants to control pain and hyperesthesia. The most important aspect of conservative treatment is *strict cage confinement* for 10 to 14 days.

Cage rest is important for dogs that have been treated with corticosteroids or other anti-inflammatory drugs. The euphoric effect promotes increased physical activity, which may cause further extrusion from an unstable, partially ruptured disc. Cervical pain aids in limiting physical activity; therefore, only dogs with severe pain are treated.

Surgery

Prophylaxis involves fenestration for removal of nuclear material from the disc itself, whereas treatment of extrusion involves exploratory decompressive techniques to remove disc material from within the vertebral canal or intervertebral foramen. A ventral approach to the cervical spine is used for fenestrations and for most decompressive procedures (ventral slot decompressions). Details of this surgical approach and others are described in Chapter 72.

Fenestration. The ventral annulus of disc spaces C2–C3 through C6–C7 is exposed by separation of the paired tendons of the longus colli muscle just caudal to their attachments on the ventral process.

Safe fenestration depends on a large ventral annular window and atraumatic removal of nuclear material. Fenestration of a partially ruptured or unstable intervertebral disc may cause dorsal extrusion of disc material and worsening of clinical signs. Efficacy of fenestration depends on complete removal of the nucleus.

Decompressive Procedures. Selection of the appropriate decompressive procedure to facilitate atraumatic removal of the compressive mass depends on the location of extruded material.

Dorsolateral extrusions are most common, followed by paramedian and dorsomedian extrusions. Each of these types of cervical disc extrusion can be accessed by a ventral slot decompression. Less commonly, intraforaminal and lateral disc extrusions may occur. These are accessible by limited dorsolateral hemilaminectomy and facetectomy.

Ventral Decompression. The ventral process of the cranial vertebra is removed with a pair of rongeurs, and the ventral annulus is excised with a number 11 blade to prepare the interspace for drilling. The slot is created using a high-speed pneumatic drill and burr. Slot dimensions do not exceed 50 per cent of the width and 33 per cent of the length of the vertebral bodies being drilled.

Remnants of the dorsal annulus fibrosus and dorsal longitudinal ligament must be carefully removed to avoid hemorrhage from the vertebral venous sinus. Adequate decompression involves removal of enough disc material and other debris to establish a clear view of the dural tube through the slot.

Limited Dorsolateral Hemilaminectomy and Facetectomy. Lateral or intraforaminal disc extrusion dictates decompression by this method rather than by the ventral slot technique. Even though the dorsolateral approach (see Chapter 72) is technically more difficult, it is the only way to gain access to the extruded disc.

Lateral disc extrusions are closely associated with both the nerve root and the vertebral artery, and removal of extruded material requires meticulous dissection.

Aftercare. From 2 to 3 weeks of confinement is optimal.

THORACOLUMBAR DISC DISEASE (pp. 1080–1086)

Incidence

Thoracolumbar lesions account for 84 to 86 per cent of the intervertebral disc problems in dogs. The most commonly affected breed is the dachshund; the Shih Tzu, Pekingese, Lhasa apso, Welsh corgi, and beagle are at significant risk. Thoracolumbar disc lesions occur most commonly between T11 and T12 and between L1 and L2.

Clinical Signs

Neurological signs associated with thoracolumbar disc lesions vary depending on anatomical location, duration, and dynamic force of compression. Back pain, nonambulatory paraparesis, and pelvic limb hyper-reflexia are most common. Although pelvic limb signs are often bilaterally symmetrical, lateralization to the right or left side may occur. Impaired urinary bladder function is common in dogs with nonambulatory paraparesis or paraplegia.

Diagnosis

A presumptive diagnosis of thoracolumbar disc protrusion or extrusion is based on signalment, history, and physical examination.

Radiographic evidence of thoracolumbar intervertebral disc extrusion may include narrowing and wedging of the space, narrowing or cloudiness of the intervertebral foramen, narrowing of the articular facet space, and calcified material within the vertebral canal. Thoracolumbar myelography is recommended.

Staging

Dogs with thoracolumbar disc lesions can be divided into four basic groups for establishing treatment guidelines (Table 75–1). Disagree-

TABLE 75-1. CLASSIFICATION OF DOGS WITH THORACOLUMBAR DISC LESIONS ACCORDING TO SEVERITY OF SIGNS

Group	Clinical Presentation	Treatment Options
I	First episode of back pain and no neurological deficits	M or F
II	Recurrent pain and/or mild to moderate paraparesis	M, F, D, D + F
III	Severe paraparesis	D or D + F
IV	Paraplegia	
	A With deep pain intact	D or D + F
	B Deep pain absent < 48 hours	D + d ± E
	C Deep pain absent > 48 hours	M or D + d ± E

M, medical therapy; F, disc fenestrations; D, decompressive surgery and mass removal; d, durotomy; E, experimental treatment (e.g., implanted oscillating field electrical stimulator).

ment exists regarding the most appropriate treatment for different stages of thoracolumbar disc disease.

Prognosis

Dogs that retain deep pain after thoracolumbar disc extrusion usually respond favorably to decompressive surgery. Once pelvic limb deep pain appreciation is lost, however, the prognosis quickly declines and rapid surgical intervention becomes critical. Durotomy is recommended for prognostic purposes in dogs without deep pain. Gross integrity of the spinal cord cannot be accurately determined without opening the dura.

Treatment

Medical Therapy

Medical treatment is reserved for animals that experience back pain or mild paresis, for animals with chronic loss of pelvic limb deep pain, and for dogs whose owners decline surgical treatment. The most important aspect of conservative treatment, especially for dogs in groups I and II, is strictly enforced cage rest for several weeks. Use of antiinflammatory drugs during this period may undermine the attempt to reduce physical activity. Nursing care is more demanding for non-ambulatory dogs in groups III and IV.

Surgery

Fenestration. The role of fenestrations in treatment of thoracolumbar disc disease remains controversial. Although some surgeons use disc fenestrations without decompression for mildly affected cases, most agree that disc fenestration does not provide spinal cord decompression.

The prophylactic benefits of disc fenestration have also been questioned. Although the lowest recurrence rates were in dogs that received disc fenestrations, protection afforded by this technique was not absolute. Dorsolateral, lateral muscle separation, and ventral abdominal paracostal/intercostal approaches to thoracolumbar disc fenestration have been described. Effectiveness of fenestration depends on the amount of nucleus pulposus removed. Prophylactic fenestration of thoracolumbar discs routinely includes T11–T12 through L3–L4.

Decompressive Procedures. Atraumatic removal of the compressive mass is the ultimate goal of these procedures. Use of methylprednisolone sodium succinate (30 mg/kg IV) is recommended because of its protective effects on the spinal cord.

Dorsal Laminectomy. This technique involves removal of the dorsal spinous processes, dorsal laminae, and variable amounts of the articular processes and pedicles of at least two consecutive vertebrae.

A significant difficulty with dorsal laminectomy in dogs has been to provide adequate exposure and decompression without predisposing to postoperative constrictive fibrosis of the spinal cord. The greater the amount of vertebral arch removed, the greater the likelihood of this problem. The *modified dorsal laminectomy* removes the caudal articular processes but leaves the major portion of each cranial articular process intact. Undercutting of the medial aspect of the pedicles provides exposure superior to the Funkquist type B laminectomy without increasing the risk of postoperative constrictive fibrosis.

Hemilaminectomy. Because the majority of thoracolumbar disc lesions involve a ventral or ventrolateral compressive mass, hemilaminectomy is preferred over dorsal laminectomy. If the disc lesion lateralizes to one side, it is imperative that the hemilaminectomy be performed on that side to enable atraumatic removal of the compressive mass. Contralateral lesions are difficult to remove without excessive cord manipulation; where the hemilaminectomy is on the wrong side, bilateral hemilaminectomy is recommended.

A durotomy is not performed except as a diagnostic aid for determination of spinal cord integrity in group IV-B and C dogs. Dorsal midline myelotomy is sometimes performed in these same patients to check for central hemorrhagic necrosis.

Aftercare. Postoperative care of dogs is similar to that described for medical treatment of dogs with thoracolumbar disc disease with one major exception: Physical therapy should be started as soon as a dog can tolerate it.

CHAPTER 76

Discospondylitis (pages 1087–1094)

Vertebral infections occur commonly in dogs but are rare in cats. Most infections involve adjacent vertebral bodies at the metaphysis and extend to the interposed disc. Various terms have been used to describe this syndrome, *discospondylitis* having gained widest acceptance in dogs.

ETIOLOGY AND PATHOGENESIS (pp. 1086–1090)

Coagulase-positive staphylococci most commonly are associated with discospondylitis. Although organisms may reach the involved disc or vertebra through foreign body migration, most infections probably originate elsewhere and spread hematogenously to the vertebrae. Potential primary sites of infection in dogs with discospondylitis include the genitourinary tract, skin, and heart. Although staphylococcal organisms have been cultured from the haircoat of affected dogs, a clear cause-and-effect relationship has not been established.

Most dogs in which staphylococci are cultured from urine also have bacteremia, suggesting that the urinary isolate could be incidental. A role for primary genitourinary tract infection is clearer in dogs with gram-negative sepsis. *Escherichia coli* is most commonly isolated. Bacterial endocarditis is another potential primary source of infection in dogs with discospondylitis. Factors that predispose dogs to discospondylitis of hematogenous origin include prior trauma, spinal surgery, and immunosuppression. Immunosuppression perhaps has the most significant role.

Clinical Findings

Discospondylitis most commonly affects large dogs. Affected males outnumber females by approximately 2:1. Certain breeds are predisposed. Any intervertebral disc space may be affected, but certain areas are predisposed. The L7–S1 disc, caudal cervical area, and midthoracic spine are affected preferentially. In addition to these sites, the thoracolumbar junction has been particularly affected in dogs at our institution. Neurological and systemic clinical signs are often noted concomitantly in dogs with discospondylitis, but either can occur separately. All signs generally progress insidiously.

DIAGNOSIS (pp. 1090–1092)

Concomitant signs of spinal cord and systemic disease should suggest a diagnosis of discospondylitis, particularly in large male dogs. The diagnosis is generally made on evaluation of survey radiographs. Collapse of the intervertebral disc is noted first, followed by bone lysis centered at the vertebral end-plates and sclerosis and spondylosis. Additional lysis can lead to marked shortening of the vertebral body and eventual instability.

In most cases, changes seen on bone scintigraphy correspond to those on survey radiographs. Leukocytosis generally is not present in dogs with discospondylitis, except when there are concomitant conditions such as vegetative endocarditis or prostatic abscesses. Biopsy is not usually performed on discospondylitis lesions because radiographic findings are generally definitive.

TREATMENT (pp. 1092–1093)

Factors in choosing a therapeutic regimen include (1) degree of neurological dysfunction, (2) results of *Brucella canis* titer and blood and urine cultures, (3) multiplicity of lesions, and (4) surgical accessibility of the lesion(s). If blood and urine cultures are negative, the causative organism is assumed to be *Staphylococcus intermedius*. β-Lactamase-resistant antibiotics such as cephradine or cloxacillin are generally effective. Dogs that fail to improve within 5 days should be reassessed.

More aggressive treatment may be required in dogs with marked neurological dysfunction. Some of these dogs have spinal cord compression that can be relieved by a hemilaminectomy or dorsal laminectomy. Lesions are curetted, and necrotic bone and disc material is removed for culture.

Considering that L7–S1 is the most common site of discospondylitis and that cauda equina involvement causes a distinct syndrome, some have chosen to discuss this entity separately. Although *B. canis* infections account for a low percentage of discospondylitis, this syndrome warrants special consideration because of its zoonotic potential and refractiveness to routine antibiotic therapy.

CHAPTER 77

Cauda Equina Syndrome
(pages 1094–1105)

Overview

ANATOMICAL FEATURES (pp. 1094–1095)

The cauda equina is a leash of nerves confined within the spinal canal of the low lumbar and sacral spine. The spinal cord terminates at L4 in large and giant breeds of dogs and at L6 in dogs less than 30 pounds. Thus, the spinal nerves in mature dogs course obliquely and caudally to exit via respective foramina. These caudally trailing nerves are referred to as the *cauda equina*. The rostral boundary of the cauda equina depends on the size of the dog. The nerves of the cauda equina include L6, L7, S1, S2, S3, and coccygeal nerves 1 through 5.

The cauda equina is enclosed within the spinal canal. Intervertebral foramina form short, restricting canals for exiting spinal nerve roots and accompanying radicular arteries and veins. Pathological disorders of the ligaments, joint capsule, osseous structures, or annular structures alter the spinal canal or foraminal diameters and result in attenuation of one or more nerve roots.

NEUROLOGICAL ASSESSMENT

Neurological signs exhibited by dogs with cauda equina attenuation are varied and may be persistent, intermittent, or progressive, depending on the cause of the disorder. All neurological signs are referable to attenuation and subsequent ischemia of trapped root(s).

Low back pain is a consistent historic feature, as is elicitation of pain by lumbosacral manipulation.

Referred pain and subsequent lameness of a rear leg (root signature) related to L6, L7, or S1 entrapment at the L6–L7 or L7–S1 spinal level is the second most common clinical sign. All these roots contribute to the sciatic nerve.

Sphincter disturbances may accompany back pain, a root signature, or paresis when the S2 and S3 roots are acutely or progressively attenuated. Urinary sphincter disturbances always precede anal sphincter disturbances in man and dogs.

Historical and clinical evaluation of tail carriage and function may assist in diagnosing cauda equina disorders.

Paresthesias and dysesthesias are manifested in dogs, predominantly with a congenital stenotic canal syndrome, as various forms of minor to major self-inflicted dermatological abrasions of the tail, perineum, genitals, or extremities.

DISC EXTRUSIONS AT L6–L7 OR L7–S1

Neurological dysfunction associated with acute extrusion of disc fragments at the L6–L7 or L7–S1 level entrapping the cauda equina occurs infrequently. Because of its infrequency, the confusing clinical picture on presentation, and difficulty in demonstrating the pathology by radiography, myelography, many go undiagnosed for prolonged periods, particularly when L7–S1 is involved.

The most frequent neurological signs are low back pain and a unilateral root signature. The onset is acute. The root signature persists

369

or is intermittent but is not induced by exercise as in congenital stenotic canal syndrome. The root signature is of sciatic origin because L7 and S1 are major contributors. Myelography often aids little in diagnosis of disc extrusion or protrusion at L6–L7 or L7–S1. Epidural myelography or combined myelography and epiduralography have been used but are often inconclusive and difficult to interpret, and they may be misleading.

Surgical treatment consists of hemilaminectomy or laminectomy with associated facetectomy providing access to the spinal canal. Decompression is achieved after removal of disc extrusion or bulging disc trapping the nerve root(s) of the cauda equina. Stabilization and fusion are not necessary.

SPONDYLOSIS (CHRONIC DEGENERATIVE DISC DISEASE; ACQUIRED STENOTIC CANAL)

Neurological dysfunction associated with spondylosis (chronic degenerative disc disease) of the L7–S1 level has been overstated with regard to degree of frequency and signs exhibited.

Spondylosis is nothing more than chronic degenerative disc disease. Despite these bony changes, there may be relatively little distortion or bulging of the disc into the spinal canal. In some instances, these degenerative changes reduce the canal diameter (acquired stenosis) and encroach on the cauda equina. If the canal is congenitally small, less protrusion is required to create neurological dysfunction.

Clinical and radiographic signs of spondylosis are most frequently observed in aging large dogs, although small dogs are also afflicted. Spondylosis of L7–S1 is frequently encountered radiographically, but only *rarely* are clinical signs present. Low back pain is the most common clinical sign and is often unassociated with leg, bladder, anal, or tail signs. Most dogs with spondylosis and pain alone respond to nonsteroidal analgesics.

When spondylosis is unresponsive to analgesics or in the event of progressive neurological dysfunction, more aggressive pursuit is justified. Neurological disturbances may consist of a root signature, progressive sciatic weakness, sphincter disturbances, or tail weakness. Radiographic evaluation demonstrates various degrees of spondylosis of L7–S1. It is important that a strong correlation of neurological and neuroradiographic features exists. Contrast studies to consider are myelography, epiduralography, or venography. Whether using myelography or combined myelography/epiduralography, stress films may help.

Although contrast studies must be used, numerous lesions will remain poorly defined. In such instances, surgical intervention is performed without objective confirmation. Depending on the neurological signs and unilateral or bilateral involvement, laminectomy or hemilaminectomy with facetectomy is performed.

LUMBOSACRAL STENOSIS (CONGENITAL SPINAL CANAL STENOSIS)

Congenital stenosis may be subdivided into the type that normally exists in achondroplastic breeds and the idiopathic type. This section discusses the pathophysiology of the stenotic canal as it relates to the nonachondroplastic breeds.

Congenital stenosis is characterized by shortening of the pedicles (lateral bony wall of canal), resulting in a decreased spinal canal diameter, thickened and sclerotic lamina and articular processes, hypertrophy and infolding of the ligamentum flavum, and sclerotic and bulbous articular facets that encroach on the dorsolateral aspect of the spinal canal. The most frequent sites in dogs are L6–L7 and L7–S1, analogous to man. Although viewed as congenital stenosis, clinical signs do not appear until middle to old age in dogs, as in man.

The neurological signs may be low back pain, exercised-induced lameness, sphincter dysfunction, self-inflicted dermatological abrasions, or severe self-mutilation of the tail, perineum, genitals, or extremities. Spinal stenosis causes not only progressive mechanical compression of the cauda equina but also vascular phenomena. Often referred to as *neurogenic intermittent claudication,* this aspect of the disease pertains to the physiological changes of the radicular arteries as they pass through stenosed intervertebral foramina and into the stenosed canal. Vessels of the cauda equina dilate greatly with exercise to provide metabolic requirements. Because of the stenotic canal, restrictions of blood flow result in root ischemia, which causes radicular pain and referred pain to the back, extremities, tail, and perineum.

The posture of an afflicted dog is noteworthy because the back is consistently flexed. The flexion is often increased with the onset of signs, which are enhanced by increased activity. With aging, intermittent back pain, neurogenic intermittent claudication, intermittent stranguria, or intermittent paresthesias intensify and become persistent.

The radiographic features are multiple and varied in intensity. Limitations exist in clearly demonstrating lesions by contrast studies. Lesions are not recognized on ventrodorsal projections. Lateral films show a narrowed canal diameter, bulbous facets, and in some instances an increased angulation (hyperflexion) of L7–S1.

Laminectomy and unilateral or bilateral facetectomy are performed. The ligamentum flavum is seen as a dorsal strap over the dural tube and ventrally and laterally positioned roots. Resection of this ligament further decompresses the cauda equina. Despite aggressive multilevel laminectomies and facetectomies, instability, deformity, and laminectomy scar have not been complicating features. Stabilization has not been used. Free fat grafts are routinely positioned over the laminectomy defect.

L7–S1 Fixation-Fusion for Cauda Equina Compression—An Alternative View*
(pages 1105–1110)

Cauda equina syndrome is impingement of the terminal nerve roots within the spinal canal. L7–S1 fixation fusion restores full function and prevents progression of the degenerative process by an early, easy, and effective surgery. It specifically treats redundant dorsal annulus fibrosus of the L7–S1 disc. The technique stretches the redundant annulus to relieve cauda equina compression, fix the vertebrae in the stretched position, and allow bone healing to fuse the vertebrae in that position.

BIOMECHANICS

When the L7–S1 disc space begins to degenerate, the distance between the end-plates of L7 and S1 diminishes, and the dorsal annulus becomes redundant and impinges on the cauda equina. It is at this stage of degeneration that L7–S1 fixation-fusion is most effective. If the degenerative process progresses to herniation of the L7–S1 nucleus

---

*Editor's note: An alternative to laminectomy is presented here.

pulposus, decompression by laminectomy and articular process removal is necessary.

PHYSICAL EXAMINATION

A patient with lower lumbar or hip pain tries to escape the extended position of the hips and lordosis of the lower lumbar spine. In cauda equina impingement, deep spinal palpation of the L7–S1 region produces pain, as indicated by yelping or aggression. Rectal palpation of the L7–S1 nerve roots is also painful in cauda equina impingement.

RADIOGRAPHIC EXAMINATION
INDICATIONS AND CONTRAINDICATIONS

L7–S1 fixation fusion is indicated for L7–S1 pain that arises from lordosis of the L7–S1 region.

SURGICAL TECHNIQUE

A foam pad is placed under the lower lumbar spine to raise the pelvis and flex the lower spine. The interarcuate space between L7 and S1 is collapsed in dogs with cauda equina. This space is reopened by surgical positioning. A vertebral spreader can assist expansion of the interarcuate space. The interarcuate space is expanded until the articular cartilage of the facets match. A cortical screw of the appropriate length is placed through a hole drilled through each caudal articular facet into the sacrum. A corticocancellous bone graft is taken from both wings of the ilium through the original skin incision. The bone graft is placed completely over the laminae from the seventh lumbar vertebra to the sacrum.

RESULTS

Once the motion at the L7 region is stabilized, the irritation to the cauda equina is rapidly reduced. Permanent fusion occurs 2 to 4 months after surgery. Because patients respond so fast to the surgery, it is recommended that they be strictly confined during the first 2 months. Patients with neurological deficits showed a return to function in 4 to 6 months.

CONCLUSIONS

CHAPTER 78
Spinal Fractures and Luxations (pages 1110–1121)

ANATOMY

Stability of the spine is due to osseous and soft-tissue components that form dorsal and ventral compartments. The dorsal compartment consists of the vertebral arch (lamina and pedicles), articular facet, joint capsule, dorsal spinous process, interspinous ligament, supraspinous ligament, and ligamentum flavum. The ventral compartment consists of the vertebral body, intervertebral disc (nucleus pulposus and annulus fibrosus), and dorsal and ventral longitudinal ligaments. Additional stability is provided to both compartments by the paraspinal musculature.

PATHOGENESIS

Pathological luxations generally occur when hereditary or congenital ligamentous instability results in a significant decrease in spinal support. The most notable example is atlantoaxial instability (see Chapter 73). Pathological fractures generally occur when the integrity of bone is compromised owing to an underlying disease process.

Traumatic fracture/luxations are induced by forces resulting in severe hyperextension, hyperflexion, compression, or rotation. They often occur at or near the junction of a movable and immovable vertebral segment.

BIOMECHANICS OF SPINAL FRACTURE/LUXATION

An understanding of the biomechanics of spinal fractures and luxations is helpful in predicting the inherent stability or instability of a traumatic fracture/luxation.

Hyperextension

Hyperextension injury results from a direct blow to the dorsal aspect of the spine. Collapse of the dorsal compartment, particularly the articular facets, generally occurs.

Hyperflexion

Pure hyperflexion injury results in wedge compression fracture of the vertebral body, often sparing the dorsal compartment.

Compression

Bursting compression fracture of the vertebral body occurs with axial load forces.

Rotation

Rotational forces seldom occur alone. Injuries resulting from rotation and flexion can be quite severe, causing disruption of the dorsal and ventral compartments.

DIAGNOSIS (pp. 1112–1113)

History and physical findings are important in diagnosis of spinal fracture/luxation and may also be helpful in classifying the type. Careful palpation of the spine may reveal the type of injury sustained. A thorough neurological examination should be performed on any patient suspected of having a spinal fracture/luxation. The presence or absence of deep pain perception has an important impact on further treatment.

Plain and contrast radiography may be required to accurately diagnose spinal fractures and luxations. Plain radiographs may be taken on awake or anesthetized patients. In any case, a complete spinal series of radiographs should be taken because 20 per cent of patients with traumatic spinal injury have spinal fracture/luxations at two locations (see Chapter 70.)

TREATMENT (pp. 1113–1114)

When considering treatment options for a patient with a spinal fracture/luxation, several factors are considered: (1) results of the neurological examination, (2) whether the fracture is pathological or traumatic, and (3) whether the fracture is stable or unstable.

If a patient has lost sensory and motor function caudal to the lesion, the prognosis is unfavorable and treatment is generally supportive. Patients with pathological fractures have an underlying disorder (localized or generalized). The cause of the underlying disorder must be determined and therapy instituted before spinal fracture/luxation repair. Physical examination findings as well as radiographic assessment of the fracture/luxation may be helpful in determining its inherent stability. If surgery is necessary, it is important to select a stabilization technique that will not further destabilize the spine.

Generally, stable fractures in patients with strong voluntary motor movements are successfully managed by conservative means, including the use of anti-inflammatory agents, body splints, and strict cage confinement. If the fracture/luxation is unstable; if the patient is non-ambulatory, paraparetic, or tetraparetic, with no voluntary motor movements; or if conservative therapy is unsuccessful, surgical management is indicated.

SURGICAL TECHNIQUES (pp. 1114–1120)

The two objectives of any surgical technique used to repair spinal fracture/luxation are decompression and stabilization.

Fractures of the Cervical Spine

Cervical spinal fractures are uncommon. Most fractures involve C2 (axis), particularly the dens or body. Fractures of the dorsal spine of the axis are approached dorsally and stabilized with orthopedic wire, monofilament or braided nonabsorbable suture material, or polymethyl methacrylate to re-establish the continuity of displaced fragments. A decompressive hemilaminectomy can be performed if fragments of bone are present in the spinal canal or if a displaced body fracture cannot be reduced.

C1–C2 body fractures/luxations, traumatic cervical disc extrusions, and atlantoaxial instability can be approached ventrally. Steinmann pins and polymethyl methacrylate should be considered for cervical spinal fractures involving the vertebral bodies of C2–C7.

Fractures and luxations rarely occur from C3 to C7. A predisposition to luxations at C5–C6 may exist. Fracture/luxations of C3–C7 may be approached dorsally or ventrally.

Fractures of the Thoracolumbar and Lumbar Spine

The thoracolumbar and lumbar spine are relatively common locations for spinal fractures in dogs and cats.

Technique Selection

The technique chosen is dictated by the location of the fracture; the size, age, and disposition of the patient; equipment available; and experience of the surgeon.

Techniques

Dorsal spinous process plating requires exposure of the dorsal spinous processes and articular facets (see Chapter 72). Metal or plastic plates are available for dorsal spinous process plating.

The advantage of dorsal spinous process plating is preserving the inherent stability provided by the articular facets and the supraspinous and interspinous ligaments.

The major limiting factors of dorsal spinous process plating are the age and size of the patient. The most common postoperative complications are fracture of the spinous processes and plate slippage.

Spinal stapling also requires exposure of the dorsal spinous processes and facet joints (see Chapter 72). An intramedullary pin is placed through a dorsal spinous process, bent 90°, laid along the lamina between the base of the spinous processes and articular processes, and secured to the base of the dorsal spinous processes with orthopedic wire. This technique is reserved for patients less than 10 kg.

Vertebral body plating (dorsal body plating) requires dorsolateral exposure of the articular facet, vertebral body, and transverse process of the lumbar vertebrae or the articular facet, vertebral body, and rib head of the thoracic vertebrae. The spinal nerve and vessels at the involved space must be severed.

Steinmann pins and polymethyl methacrylate require exposure of the dorsal spinous processes, articular facets, and transverse processes bilaterally (see Chapter 72). Two Steinmann pins are placed into the vertebral bodies on each side of the fracture/luxation. Steinmann pins are driven so they exit 2 to 3 mm from the ventral aspect of the vertebral body, are cut leaving 1.5 to 2 cm exposed dorsally, and notched with a pin cutter. The polymethyl methacrylate forms around the notched pin and helps prevent pin migration. If a laminectomy is not performed, polymethyl methacrylate is simply applied as a circular mass, incorporating the Steinmann pins as well as the articular facets and adjacent dorsal spinous processes. If a laminectomy is performed, the exposed spinal cord is covered with an autogenous fat graft, and the polymethyl methacrylate is molded into the shape of a doughnut.

In some instances (generally thoracolumbar fractures or luxations in large, hyperactive dogs), a combination of the previously described techniques should be considered.

Fractures of L6, L7, and S1

Fractures and luxations of the caudal lumbar and sacral vertebrae are relatively common because of the static-kinetic relationship of the sacral and lumbar segments.

Because of the increased shearing forces present in the lumbosacral region, caudal lumbar and lumbosacral fracture/luxations are difficult to stabilize. Techniques successfully used to treat L7–S1 fracture/luxations include transilial pinning; transilial pinning with Lubra plate support, pins, and polymethyl methacrylate; transilial pinning with external skeletal fixation; and spinal stapling.

Techniques
Sacral and Sacrococcygeal Fractures

S2–S3 sensory examination and evaluation of anal and bladder function are considered when performing a neurological examination on patients with sacral and sacrococcygeal fracture/luxations.

A dorsal approach to the sacroiliac junction can be used to expose fractures of the sacral wing (see Chapter 72). Once reduced, the fracture can be stabilized with a lag screw inserted through the ilium and sacral fragment and into the sacral body. A parallel Kirschner pin is inserted to provide rotational stability.

Coccygeal Fractures
POSTOPERATIVE TREATMENT (p. 1120)

CHAPTER 79

Intracranial Surgery (pages 1122–1135)

INDICATIONS (pp. 1122–1124)
Craniocerebral Trauma

Indications for craniotomy include evacuation of hematomas (epidural, subdural), hemostasis, decompression of skull fractures, removal of foreign bodies, and decompression for uncontrolled progressive cerebral edema. Subdural hemorrhage is rare in small animals. Epidural hemorrhage, caused by meningeal arterial laceration, occurs with all skull fractures.

Uncontrolled cerebral edema is progressive cerebral edema unresponsive to repeated therapy for the edema or the underlying cause. Depressed skull fragments lacerate underlying parenchyma and precipitate elevated intracranial pressure.

Intracranial Masses

Intracranial masses include tumors (primary, metastatic), vascular malformations (hamartoma, arteriovenous shunt, aneurysm), epidermoid inclusion bodies, abscess, and granuloma. The more common brain tumors of dogs are meningiomas, gliomas (oligodendroglioma, astrocytoma), and undifferentiated sarcomas. Meningiomas are the most common brain tumors in cats. Metastatic brain tumors are uncommon.

Hydrocephalus

Unfortunately, hydrocephalus in small animals is infrequently diagnosed at the time when shunting could provide the maximum benefit.

Olfactory Tractotomy
DIAGNOSTIC METHODS (pp. 1124–1126)
Minimum Data Base

A thorough history, physical examination, neurological examination, analyses of blood and urine, and electrocardiography are components of the presurgical data base.

Electrodiagnostics

An electroencephalogram (EEG) can be helpful in diagnosing certain intracranial diseases such as hydrocephalus and focal lesions but is relied on less frequently in an age of advanced imaging techniques.

Brain mapping is being used extensively in human neurology and neurosurgery and is beginning to be used in animals. The brain-stem auditory evoked response (auditory brain-stem response) test has been used to diagnose brain-stem diseases.

Cerebrospinal Fluid Tap/Analyses

Results of complete cerebrospinal fluid (CSF) analyses* have been cited as the most productive diagnostic test in dogs with intracranial neoplasia, apart from advanced imaging.

Radiography

Skull radiographs contribute infrequently or provide redundant supportive data in the diagnosis of intracranial disease.

Advanced Imaging Techniques

Nucleotide brain imaging can be used to identify focal intracranial masses but does not differentiate between inflammatory and neoplastic processes. MRI produces the clearest image of the brain parenchyma, but bone is poorly defined. Ultrasonography is useful in the operating room to locate a subcortical lesion.

PREOPERATIVE CONSIDERATIONS (pp. 1126–1128)

The Patient

The most basic principle to consider is the Monro-Kellie doctrine: The contents of the cranial vault are blood, CSF, and parenchyma; an increase in any component results in a net decrease of the other two. How any pre-existing condition, the type of anesthesia, surgical manipulations, location of the surgery, fluid therapy, and any medications may influence the principles of the Monro-Kellie doctrine is paramount in the operative management of patients.

Medications

The debate continues about the need for prophylactic antibiotics as a routine protocol in intracranial surgery, as well as the efficacy and the type of antibiotic. The use of corticosteroids in head trauma is controversial; they are almost always included in the preoperative regimen for craniotomy.

Diuretics are often used for craniotomy. Fluid therapy is essential during anesthesia but should be reduced to two-thirds maintenance after surgery. Anticonvulsant therapy is instituted or continued after craniotomy.

General Health of the Animal

Anesthesia (see Chapter 168)

Instrumentation

Components of a general surgery pack, an assortment of rongeurs (Lempert, Ruskin, Kerrison, and others), Derf needle holders, micro-curettes, and self-retaining (Weit-laner, Gelpi) and hand-held retractors (Army-Navy, Senn) are included in the basic neurosurgery pack. Many

---

*CSF pressure recording, cell count, cytological evaluation, total protein determination, CSF protein electrophoresis.

specialty instruments are available. Optical loupes are sufficient for most procedures; however, as the field of veterinary neurosurgery advances, use of the operating microscope will become more common.

SURGICAL PROCEDURES (pp. 1128–1132)

Patient Positioning

Most craniotomies are performed with the animal in sternal recumbency. The head is supported in a custom-made or commercially available head stand. The cavernous sinus can be approached with the animal in lateral recumbency. Dorsal recumbency is also used for a ventral aboral craniectomy.

Monitoring

Routine anesthetic monitoring, including heart and respiratory rates and rhythms, can help determine the depth of anesthesia. Because of the direct correlation between carbon dioxide pressure and cerebral blood flow, arterial blood gas or end-expiratory carbon dioxide analyses are helpful.

The importance of understanding, assessing, and controlling intracranial pressure dynamics cannot be overemphasized; monitoring intracranial pressure during the craniotomy is perhaps the best method of monitoring patients.

Surgical Approaches to the Brain (pp. 1129–1132)

Rostrotentorial (Lateral) Craniotomy

Extended Rostrotentorial Craniotomy

Bilateral Rostrotentorial Craniotomy

Transfrontal Craniotomy

Caudotentorial (Suboccipital) Craniectomy

Ventral Craniectomy

INTRACRANIAL SURGICAL TECHNIQUES (pp. 1132–1133)

Tissue Handling

High-speed surgical drills and craniotomes create heat, which should be dissipated by frequent or constant lavage with lactated Ringer's solution or saline. Surgical sponges contain lint and should not be used in handling brain parenchyma. Surgical gloves should be free of talc. Incisions through the brain parenchyma are made through the less vascular gyri and not the sulci. Dissection is performed slowly; retraction requires a wide-blade spatula.

Tumor Resection

When attempting removal of a mass, the capsule should remain intact whenever possible. The vasculature is identified and ligated, and surrounding brain tissue thought to be involved in a neoplastic process is removed by gentle suction.

Surgical Treatment of Hydrocephalus

Ventriculoatrial and ventriculoperitoneal shunts have been placed in dogs. The advantages of the ventriculoperitoneal shunt make it the preferred method.

Closure

Closure begins with replacement of the dural flap. The bone flap is replaced with wire sutures or large monofilament suture placed through the preplaced holes in the skull and flap. Cranioplasty is seldom necessary in dogs because of the thick temporal muscle covering.

COMPLICATIONS (pp. 1133–1134)

Increased intracranial pressure during surgery and postoperatively is the most common and consequential complication of craniotomies. Poor anesthetic management can precipitate many factors that contribute to increased intracranial pressure.

Seizures are a common sequel to postoperative craniotomy, resulting from formation of scar tissue or from cerebral vasospasm, which occurs in association with the presence of subarachnoid hemorrhage.

Infection can be devastating. Prophylactic antibiotic regimens are frequently used. Cefazolin sodium (20 mg/kg IV and IM preoperatively and every 6 hours thereafter for 36 hours) has been effective.

POSTOPERATIVE CARE (p. 1134)

Postoperative Monitoring

Twenty-four-hour daily monitoring should be available for at least the first 3 to 5 days after surgery for craniotomy patients.

Fluid Therapy and Alimentation

Intravenous fluids are often given but should not exceed two-thirds the normal daily maintenance (approximately 40 ml/kg). Higher amounts may contribute to development or exacerbation of cerebral edema. Animals without difficulty in eating should be provided up to twice the normal caloric requirements during the first 1 to 2 weeks of the recovery.

Nursing Care and Rehabilitation

The surgical site is dressed with sterile nonadhesive pads and gauze wrapping, then covered with orthopedic stockinette with ear holes pulled over the head. Whenever possible, animals should have supervised outside excursions at least twice daily, and visits from owners are usually encouraged.

CHAPTER 80

Peripheral Nerve Surgery

(pages 1135–1141)

MORPHOLOGY AND PATHOPHYSIOLOGY

Axons, the basic units of peripheral nerves, are extensions of nerve cell bodies in or near the spinal cord. The endoneurium is the loose interstitial tissue that surrounds and separates the axon and Schwann cell units. The next connective tissue layer is the perineurium, a tough fibrous sleeve that encases bundles of nerve fibers. The perineurium is very important as a diffusion barrier to keep out foreign substances while maintaining an internal environment similar to that of the central nervous system. The entire nerve is surrounded by epineurium. Collagen, which provides strength to a repaired nerve, is produced by fibroblasts in the epineurium.

When a nerve is traumatized, any disruption of the endoneurium permits the regenerating axons to grow into unorganized fibrous tissue. As the axons grow in a disorderly fashion, a nodular enlargement, or neuroma, is formed. The degree of continuity of the endoneurium, perineurium, and epineurium relates directly to the regenerative ability of the nerve. Neurapraxia is the mildest degree of trauma, representing only a transient interruption in function. No degenerative changes occur, and full return of function can be expected. With axonotmesis, the next degree of nerve injury, some axons are disrupted, but the endoneurial tubules and connective tissue elements remain intact. Regrowth of axons is spontaneous, but the time until return of function depends on the extent of injury and the distance from denervated endorgans.

Neurotmesis, the most severe injury, is severance and complete separation of all nerve structures with a gap between the severed nerve ends (e.g., with laceration). Separation and malalignment of the nerve ends eliminate spontaneous recovery.

FACTORS INFLUENCING HEALING AND REGENERATION

The wounding mechanism determines the extent of nerve disruption and also may dictate treatment. Regeneration of the end-organ and ultimate functional return are decreased by excessive delays in reinnervation.

Young patients exhibit a much more rapid and complete regeneration of traumatized nerves than do older patients. One of the most important factors in the final result is the technique of the surgeon. Inflammation and fibroplasia, both deterrents to axon regeneration, result directly from improper surgical techniques. Because regrowth of axons starts soon after the initial injury, early primary surgical repair eliminates delay in reinnervation that otherwise might prevent early and rapid regrowth of axons.

GENERAL CONSIDERATIONS

Because both nerve segments usually retract after complete laceration, the ends may be separated by several centimeters. Thus, it is important that the initial skin incision be of adequate length and extend an equal distance proximally and distally from the injury site.

If surgical exploration is delayed, the nerve ends may be embedded in scar tissue or adherent to other structures. In nearly all cases, débridement of the nerve ends is needed before surgical anastomosis. The nerve ends must be trimmed evenly to permit flush contact when sutured. Each transection must be perpendicular to the long axis of the nerve for optimal identification of the fascicular pattern and so that the débrided ends make contact.

Surgical exposure of the nerve can be accomplished with standard instruments, but to manipulate and suture nerves appropriately one needs microsurgical scissors, microneedle holder, fine-tipped jeweler's forceps, and tissue forceps with microfine teeth (0.12 mm). Magnification is needed for adequate observation of nerve structures.

BASIC PRINCIPLES OF NERVE REPAIRS

Many methods for suturing or repairing traumatized peripheral nerves have been described, but no single technique is superior. The neurorrhaphy is completed as soon as possible after the injury.

During débridement of nerve ends, bleeding denotes an adequate blood supply. Blood clots and hematomas promote detrimental scar formation at the surgical site.

Failure to match the fascicles in the two segments prevents regenerating axons from reaching their appropriate end-organs. Both longitudinal and circumferential tension at the repair site stimulate detrimental scar formation.

The suture material for nerve repair should be nonreactive so that it will not incite foreign body scar formation. The smallest number of the smallest practical size sutures is used for neurorrhaphy.

EPINEURIAL NERVE REPAIR

A majority of nerve injuries are suitable for epineurial suture techniques, especially those in which loss of nerve tissue is minimal. The injured nerve is exposed surgically, and necessary débridement is performed.

Precise anatomical detail of the nerve ends should be kept in mind during the repair procedure. Matching longitudinal blood vessels in the epineurium helps ensure rotational alignment. No portion of the nerve except the epineurium is grasped with forceps. Rarely are more than six or seven sutures required in an epineurial neurorrhaphy without tension, and four or five sutures usually are adequate.

PERINEURIAL (FASCICULAR) NERVE REPAIR (p. 1139)

Perineurial, or fascicular, nerve repairs require greater magnification and are more tedious to perform than epineurial neurorrhaphies. I do not use or recommend this technique when the injured nerve contains many small fascicles, and rarely is it indicated in companion animals.

NERVE GRAFTS

Management of traumatized nerves in which nerve tissue has been lost is a difficult clinical problem. Nerve tissue may be lost as a result of the original trauma or from débridement required to eliminate fibrotic areas. Nerve grafting involves interposing an avascular segment that loses all endoneurial elements and requires two separate neurorrhaphies for regenerating axons to cross.

Free autogenous donor nerve segments are used for the grafts. Numerous small nerve segments are used for grafts because the smaller diameter across which vascular ingrowth must occur allows circulation to be restored more quickly to the entire graft. Optimal graft survival requires a healthy vascular wound bed without excessive scar tissue. I prefer the caudal cutaneous sural nerve as the donor nerve for autogenous grafts. The sural is a branch of the tibial nerve and extends from the popliteal region distally beyond the calcaneus. Suturing nerve grafts is similar in technique to perineurial fascicular repairs. It is essential that all suture lines be without tension.

POSTOPERATIVE CONSIDERATIONS (p. 1141)

The severity of the original injury and the type of neurorrhaphy performed dictate the amount of postoperative limb protection and immobilization.

It is imperative to protect insensitive or anesthetized portions of the limb during reinnervation to prevent self-mutilation. Functional recovery of the limb can be enhanced by strict adherence to conscientious general nursing and wound care principles.

PROGNOSIS

It is impossible to provide the owner of a dog or cat with an accurate prognosis for the degree of functional recovery after repair of a traumatized nerve.

Eye and Adnexa

CHAPTER 81

Principles of Ophthalmic Surgery (pages 1142–1156)

Meticulous attention to detail is essential to success in ophthalmic surgery. Failure to attend to seemingly minute pharmacological pre-operative, procedural, or postoperative details may cause unnecessary complications with intraocular or corneal surgery.

ANESTHESIA

PREOPERATIVE PREPARATION

Pharmacological Preparation

Anti-inflammatory Agents

The canine eye rapidly becomes inflamed during or after ocular surgical procedures. Corticosteroids are frequently used both systemically and topically to reduce miosis and postoperative inflammation.

Complications with steroids include slower wound healing and decreased resistance to bacterial and fungal infections. To reduce these complications, use of preoperative antibiotics and disinfecting solutions to reduce conjunctival bacterial numbers is recommended. Topical corticosteroids reduce serum cortisol and suppress adrenocorticotropic hormone response. Long-term use in healthy dogs produces few effects.

Prophylactic antibiotics are bactericidal and are changed regularly during the preoperative and postoperative periods.

Prostaglandins are important mediators of ocular inflammation, including protein release during intraocular surgery. Inhibitors of prostaglandin synthetase reduce vascular permeability when administered preoperatively. In dogs, acetylsalicylic acid (30 mEq/kg PO every 8 hours for 40 hours before surgery) reduces aqueous protein concentrations. Topical indomethacin (1 per cent) and flurbiprofen are particularly useful preoperatively to reduce protein release during surgery. Flunixin meglumine (0.5 mg/kg) is used systemically as a preoperative prostaglandin inhibitor and analgesic.

Osmotic Agents

Mannitol is widely used to reduce loss of vitreous during intraocular surgery. Potential interaction between mannitol and methoxyflurane resulting in pulmonary edema was not reproducible experimentally.

Antibacterials

Preoperative preparation for several days with a broad-spectrum bactericidal antibiotic and povidone-iodine solution (diluted 1:25 with saline) immediately before surgery during preparation is advised.

The periocular area is carefully clipped and cilia on the upper lid are removed.

1. Gross contamination is removed with gauze sponges soaked in sterile saline.

2. The periocular area is scrubbed with povidone-iodine solution diluted with saline.

3. The corneal and conjunctival surfaces are irrigated with balanced salt solution or saline, and a drop of broad-spectrum antibiotic solution may be instilled.

4. A final preparation of ethyl alcohol followed by povidone-iodine solution may be used.

Draping

Three field drapes are placed around the eye and fastened with small towel clamps. A fenestrated drape with a 3-cm eccentrically placed hole or an adhesive drape may be used. Full aseptic precautions are used for intraocular surgery. Starch powder is removed from surgical gloves with sterile saline.

SURGICAL EQUIPMENT AND SUPPLIES (pp. 1144–1148)

Illumination and Magnification

Ophthalmic surgery is performed in a semidarkened room with a focal light. For adnexal surgery, a standard operating light is suitable, but for finer procedures, a focal or head-mounted light source is desirable.

Surgical procedures involving cilia, lacrimal puncta, or globe usually require magnification. A loupe as used in ocular examination (2.5 to 4.0 ×), and a focal length of 20 to 30 cm is recommended. For more intricate procedures, an operating microscope is essential.

Hemostasis

Methods of hemostasis used in ophthalmic surgery include pressure with a cotton-tipped applicator; ligation of vessels, especially in lid and orbital surgery; electrocautery; electrohemostasis; and the use of 1:10,000 epinephrine solution. Electrocautery may be applied by small hand-held disposable battery-powered units. Electrohemostasis units are not to be used for epilation.

Cryotherapy

Cryotherapy is used for selective destruction of neoplasms, removal of luxated lenses, treatment of distichiasis and trichiasis (microcryoepilation), and destruction of parts of the ciliary body in control of glaucoma. Microcryoepilation and cyclocryotherapy are major advances in veterinary ophthalmic surgery. General cryosurgical equipment may be used for periocular tumors, but for small lesions or for use on the globe, ophthalmic cryosurgical units are necessary.

Suture Materials and Needles

The principles of selection of ophthalmic suture material are:

1. The suture should be as fine as possible.
2. Suture materials that touch the cornea are soft and pliable.
3. Chromic gut is not used in the cornea. For buried sutures, in subcutaneous sites, and in the cornea, polyglycolic acid (Dexon), po-

lyglactin 910 (Vicryl), modified polyglycolic acid (Maxon), and polydioxanone (PDS) sutures have many advantages.

4. Absorbable materials should be used with caution as the sole
suture in a major corneal or scleral wound when nonabsorbable materials are available.

Fine, nonirritant suture materials limit postoperative inflammation.

Surgical Needles

For corneal suturing, a micropoint spatula GS-9 (Ethicon) or cutting
micropoint G-1 needle is recommended. For eyelids and the third
eyelid, a cutting PS-2 needle is recommended.

Scalpel Blades

Three systems are commonly used:

1. Beaver handle with number 64 or 65 blade.
2. Standard number 3 handle with number 11 and 15 blades.
3. Special-purpose blades. These have generally replaced the broken edge of razor blades once used.

CARE AND STERILIZATION OF OPHTHALMIC
INSTRUMENTS (p. 1149)

PREVENTION OF SELF-TRAUMA (pp. 1149–1150)

Prevention of self-trauma is important, especially when a cycle of
scratching has been established. Various methods are available.

1. An Elizabethan collar is recommended for all external
ophthalmic surgical procedures.
2. Bandaging dewclaws.
3. Bandaging the eye.
4. Appropriate cycloplegics for ciliary spasm. Topical anesthetics
are not used.
5. Tranquilization in severe cases.
6. Postoperative analgesia (e.g., butorphanol).

EXPOSURE AND FIXATION OF THE GLOBE

Exposure and control of the globe are prerequisites for successful
ophthalmic surgery. The eye deviates in an inferomedial direction
under general anesthesia (reversed Bell phenomenon) in animals. The
third eyelid also restricts exposure.

Exposure

For short procedures, a lid speculum is useful. For major procedures,
the Castroviejo and Maumenee-Park speculae are recommended.

Canthotomy

A lateral canthotomy greatly improves exposure of the eye. The lateral
canthus is incised with straight Mayo scissors up to but not including
the orbital ligament. The area should *not* be crushed with hemostats.
After the ophthalmic procedure is completed, the incision is closed in
two layers. The first layer of simple interrupted sutures of 6-0 polyglactin 910 or polyglycolic acid apposes the conjunctiva underlying
the incision. The second layer of simple interrupted sutures of 4-0 or

6-0 silk or nylon closes the skin. In the second layer, the first suture is placed at the junction of the upper and lower lids and emerges from the lid margin in the same way as the suture used to close a lid laceration.

Fixation

Scleral Fixation Sutures

Scleral fixation sutures are invaluable but must be placed partially through the sclera. A suture of 3-0 or 4-0 silk with a swaged cutting needle is placed 1 to 2 mm from the limbus and is tagged lightly with either a small hemostat or serrefines. Subconjunctival hemorrhage is frequent with scleral fixation sutures.

OPHTHALMIC SURGICAL INSTRUMENTS (p. 1156)

CHAPTER 82
Eyelids (pages 1157–1177)

ANATOMY (p. 1157)

The eyelids are thin, mobile folds of skin that normally cover the eyes. In cross section, the lids are composed of the external epidermal surface, the orbicular muscle, the tarsal plate, the tarsal glands, and the palpebral conjunctiva. Openings of the tarsal glands (20 to 40 per lid) can be seen on the surface of the lid margins. Tarsal glands secrete a phospholipid-rich sebaceous material that forms the superficial lipid layer of the tear film. The tarsal plate is a poorly defined fibrous sheet that supports the lids and is continuous with the orbital septum, which is attached to the orbital periosteum. The cilia in dogs are found on the outer surface of the upper lid margin. Dogs have no cilia on the lower lid, and cats have no cilia at all.

Muscles of the Eyelids

The orbicular muscle lies anterior to the tarsal plate and encircles the palpebral fissure. It is innervated by the palpebral nerve, a branch of the facial nerve (cranial nerve VII) and functions as a sphincter to close the lids. The superior palpebral levator is innervated by the oculomotor nerve (cranial nerve III).

DIFFERENTIAL DIAGNOSIS OF EYELID DISEASE (p. 1157)

CONGENITAL ABNORMALITIES OF THE EYELIDS REQUIRING SURGICAL CORRECTION (pp. 1157–1160)

Ophthalmia Neonatorum

The lids in newborn puppies normally separate at 10 to 15 days. In some puppies but rarely in other species, an acute purulent conjunctivitis occurs before lid separation. The lids are swollen, and a purulent exudate is observed from the medial canthus or nares. It is imperative to open the lids surgically as soon as possible to prevent corneal damage.

Colobomas

A coloboma, or agenesis of the eyelid, is a defect in the lid margin. In cats, the defect usually involves the lateral portion of the upper lid and can result in entropion, trichiasis, blepharospasm, or secondary keratitis. Surgical correction of the defect using a horizontal pedicle graft is usually required if the lesion is causing clinical signs.

Narrow Palpebral Fissure

A narrow palpebral fissure is congenital in the chow chow, Kerry blue terrier, collie, Shetland sheepdog, and bull terrier. If the condition is associated with concomitant microphthalmia, surgical correction may not be necessary. In a dog with a normal-sized globe, this condition may result in entropion (inversion of the lid margins). Enlargement of the palpebral fissure by performing a canthotomy and canthoplasty usually corrects the entropion.

Large Palpebral Fissure (Macropalpebral Fissure)

Too large a palpebral fissure, in the presence of a normal-sized globe, can result in ectropion (eversion of the lid margins). Although the condition rarely causes ocular disease, certain breeds, such as the English bulldog, spaniel, and hounds, may require shortening of the fissure. The procedure may also be indicated in cases of phthisis bulbi or endophthalmos secondary to loss of orbital fat.

The procedure performed to shorten the palpebral fissure is a permanent tarsorrhaphy. The amount of tissue to be removed varies with each individual. Between one-quarter and one-third of the margins can usually be closed without causing an unacceptable cosmetic appearance. In performing a medial tarsorrhaphy, care must be taken not to remove or occlude the puncta of the nasolacrimal system.

CONGENITAL AND ACQUIRED EYELID DISEASES
(pp. 1160–1168)

Entropion

Entropion is an inversion of the eyelid margin in which the eyelashes rub the cornea. This condition often results in a superficial irritation of the conjunctiva and cornea. Chronic ocular discharge and blepharospasm are commonly seen. If not surgically treated, the condition can lead to vascularization, pigmentation, and possible ulceration of the cornea. Three commonly accepted etiologies are congenital, spastic, and acquired.

Congenital Entropion

Congenital entropion is usually a bilateral condition that is commonly noted in dogs. The lower lateral lid is most frequently affected, followed by the upper lid and, infrequently, the medial lower lid. The chow chow, bloodhound, Labrador retriever, English bulldog, Doberman pinscher, Chesapeake Bay retriever, Saint Bernard, rottweiler, poodle, Irish setter, and Sharpei are predisposed to entropion.

Surgical correction is satisfactory in most cases. It is wise to postpone entropion correction until the dog is 4 to 6 months of age and its facial features have matured. Sharpei puppies as young as 3 weeks of age often may require surgical intervention to prevent severe corneal disease. The preferred method is "lid tacking." Permanent correction of entropion is often necessary at a later date.

Surgical Correction

The technique that provides the most consistent result is a modified Holtz-Celsus procedure involving excision of a half-moon-shaped flap of skin 2 to 3 mm from the lid margin. The skin excision is 3 to 4 mm wider than the affected area of lid.

Immediately after surgery, the lids should be in a normal position. During the first few days of recovery, the lids appear to be slightly overcorrected, but as the swelling subsides, they return to normal. Postoperative treatment consists of placing an antibiotic ointment in the eye and on the wound twice a day. A plastic Elizabethan collar is placed on the animal to prevent self-injury. Sutures are removed 10 to 14 days after surgery.

The two major reasons for failure to achieve a good cosmetic result are (1) not making the incision close enough to the lid margin and (2) placing the sutures too far apart.

Spastic Entropion

Spastic entropion is usually unilateral and can occur at any age. The cause of the lid inversion is spasm of the orbicular muscle secondary to ocular irritation. The etiology includes conjunctivitis, foreign bodies, keratoconjunctivitis sicca, trichiasis, distichiasis, ectopic cilia, and corneal ulceration. One diagnostic method to help differentiate spastic from congenital or acquired entropion is to place several drops of topical anesthetic on the eye. If the entropion resolves spontaneously, it was most likely spastic in character.

If the entropion persists once the underlying cause has been corrected, one can use a soft contact lens or a temporary tarsorrhaphy to reduce further irritation. Sutures for both of these procedures are removed in 2 to 3 weeks. If all else fails, a standard entropion correction cures the condition.

Acquired Entropion

Entropion is a common sequel to endophthalmos from loss of orbital fat or temporal muscle atrophy. An abnormally small globe with normal lids, as seen with phthisis bulbi or microphthalmos, can also result in entropion. Surgical correction of this type of entropion is performed by a lateral canthoplasty to shorten the palpebral fissure by separating the skin from the orbicular muscle of the eye at the lateral canthus with a small scalpel. A triangular flap of skin, in proportion to the amount of closure required, is removed from the upper lid. A flap from the lower lid is sutured into the defect in the upper lid. This procedure has the advantage of providing a palpebral fissure proportionate to the globe size while correcting the acquired entropion.

Medial Entropion and Facial Folds

In poodles, Pekingeses, and pugs, the lid margins at the medial canthus may be slightly inverted. The lacrimal puncta are slightly compressed, and epiphora may be the only presenting sign. Medical therapy using 25 mg of oral tetracycline once a day often eliminates the staining of the tears on the facial fur of these patients and obviates surgical intervention. Brachycephalic breeds such as the Pekingese and pug often have a combination of medial entropion and prominent facial folds. One or both of these conditions can cause keratitis and eventually pigment infiltration of the cornea from the medial limbus. In older dogs (7 to 8 years and older) in which the pigment has infiltrated only one-fourth or less of the cornea and no visual loss is observed, surgery is generally not necessary. In younger dogs with progressive pigmentary keratitis, close examination usually reveals the cause of the irritation, which may require surgical intervention.

Removal or reduction of the nasal folds is indicated when the hairs on the folds rub on the cornea. The nasal folds must usually be reduced to at least half their original height. Concurrent superficial keratectomy for pigmentary keratitis is unnecessary, because correction of the medial entropion or nasal folds stops the physical irritation to the cornea. Pigmentation decreases with time and *judicious* use of corticosteroids.

Combined Entropion-Ectropion (pp. 1164–1165)

Ectropion

Ectropion, or eversion of the lid margin, is a common finding in the Saint Bernard, bloodhound, American cocker spaniel, basset hound, and bulldog. It is usually congenital and generally involves the lower eyelids but can result from scarring. Most dogs do not require surgical correction. Only those experiencing chronic keratitis or conjunctivitis that is unresponsive to medical therapy are considered for surgery.

The Wharton-Jones blepharoplasty (V-Y technique) is the simplest and most commonly used technique. In severe cases in which the V-Y technique will not correct the ectropion, a modification of the Kuhnt-Szymanowski technique can be used.

EYELID TUMORS (pp. 1168–1172)

Eyelid tumors are common in dogs. Tarsal gland adenomas are the most frequent. Tarsal gland adenoma is clinically benign, and surgical excision is usually curative. Cryosurgery using liquid nitrogen can also be used to treat these tumors.

Excision of Eyelid Tumors

A full-thickness eyelid resection is the simplest procedure used in lesions that involve up to one-third of the lid margin on either the upper or lower lid. Immobilizing the lesion with a Desmarres chalazion clamp or using hemostats to crush along the proposed incisions decreases bleeding.

Tumors that require excision of one-third or more of the eyelid require more extensive restoration techniques. For lesions that do not involve the full thickness of the eyelid, partial-thickness tissue advancement may be used. If the majority of the lower lid is removed, a mucocutaneous flap from the lower lip can be used for restoring the lid. The use of a mucocutaneous subdermal plexus flap has several advantages over other procedures. It can replace extensive areas of eyelid and provides a new mucous membrane to replace the palpebral conjunctiva.

Alternative methods for removing small tumors of the eyelid include electrocautery and cryosurgery. Electrocautery may be contraindicated if microscopic examination of the excised tissue is desired, because it coagulates small tumors and alters their histological architecture.

Cryosurgery

Cryosurgery is an alternative to excision of eyelid tumors. Only liquid nitrogen is used as the cooling agent. General anesthesia is recommended.

The most commonly used cryosurgical technique for removing eyelid tumors is the freeze-thaw-refreeze method. Liquid nitrogen is sprayed on the center of the mass. The tissue is allowed to thaw to 32°F (0°C) and is then refrozen. Depigmented hair grows into the previously frozen area, and the resulting white spot may be objectionable in black or dark-colored animals.

EYELASH-RELATED DISEASES (pp. 1172–1175)

Distichiasis, districhiasis, trichiasis, and ectopic cilia all result in corneal irritation or ulceration. In the cocker spaniel, distichiasis (cilia emerging from the tarsal [meibomian] gland openings) and distichiasis (more than one cilium emerging from the gland opening) are common findings. Many of these dogs have few or no adverse effects from the presence of these cilia and do not require surgical treatment.

Surgical Correction

Manual epilation can be accomplished using either cilia forceps or jeweler's forceps. This method may be useful when a corneal ulcer has developed in a dog that has had distichiasis without complications for years. Once the cornea becomes ulcerated, the distichiasis may prevent healing by mechanically rubbing the loosely adhered, healing epithelium. Manual epilation yields only temporary results but often relieves the irritation long enough for the cornea to heal before the cilia grow back.

Electroepilation can be used to treat distichiasis permanently when only five or six cilia are present on each lid. To permanently destroy the hair follicle in the tarsal gland, a thin wire (25 gauge or less) is passed down the hair shaft and current is applied until the cilia can be removed with little tension. A transconjunctival *en bloc* resection of the hair follicles or destroying them with electrocautery has been used in selected cases.

Microcryoepilation

The tarsal gland is not permanently damaged, and if done with precision, the procedure yields excellent results. The only complications are temporary and include conjunctivitis and occasional depigmentation of the eyelid margin.

Ectopic Cilia

Ectopic cilia originate from the tarsal gland and penetrate the conjunctiva. Superficial corneal ulceration is a common finding associated with ectopic cilia, and the condition should be suspected when any small ulcer fails to heal with medical therapy, especially in a young dog. Unlike distichiasis, ectopic cilia usually involve one individual cilium rather than a row and may be very difficult to locate. Simple *en bloc* excision is the preferred treatment.

CHALAZION (pp. 1175–1177)

A chalazion is an accumulation of secretory products in a blocked tarsal gland. It is common in dogs and is usually recognized as a painless swelling 4 to 6 mm from the lid margin. A chalazion must be differentiated from a tarsal gland adenoma, which becomes more invasive, and a hordeolum, which contains purulent material. The treatment of choice for chalazion is incision and curettage. Attempts to express a chalazion manually should be avoided, because rupture of the gland may lead to lipid granulomas in the surrounding tissue as a result of the release of inspissated material.

HORDEOLUM

A hordeolum is a bacterial infection (usually *Staphylococcus aureus*) of either the lash follicle and associated gland of Zeis (external hordeolum) or the tarsal gland (internal hordeolum). A hordeolum is characterized by marked inflammation of the surrounding tissue. External hordeolums are usually raised, painful pustules on the external lid margin. Treatment consists of incising the lesions with the tip of a scalpel or the point of an 18-gauge needle. Hot packing and topical and systemic antibiotics may also be used, depending on the severity of the disease.

LACERATIONS (p. 1177)

A full-thickness laceration of the eyelid is best repaired using a simple two-layer technique. If the wound is near the medial canthus, the nasolacrimal puncta and canaliculi are examined to ensure that they are not involved in the wound.

CHAPTER 83

Conjunctiva (pages 1178–1184)

ANATOMY AND PHYSIOLOGY

Conjunctiva is the richly vascularized ocular mucous membrane that covers the inner aspects of the upper and lower eyelids, both sides of the third eyelid, and the anterior portion of the globe.

The conjunctiva is supplied by blood vessels originating from the anterior ciliary arteries. Conjunctival vessels are distinguished from episcleral vessels because they are superficial, branch extensively, and are movable within the conjunctiva. Episcleral vessels are deeper, radiate from the limbus with little branching, and do not move with shifting of the conjunctiva.

The conjunctival mucosa allows smooth, friction-free movements between the globe, the third eyelid, and the eyelids. The epithelium is covered by a layer of mucus produced by epithelial goblet cells. This mucus also traps particulate material and debris and contains immunoglobulin A. Aggregates of lymphoid cells are prevalent in the substantia propria of the conjunctiva.

SURGICAL CONSIDERATIONS
Conjunctival Healing

Because of the high density of vessels and lymphatics within the conjunctiva, edema (chemosis) occurs quickly after conjunctival insult. Primary healing of mucosal lesions results as epithelial cells divide and slide rapidly (i.e., in 24 to 36 hours) to cover small defects. Large denuded areas heal by granulation in 4 to 7 days.

CONGENITAL DISORDERS (pp. 1178–1179)
Dermoid

Dermoids are congenital ocular tumors with characteristic growth of hair. They commonly occur on the epibulbar surface and conjunctiva between the limbus and the lateral canthus. Dachshunds and Saint Bernards have higher incidences. In cats, Burmese are more commonly affected. Clinically significant dermoids are removed surgically by conjunctivectomy, keratectomy, or eyelid reconstruction.

Lacrimal Caruncle Trichiasis

Hairs growing from the lacrimal caruncle may cause epiphora, mild conjunctivitis, or superficial medial keratitis. The term *aberrant dermis* has been used to describe the more prominent forms of lacrimal caruncle trichiasis in brachycephalic dogs.

Clinical signs are resolved by removing caruncle tissue containing the follicles of offending cilia. In brachycephalic dogs, removal of lacrimal caruncle hairs may be combined with a permanent medial tarsorrhaphy.

INFLAMMATORY DISORDERS (pp. 1179–1181)

Symblepharon

As conjunctival ulcerations heal, fibrosis of two apposing ulcerated areas may cause permanent adhesions (symblepharon). Feline herpesvirus is the most common cause of extensive conjunctival adhesions.

Adhesions of palpebral and bulbar conjunctiva may reduce or obliterate the conjunctival fornices, and scarring of the lacrimal puncta may cause persistent epiphora. Extensive symblepharon may occur between the cornea and the palpebral or third eyelid bulbar conjunctiva, resulting in considerable corneal scarring. Symblepharon may result in reduced ocular mobility, including immobility of the third eyelid and various degrees of enophthalmos.

Once symblepharon has occurred, treatment involves surgical dissection of the adhered surfaces. After surgery, topical treatment with antibiotic ophthalmic ointment several times daily for 14 days and regular separation of affected surfaces is recommended to discourage additional adhesions.

In more severe cases of symblepharon, conjunctivectomy and superficial keratectomy, combined with grafting of adjacent healthy conjunctiva or application of overlays to prevent adhesions, provide means of restoring or improving ocular function.

Follicular Conjunctivitis

Abnormal conjunctival lymphoid follicles, or *follicular conjunctivitis,* occur as a nonspecific immunological response to ocular surface antigens. In dogs, this condition usually occurs in animals younger than 18 months and is characterized by a mildly inflamed conjunctiva and mucoid ocular discharge. Treatment of follicular conjunctivitis in dogs consists of topical or intralesional (subconjunctival) corticosteroids. In cats, follicular conjunctivitis is most often associated with subacute or chronic stages of chlamydial infections, and affected eyes are treated with topical tetracycline.

CONJUNCTIVAL TUMORS (pp. 1181)

Neoplasia

Types of Conjunctival Neoplasia

The conjunctiva is an uncommon site for primary tumors.

Of primary conjunctival neoplasms in dogs, hemangiosarcomas are more common. The anterior surface of the third eyelid and bulbar conjunctiva are the usual sites. Hemangiomas are typically small, raised telangiectatic lesions. Conjunctival hemangiosarcomas may appear similar but are larger, broader-based tumors characterized by aggressive behavior. Ocular squamous cell tumors, which often involve both the eyelids and conjunctiva, occur more frequently in cats than dogs.

Papillomas, presumably of viral origin, may arise from the conjunctiva of dogs. Limbal melanocytomas are more common than primary conjunctival melanomas but originate from scleral melanocytes. Limbal melanocytomas are typically noted as elevated pigmented lesions at the dorsolateral limbus and are static or grow slowly. A breed predisposition occurs in German shepherds.

Therapeutic Procedures for Conjunctival Neoplasia

Local Excision. Masses localized to the bulbar conjunctiva are readily removed. Small conjunctival wounds from local tumor excision generally do not require suturing. Palpebral tumors may require full-thickness eyelid resection.

Conjunctival Reconstruction. Undermining and sliding of adjacent conjunctiva usually facilitates closure of wounds greater than 5 mm in diameter.

Cryosurgery. Freezing of non-neoplastic proliferative conjunctival lesions with a probe cooled with nitrous oxide or liquid nitrogen is also effective.

Radiation Therapy. After surgical excision, beta radiation (5,000 to 10,000 cGy/site) from a strontium 90 applicator may be used. Beta radiation application is unsuitable as the sole treatment for most ocular surface neoplasms.

Therapy for Specific Conjunctival Neoplasms

With papillomas, adenomas, and mastocytomas, surgical excision alone is usually curative. With squamous cell carcinomas or adenocarcinomas, excision plus ancillary treatment with local radiation therapy is recommended. Chemotherapy results in regression of conjunctival lymphosarcoma.

TRAUMA

Punctures/Lacerations

Because the conjunctiva repairs rapidly, many lacerations and punctures heal spontaneously without suturing. Whether or not the conjunctiva is sutured, broad-spectrum antibiotics are applied topically three or four times daily and systemic antibiotics are administered for 1 week to prevent opportunistic infections.

Traumatically induced subconjunctival hemorrhage resorbs spontaneously in 7 to 14 days depending on the amount of blood present and the area involved. When conjunctival hemorrhage occurs with no evidence of puncture or without a history of trauma, a systemic clotting disorder is considered.

Conjunctival Biopsy

Biopsy of the conjunctiva is indicated for differentiating inflammatory from neoplastic diseases and in suspected preocular goblet cell (mucin) deficiency. Conjunctival biopsy is performed with the patient under local anesthesia. Defects resulting from conjunctival biopsy that are less than 4 × 4 mm heal uneventfully with topical antibiotic treatment.

The Lacrimal System (pages 1184–1194)

The lacrimal system produces and removes tears. There is a coordinated secretion of glandular products that combine to form the precorneal tear film. This film is distributed across the cornea and performs several important functions. A substantial portion of tear volume is lost through evaporation, and the remainder is removed through drainage channels.

ANATOMY OF THE LACRIMAL SYSTEM

The lacrimal glands are responsible for producing most of the tears. Lacrimal glands are located in the orbit between the globe nasally and orbital ligament and zygomatic process of the frontal bone temporally. The ducts in dogs (3 to 20) are not visible but open through the conjunctiva in the superior temporal fornix.

The gland of the third eyelid is an accessory lacrimal gland encompassing the stem of the cartilaginous shaft in the third eyelid. In dogs, 29 to 57 per cent of the serous tear component is produced by this gland.

The tarsal glands are perpendicular to the margin of the eyelid. The secretion is a lipid-laden sebaceous material, which can be manually expressed on the margin of the eyelid as a cream-colored exudate. The upper and lower eyelids each have a small opening, the lacrimal punctum—the beginning of the lacrimal drainage system. The puncta are 2 to 5 mm from the nasal canthus. After entering a punctum, the tears pass into the upper or lower canaliculus. The lacrimal sac at the confluence of the canaliculi is not always a distinct structure in animals, as it is in man.

The nasolacrimal duct begins at the lacrimal sac. The duct continues rostrally through the bony channel of the lacrimal bone and into the lacrimal sulcus of the maxilla. The duct emerges from the bony capsule at the conchal crest, adjacent to the second premolar tooth, or at the infraorbital canal. An accessory opening is present at the root of the upper canine tooth in approximately 50 per cent of dogs. The duct makes an abrupt 90° turn 2 mm from the orifice and opens onto the floor of the nasal cavity at the junction of the ventral and lateral walls, approximately 1 cm inside the opening of the external nares.

TEAR MOVEMENT

The flow of tears begins in the lacrimal gland, passes across the cornea, blends with other secretory components, and pools in the lacrimal lake. The heavy, oily secretions from the tarsal glands help to prevent spillage of tears onto the face and direct the tears toward the lacrimal lake.

EPIPHORA AND LACRIMATION

Epiphora is an overflow or spillage of tears onto the face as a result of impaired outflow apparatus. Lacrimation is increased production of tears that may result in tear overflow when the production exceeds the capacity for drainage and evaporation.

CONGENITAL ANOMALIES OF DRAINAGE
(pp. 1185–1188)

Absence of the Punctum

Cocker spaniels, golden retrievers, Samoyeds, toy poodles, miniature poodles, and Bedlington terriers, as well as Persian cats, may lack one or more puncta. If either the upper or lower punctum is present, epiphora may not exist. If only the lower is absent, epiphora is more likely than if only the upper is absent, because the lower punctum is more important in removing tears. Epiphora may still be present when the drainage system does not have adequate functional capacity, even though the punctum is open and patency is established.

If a new punctal opening is established and is not satisfactory, a monofilament nylon suture may be passed. A larger polyethylene catheter is threaded over the monofilament nylon and pulled through the nasolacrimal system. The nylon guide is removed, and the tubing is sutured in place at the nasal canthus and on the hair-bearing skin just posterior to the planum nasale.

Congenital Membrane

A conjunctival membrane or flap may be present over the punctum, providing partial or complete obstruction.

Stenotic Punctum

Stenotic puncta are occasionally found in Manx and Persian cats. A lacrimal dilator, a blunt, taper-point instrument, may be introduced through the small punctum and gradually advanced into the canaliculus. Additionally, the punctum may be enlarged by excision.

Atresia of Canaliculi or Lacrimal Duct

The canaliculi or nasolacrimal duct may be obstructed by a membrane owing to failure of the facial fissure to close properly.

Tear Staining Syndrome

The tear staining syndrome is a poorly defined clinical entity of chronic facial moisture and secondary staining of facial hairs. The nasolacrimal system is patent when flushed, but a functional blockage exists.

Medical Treatment of Tear Staining

Palliative management with topical creams and pastes to protect the facial hair and skin has been uniformly unsuccessful. One medical approach is based on a theory that tetracyclines may bind with circulating porphyrins or lactoferrin-like pigments and prevent hair staining. The face remains wet, but the hair is not stained; therefore, the tear staining is less noticeable.

Surgical Treatment of Tear Staining

The gland of the third eyelid is not responsible for epiphora; the benefit derived by removing the gland is a reduction of the total tear volume. Surgical removal of the gland of the third eyelid effectively reduces the tear volume by up to 50 per cent. This relatively simple procedure *should not be attempted* unless the Schirmer test values are known to exceed 20 mm in 60 seconds.

Hair may be observed growing from the nasal canthal conjunctiva and third eyelid. If this leads to facial staining and constant moisture on the face, the offending tissue may be excised or removed by cryoepilation.

ACQUIRED ANOMALIES OF TEAR OUTFLOW
(pp. 1188–1189)

Spastic Entropion

Proper eyelid position and function are essential for even distribution and removal of excessive tears. Orbicularis muscle spasm produces a spastic entropion, which is treated early.

Cicatricial Entropion

Scar tissue must be freed and the eyelid function restored to regain normal function.

Blepharitis

Swelling of the eyelids alters eyelid and lacrimal function.

Conjunctivitis

Acquired occlusion of the punctum may result in epiphora. In cats with herpesvirus infection, symblepharon may be extensive.

Folliculosis

Extensive follicle formation may inhibit tear flow and occlude the punctum. Increased lacrimation or epiphora may be associated with folliculosis in young dogs. Appropriate treatment of the follicles eliminates the tearing.

Autoimmune Disease

Autoimmune erosions of the mucocutaneous junction, as in the pemphigoid diseases, may be associated with closure of the punctum and epiphora. Each condition must be correctly diagnosed and treated specifically.

ACQUIRED OCCLUSION OF THE CANALICULI, SAC, OR NASOLACRIMAL DUCT (pp. 1189–1190)

Upper Respiratory Infections

Upper respiratory infections in cats and chronic bacterial infections can extend into the canaliculus and sac. Repeated flushing with antibiotic-steroid combinations is indicated.

Dacryocystitis

Dacryocystitis is inflammation of the nasolacrimal sac characterized by epiphora and persistent conjunctivitis. Typical infections in small animals result in epiphora with a mucoid to mucopurulent discharge from the lower punctum. Digital pressure may result in extrusion of material from the upper and lower puncta. Pain may be evident but only in a few patients can a detectable swelling of the sac be seen. The treatment for dacryocystitis is the establishment of patency of the outflow system by mechanical flushing and removal of any foreign material and debris.

Mucocele

Mucocele of the lacrimal sac is rare. Facial swelling by a fluctuating mass over the lacrimal sac with minimal pain and an absence of signs of infection suggests a mucocele.

Lacerations

If only the punctum is damaged, it is unlikely that sufficient scarring will occur to produce epiphora. If the canaliculus is lacerated, however, surgical repair is indicated.

SURGICAL CREATION OF A NEW DRAINAGE APPARATUS (pp. 1190–1191)

Dacryocystorhinostomy

Dacryocystorhinostomy may be used in patients with a patent canaliculus but an obstruction of the sac or canal.

In dogs and cats, the largest polyethylene tubing that can pass through the punctum and canaliculus is threaded through the new bony canal and sutured in place as described for dacryocystitis. The catheter is left in place for at least 4 months to ensure continued patency.

Conjunctivorhinostomy

A small Steinmann pin is directed ventromedially into the orbital rim toward the nasal cavity. The pin is aimed at the ipsilateral external nares, with the shaft of the pin. Either polyethylene or Silastic tubing may be used in lengths of 2.5 to 3.8 cm. A flanged end or rim is applied to the tubing and is used to suture the tubing in place at the mucocutaneous junction of the nasal canthus.

A topical antibiotic-steroid ointment is applied three times daily for 3 to 4 days and then once daily until the tubing is removed. The tube is flushed at least once weekly. The actual relief of epiphora is usually not noticed until after the final tube is removed.

Only an experienced ophthalmic surgeon should attempt any of these procedures.

DEFICIENCY OF PRECORNEAL TEAR FILM (pp. 1191–1194)

Surgical Treatment

Punctal Occlusion

This technique is of no proven value.

Parotid Duct Transposition

Parotid duct transposition is recommended for dogs and cats without measurable tear volume and for chronic keratoconjunctivitis sicca that has not responded to medical treatments. Before surgery, medical treatment is necessary to ascertain complete loss of lacrimal function. The function of the parotid salivary gland is evaluated by stimulating salivation and observing saliva flowing from the duct opening. Only an experienced surgeon should perform this procedure.

Surgical Technique. Immediate postoperative care consists of systemic and topical antibiotic therapy for 5 days. Several small meals during each day stimulate the parotid flow (a small blood clot can be milked from the duct through the skin on the first postoperative day). The major postoperative complication is failure of the duct to function. This usually results from twisting the duct during surgery. Preoperative catheterization and careful placement of the transposed duct reduce the likelihood of this complication. Uncontrolled conjunctival infections may also lead to fibrosis and closure of the duct. If a duct fails to function, it should be catheterized and evaluated for patency. If a stricture is found, the duct is surgically exposed and examined.

Complications of Parotid Duct Transposition. Immediate complications of parotid duct transposition include a nonfunctioning parotid gland, twisting or kinking of the duct, bending around a vessel or nerve, and suturing through the duct. Delayed complications include slippage of papilla into subcutaneous tissues, stricture formation, skin maceration, and solid deposits on the cornea and eyelids.

Skin infections resulting from maceration by saliva are a potential problem, and it may be necessary to apply petrolatum or other ointment around the eyelids to protect the skin. Another potential complication is the appearance of chalklike deposits on the eyelid margins and on and in the cornea. Periodic use of mucolytic agents (acetylcysteine) or 1 per cent EDTA solution slows the accumulation of these deposits.

CHAPTER 85

Third Eyelid (pages 1195–1201)

ANATOMY AND PHYSIOLOGY (p. 1195)

The third eyelid is a triangular structure that arises from the anterior ventromedial aspect of the orbit. A T-shaped hyaline cartilage supports the third-eyelid gland, connective tissue stroma, and conjunctiva that covers the anterior (palpebral) and posterior (bulbar) surfaces. A seromucous gland surrounds the base of the cartilage and provides a significant portion of the basal tear secretion in dogs. The position of the third eyelid depends on normal size and position of the globe and sympathetic tone of smooth-muscle fibers within the orbital fascia.

The third eyelid protects the globe and secretes and distributes tears. When the retractor bulbi muscle retracts the globe, the third eyelid passively covers the eye and serves as a protective barrier. Free border of the third eyelid is usually pigmented.

PATHOPHYSIOLOGY—SURGICAL IMPLICATIONS

Because of the contribution of the third eyelid to production and distribution of preocular tear fluid, every effort *must* be made to preserve its integrity. If the third eyelid is removed, chronic keratoconjunctivitis with or without keratoconjunctivitis sicca often results.

CONGENITAL/DEVELOPMENTAL DISORDERS

Cartilage Eversion

Defective cartilage allows the third eyelid to roll toward or, more commonly, away from the globe. A predisposition is noted in large canine breeds (e.g., Great Danes, Saint Bernards, Newfoundlands, and German shorthaired pointers).

Treatment is removal of the scrolled portion of the cartilage from the posterior side while the anterior conjunctival surface, the leading margin, and the gland are left intact. Care is taken to remove only the defective portion of the cartilage.

Protrusion of the Gland of the Third Eyelid

Gland protrusion "haws" or "cherry eye" is seen in puppies and dogs usually less than 1 year of age. A breed predisposition is noted in beagles, American cocker spaniels, Boston terriers, poodles, and brachycephalic breeds.

Clinical problems associated with gland prolapse include ocular discharge, conjunctivitis, and the cosmetic concern of a pink mass being visible in the medial canthus. Definitive treatment of third-eyelid gland prolapses is surgical. Manual replacement of a prolapsed gland followed by medical therapy usually produces a temporary response only.

Replacement Techniques

A number of replacement techniques have been described. Most involve inverting the gland and using suture to anchor the gland to adjacent fibrous tissue. Less invasive techniques are generally simpler to perform but may be less likely to accomplish permanent replacement, particularly in cases of chronic gland prolapses.

The Blogg technique involves dissecting the gland free and suturing it to the ventral epibulbar fascia. Gross modified the technique by anchoring the gland to the ventral equatorial sclera. Each of these procedures involves dissection on the posterior aspect of the third eyelid. The most serious potential complication of these procedures is globe penetration.

Kaswan and Martin developed a technique that is primarily performed on the anterior side of the third eyelid. This technique also avoids postoperative contact of suture material with the cornea. A 3-0 monofilament suture is placed through the periosteum of the orbital rim and passed through the base of the third eyelid into the gland.

Slatter recommends modifying Kaswan's technique by extending dissection ventrally to expose the zygomatic periosteum after making the initial incision. This more extensive exposure allows precise placement of the nylon anchor suture into the periosteum. Precise suturing in this procedure produces a highly reliable method of gland prolapse repair.

INFLAMMATORY DISORDERS (pp. 1198–1200)

Follicular Conjunctivitis

Lymphoid follicles are normally present on the bulbar side of the third eyelid. The presence and hypertrophy of lymphoid elements on the anterior side of the third eyelid occur as a nonspecific ocular surface response to chronic antigenic stimulation. Mucoid discharge, mild epiphora, and a red cobblestone appearance of the anterior surface of the third eyelid are characteristic. Treatment is aimed at removing stimulating antigens.

Plasmacytic Infiltrates

In German shepherds, thickened, hyperemic third eyelids with bilateral third-eyelid protrusions occur as a result of diffuse plasmacytic infiltration of the conjunctiva (plasmacytoma).

Variable responses result from local and systemic corticosteroids used either separately or in combination. Preliminary indications are that topical 1 to 2 per cent cyclosporine in oil is promising as a safe and effective treatment.

Pseudotumors

Proliferative granulomatous lesions of the third eyelids in dogs may accompany similar lesions of the eyelids, conjunctiva, or cornea. These appear as smooth, raised, usually pink lesions on the leading edge or anterior surface of the third eyelid. Collies are more frequently affected. (See the section on proliferative keratoconjunctivitis in Chapters 83 and 86.)

NEOPLASIA (p. 1200)

Squamous cell carcinoma is the most common tumor of the third eyelid. Most third-eyelid neoplasms, including squamous cell tumors, arise from the conjunctiva.

Local Excision with Partial Removal of Third Eyelid

If the neoplasm involves only the leading edge of the third eyelid, local excision may be accomplished. Removal of the mass and repair of the third eyelid conjunctiva over the remaining cartilage and gland usually allow functional and cosmetic healing of the third eyelid.

Total Excision with Reconstruction of Third Eyelid

Extensive neoplastic invasion is one of the rare indications for complete surgical removal of the third eyelid. To replace lost tissue, a buccal mucosal graft may be constructed. A similar technique may also be used for traumatic avulsions or iatrogenic causes (prior removal) of the third eyelid. Slatter reports a survival rate of approximately 65 per cent using the mucosal grafting technique.

TRAUMA (p. 1200)

Punctures and Lacerations

Third-eyelid lacerations are most commonly encountered as a result of claw punctures due to cat-scratch injuries. Small superficial punctures or partial-thickness lacerations involving only mucosa do not require suturing. Linear lacerations, particularly those involving the third-eyelid margin, are sutured with 6-0 or 7-0 absorbable suture.

If the cartilage is torn, it is generally not trimmed unless jagged edges are present. Repairing lacerated conjunctiva over torn cartilage usually allows functional and cosmetic healing of the third eyelid.

When linear lacerations involving the third-eyelid cartilage occur parallel to the free margin and very near it, a primary repair may not be possible and a small strip of marginal tissue may be removed. It is extremely important that the leading edge of the third eyelid be left smooth.

PROMINENT THIRD EYELID

Congenital and acquired diseases or conformational variations may cause protruding, conspicuous third eyelids. Protruding third eyelids are often associated with breed-related enophthalmos, which is frequently seen in larger canine breeds (e.g., Doberman pinschers and Great Danes).

Changes in orbital volume can have a profound effect on third-eyelid position. An anterior shift in globe position from an increase in orbital contents or a posterior shift from reduction of orbital contents causes third-eyelid protrusion. Dehydration or emaciation with subsequent loss of retrobulbar tissue volume may cause third-eyelid protrusion. Ocular pain may also stimulate retraction of the eye with third-eyelid prominence.

Sympathetic denervation (Horner's syndrome) of periocular tissues is associated with prominence of the third eyelid(s). In cats, a syndrome of bilateral third-eyelid protrusion (haws syndrome) is associated with loss of sympathetic tone in both third eyelids.

CHAPTER 86

Cornea and Sclera (pages 1202–1225)

Knowledge of normal unique corneal reactions is necessary for acceptable surgical results.

ANATOMY (pp. 1202–1204)

The cornea is the transparent anterior window in the fibrous coat of the eye, the sclera is the posterior opaque part, and the limbus is the transition zone between. The cornea has five layers: the precorneal tear film, epithelium and basement membrane, stroma, Descemet's membrane (basement membrane of the endothelium), and endothelium. The outer superficial layer serves two functions: (1) to increase surface tension and bind the precorneal tear film to the corneal surface and (2) to limit evaporation of the aqueous layer beneath. The middle, or aqueous, layer is mostly water and has the following functions:

1. It flushes foreign material from the conjunctival sac.
2. It lubricates passage of the lids and third eyelid over the epithelium.
3. It serves as a medium for passage of oxygen, inflammatory cells, and immunoglobulins A and G to the cornea.
4. It provides a smooth corneal surface for greatest optical efficiency.

The corneal epithelium is composed of simple stratified squamous and nonkeratinized cells, attached to its basement membrane by hemidesmosomes. Regular spacing of stromal collagen fibrils maintains corneal transparency and distinguishes the stroma from collagen in scar tissue and sclera.

Descemet's membrane is the basement membrane of the endothelium. In a descemetocele in which the overlying stroma has been destroyed, Descemet's membrane often protrudes dramatically because of its elasticity. After rupture, the endothelium secretes a new membrane to fill small defects. The Descemet's membrane does not stain with fluorescein, and its presence as a dark, transparent bulge in the center of a corneal ulcer or wound signals impending rupture.

The endothelium is one cell thick and has a limited ability to replicate depending on age and species. With advancing age, the number of endothelial cells decreases. The endothelium is extremely susceptible to osmotic and traumatic damage during surgery.

The sclera is composed of collagen fibers and fibroblasts. Scleral collagen fibrils differ from corneal fibrils in their considerable variation in diameter and absence of regular fixed spacing between them.

PHYSIOLOGY (pp. 1204–1205)

The cornea is the most powerful refractive component of the eye. The cornea but not the sclera is transparent owing to the following features:

1. Lack of blood vessels and few stromal cells
2. Lack of pigment
3. Control of water content
4. A smooth optical surface provided by precorneal tear film
5. A high mucopolysaccharide content
6. Orderly arrangement of collagen fibrils of uniform diameter and spacing

Glucose metabolism is the most important source of energy. The endothelium receives most of its oxygen from aqueous, whereas the rest of the avascular cornea receives oxygen mainly from the atmosphere via the precorneal tear film and from limbal and conjunctival capillaries.

Water enters the cornea under the influence of intraocular pressure and the hydrophilic character of stromal collagen and mucopolysaccharides. Endothelial and epithelial barriers limit entry of water into the cornea. Water leaves by evaporation from the anterior corneal surface. The corneal state of relative dehydration is important to transparency.

Elevated intraocular pressure and endothelial damage cause corneal edema and opacity. In scars, irregular size and arrangement of collagen fibrils cause opacity. Removal of epithelium allows entry of water from tears into the stroma and causes gross corneal swelling.

PATHOLOGICAL RESPONSES (p. 1205)

The normal cornea is avascular. Penetration of new vessels and immunoglobulins into the cornea is impeded by the compact stromal tissue. These features make corneal pathological reactions sluggish, chronic, and intractable. Changes that would be mild in other tissues may greatly alter transparency and are more significant in the cornea. The corneal epithelium forms an effective barrier against exogenous influences. Bacteria rarely cause primary keratitis in dogs and cats.

NORMAL CORNEAL HEALING (pp. 1205–1206)

Epithelium

The regenerative capacity of the epithelium is great. Within a short time, cells around a lesion slide over the defect. An entirely denuded cornea can be re-epithelialized in 4 to 7 days.

Stroma

Superficial stromal defects are filled by epithelial facets. Deeper defects are covered initially by epithelium, with regeneration of stroma from beneath. Uncomplicated stromal wounds heal without vascularization, but infected or destructive lesions heal with vascularization.

Avascular Stromal Healing

Edema formation begins immediately after stromal injury. Within 1 to 2 days, neutrophils from tears and limbal blood vessels infiltrate the wound under chemotactic influences. Keratocytes adjacent to the wound die. Keratocytes transform into fibroblasts, migrate to the damaged area, and produce collagen and mucopolysaccharides of corneal ground substance. Macrophages invade the lesion, remove cellular debris, and subsequently transform into keratocytes. The collagen fibrils of regenerated stroma are irregular, causing opacity. Within weeks to months, the density of the scar decreases. A sutured full-thickness corneal wound depends on mechanical support by sutures for 16 days.

Vascular Stromal Healing

Cellular infiltration is more extensive than in avascular healing. Blood vessels originating from the limbal vascular plexus invade the area. Granulation tissue is laid down and forms a denser scar than in avascular healing. Blood vessels eventually collapse but do not disappear.

Endothelium and Descemet's Membrane

Descemet's membrane is elastic and retracts and curls when damaged, exposing corneal stroma. Neighboring endothelial cells slide in to cover the area, and a new Descemet's membrane is laid down.

CORTICOSTEROIDS AND CORNEAL HEALING (p. 1206)

Corticosteroids inhibit epithelial and endothelial regeneration, infiltration with inflammatory cells, and fibroblastic activity. The tensile strength of the healing wound is lessened, collagenases are potentiated many times, and the risk of infection is greatly increased. If topical corticosteroid therapy can be delayed for 7 days after wounding, fibroblastic activity will be well under way and wound healing will be much less impeded.

INTERPRETATION OF CORNEAL PATHOLOGICAL REACTIONS (pp. 1206–1209)

Edema

Corneal edema results from excess fluid in the stroma. It distorts the collagen lattice, causing opacity. Edematous cornea is hazy gray to blue. The condition is usually reversible if the underlying cause is removed. Chronic edema may cause corneal vascularization or, less commonly, bullous keratopathy. Corneal edema may be cleared temporarily for examination by topical application of hypertonic solutions (e.g., 5 per cent sodium chloride, 40 per cent glucose, or 50 per cent glycerin).

Vascularization

There are no blood vessels in normal cornea. Vascularization may be induced by different stimuli, including stimulated lymphocytes or their elaborated lymphokines.

Corneal vascularization may be superficial or deep. Superficial vessels are continuous with the conjunctival circulation at the limbus and are brighter red than deep vessels. Deep vessels are continuous with the ciliary circulation and disappear from view at the limbus. The timing sequence of corneal vascularization is important both for diagnostic evaluation of corneal lesions and during postoperative assessment.

In complicated stromal lesions, vessels may not collapse and further vascularization and granulation occur. Vascularization is a beneficial response, but vessels result in decreased transparency, ingrowth of pigment, and occasionally transport of antibodies and inflammatory cells that decrease corneal transparency. Control of vascularization is often attempted with topical corticosteroids or beta radiation.

Scar Formation

Corneal stromal repair results in disorganized collagen fibrils of uneven diameter, causing loss of transparency. Scars increase in transparency with time, but in dogs, pigmentation and lipid deposition may occur. The deeper the initial injury, the more dense and permanent the resulting scar and the less the tendency for clearing. Corneal opacities are termed *nebula, macula,* and *leukoma.* If the stroma is destroyed full thickness and a bare Descemet's membrane bulges forward, the lesion is called a *descemetocele.* Descemetoceles frequently form after unremitting ulceration, and if untreated, the membrane either ruptures, with loss of aqueous and collapse of the anterior chamber, or becomes surrounded by scar tissue. If the iris is carried out through the wound, an iris prolapse exists.

Opacity may be limited by corticosteroids, provided that (1) infection has been controlled, (2) an epithelial covering can be demonstrated with fluorescein, and (3) the structural integrity of the cornea is not compromised.

Pigmentation

Pigmentation is a nonspecific response to corneal inflammation. Stromal melanin originates from proliferation of normal limbal melanoblasts that migrate into the cornea along with blood vessels. Epithelial pigmentation is more common in chronic corneal diseases, especially when continuous exposure or irritation is present. Removal of the stimulus usually prevents progression of pigmentation. Stromal pigmentation usually is associated with more severe corneal disease and vascularization. In cats, melanin pigmentation must be distinguished from focal corneal necrosis in which the color may be due to necrotic tissue and keratin. Pigmentation itself is not normally treated unless vision is threatened. The underlying cause is removed whenever possible.

GENERAL PRINCIPLES OF SURGICAL MANIPULATION OF CORNEA (pp. 1209–1211)

Grasping the cornea often requires toothed forceps that allow wound edges to be held. When corneal stroma is cut *with scissors,* the resulting cut has an S-shaped profile. This distortion of incision shape can be minimized by preliminary reduction of the tissue thickness to be cut. *Corneal suturing* requires precise placement and guidance of the needle. In full-thickness wounds, sutures are placed deeply but not totally through the stroma.

SURGICAL PROCEDURES (pp. 1211–1218)

Treatment of Corneal Injuries

With a penetrating wound of the globe, pressure may cause further intraocular damage. A third-eyelid flap is initially placed over the eye to prevent further damage until skilled assistance is available. One of the most common causes of severe endophthalmitis and secondary glaucoma leading to enucleation in dogs is unsuspected damage to the lens and its capsule after a perforating injury.

Equipment (p. 1211)

Closure of a Corneal Wound

1. The corneal endothelium is exquisitely sensitive to trauma. It must not be touched with instruments.
2. The edges of corneal wounds are not débrided.
3. If the wound is fresh, an attempt is made to replace protruding iris with an iris repositor.
4. Blood and fibrin clots in the anterior chamber are carefully removed.
5. Partial-thickness rather than full-thickness sutures are used.
6. The cornea is sutured with simple interrupted sutures placed about 1 mm apart.
7. After partial closure, the anterior chamber is reconstituted with balanced salt solution or a small air bubble.

The prognosis for a corneal wound depends on its initial depth and severity.

Removal of Corneal Foreign Bodies

Corneal foreign bodies are removed to limit pain, reduce infection, and prevent vascularization and scarring. Many can be flushed off with physiological saline. Small embedded foreign bodies are removed with a *foreign body spud.* Deeply embedded foreign bodies may require an incision in the overlying epithelium and stroma. Foreign body extractions are performed with the utmost care. Inappropriate attempts at removal may result in penetration into the anterior chamber or corneal damage with more severe vascularization and scarring.

After suture removal, a topical broad-spectrum antibiotic (applied four times a day) and atropine are administered to control infection and ciliary spasm due to secondary uveitis.

Superficial Keratectomy

Keratectomy is removal of the corneal epithelium or stroma. Because the stroma does not regenerate, the number of successive keratectomies that can be performed on the same site is limited to two or three. The safety of performing a successive keratectomy can be determined by measuring the corneal thickness by ultrasonic pachymetry. Use of an operating microscope greatly improves the safety and results of this procedure. Indications include:

1. Removal of neoplasms
2. Treatment of specific keratopathies, chronic superficial erosion syndrome, and focal corneal necrosis
3. Débridement of any superficial epithelial corneal wound

Penetrating Corneoscleral Allograft

Replacement of continuous cornea and sclera from a donor of the same species is a treatment for canine epibulbar melanomas when the tumor infiltrates the cornea or sclera.

Corneoscleral Transposition

Corneoscleral transposition is partial replacement of the cornea by the adjacent sclera to fill a defect resulting from removal of a lesion. Alternatives to this technique include penetrating keratoplasty, autogenous lamellar corneal transplantation, penetrating corneoscleral allograft, and conjunctival pedicle graft.

CORNEAL DISORDERS OF SURGICAL IMPORTANCE
(pp. 1218–1224)

Superficial Corneal Erosion

Superficial corneal erosion is most common in boxers and corgis. Affected dogs usually have a history of blepharospasm and epiphora resistant to treatment for weeks to months.

Clinical Signs

Unilateral chronic blepharospasm, epiphora, and photophobia are common. The lesions are due to separation of the epithelium from the basement membrane secondary to a defect in hemidesmosomes or in the layers of the basement membrane.

Some may be due to mild endothelial dysfunction with diffuse, persistent corneal edema. Affected areas are usually 3 to 4 mm in diameter, have a ragged outline, cause pain, and stain with fluorescein.

Treatment

If the lesion is discovered early, débridement and placement of a dissolving collagen shield, followed by topical antibiotics and hyperosmotic solutions, constitute the first treatment. For refractory cases, superficial keratectomy is the treatment of choice. The cornea is covered with a third-eyelid flap and treated as for a superficial ulcer.

Superficial Pigmentary Keratitis

Superficial pigmentary keratitis occurs frequently in Pekingeses, pugs, and similar breeds. It is a nonspecific, chronic low-grade keratitis with pigmentation of the superficial stroma and epithelium due to prominent exposed globes and a large palpebral fissure (euryblepharon) with chronic exposure of the cornea, distichiasis, and nasal fold trichiasis. Therapy aims at correction of causative factors to prevent progression of pigmentation.

Pseudopterygium and Symblepharon

Pseudopterygium is an adhesion of the conjunctiva to the cornea. When palpebral conjunctiva adheres, the condition is termed *sym-*

blepharon. Its most common cause is feline herpesvirus infection in young cats. With more extensive adhesions, reconstructive surgery may be needed to achieve a continuous conjunctival epithelial cover over the sclera or inside the eyelid.

Ulcerative Keratitis

A corneal ulcer is present when corneal epithelium and a variable amount of stroma are missing. Small acute ulcers heal rapidly.

Progression

Corneal ulcers may progress to involve deeper layers (see the upper box on page 408). In treating corneal ulceration, the most important steps are to determine and remove the causes, to prevent progression, and to create an ideal environment for healing (see the lower box on page 408).

All corneal ulcers have the potential to evolve to perforation and endophthalmitis if not treated.

In chronic or infected ulcers, proteases may speed progression ("melting") of a simple ulcer to perforation and iris prolapse, sometimes within 24 hours. Proteases are produced by epithelium, bacteria (*Pseudomonas* spp. especially), neutrophils, and possibly stroma.

Diagnosis

Corneal ulcers are frequently invisible even with good lighting. All red and painful eyes must be stained with fluorescein and the intraocular pressure measured if fluorescein negative. The clinical handling of a corneal ulcer is summarized in Table 86–1.

The following combination of antibiotics, atropine, antiprotease agents, and base is commonly and effectively used:

Acetylcysteine 20 per cent 6 ml
Atropine ophthalmic solution 1 per cent 6 ml
Gentamicin 1.5 ml
Artificial tear solution to 25 ml

In deep ulceration, descemetoceles, and perforated ulcers, systemic antibiotic therapy is used.

Surgical Therapy

Mechanical support for ulcers often is warranted. Tarsorrhaphy, third-eyelid flaps, direct suturing of descemetoceles, and conjunctival flaps have been used successfully.

In uncomplicated ulcers, coverage with a third-eyelid flap should be maintained for 7 to 10 days. If any of the following signs appear, the flap is removed and the cornea examined:

1. Purulent discharge
2. Sudden voluminous watery discharge
3. Hemorrhagic discharge
4. Sudden, painful blepharospasm

Flaps usually relieve much of the discomfort of painful corneal lesions. Deep ulcers may be treated with third-eyelid flaps or conjunctival grafts. With descemetoceles, third-eyelid flaps are insufficient to prevent rupture. During the healing of any ulcer, corneal vascularization and scar formation may occur.

Conjunctival Pedicle Grafting

Conjunctival pedicle grafting is effective in saving the integrity of the eye in severe ulceration, with or without perforation. Conjunctival

Superficial ulceration → Deep ulceration → Descemetocele → Iris prolapse → Endophthalmitis

Diagnosis of corneal ulcer

1. Determination of etiology → Specific therapy to eliminate etiology (e.g., antibiotics, correction of entropion)

2. Steps to prevent progression → Specific drugs (e.g., protease inhibitors) or surgical techniques

3. Procedures to maintain corneal integrity and produce optimal healing conditions → Third-eyelid flap, conjunctival flap, tarsorrhaphy, corneoscleral transposition, corneal suturing

TABLE 86–1. TREATMENT OF CORNEAL ULCERATION

Type of Ulcer	Phase 1	Phase 2	Phase 3
Simple superficial ulcer	Topical antibiotics Correction of lid defects (e.g., entropion, cilia) Topical atropine	Rarely necessary	Rarely necessary
Uncomplicated deep ulcer	Topical antibiotics Topical atropine	Antiprotease agents Débridement	Third-eyelid flap Tear replacement
Complicated deep ulcer	Topical, subconjunctival, and systemic antibiotics (subpalpebral lavage) Topical atropine	Antiprotease agents Débridement (surgical)	Conjunctival or third-eyelid flap, conjunctival pedicle graft Tear replacement
Descemetocele	Topical, subconjunctival, and systemic antibiotics (subpalpebral lavage) Topical atropine	Antiprotease agents	Conjunctival or third-eyelid flap Tear replacement or corneoscleral transposition, conjunctival pedicle graft
Iris prolapse	Topical, subconjunctival, and systemic antibiotics (subpalpebral lavage) Topical atropine	Antiprotease agents	Resection or replacement of prolapsed iris Conjunctival or third-eyelid flap, conjunctival pedicle graft Suture lacerations Reconstitution of anterior chamber

grafts are effective against enzymatic corneal melting, infection, and pain. Magnification with loupes or an operating microscope is necessary.

The pedicle is prepared from dorsolateral or dorsomedial bulbar conjunctiva. The graft is sutured to firm corneal stroma around the recipient bed with simple isolated sutures. In large grafts and perforated, leaking ulcers, one suture is placed through the middle of the pedicle into the dorsal rim of the ulcer, taking care not to strangulate vessels in the pedicle. In melting ulcers, the graft edges must cover all of the devitalized stroma and are sutured into viable stroma around the lesion.

Aftercare includes daily cleaning of the eye with warm, wet compresses. Medications include topical antibiotic solution (three to four times daily), topical atropine solution (three times daily), and possibly systemic antibiotics and anti-inflammatory drugs.

Patients are re-evaluated 2 to 4 days after surgery and then weekly or as indicated. After 1 to 3 weeks, topical corticosteroid therapy is added to the regimen to decrease corneal neovascularization and scarring. Systemic antibiotics are given for 7 to 10 days with corneal perforation. The graft is left in place for several months to allow for corticosteroid treatment of keratitis under protection of the vascularized graft.

Conjunctival flaps covering parts or all of the cornea (360° flaps) are prepared by undermining the conjunctiva from the limbus peripherally and suturing it to the cornea or to conjunctiva from across the eye.

Dermoids (Dermolipoma)

Dermoids usually afflict both conjunctiva and cornea. Those involving the cornea are removed by superficial keratectomy with local conjunctivectomy.

Feline Focal Corneal Necrosis

Focal corneal necrosis occurs most commonly in Persian and Siamese cats. It consists of brown to black areas of necrotic stroma tightly attached to the cornea.

Clinical Signs

Clinical signs include (1) a slowly progressive, focal, brownish-black corneal lesion, often of several months' duration; (2) corneal vascularization; (3) epiphora; and (4) pain and blepharospasm.

Treatment

Before treatment is attempted, the lesion should have ceased to enlarge, because a nonprogressive lesion is less likely to recur postoperatively. If herpetic keratitis is present, the lesion must be quiescent. The necrotic material is removed by superficial keratectomy before healing occurs. The use of an operating microscope is recommended because the lesion often is deep. Topical corticosteroids should not be used at any stage because of the frequency of herpesvirus as the cause.

ADVANCES IN CORNEAL SURGERY AND THERAPEUTICS (pp. 1224–1225)
Viscoelastic Substances

Sodium hyaluronate is used during intraocular procedures to facilitate dissection, protect the corneal endothelium, and prevent adhesions between tissues.

Hydrophilic Contact Lenses

Hydrophilic contact lenses may be used to cover corneas with severe bullous keratopathy or persistent epithelial erosions. They can also be used to deliver drugs to the cornea in high concentrations. A dissolving collagen lens is available for similar coverage and application of drugs. This lens or shield is never used to cover deep ulcers or in the presence of uncontrolled infection.

CHAPTER 87

Iris and Ciliary Body (pages 1226–1231)

Indications for surgical manipulation of the iris and ciliary body are infrequent.

SURGICAL ANATOMY AND PHYSIOLOGY

The iris and ciliary body consist of two-layered epithelium of neuroectodermal origin. The iris epithelium is heavily pigmented with melanin in both layers. The bilayered posterior iris epithelium is pigmented even in blue-eyed individuals. The stromal melanin gives the iris its characteristic color. The pupillary sphincter constricts to produce miosis.

Ciliary body landmarks include the junction between the pars plana of the ciliary body and the peripheral retina; this area in dogs is located 8 mm posterior to the limbus superiorly and temporally but only 4 mm inferiorly and nasally. Iridocyclectomy extending posterior to the ora may cause peripheral retinal dialysis and detachment. The ciliary epithelium produces aqueous humor. The zonules arise from both the pars plana and the pars plicata of the ciliary body.

Fibrinous exudation from the iris vasculature and miosis are frequent surgical complications that can be minimized by preoperative treatment with systemic and topical antiprostaglandins. Intracameral application of agents such as epinephrine (1:100,000) and heparin (2 units/ml) can help maintain mydriasis and inhibit fibrin clot formation.

SPHINCTER IRIDOTOMY

The most common indication for sphincter iridotomy is enlargement of the pupillary aperture during cataract surgery. If the pupil constricts before lens extraction or is less than 3 mm after extraction, a one- to four-quadrant sphincterotomy is performed as necessary to enhance exposure or achieve at least a 5-mm pupil. Incision with scissors is less traumatic and more readily controlled.

PUPILLARY MEMBRANECTOMY

The formation of opaque pupillary iridocapsular membranes is one of the more common complications of extracapsular cataract extraction in dogs. If extensive, these membranes may impair vision or block the flow of aqueous, precipitating secondary glaucoma. In an aphakic animal, membranectomy is a simple and effective secondary procedure that frequently allows the patient to see. When available, a neodymium:yttrium-aluminum-garnet (Nd:YAG) laser is ideally suited to the incision of such membranes.

EXCISIONAL PROCEDURES FOR TREATMENT OF ANTERIOR UVEAL NEOPLASIA (pp. 1227–1229)

The therapeutic approach required for management of an anterior uveal mass is based on an accurate diagnosis. In cats, iritis may mimic neoplasia, with a nodular appearance unassociated with classic signs of flare and miosis. In such cases, a positive response to systemic and topical corticosteroids is usually diagnostic. For masses that are clearly neoplastic, a thorough systemic evaluation is necessary to differentiate primary ocular neoplasia from neoplasia that has metastasized from a distant site. The risks of a surgical procedure on an eye with a potentially malignant tumor must be weighed against the advantages of preserving a cosmetic, visual globe. Ocular melanomas in cats are often highly malignant, with widespread and fatal metastases. Limbal melanomas are consistently benign, although they may be locally invasive. The preferred treatment for limbal melanomas is partial excision and cryotherapy; iridocyclectomy is indicated only if the base of the iris is involved to a depth of more than 3 mm.

IRIDECTOMY (p. 1229)

Sector iridectomy is indicated for excisional biopsy of iris neoplasia.

IRIDOCYCLECTOMY

Partial excision of the iris and ciliary body is used infrequently for anterior uveal tumors. Anterior uveal malignant melanomas and ciliary body adenocarcinomas are usually diagnosed only when they have been present for some time and have extended into the aqueous outflow pathways or posteriorly into the choroid, retina, or deep sclera. The ideal surgical candidate has an uninvolved iridocorneal angle on gonioscopic examination, a discrete, well-defined lesion confined to the iris or ciliary body, and no secondary uveitis or glaucoma. The maximum tolerable extent of uveal excision is 45° to 60°. The possibility of residual neoplasm with the potential for metastasis is high.

REMOVAL OF ANTERIOR UVEAL CYSTS

Cysts of the iris and ciliary body epithelium may be attached to the ciliary processes or pupillary margin or may be free in the anterior chamber. These are distinguished by their regular margins and transparency. They may be aspirated if they become excessively large, if they contact the corneal endothelium, when a large number of cysts occlude the iridocorneal angle, resulting in glaucoma, or if vision is reduced.

A laser is ideally suited to the disruption of this avascular uveal tissue. An alternative surgical technique involves the use of two needles as described for a membranectomy.

CHAPTER 88

The Lens (pages 1231–1240)

Surgery of the lens is limited to extraction, which is indicated when visual impairment is due to opacification, when the lens is dislocated, and when lens-induced uveitis does not respond to medical therapy.

EMBRYOLOGY (p. 1231)

ANATOMY

A fully developed lens is composed of anterior and posterior capsules, anterior epithelium, and elongated cells (fibers). The lens is bounded by the anterior and posterior chambers and iris anteriorly and the vitreous posteriorly. Firm vitreolenticular adhesions are present.

The anterior lens capsule is thicker (about 50 μm) than the posterior capsule (about 4 μm). The capsule has elastic properties that permit alteration in lens shape owing to the effect of the ciliary muscle, which exerts traction on the lens capsule via the zonular fibers during accommodation.

The adult nucleus is continuously formed throughout life. As the cortical fibers are compressed concentrically, they become relatively dehydrated; in older animals, this process commonly results in nuclear sclerosis.

PHYSIOLOGY AND BIOCHEMISTRY

The lens refracts light, controlled to some extent by the process of accommodation. Most refraction in the eye takes place at the cornea. The lens in humans and some animals has the ability to change shape, thus allowing focus adjustments for objects at various distances. This process, called *accommodation,* requires a pliable lens and capsule, intact zonular fibers, and a functional ciliary muscle. Maintaining lens transparency is a primary function of the anterior lens epithelium and intact lens capsule.

IMMUNOLOGY

The lens is immunologically unique. If lens protein is exposed to the immune system, it is recognized as a foreign substance. Lens protein is sequestered and potentially antigenic for the following reasons: (1) The lens capsule is formed before the immune system develops; lens protein is thus never recognized as "self." (2) The lens is avascular. (3) The lens is enclosed by a capsule that is impermeable to cells and large molecules.

Lens protein may be exposed to the body by leakage through the lens capsule during liquefaction and resorption of a cataract, traumatic lens rupture, or extracapsular lens extraction. Leakage of soluble lens protein from a hypermature cataract may result in mild to moderate anterior uveitis. Acute traumatic lens rupture may result in severe intraocular inflammation. If most of the lens material is successfully removed, the resultant inflammation is mild and responsive to anti-inflammatory therapy. Intracapsular lens extraction results in minimal inflammation relative to other manipulations of the globe.

ROLE OF THE LENS IN AN ANIMAL'S VISION

Accommodation is poorly developed in domestic animals. Mature cataracts result in functional blindness. Successful cataract extraction allows restoration of functional vision—the ability to recognize people and objects.

CATARACTS (pp. 1232–1233)

Cataracts are a nonspecific disease that results in opacification of the lens fibers or capsule. Cataracts may be characterized clinically according to stage of development, location within the lens, age of the animal at the time of development, and etiology.

Stages of Development

Incipient. Focal opacification of the lens or its capsule. An affected animal can still see well.

Immature. Opacity is more or less diffuse. Fundic reflex is present, and the animal may experience some visual impairment.

Mature. Total dense opacification of the lens with absence of the fundic reflex. Visual function is significantly impaired. Cataract surgery is recommended at this stage.

Hypermature. Lens protein liquefies and may leak through the capsule. If leakage is extensive with significant resorption of protein, the lens capsule becomes wrinkled. Uveitis may result from leakage of lens protein.

Location

Cataracts may be capsular, subcapsular, cortical, nuclear, or axial or equatorial and anterior or posterior.

Age of the Animal

Congenital. Present at birth, congenital cataracts may be inherited or noninherited; inherited congenital cataracts are most commonly encountered in miniature schnauzers.

Developmental. A developmental cataract is an inherited bilateral cataract that occurs after birth, usually in young animals.

Senile. Senile cataracts occur in aged animals and precede or accompany nuclear sclerosis.

Etiology

Cataracts may occur secondary to ocular diseases, including uveitis, retinal degeneration, lens dislocation, and glaucoma. They may occur in association with diabetes mellitus and Cushing's disease, secondary to blunt or penetrating trauma.

CATARACT SURGERY (pp. 1233–1238)

Cataracts are a surgical disease. Extracapsular lens extraction is routinely performed for the majority of cataract extractions owing to the strong hyaloideocapsular ligament. With the extracapsular technique, the posterior lens capsule and vitreous face are not disturbed. Cataract extraction is a most successful and rewarding procedure.

Selection of Patients

The objective of cataract surgery is to restore functional vision. Functional vision is not significantly impaired until bilateral cataracts approach maturity. When the animal is constantly bumping into objects and is unable to maintain its normal life-style and personality, cataract extraction should be considered.

To evaluate the neural visual components, history, ophthalmoscopy, visual function tests, and electrophysiology should be used in combination.

Inherited retinal degenerations are the primary cause of failure in technically successful cataract surgery. The problem is complicated by the fact that breeds with a high incidence of inherited retinal degeneration, such as the miniature and toy poodle and the Irish setter, also have primary genetic cataracts unassociated with retinal disease.

Pupillary responses are unreliable as the sole method of assessing peripheral and central vision potential. These responses may persist in the presence of well-advanced retinal degeneration. Iris atrophy is frequently observed in miniature poodles and results in the absence of pupillary reflexes. Normal pupillary reflexes provide minimal information.

Without exception, visual and ophthalmoscopic changes in inherited retinal degeneration precede associated cataract development. If inherited retinal degeneration is present, a history of initial nyctalopia (night blindness) may be elicited. Critical ophthalmoscopy performed while the cataracts are still immature, rather than waiting until the fundus cannot be critically examined, is beneficial.

Generally, if a fundic reflex can be obtained, some vision should be present and should change minimally with alterations in ambient light if the retina is healthy. Electroretinography should be performed on all patients with cataracts and unobservable fundi; in those breeds with predisposition to inherited retinal degeneration, electroretinography is a prerequisite to cataract surgery.

Dogs between 1 and 3 years of age with inherited developmental cataracts may undergo spontaneous resorption of their cataracts. We prefer to manage these animals with topical application of 1.0 per cent atropine sulfate to enhance peripheral vision and corticosteroids to temper the uveitis. Surgical success rates in animals with previous uveitis are somewhat lower than in those with uncomplicated cataracts.

Thorough multisystem evaluation should be performed before cataract surgery.

Philosophies of Cataract Surgery

The procedure for cataract removal, when performed with appropriate preoperative treatment and instrumentation, is not difficult. However, the incidence of intraoperative or postoperative complications is high compared with other procedures, and these complications frequently have disastrous effects on the visual outcome. An experienced cataract surgeon, using an operating microscope and having the instrumentation necessary to perform vitrectomy, should anticipate success rates of 90 to 95 per cent.

Routine Procedures and Techniques

Adequate preoperative preparation minimizes intraoperative and postoperative complications. Pretreatment with antiprostaglandins and topical antibiotic-corticosteroids and mydriatics minimizes intraoperative miosis.

Two general approaches are available for the extraction of cataractous lenses: manual extracapsular extraction and phacoemulsification. Stable deep anesthesia and smooth recovery are important. Quiet recovery minimizes the likelihood of self-inflicted trauma.

Phacoemulsification uses ultrasonic energy to disrupt and liquefy the cataract, which is simultaneously aspirated. This technique represents the optimum in formed chamber surgery and greatly facilitates total cortical removal. The technique involves a smaller incision, formed chamber needle capsulectomy or capsulotomy, and disruption and aspiration of the cataract.

Postoperative care is critical and is aimed at reducing inflammation and maintaining pupil size. Topical 1.0 per cent atropine sulfate, 2.5 per cent phenylephrine, and antibiotic-corticosteroid solutions are applied as required to control pupillary size and inflammation. Bandages, Elizabethan collars, sedation, and analgesics are not routinely used because the surgery is tolerated well. Patients should be re-examined frequently after surgery.

Complications

Operative complications include miosis, hemorrhage, posterior capsular tears with vitreous presentation, and posterior capsular opacity.

Vitreous presentation occurs when the posterior capsule or zonules are unintentionally disrupted or in the presence of lens subluxation. Vitreous must be removed from the anterior chamber to reduce the likelihood of disastrous sequelae, including corneal edema associated with vitreous touch, pupillary block glaucoma, and retinal detachment. Vitrectomy is performed until the anterior chamber is completely free of vitreous and the iris plane assumes a concave appearance.

If the cataract has been present for some time, the posterior capsule may be translucent or opaque at the time of surgery. If the fundus cannot be readily observed at surgery, the capsule is incised or removed.

Postoperative complications include (1) pupillary membrane with or without pupillary occlusion and secondary glaucoma, (2) corneal edema, (3) glaucoma without pupillary obstruction, and (4) retinal detachment. Although focal opacification of the posterior capsule and synechiae of the iris to the posterior capsule are common, functional vision persists around the secondary cataract if a pupil is maintained. Scarring of the limbal cornea in the area of incision is expected and is of no consequence.

LENS DISLOCATION (pp. 1238–1240)

Lens dislocation can be complete (luxation) or partial (subluxation, with some intact zonules remaining). The lens may dislocate into the anterior chamber (anterior luxation) or the vitreous (posterior luxation) or may remain within the retropupillary space (subluxation). The condition is a spontaneous bilateral problem in the terrier breeds, most likely related to inherited zonular weakness. Obstruction of aqueous flow from the posterior to anterior chamber by the dislocated lens or displaced vitreous frequently causes secondary glaucoma.

Lens extraction is recommended in all cases of anterior lens luxation and subluxation associated with clinical disease (glaucoma or anterior uveitis). Intracapsular extraction is the technique of choice for a primary dislocated lens.

Anterior lens luxation is a nonelective surgical procedure owing to the potential for damage to the corneal endothelium or glaucoma as a result of pupillary block. Preoperative topical pilocarpine may maintain a small pupil, which traps the lens in the anterior chamber and facilitates extraction. If the intraocular pressure is significantly elevated (greater than 40 mm Hg), intravenous mannitol is given at 1 mg/kg 1 hour before surgery to minimize vitreous presentation and spontaneous choroidal hemorrhage.

Exposure of the anterior chamber and approach to it are identical to those used during extracapsular lens extraction. Postoperative complications include corneal edema, pupillary membrane, persistent glaucoma, and retinal detachment. Continued elevation of pressure uncontrollable by medication is an indication for further surgical intervention.

Retinal detachment is the most common and discouraging of complications. The majority of detachments occur 2 to 4 weeks postoperatively and are associated with peripheral tears of the retina.

CHAPTER 89

Surgery of the Vitreous and Retina (pages 1241–1245)

"Open sky" anterior vitrectomy is a commonly performed, essential technique in the treatment of anterior vitreous presentation with rupture of the anterior hyaloid membrane that may occur during removal of dislocated or cataractous lenses. Otherwise, vitreoretinal surgery is undeveloped in veterinary ophthalmic surgery for two reasons. First, the number of animals with posterior segment disease that would benefit by manipulative intervention is low. Second, surgery in the posterior segment requires instrumentation not readily available and skills not highly developed by most veterinary ophthalmic surgeons.

VITREOUS (pp. 1240–1243)

Surgical Anatomy and Physiology

The vitreous is a transparent hydrated connective tissue consisting of collagen and mucopolysaccharides, primarily hyaluronic acid, that fills the posterior segment of the globe.

Collagen fibrils within the vitreous are continuous with Müller cell processes, which form the internal limiting membrane of the retina. Firm areas of attachment to adjacent structures occur at three locations: the peripheral posterior lens capsule (hyaloideocapsular ligament), the ora ciliaris retinae (vitreous base), and the margin of the optic nerve.

Development of Vitrectomy

Removal of opaque vitreous was first performed in man using an approach through the pars plana. Modifications have been used to clear vitreal opacities, to treat retinal detachment by reducing traction and removing vitreous sequestered behind the detachment, to remove posterior segment foreign bodies, and to prevent anterior vitreal prolapse in aphakic eyes.

Techniques of vitreous removal have involved use of cellulose sponges with transection of fibrils using scissors. Mechanized suction cutters, either rotating or oscillating, minimize retinal traction. Controversy has existed over proper replacement of vitreous with a substance of similar properties. Balanced salt solution is most practical for use in veterinary ophthalmology.

Pathophysiology and Indications

Any process altering the volume or structure of the vitreous may cause retinal detachment. Syneresis, or liquefaction, of the vitreous can occur as a result of senile changes or inflammation. Postinflammatory scarring, or cicatrization, can result in the formation of traction bands that separate the inner retina from the underlying pigmented epithelium.

Vitreal surgery in animals is rarely a primary or elective procedure. Asteroid hyalosis is unlikely to significantly affect functional vision. Vitreous or subretinal aspiration may be performed as a diagnostic tool. Vitrectomy may be used to remove persistent hyperplastic primary vitreous. The most frequent indication for vitrectomy occurs during intracapsular extraction of a dislocated lens in which some degree of vitreal prolapse is expected owing to the firm attachment of the posterior lens capsule to the anterior hyaloid membrane.

Vitreous in the anterior chamber is removed because (1) it can physically obstruct circulation of aqueous through the pupil and iridocorneal angle; (2) it provides a scaffolding for growth of membranes and adhesions; and (3) when in contact with corneal endothelium, it causes endothelial dysfunction and corneal edema.

Techniques

Vitreous Aspiration

Aspiration of liquefied vitreous can be performed through the pars plana. These techniques are not recommended unless a suction cutting machine is not available.

Pars Plana Vitrectomy

Pars plana vitrectomy is uncommonly used. The globe is entered over the pars plana ciliaris, 6 to 8 mm behind the limbus; an anterior approach may result in ciliary trauma and hemorrhage or damage to the lens.

Anterior Vitrectomy

Once formed vitreous is present in the anterior chamber, anterior vitrectomy is necessary. Cellulose sponges absorb the liquid components and adhere to formed vitreous, facilitating gentle elevation.

Vitreophages combine controlled suction with atraumatic tissue resection via a rotating or guillotine-like blade within an aspirating needle. These instruments markedly reduce the time required for vitrectomy, minimize traction on the retina, and are particularly applicable when more than a small amount of vitreous must be removed. Limitations of this technique are as its name implies—the open sky anterior vitrectomy does not allow observation or control much beyond the equator.

Complications

Complications of vitrectomy may occur at surgery or in the postoperative period.

Complications of anterior vitrectomy associated with canine lens removal include corneal edema, retinal detachment, and glaucoma. Excessive manipulation and traction on the vitreous can lead to retinal detachment. During pars plana vitrectomy, failure to cut cleanly through the vitreous base may push the vitreous ahead of the needle, the resulting traction producing retinal dialysis and detachment. Hemorrhage may result from cutting fibrovascular membranes.

RETINA (pp. 1243–1244)

Repair of retinal detachments requires an understanding of the pathophysiology of the posterior segment.

Pathophysiology and Indications

Retinal detachments are (1) rhegmatogenous—that is, associated with a retinal tear or hole through which, when combined with vitreous traction and liquefication, vitreous enters; (2) tractional, in which neurosensory retina is pulled off the retinal pigment epithelium; or (3) exudative/hemorrhagic, in which the primary disease involves the choroidal vasculature or retinal pigment epithelium to allow plasma transudate, exudate, or hemorrhage to accumulate between the photoreceptors and retinal pigment epithelium. Separation of photoreceptors from their source of nutrition (the choriocapillaris) and their photopigment recycling factories (the retinal pigment epithelium) initiates photoreceptor degeneration. Prognosis for vision depends on duration. It is not likely that reattachments will result in vision if the detachment is prolonged.

Indications for surgical reattachment include a rhegmatogenous detachment or a tractional detachment.

Techniques

Tractional detachments require pars plana vitrectomy as well as appositional techniques. Rhegmatogenous detachments are repaired by the drainage of subretinal fluid, apposition of neurosensory retina to retinal pigment epithelium at the hole or tear, and creation of chorioretinal adhesions adjacent to the defect.

CHAPTER 90

Orbit (pages 1245–1263)

The orbit is the bony cavity surrounding the eye. Orbital surgery should not be attempted without a thorough understanding of orbital anatomy.

The dorsolateral wall of the orbit is formed by the orbital ligament between the zygomatic process of the frontal bone and the frontal process of the zygomatic bone. The soft-tissue contents of the orbit are enclosed by the periorbita. The periorbita also surrounds the extraocular muscles and forms Tenon capsule, which blends with the sclera and conjunctiva near the limbus. The periorbita is continuous with the periosteum of the facial bones around the orbital rim, the orbital septum, and the dura of the optic nerve at the optic foramen. The lacrimal gland lies beneath the orbital ligament on the dorsolateral surface of the globe.

PATHOLOGICAL MECHANISMS (pp. 1248–1250)

The orbit is a confined space. Changes in the volume and contents of the orbit affect the position of the globe in relation to the orbital rim, the face, and the other eye. The periorbita and extraocular muscles provide three possible compartments: (1) within the muscle cone, (2) outside the muscle cone but within the periorbita, or (3) within the bony walls of the orbit but outside the periorbita.

Space-occupying lesions displace normal orbital contents, causing protrusion of the third eyelid rostrally, exophthalmos, and swelling behind the last upper molar (Fig. 90–1). Accurate differentiation between exophthalmos and buphthalmos is essential (see Chapter 91).

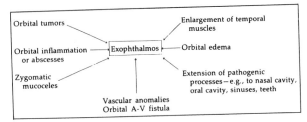

Figure 90–1. Mechanisms of exophthalmos.

The position of space-occupying lesions alters the direction in which the globe is displaced and is useful in localizing a mass. Exophthalmos leads to increased evaporation of the precorneal tear film with exposure keratitis, ulceration, and conjunctivitis.

The proximity of the paranasal sinuses, teeth, zygomatic gland, and vertical ramus of the mandible to the orbit influences the extension of disease processes in these structures. Orbital infection or cellulitis can be caused by infections of the roots of the molar teeth or foreign body penetration of the ventral orbit. A discharging fistula beneath the eye is also a common sign of abscessed tooth roots. When the mouth is opened, the vertical ramus of the mandible moves forward, pressing on the orbital contents and causing pain if cellulitis or abscess is present.

DIAGNOSTIC METHODS AND SIGNS OF ORBITAL DISEASE (pp. 1250–1252) (Table 90–1)

The most common sign of orbital disease is displacement of the third eyelid and globe. Other signs include chemosis, conjunctival erythema, periorbital swelling, pain on opening the mouth if inflammation is present, neurological deficits including blindness, and posterior indentation of the globe.

Thorough diagnostic evaluation can help differentiate surgical disease from nonsurgical disease and permit more directed surgical approaches. Thorough palpation, complete cranial nerve evaluation, ocular examination (including the fundus), and examination of the oral cavity and nasal passages represent a preliminary evaluation of the orbit, orbital contents, and contiguous structures.

Palpation of the orbit is essential; the bony orbital rim and ventral orbit (via the oral cavity) may be palpated directly. The posterior orbit may be palpated by using the globe as an extension of the palpating finger (ballottement). Inability to retropulse the globe or retropulsion in an abnormal direction may suggest the location and extent of retrobulbar lesions.

If fundus indentation is "fixed in the fundus," it moves within the extraocular muscle cone. If it "rolls" across the fundus as the eye moves, the lesion usually is outside the cone. Elevation and palpation of the base of the third eyelid may localize the lesion to the third eyelid. Ultrasonography and fine-needle aspiration often result in a specific diagnosis. Exploratory orbitotomy is reserved for therapeutic purposes if possible.

ORBITAL DISORDERS (pp. 1252–1254)

Orbital Inflammation

Orbital inflammation may be diffuse, with or without abscessation, or may be localized, involving masticatory muscles, extraocular muscles, or other specific orbital structures. Diffuse cellulitis is often associated with a foreign body or infection introduced locally or by hematogenous spread.

Clinical signs of orbital inflammation include pyrexia, chemosis, protrusion of the third eyelid, conjunctival congestion, decreased or painful retropulsion of the globe, pain on opening the mouth, variable exophthalmos, fluctuating red swelling in the oral mucous membrane behind the last upper molar tooth, periorbital swelling, and anorexia.

It is often impossible to distinguish orbital cellulitis from abscess. Orbital inflammation is distinguished from other causes of exophthalmos by its acute onset, pain, pyrexia, and the frequent occurrence of leukocytosis with neutrophilia. Accurate diagnosis should be pursued vigorously, because major differential diagnoses include aggressive neoplasia and systemic mycoses, which require early and specific treatment.

Treatment

Cellulitis and abscesses are treated by ventral drainage to the oral cavity and systemic and local antibiotics. Exploratory orbitotomy may occasionally be required if response to therapy is poor or to locate foreign bodies.

Zygomatic Mucocele

A mucocele is a leakage of saliva from a gland or duct with inflammation and fibrosis. Mucocele of the zygomatic salivary gland beneath the eye occurs spontaneously in dogs.

Clinical signs include protrusion of the oral mucous membrane behind the last upper molar, the presence of a mass in the ventral conjunctival fornix, protrusion of the third eyelid, exophthalmos, and painless orbital swelling. Treatment is resection of the gland and mucocele.

Orbital Emphysema

Air may enter the orbit from the paranasal sinuses after trauma, from the nasolacrimal duct after enucleation, or from an erosion of the wall of an adjacent sinus. Air is palpable as crepitus beneath the conjunctiva or periocular skin.

SURGICAL PROCEDURES

Enucleation

Enucleation is removal of the globe and the third eyelid. It is indicated for intraocular neoplasia, severe perforating ocular trauma, uncontrollable endophthalmitis or panophthalmitis, and intractable glaucoma when other treatment methods have failed. Cryotherapy, intrascleral prostheses, and laser therapy have almost eliminated the need for enucleation in glaucoma therapy. In dogs and cats, the lateral subconjunctival technique gives excellent results.

Lateral Subconjunctival Enucleation

Postoperative swelling is common but usually resolves in 3 to 4 days. With enucleation, orbital fat and extraocular muscles are retained, making the defect after healing more cosmetic than after exenteration. A number of techniques have been used to reduce the orbital defect. Silicone prostheses are the latest to gain acceptance.

TABLE 90–1. SUMMARY OF ORBITAL DISEASES*

Type of Disorder	Condition	Clinical Signs
Developmental abnormalities	1. Shallow orbit (brachycephalic breeds)	1. Exophthalmos, exposure keratitis, corneal ulceration, pigmentation
	2. Microphthalmos, anophthalmos	2. Small or absent globe, narrow palpebral fissure, prominent third eyelid, epiphora, blindness
	3. Hydrocephalus with orbital malformation	3. Exotropia, hypotropia, poor vision
	4. Euryblepharon	4. Long palpebral fissure resulting in apparent exophthalmos
	5. Orbital arteriovenous fistula	5. Exophthalmos, fremitus, pulse detectable (''exophthalmos pulsans'')
Trauma	1. Hemorrhages	1. Subconjunctival and episcleral hemorrhages; retrobulbar hemorrhage with exophthalmos or proptosis
	2. Penetrating foreign bodies (grass awns, needles, etc., from mouth)	2. Discharging sinus fluid through the conjunctiva, periocular skin, buccal mucosa; pain on opening mouth
	3. Orbital fractures	3. Pain, crepitus; skin abrasions, displacement of globe
Infections	1. Bacterial, fungal	1. Ocular discharge usually secondary to penetrating foreign bodies from conjunctiva or oral cavity; sinusitis, rhinitis, or infections of roots of teeth
	2. Parasites *(Dirofilaria immitis; Pneumonyssus caninum)*	2. Granulomatous lesions due to wandering larvae, e.g., *Dirofilaria* (rare), or extension of infection from nasal cavity *(Pneumonyssus)*

Neoplasia	1. Primary orbital neoplasms—sarcoma, meningioma, adenocarcinoma from nasal cavity, lymphosarcoma in cattle	1. Exophthalmos, exposure keratitis, strabismus, displacement of globe
	2. As for (1), plus nasal or neurological signs	
Miscellaneous conditions	1. Zygomatic mucocele	1. Exophthalmos, strabismus, swelling in any part of orbit or behind upper last molar tooth
		2. Discharging fistula beneath eye in dogs
	2. Infections of roots of teeth (especially carnassial)	
	3. Dehydration	3. Enophthalmos, protrusion of third eyelid
	4. Eosinophilic myositis	4. Exophthalmos, pain with dysphagia in acute stage; enophthalmos potentiated by opening mouth in chronic stage when temporal muscles have atrophied
	5. Horner's syndrome	5. Enophthalmos, miosis, ptosis, protrusion of nictitating membrane, ipsilateral sweating in horses, dermal vasodilation, and hypothermia

*Reprinted with permission from Slatter D: *Fundamentals of Veterinary Ophthalmology.* W.B. Saunders, Philadelphia, 1990. Modified from Smith JS: Diseases of the orbit. *In* Kirk RW (ed): *Current Veterinary Therapy VI.* W.B. Saunders, Philadelphia, 1977.

All enucleated globes should be examined histologically, because the clinical reason for enucleation is frequently inaccurate. Foreign materials should not be placed in the orbit before closure.

Exenteration

Exenteration is removal of the globe, adnexa, and orbital contents. Transpalpebral exenteration differs from enucleation in that the lids are incised initially and the plane of dissection is outside the extraocular muscles rather than adjacent to the sclera. Orbital contents are removed with this method. Orbital implants are contraindicated after this procedure.

Evisceration

Evisceration is removal of the contents of the globe. It is performed before insertion of an intrascleral prosthesis in the treatment of advanced glaucoma.

Orbitotomy

There are a number of approaches to the orbit.

1. Dorsal, nasal, and temporal transconjunctival approach, for lesions anterior to the equator of the globe
2. Limited orbitotomy with transection of the orbital ligament for lesions posterior to the globe
3. Dorsal orbitotomy for exposure of the dorsal and medial orbit
4. Complete orbitotomy with zygomatic arch resection for extensive orbital exposure

Dorsal Conjunctival Approach

The dorsal conjunctival approach is used for lesions either inside or outside the muscle cone. A perilimbal incision is made through the conjunctiva, and dissection is continued either above or beneath the insertions of the dorsal rectus and dorsal oblique muscles, depending on the site of the lesion in relation to the muscle cone.

Nasal and Temporal Transconjunctival Approaches

Nasal and temporal transconjunctival approaches may be used for lesions located nasally or temporally and anterior to the equator. An inferonasal approach is useful for periorbital epidermoid cysts, masses, or foreign bodies involving the base of the third eyelid.

Partial Orbitotomy with Orbital Ligament Transection

Partial orbitotomy with orbital ligament transection is useful for removal of zygomatic mucoceles and lesions in the lateral orbit of a dog. Transecting the short ligament in cats seldom improves exposure.

Lateral Orbitotomy with Zygomatic Arch Resection

Lateral orbitomy with zygomatic arch resection is an extensive and time-consuming approach. It affords excellent exposure of deeper orbital structures and is indicated for removal of neoplasms and foreign bodies and for diagnostic and experimental procedures.

Dorsal Orbitotomy
OCULAR PROSTHESES (p. 1262)

Prostheses for ocular use in animals are of three types: intraorbital, intrascleral, and extrascleral.

Orbital Prosthesis

Implantation of a silicone prosthesis after enucleation or exenteration reduces the facial distortion caused by removal of orbital contents. Extrusion of the prosthesis is rare.

Intrascleral Prosthesis

An intrascleral silicone prosthesis is used in dogs and cats in the treatment of chronic intractable glaucoma in blind, painful eyes. In buphthalmic eyes, the sclera and cornea shrink to conform to the size of the prosthesis. Complications of the technique are minimal.

Extrascleral Prosthesis

An extrascleral prosthesis is a porcelain or acrylic hemisphere that is manufactured to fit over the surface of a phthitic or deformed eye. An eye is painted on the surface of the prosthesis after it has been accurately fitted.

CHAPTER 91

Glaucoma (pages 1263–1276)

Glaucoma is an important therapeutic enigma in dogs because of its relatively high incidence in certain breeds (Table 91–1) and in cats because the subtle signs usually result in presentation late in the disease. Because various conditions may precipitate glaucoma, a thorough examination should be performed on the normal and the affected eye.

Glaucoma is defined as an elevation in intraocular pressure (IOP)

TABLE 91–1. BREED PREDISPOSITION AND USUAL FORMS OF GLAUCOMA

American cocker spaniel	Closed angle
Bouvier des Flandres	Closed angle
Basset hound	Closed angle
Chow chow	Closed angle
Samoyed	Closed angle
Siberian husky	Closed angle
Norwegian elkhound	Closed and open angle
Brittany spaniel	Closed angle
Beagle	Open angle
Miniature and toy poodle	Open and closed angle
Welsh springer spaniel	Closed angle
Wire- and smooth-haired fox terrier	Lens displacement ± closed angle
Sealyham terrier	Lens displacement

that is accompanied by impaired ocular function. In view of the advanced state of nerve fiber loss that is present in animals before visual signs are manifested, it is obvious why it is difficult to keep animals seeing when presented with this complaint.

The reported upper limit of normal IOP is 27 to 30 mm Hg, as measured with a Schiøtz tonometer and using the human conversion tables. Two separate conversion tables for the Schiøtz tonometer have been calculated, one for dogs and one for cats (Tables 91–2 and 91–3). The IOP should not vary more than 5 mm Hg between eyes of the same dog.

TABLE 91–2. CALIBRATION TABLE FOR SCHIØTZ TONOMETRY IN DOGS

Schiøtz Scale Reading	IOP (mm Hg) 5.5 g wt.	IOP (mm Hg) 7.5 g wt.	IOP (mm Hg) 10.0 g wt.
0.5	46	61	75
1.0	44	59	73
1.5	43	56	70
2.0	40	53	66
2.5	33	47	61
3.0	26	40	55
3.5	23	35	49
4.0	21	32	44
4.5	20	29	41
5.0	19	27	38
5.5	18	26	36
6.0	17	24	33
6.5	16	23	31
7.0	15	22	30
7.5		20	28
8.0	14	19	27
8.5	13		25
9.0		18	24
9.5	12	17	23
10.0		16	22
10.5	11	15	21
11.0			20
11.5	10	14	19
12.0		13	18
12.5			17
13.0		12	16
13.5	8	11	15
14.0			
14.5		10	14
15.0	7		13
15.5		9	12
16.0			
16.5	6	8	11
17.0			10
17.5		7	
18.0	5		9
18.5		6	
19.0			8
19.5			7
20.0		5	

IOP, intraocular pressure.

From Pickett P, et al: Calibration of the Schiøtz tonometer for the canine and feline eye. Transactions of the 19th Annual Scientific Program of the American College of Veterinary Ophthalmologists *19:*47, 1988.

TABLE 91-3. CALIBRATION TABLE FOR SCHIØTZ TONOMETRY IN CATS

Schiøtz Scale Reading	IOP (mm Hg) 5.5 g wt.	IOP (mm Hg) 7.5 g wt.	IOP (mm Hg) 10.0 g wt.
0.5	44	73	
1.0	42	71	
1.5	40	68	
2.0	37	65	80
2.5	33	61	76
3.0	30	56	71
3.5	27	48	66
4.0	25	42	61
4.5	24	37	56
5.0	22	34	51
5.5	21	31	47
6.0	20	29	44
6.5	18	27	40
7.0		25	37
7.5	17	24	35
8.0	16	22	33
8.5	15	21	31
9.0	14	20	29
9.5	13	19	27
10.0		18	25
10.5		17	23
11.0	12	16	22
11.5	11	15	20
12.0		14	19
12.5	10	13	18
13.0		12	17
13.5	9		15
14.0		11	14
14.5	8	10	13
15.0			12
15.5		9	11
16.0	7	8	10
16.5			9
17.0	6	7	8
17.5		6	7
18.0			6
18.5	5	5	5
19.0			
20.0			

IOP, intraocular pressure.
From Pickett P, et al: Calibration of the Schiøtz tonometer for the canine and feline eye. Transactions of the 19th Annual Scientific Program of the American College of Veterinary Ophthalmologists *19:*47, 1988.

ANATOMY AND PHYSIOLOGY

Aqueous humor is produced continuously by the ciliary processes and leaves the eye mainly via the iridocorneal angle. In relation to external landmarks, the ciliary processes are 4 mm posterior to the limbus dorsally and 3 mm in the remaining regions. Aqueous produced in the posterior chamber flows through the pupil and leaves mainly through the iridocorneal angle.

CLINICAL SIGNS AND DIAGNOSTIC TECHNIQUES
(pp. 1265–1268)

The signs of glaucoma are generally pressure dependent. It is not until the IOP reaches the mid-40s that typical external signs of vascular injection, pupillary dilation, and corneal edema appear.

Increased Intraocular Pressure

All signs of glaucoma are nonspecific, necessitating an objective means of measurement of IOP. An accurate objective measurement is required for monitoring the response to therapy when an obvious hypotony does not develop.

Tonometry is the measurement of intraocular tension. The most practical instrument for tonometry in dogs is the Schiøtz tonometer, which measures the amount of corneal indentation that a plunger with a given weight produces. Applanation tonometry measures the force necessary to flatten or applanate the cornea over a given surface area of a plunger.

Dilated Pupil

The pupil dilates at about 45 to 50 mm Hg. Mydriasis is neither a sensitive nor specific sign of glaucoma.

Conjunctival and Episcleral Vascular Injection

Various degrees of vascular injection are present in most cases of canine glaucoma. Vascular injection occurs before pupil dilation and is similar to that in intraocular inflammation. Large conjunctival veins that bend near the limbus and drain the episcleral and scleral plexus are selectively injected.

Corneal Pathology

Corneal opacification occurs with increased IOP by disruption of the normal corneal stromal lamellar arrangement, resulting in light scattering, and from corneal edema. Stretching of the globe frequently results in breaks (Descemet streaks) that are permanent and specific for glaucoma. Chronic corneal edema combined with lagophthalmos and decreased corneal sensation usually results in a degenerative pannus or a superficially scarred cornea. Corneal scarring may significantly alter Schiøtz tonometer readings.

Fundus Abnormalities

With higher pressure, retinal vascular attenuation, optic disc hemorrhages, and papilledema may be visible. In chronic IOP elevations, peripapillary or diffuse hyper-reflectivity of the tapetum and attenuation of the retinal vessels may be seen. The optic nerve usually develops cupping, loss of myelin, and change in color to grayish white in ic cases.

Pain

with primary glaucoma have epiphora but lack blepha-
lar pain that is recognized by the owner. Once the IOP
rmal, it is common for owners to comment on how
appears. Pain with glaucoma is usually manifested

as sleepiness, depression, irritability, and reduced playfulness. Pain should be considered present even if it is not a complaint.

Decreased Vision or Blindness

Increased IOP for 2 to 4 hours to a few days may cause loss of vision in acute high-pressure glaucoma, or an insidious loss may occur with modest elevations of IOP or pressure that has gradually increased. One of the frustrations of treating glaucoma is late presentation for therapy. Client education and experience usually result in earlier presentation of the second eye in patients with primary glaucoma.

Buphthalmos

Enlargement of the globe is a typical and specific but not sensitive sign of canine glaucoma. Once significantly stretched, the globe remains large even after the IOP returns to normal.

Luxated Lens

Various degrees of lens luxation are commonly associated with glaucoma, and it is often difficult to determine cause and effect. Signs of subluxation are an aphakic crescent, iridodonesis, and alterations in depth of the anterior chamber and vitreous strands. Lens luxation into the anterior chamber may precipitate glaucoma or may turn chronic glaucoma into an acute syndrome.

Aqueous Flare

Increased aqueous protein and pigment clumps may be observed in many forms of glaucoma.

CLASSIFICATION AND PATHOGENESIS OF GLAUCOMA
(pp. 1268–1269)

Glaucoma is divided into two broad categories, primary and secondary, and these in turn are each subdivided according to the gonioscopic findings of an open or closed angle. Primary glaucoma is glaucoma not caused solely by acquired intraocular lesions. Most cases of primary glaucoma in dogs are associated with bilateral closed angles. In severe goniodysgenesis, a sheet of iris-like tissue replaces the pectinate ligament. On close inspection of closed angles in normotensive eyes, flow holes can be observed near the corneal insertion of the obstructing sheet. These holes are presumably more prone to obstruction, and if obstruction occurs suddenly, an acute syndrome may develop. If slowly progressive closure occurs, an insidious onset of glaucoma results. Primary open-angle glaucoma is relatively rare in dogs.

Feline glaucoma is more subtle and consequently is presented in the late stages. Secondary glaucoma associated with inflammation is the most common form. Secondary glaucoma is associated with acquired diseases that alter fluid dynamics at the pupil or angle and may vary from inflammation to neoplasia.

EMERGENCY THERAPY (pp. 1269–1271)

All recently functional eyes should be treated with emergency medi[cal] therapy to reduce IOP whether surgery is planned or not. A delay [of] several hours may be critical, considering the high IOPs that are o[ften] present.

Systemic Therapy

Emergency therapy is administration of osmotic diuretics. Osmotic diuretics create a hyperosmolar vascular space, which withdraws extravascular fluid into the vessels. Water is restricted for 2 to 3 hours so that the drug effect is not neutralized.

Mannitol and glycerol are routinely used. Mannitol, 1 to 2 g/kg, is given by slow push intravenous injection over 5 minutes or by slow intravenous drip. The hypotensive effect occurs in about 15 to 30 minutes and usually lasts for 4 to 6 hours, although some patients have a prolonged response for up to 48 hours. Repeat injections of mannitol can be given, but dehydration may reach critical levels. Caution should be used in animals with cardiac disease.

Orally administered glycerol (glycerin) lowers the IOP within 15 to 30 minutes. A dose of 1 to 2 g/kg PO may cause gastric irritation and vomiting, but it is nontoxic and does not induce diuresis like mannitol.

Carbonic anhydrase inhibitors (CAIs) are the second type of drug used (Table 91–4). CAIs decrease aqueous secretion by about 40 to 50 per cent and have a minimal effect on the facility of outflow. Intravenous acetazolamide is available and may produce a recognizable reduction in pressure after 10 minutes. Some patients do not tolerate any of the products at therapeutic doses, but intolerance to one does not imply intolerance to all. The primary side effects noted are panting, vomiting, anorexia, and acidosis. Vestibular signs of nystagmus and circling and apparent paresthesias have also been noted.

Topical Therapy

Epinephrine decreases aqueous formation and increases outflow facility. The main indication for use of epinephrine is open-angle glaucoma.

The use of miotics in emergency therapy is restricted to direct-acting agents such as pilocarpine. The more potent cholinesterase inhibitors are avoided because of their systemic toxicity if used frequently, as well as their potentiation of bleeding and inflammation if surgery is performed. The mydriasis of glaucoma is not overcome with miotics until the pressure is lowered.

Pilocarpine solution 2.0 per cent is the most efficient concentration with no additional benefits resulting from the higher concentrations. Although minimal ocular effects are noted while the IOP is elevated, pilocarpine is given to be present when the pressure is lowered. Administration at 30-minute intervals for two treatments and then at 6-hour intervals delivers adequate drug concentration without complicating systemic side effects.

Timolol maleate, betaxolol, and levobunolol are beta-adrenergic blockers. A significant lowering of IOP has not been noted in normal dogs given commercial concentrations.

Emergency medical therapy consists of an osmotic diuretic, a CAI (oral or intravenous), and topical pilocarpine. Once the IOP is lowered,

BLE 91–4. CARBONIC ANHYDRASE INHIBITORS FOR GLAUCOMA THERAPY

ug	Dose (mg/kg)	Frequency of Administration
de	10–30	BID to TID
nide	2–4	BID to TID
	2–4	BID to TID

maintenance therapy with a CAI and pilocarpine is continued to determine the chronic response to therapy. Most cases of acute high-pressure glaucoma are associated with closed angles or mechanical obstructive phenomena and respond poorly to chronic medical therapy. Persistence with medical therapy simply delays the inevitable surgical procedure, allowing more ocular damage to occur from erratic control. Owners should be forewarned so that the decision for surgery can be made early in the course of therapy.

SURGICAL THERAPY (pp. 1271–1275)

Before surgical procedures are attempted on a glaucomatous eye, a thorough ophthalmic examination must be performed to determine the cause of the glaucoma and select the most rational therapy and prognosis. Selection of therapy may depend on restoration of vision as opposed to cosmetic appearance and pain relief alone.

Surgical therapy is categorized into those procedures that increase aqueous outflow, those that decrease aqueous production, and salvage procedures used to relieve pain and provide a cosmetically acceptable eye. Salvage procedures are not acceptable for a potentially functional eye.

Surgical procedures such as iridencleisis, corneoscleral trephination, cyclodialysis, sclerectomy, anterior chamber implantation of aqueous shunts, and combinations of these procedures have been used to overcome the angle obstruction. The success rate has been reported to be 30 to 50 per cent, and few surgeons persist with these procedures.

Luxated Lens Removal

The role of lens displacement and lens luxation in canine glaucoma is not understood. Lens displacement may produce glaucoma, may be the result of glaucoma, or may be an exciting event in precipitating glaucoma. Removal of a displaced lens may simplify or eliminate the need for medical management if the drainage angle remains partially open. Anteriorly luxated lenses should be removed from eyes that are still functional. Removal of a luxated lens is an intracapsular procedure. Postoperative management is similar to that for routine cataract extraction. Retinal detachments are relatively common after intracapsular extractions with vitreous loss.

Procedures That Decrease Aqueous Production

Methods of damaging the ciliary body are cyclodiathermy, cyclocryotherapy, laser ablation, focused ultrasound, and chemical ablation.

Cyclodiathermy is the application of intense heat within the ciliary body. This technique produces severe postoperative inflammation and is unpredictable, frequently resulting in phthisis bulbi. Trans-scleral application of a laser at 8 J per site has been used to produce necrosis of the ciliary body. The expense of this form of laser precludes its wide availability.

Cyclocryotherapy or cold applications to the ciliary body also destroy the ciliary epithelium and decrease aqueous production. The cryogen used for freezing the ciliary epithelium is liquid nitrogen. Repeat freeze-thaw cycles in a given location are no more effective than single freezes and result in more severe postoperative chemosis. Overzealous cryotherapy may occasionally result in phthisis bulbi. After cryotherapy, marked conjunctivitis, chemosis, and uveitis occur. A subconjunctival injection of 0.5 to 1.0 mg of dexamethasone is administered at the end of the cryotherapy, and topical antibiotic-steroids are administered for 10 to 14 days.

The IOP may gradually increase as ciliary epithelium regenerates. If IOP increases, medical management may control the pressure. Cyclocryotherapy with liquid nitrogen has been more successful than nitrous oxide in controlling IOP in patients requiring repeat freezing.

Cyclocryotherapy is advantageous over filtering procedures because it is noninvasive, easily repeatable, less expensive, technically easier, and more successful. Success rates as high as 90 per cent have been reported, but cats do not respond as well as dogs to cyclocryotherapy. Prophylactic cryotherapy on an eye with ocular hypertension but no clinical signs of glaucoma is not recommended.

Cyclocryotherapy is useful for narrow-, closed-, and open-angle glaucoma. Glaucoma secondary to uveal inflammation responds but with a lower success rate than primary glaucoma.

Salvage Surgical Procedures for Glaucoma

Ocular Prosthesis

Ocular evisceration and insertion of a prosthesis are indicated in chronically blind, painful eyes that do not have an ocular tumor, infection, or deep corneal ulcer. Preservation of a nearly normal eye is very desirable to most owners, who invariably elect the prosthesis over enucleation. If the globe is greatly enlarged, the contralateral normal eye is measured for the size of implant.

Once all intraocular contents are removed, the black sphere is positioned with a sphere introducer. The ocular contents should be submitted for histopathological examination in patients that have not had clear media.

Postoperative complications include extrusion of the implant through a central corneal ulceration, recurrence of an unsuspected ocular tumor around the implant, and extrusion due to intraocular infection. Despite occasional failures, the prosthesis is a viable alternative to enucleation for a painful glaucomatous globe.

Enucleation

Enucleation is indicated mainly in glaucoma associated with an intraocular tumor or overwhelming infection. The low cost and high efficacy of cyclocryosurgery and intraocular implants make enucleation the last choice of all the surgical procedures available for treating canine glaucoma.

SUMMARY

Most cases of glaucoma cannot be adequately or consistently controlled with medical therapy and require surgery. The type of surgical procedure selected depends on the equipment available, whether return of vision is a goal, the cause of glaucoma, and the surgeon's preference. Cyclocryotherapy is the procedure of choice.

CHAPTER 92

Ocular Emergencies and Trauma (pages 1276–1292)

EVALUATION OF THE TRAUMATIZED EYE (pp. 1276–1277)

Ocular emergencies include corneal abrasion or chemical irritation, lid laceration, corneal foreign body, acute infectious keratitis, corneal or scleral laceration, contusion and penetrating intraocular injury, proptosis of the globe, endophthalmitis, and acute glaucoma.

  1. Obtain an adequate history from the owner.
  2. Examine the eye for any discharge, blepharospasm, or photophobia. If a severe corneal ulcer, laceration, or penetrating wound is present, the animal is anesthetized and preparations are made for surgery before examination.
  3. Note the position of the globe within the orbit and the presence of exophthalmos or proptosis.
  4. Note swelling, contusions, or lacerations of the lids and whether the lids cover the cornea.
  5. Palpate the orbital margins for fractures, crepitus, air, and cellulitis.
  6. Examine the conjunctiva for hemorrhage, chemosis, lacerations, or foreign bodies and the superior and inferior conjunctival cul-de-sacs for foreign bodies.
  7. Examine the cornea for opacities, ulcers, foreign bodies, abrasions, or lacerations.
  8. Record pupil size, shape, and response to light.
  9. Examine the anterior chamber and note its depth and the presence of hyphema, iridodonesis, or iridodialysis.
  10. If indicated and if the cornea is undamaged, measure intraocular pressure.
  11. Dilate the eye with 1 per cent tropicamide drops and examine the fundus.

OCULAR EMERGENCIES (pp. 1276–1291)

Differential Diagnosis

Acute Vision Loss

The differential diagnosis includes:

  1. Massive vitreous or retinal hemorrhage from any cause (no pain)
  2. Bilateral optic neuritis or retrobulbar optic neuritis (painful)
  3. Retinal detachment (no pain)
  4. Severe anterior or posterior uveitis (painful)
  5. Severe keratitis with blepharospasm (painful)
  6. Acute congestive glaucoma (painful)

Asymmetry of Pupils

Pupillary asymmetry may be caused by any of the following:

  1. Traumatic uveitis with miosis of the pupil
  2. Horner's syndrome—miosis of the ipsilateral side
  3. Intraorbital trauma to ciliary nerves or ganglia—mydriasis.

4. Optic neuritis or optic nerve avulsion—mydriasis with acute vision loss
5. Iridodialysis and rupture of iris sphincter—mydriasis
6. Unilateral use of topical mydriatic or miotic drugs
7. Diffuse central neurological disease—increased cerebrospinal fluid pressure

Chemical Burns

Chemical irritation of the eye may result from accidental contact with a noxious agent.

Immediate first aid is aimed at removing the offending chemical from the eye with irrigation using large amounts of water or saline.

In general, acidic compounds are less dangerous than basic compounds. Acidic compounds denature surface proteins and stop their penetration, whereas basic compounds destroy protein and penetrate deeper ocular structures.

Lid Injuries

Lid contusions and lacerations are most commonly associated with bite wounds or vehicular trauma. Careful primary repair is undertaken to ensure adequate physiological and cosmetic results.

Meticulous repair of lid lacerations is important if good cosmetic and physiological results are to be obtained. Lacerations of the lid margin *without* lid avulsion that are presented 24 to 48 hours after injury and are grossly contaminated should not be immediately operated on but carefully cleaned, the eye evaluated for further injury, the lids treated with topical antibiotics, and systemic infections controlled. The animal can undergo surgical repair of the lid in 5 to 7 days.

Although avulsions may be grossly contaminated and 24 to 48 hours old, they are carefully cleaned, minimally débrided, and resutured to restore adequate circulation.

Treatment

The lid laceration is lavaged with sterile saline, and any foreign material removed aseptically. All hair is carefully clipped and irrigated from the wound, and a 1 per cent povidone-iodine solution is applied around the wound margins but not in the wound itself.

A minimum of two suture layers gives well-approximated lid closure.

Lacerations of the lids near the medial canthus can present difficult problems if a canalicular laceration is also present. For repair of canalicular defects, see Chapter 84.

Corneal Foreign Bodies

Blepharospasm, photophobia, pain, keratitis, and secondary uveitis may develop. The foreign body may penetrate the corneal stroma and enter the anterior chamber.

In all cases of corneal foreign bodies, removal of the foreign body is the most effective treatment. If a foreign body is embedded in the cornea, the epithelium may have to be carefully incised to remove it.

Acute Infectious Keratitis

Infectious keratitis is an ocular emergency because of the rapidity with which certain forms of infection spread, destroy the corneal stroma, and result in corneal perforation, endophthalmitis, and loss of the affected eye.

Clinical Diagnosis

The following may signal active keratitis associated with microbial infection: (1) rapidly developing keratitis in a previously normal eye; (2) loss of corneal epithelium accompanied by stromal cellular infiltrates and stromal edema; (3) mucopurulent stromal necrosis; and (4) secondary anterior uveitis with possible hypopyon.

Confirmation of Infectious Keratitis

Corneal and conjunctival cultures can quickly confirm a diagnosis of infectious keratitis.

Corneal scrapings are made with the Kimura platinum spatula. The slides are stained with Gram and Giemsa stains. New methylene blue stain can be used for immediate evaluation of cytological detail.

Treatment

The initial selection of antibiotics is based on the results of Gram staining. It can generally be assumed that gram-positive infections are caused by penicillin-resistant *Staphylococcus* spp. and gram-negative rod infections are caused by *Pseudomonas* spp.

The treatment for gram-positive infections includes subconjunctival therapy with 75 mg cefamandole or 100 mg cefazolin; topical treatment is a concentrated solution of gentamicin and cefazolin if it can be applied frequently. In severe cases, systemic therapy is provided with intravenous methicillin or ampicillin.

Infection with gram-negative rods can be treated subconjunctivally with 20 mg gentamicin, 20 mg tobramycin, and topically with fortified gentamicin drops or gentamicin ointment. In many cases, topical fluoroquinolone (Ciprofloxacin) drops have replaced the previously discussed antibiotics in the treatment of infectious keratitis.

Pseudomonas Infections

Keratitis produced by *Pseudomonas aeruginosa* is a rapidly spreading and destructive corneal disease. *Pseudomonas* produces proteolytic enzymes and additionally may stimulate collagenase production, which causes the rapid spread of infection and the destruction of corneal stroma with perforation.

The new fluoroquinolone Ciprofloxacin is highly effective against a broad spectrum of gram-positive and gram-negative organisms including *P. aeruginosa*.

Additional Treatment

Additional treatment measures include:

1. The animal is hospitalized whenever possible.
2. Pain associated with secondary uveal inflammation is controlled with atropine (1 to 4 per cent).
3. If the cornea appears soft, acetylcysteine drops may be used (two drops every 2 hours for the first 24 to 48 hours).
4. Careful cleaning to remove necrotic corneal tissue.
5. Self-multilation is prevented by an Elizabethan collar.
6. Pain is relieved with systemic agents.
7. When extensive loss of corneal stroma may result in imminent

perforation, a conjunctival or third-eyelid flap may be placed over the cornea.

Corneal Lacerations

Management of Small Corneal Lacerations

Tissue adhesive in the form of a cyanoacrylate monomer can be used for closure of corneal perforations measuring less than 2 mm.

Corneal lacerations or perforations greater than 2 to 3 mm in diameter are best managed by surgical intervention.

Complicated Corneal Lacerations

Complicated corneal lacerations are accompanied by iris prolapse, hyphema, cataract formation, luxation of the lens, or loss of vitreous. If examination of the eye reveals a damaged lens with rupture of the anterior lens capsule, extraction of the lens via an extracapsular approach may be indicated. If the corneal wound is small, the wound is first closed and a limbal or corneal section made to extract the lens. Incarceration or prolapse of uveal tissue in corneal wounds presents a difficult surgical problem. If the wound is small and the iris prolapse is small and of short duration, the iris may be repositioned. If the surgeon cannot effectively replace a prolapsed iris or if the iris is excessively contaminated and necrotic, it is excised. When a corneal laceration is attended by prolapse of the iris, lens, vitreous, and ciliary processes, a decision must be made whether, under these circumstances, it is better to perform immediate enucleation. If there is any chance of saving the eye, repair can be attempted and enucleation performed if necessary in 10 days to 2 weeks.

Contusion and Penetrating Injury

Severe ocular contusions are caused by injury resulting from sudden acceleration or deceleration imparted by a blunt force. A number of factors determine the effect of this form of trauma on the eye: (1) impact of the force on the globe at the point of injury, (2) contrecoup impact in direct line with the force but on the opposite side of the globe, and (3) indirect force when the globe is pushed or "hurled" against the orbital contents.

Fractures of the orbital floor, as in man, are not seen. However, fractures of the zygomatic arch or maxillary, frontal, or lacrimal bones can occur. Therefore, animals with concussive ocular injuries are radiographed to evaluate damage. Hyphema is blood in the anterior chamber of the eye. Simple hyphema usually resolves spontaneously in 7 to 10 days and does not cause vision loss. Loss of vision following hyphema is associated with secondary ocular injuries, including glaucoma, traumatic iritis, cataract, retinal detachment, endophthalmitis, and corneal scarring.

Retinal and vitreous hemorrhage associated with trauma usually resorbs spontaneously over a 2- to 3-week period. Unfortunately, vitreous hemorrhage can produce vitreous traction bands as it organizes, eventually leading to retinal detachment. Extensive retinal hemorrhage may be associated with scarring and glial proliferation as the blood resorbs.

Several basic principles are significant in the management of traumatic hyphemas in animals. Traumatic uveitis is also present after concussive or penetrating intraocular injury with hyphema. Bleeding usually stops spontaneously. Very little can be done to control intraocular bleeding. Animals are confined and kept as quiet as possible.

Rebleeding may occur within the first 5 days after injury. Secondary uveal inflammation is controlled. Intraocular pressure is monitored. If pressure increases, an oral carbonic anhydrase inhibitor is administered. The animal is repeatedly observed for the initial 5 to 10 days during resorption of blood. After 5 to 7 days, blood in the anterior chamber changes from bright red to bluish black. If total hyphema persists and elevated pressure is evident despite medical therapy, surgical intervention is indicated.

Surgical Intervention

If the blood has formed a firm, well-organized clot, it can be removed. Sophisticated anterior chamber irrigating and vitreous cutting units using microsurgical handles and needles are available. Surgical intervention and blind probing of the anterior chamber in an attempt to remove blood or blood clots may cause *serious* surgical complications, such as rebleeding, luxated lens, extensive iris damage, and damage to the corneal endothelium.

Ocular Foreign Bodies

Periorbital, scleral, or corneal punctures or lacerations may be due to penetrating foreign bodies.

A foreign body entering the eye may follow one of several trajectories, depending on its velocity and angle of entry. It may penetrate the cornea and fall into the anterior chamber or become lodged in the iris, or it may penetrate the anterior capsule of the lens, producing a cataract. Some metallic high-speed foreign bodies may perforate the cornea, iris, and lens to lodge in the posterior wall of the eye or in the vitreous or may pass entirely through the eye and remain within the orbit. Direct observation is the best means of locating a foreign body. Examination with a biomicroscope or indirect ophthalmoscope may prove invaluable. In addition to radiography, the more refined technique of ultrasonography may be used to locate foreign bodies. This technique is most valuable in evaluating the extent of intraocular damage in the presence of extensive corneal edema or secondary cataract formation.

Intraocular penetration by a foreign body always warrants a guarded prognosis. Chalcosis is produced by retention of copper or its alloys of bronze or brass and results in rapid inflammation, hypopyon, and localized abscess formation. Retained foreign bodies of iron and steel may lead to repeated episodes of ocular inflammation and siderosis. When considering removing any foreign body from an eye, the dangers of leaving the foreign body in the eye must be weighed against the dangers of surgical removal.

Proptosis of the Globe

Proptosis of the globe secondary to trauma is common in brachycephalic animals. The proptosed globe must be protected against further exposure and drying. This can be accomplished by using sponges soaked in cold hypertonic 10 per cent dextrose to reduce edema and prevent corneal drying.

Proptosis of the globe results in several pathological phenomena that must be considered in establishing treatment and prognosis. (1) Occlusion of the vortex and ciliary veins of the eye by the lids produces venous stasis and a form of congestive glaucoma. (2) Proptosis results in marked exposure keratitis and corneal necrosis. (3) Proptosis of the globe can be associated with iritis, chorioretinitis, retinal detachment, luxation of the lens, and avulsion of the optic nerve. An attempt is made to replace most proptosed globes. Postoperative treatment is designed to control traumatic iritis and the extensive corneal damage that is associated with proptosis and exposure. Extraocular muscle injury and the resultant strabismus are common after proptosis. The most frequent deviation observed is upward and outward, suggesting possible paralysis or rupture of the medial rectus, dorsal oblique, and ventral rectus muscles or an overaction of the lateral or dorsal rectus muscle. In most cases, a relatively normal visual axis returns in 3 to 4 months after the initial injury.

Endophthalmitis

Endophthalmitis (inflammation of the eye and its contents) is more severe than uveitis, and an infectious agent is often associated with this inflammatory reaction.

Signs of endophthalmitis include extreme pain, very deep scleral vascular engorgement, corneal edema with large numbers of cells and proteins in the anterior chamber, large amounts of vitreous exudate, systemic signs (e.g., anorexia and pyrexia), and neutrophilia.

Treatment

If very severe structural damage is not evident and the cornea has not been ruptured with intraocular tissue loss, treatment may be attempted.

Initial Therapy. The intraocular antibiotic regimen for the endophthalmitis is as follows:

1. Intraocular gentamicin, 0.1 mg, and cephaloridine, 0.25 mg
2. Subconjunctival gentamicin, 25 mg, and cephaloridine, 1 mg, or methicillin, 100 mg
3. Topical gentamicin ophthalmic ointment
4. Cephaloridine intravenously

Intraocular aspiration is repeated at 48 hours, and if bacteria are still evident and culture positive, the intraocular antibiotic regimen is repeated.

ACUTE ELEVATION IN INTRAOCULAR PRESSURE—GLAUCOMA (pp. 1291–1292)

Glaucoma is an ocular emergency because uncontrolled elevated intraocular pressure causes irreversible damage to the ganglion cells of the retina and optic nerve, resulting in irreversible vision loss. This damage can take place within 24 to 48 hours of the onset of acute pressure elevation.

In the initial treatment of acute congestive glaucoma, it is important to consider the differential diagnosis of the major problems producing secondary narrow-angle glaucoma.

Anterior Uveitis

Uveitis is one of the most common causes of glaucoma. It rapidly produces a plasmoid aqueous, which can lead to blockage of the trabecular meshwork with fibrin and cells, secondary broad-based anterior synechia, and elevations in intraocular pressure. Cyclytis is a diagnosis that often remains undetected until the zonular ligaments supporting the lens are broken and the lens subluxates or luxates. Cyclytis and lens luxations are primarily encountered in terriers and small breeds of dogs.

Basset hounds with acute congestive unilateral glaucoma have active severe uveitis that has caused decompensation of a poorly formed anterior drainage angle and secondary glaucoma. Animals with acute lens subluxation or luxation into the anterior chamber and secondary anterior uveitis and cyclitis can be helped by surgical removal of the lens and control of underlying intraocular inflammation.

Treatment

Initial treatment in acute elevations of intraocular pressure is mannitol, 1 g/kg IV given slowly. Glycerin 50 to 75 per cent can also be given (8 to 12 ml to a 15-kg dog every 8 hours).

Carbonic anhydrase inhibitors can be used to decrease the production of aqueous fluid. An initial loading dose can be achieved with acetazolamide, 250 to 500 mg by intravenous bolus to a 15- to 20-kg dog. The initial loading dose can be followed with oral dichlorphenamide, 50 mg/20 kg every 8 hours. Dichlorphenamide produces fewer serious side effects, including vomiting, diarrhea, panting, and weakness, than other carbonic anhydrase inhibitors. Further appropriate therapy, such as treatment for uveitis, lens removal, cyclocryotherapy, or intraocular implant, can be undertaken.

Reproductive System

CHAPTER 93
Ovary and Uterus
(pages 1293–1308)

ANATOMY (pp. 1293–1294)

PHYSIOLOGY OF THE OVARIAN CYCLE
(pp. 1294–1295)

Ovarian Cycle in the Bitch

The ovarian cycle in a bitch is monestrous, with considerable individual variation in the extent and timing of hormonal changes. The interval between cycles varies among breeds, ranging from 4 to 13 months and averaging 7 months. Generally, smaller breeds have shorter cycle lengths than larger breeds. Puberty begins in most dogs at 6 to 9 months of age.

Proestrus

Proestrus averages 5 to 9 days, ranging from 2 to 22 days. Ovarian follicles produce estradiol as they develop. Hormonal changes from proestrus to estrus reflect the transition from the follicular phase to the luteal phase of the cycle. After ovulation, the follicles form corpora lutea, which secrete progesterone.

Estrus

Behavioral estrus occurs when a bitch stands firmly for a male, usually with reflex tail deviation, and permits copulation. Behavioral estrus lasts 6 to 12 days, varying from 2 days to more than 3 weeks. The period of fertility is assessed better by vaginal cytological study, vaginoscopy, and hormonal assay than by behavior.

Metestrus

The period after estrus is described by loss of estrus behavior and vaginal cornification, vaginal crenulation, and reappearance of leukocytes in the vaginal smear. The duration of metestrus varies, depending on criteria used. The increase in progesterone during the first part of the luteal phase promotes growth and development of uterine mucosa and mammary epithelium.

The term *diestrus* has been substituted for *metestrus*.

Anestrus

Anestrus is the transition from one cycle to the next and is characterized by low progesterone levels.

Pseudopregnancy

Overt pseudopregnancy, or pseudocyesis, occurs when mammary development and behavior are indistinguishable from that of late pregnancy or lactation.

Ovarian Cycle in the Queen

An adult queen is seasonally polyestrous. A queen does not ovulate spontaneously; ovulation usually occurs 24 to 30 hours after copulation. Proestrus is not routinely observed in queens. Proestrus usually lasts 12 to 48 hours. Estrus begins when a queen allows a male to mount and ends when this behavior ceases.

DISORDERS OF THE OVARY AND UTERUS (pp. 1295–1303)

Diagnostic Techniques

Abdominal Palpation

Pregnancy Determination. Abdominal palpation is frequently used to diagnosis pregnancy in dogs and cats.

Radiography is useful in diagnosing pregnancy after fetal skeletal ossification during the last 15 days of gestation. Radiographs taken after pneumoperitoneum may delineate uterine swellings as early as 30 to 35 days of pregnancy. Using ultrasonography, pregnancy can be diagnosed in dogs as early as 28 days after breeding. Ultrasonography is also useful for identifying the origin of soft-tissue masses on caudal abdominal radiographs (e.g., enlarged uterus or uterine stump).

Exploratory Laparotomy

If the ovaries are not grossly enlarged, the ovarian bursa is first incised to expose the ovaries. Uterine biopsy and culture samples can be taken.

Acquired Ovarian Lesions

Ovarian Cysts

Follicular cysts develop from graafian follicles. Clinical signs associated with follicular cysts have been reported as prolonged estrus with bloody vaginal discharge, cystic mammary hyperplasia, and genital fibroleiomyomas. In cats, cysts from atretic follicles can be functional. *Lutein cysts* form from the corpus luteum after ovulation. They may also be associated with cystic endometrial hyperplasia or pyometra. *Parovarian cysts* originate from the remnants of either mesonephric (wolffian) or paramesonephric tubules and ducts. They are more frequently encountered in dogs than cats.

Ovarian Tumors (see Chapter 159)

Ovarian tumors are uncommon in dogs and cats. They occur more frequently in older, nulliparous bitches.

Sex cord-stromal tumors of the ovary are divided into two main groups: granulosa-theca cell tumors, which are the most common canine ovarian tumors, and Sertoli-Leydig cell tumors. Granulosa cell tumors are composed of cells that differentiate to female-type cells. Bitches with granulosa cell tumors may show signs of elevated levels of estrogen (e.g., hyperplasia and cornification of the vaginal epithelium).

Sertoli-Leydig cell tumors are composed of cells that differentiate into male-type cells. Surgical therapy is ovariohysterectomy.

Papillary cystadenomas and cystadenocarcinomas occur only in bitches. Bitches with cystadenocarcinomas may have irregular estrous cycles, cystic endometrial hyperplasia, or ascites. Because even a confined papillary cystadenocarcinoma frequently is marked by peritoneal implantation and lung metastasis, prognosis is poor. *Germ cell tumors,* including teratomas and dysgerminomas, originate from primordial germ cells of the gonads.

Congenital Anomalies of the Uterus

Agenesis of one uterine horn may be accompanied by unilateral renal agenesis. Other congenital abnormalities of the uterus include hypoplasia, agenesis, atresia, segmental aplasia, septate uterine body, double cervix, and cornual fusion.

Acquired Diseases of the Uterus
Pyometra

The term *pyometra* describes a pus-filled uterus and associated ovarian changes and extragenital disorders. Pyometra is one stage of the *cystic hyperplasia-pyometra complex.* Type I is cystic endometrial hyperplasia, which occurs in middle-aged dogs and is not related to the ovarian cycle. Type II occurs only during diestrus when the cervix is relaxed and patent. In type III, cystic endometrial hyperplasia is accompanied by an acute inflammatory reaction of the endometrium. Bitches found to have pyometra usually have type III uterine changes. Affected dogs usually present within 8 weeks of their last estrus. In chronic endometritis, type IV, the cervix can be either open or closed. If the cervix is open, chronic vaginal discharge occurs. If the cervix is closed, the uterus is greatly distended and the uterine walls may be thin.

Long-acting progestational compounds administered to intact bitches cause endometrial hyperplasia with progression to pyometra in some animals. Short-term progestational compounds, administered when endogenous estrogen concentrations are high, may also cause pyometra.

Because cats do not ovulate spontaneously, a progesterone-dependent disease like pyometra should occur only after sterile matings. However, pyometra is encountered in unbred cats. Even though infection is not the primary cause of pyometra, it is usually present. The most common bacterium cultured from the uterine contents of dogs with pyometra is *Escherichia coli.* Rarely, the uterus is sterile, as determined by aerobic bacterial culture, but anaerobic infections may be present. Bacteria have been isolated from 68 to 85 per cent of uteri of cats with pyometra.

Pyometra is a polysystemic disease. Leukocytosis, anemia, hypoalbuminemia, hyperglobulinemia, increased alkaline phosphatase levels, azotemia, and acidosis all can occur to various degrees. From 20 to 25 per cent of dogs and 12 per cent of cats with pyometra are azotemic. Glomerular filtration rate is often reduced even in dogs that are not azotemic. Dogs with pyometra have decreased urine-concentrating ability, although diluting ability may be retained. The reduction in glomerular filtration rate is a functional abnormality not correlated with structural damage in the glomerulus. The rate of urinary tract infection is at least 22 per cent and may be as high as 69 per cent. Alkaline phosphatase concentrations may be increased.

Some dogs with pyometra may have respiratory alkalosis, but the most important acid-base disturbance associated with pyometra is metabolic acidosis. Rupture of the uterus produces peritonitis and sepsis, with accompanying hypoglycemia and leukopenia. Dogs that are septic are treated as described in Chapter 99 for dogs with prostatic abscesses.

Diagnosis. The diagnosis of pyometra can usually be made from the clinical history, physical examination, and laboratory values. Pyometra is considered in any ill diestrual bitch or queen.

The type and severity of clinical signs depend on patency of the cervix, duration of the illness, and associated extragenital disease. In dogs, the most frequently reported signs include anorexia, polydipsia, depression, vaginal discharge, vomiting, and diarrhea.

Signs of pyometra in cats are more subtle than in dogs. An enlarged uterus may be felt during abdominal palpation. Care must be taken to avoid rupturing a distended uterus.

Laboratory findings are not pathognomonic for pyometra. Total leukocyte count is usually greater than 15,000, although some animals have a normal count and even leukopenia. A left shift that may be degenerative is common. The hematocrit may be decreased, but the severity of the anemia can be masked by dehydration.

Renal function is carefully evaluated. Urine for bacterial culture and urinalysis is obtained by cystocentesis during surgery. Because 30 per cent of dogs with pyometra have urinary tract infection, follow-up diagnosis and treatment are important.

When radiographic examination is necessary for confirmation, abdominal preparation such as enemas or withholding food is not recommended.

Treatment. The usual treatment for pyometra is ovariohysterectomy. Broad-spectrum antibiotics are administered intravenously at the time of anesthetic induction and continued for 7 to 10 days after surgery. Corrective therapy for fluid deficits, acidosis, and sepsis is started before surgery and continued as needed during and after surgery (see Chapter 99 for treatment of sepsis). In a sick animal, surgery is not postponed for more than a few hours because the diseased uterus continues to contribute to bacteremia and septicemia.

If renal function is impaired before surgery, 20 per cent mannitol (0.25 to 0.5 g/kg IV) is administered. The recommended method for handling the uterine body is the classic triple-clamp method with individual ligation of the uterine arteries. The ligatures are placed on the cranial cervix to avoid leaving any uterine body. The uterus is isolated from the abdomen with laparotomy sponges before it is severed, to prevent abdominal contamination. The small amount of exposed uterus is lavaged and suctioned to remove residual pus.

Medical therapy for pyometra is directed at lowering the progesterone concentrations, eliminating bacteria, and opening the cervix. Several investigators have reported the use of prostaglandin F_2 in dogs and cats. At this time, the drug has not been approved for use in dogs or cats.

Hydrometra and Mucometra

Hydrometra and mucometra are sterile accumulations of fluid within the uterus from endometrial gland secretions under progesterone stimulation.

Subinvolution of Placental Sites

Normal involution of the uterus is complete by 12 weeks after parturition. With subinvolution of placental sites, a disturbance in the normal postparturient placental degeneration and endometrial reconstruction takes place.

Subinvolution of placental sites causes persistent serosanguineous vaginal discharge 7 to 12 weeks after parturition. It usually occurs in bitches less than 2½ years of age after the first or second whelping. Severe anemia may develop. Abdominal palpation may reveal discrete, firm, spherical enlargements of the uterine horns.

Spontaneous remission usually occurs, and bitches with subinvolution of placental sites rarely require medical or surgical therapy. If bleeding continues and anemia is worsening, ovariohysterectomy is recommended.

Metritis

Acute metritis occurs most commonly in the immediate postpartum period and is usually associated with dystocia, obstetrical manipulations, or retained placentas or fetuses. Acute metritis may also develop after a normal whelping or following contaminated artificial insemination. Mastitis may also be present.

Ovariohysterectomy is recommended. Supportive therapy may be necessary before surgery. The puppies or kittens are weaned and hand-fed. Medical treatment can be attempted for a breeding animal that is not too sick. Antibiotics are instilled into the uterus daily until there is no uterine discharge, white blood cell count is normal, and temperature is normal.

Uterine Prolapse

Prolapse of the uterus is infrequent in dogs and cats. One horn or the entire uterus can prolapse during prolonged labor or up to 48 hours after parturition, when the cervix is extremely dilated.

If the animal is in good physical condition and the uterus is healthy, manual reduction can be attempted. General anesthesia or epidural anesthesia is usually necessary. The uterus is cleaned with warm saline followed by an antibiotic wash and lubricated with a water-soluble jelly. Gentle manipulation with gloved fingers, a sterile smooth syringe plunger, or a long glass tube may assist reduction.

Extensive uterine devitalization necessitates ovariohysterectomy after reduction of the prolapse. If reduction of the uterus is impossible, the uterus is amputated and the stump is reduced. Gentle traction on the uterine horns may expose the ovaries.

Uterine Neoplasia (see also Chapter 159)

The incidence of uterine tumors in dogs is 0.3 to 0.4 per cent of canine tumors. Leiomyoma is the most frequent tumor. In cats, endometrial carcinoma is the most frequently reported malignant uterine tumor.

OVARIOHYSTERECTOMY (pp. 1303–1306)

Indications

Elective sterilization is the most common indication for ovariohysterectomy. The customary age for spaying dogs and cats is around 6 months, either just before or after their first estrus. Ovariohysterectomy before the first ovarian cycle decreases the incidence of mammary gland tumors to less than 0.5 per cent. At some humane society shelters, pups and kittens are neutered at 8 to 12 weeks of age, with no reported adverse effects. After very early ovariohysterectomy, there may be a greater potential for hypoplasia of the vagina and vulva, leading to perivulvar dermatitis.

Procedure

Complications

Hemorrhage is reported as the most common cause of death after ovariohysterectomy. Operative hemorrhage may be caused by rupture of the ovarian vessels when the suspensory ligament is stretched or by tearing the vessels in the broad ligament. The uterine vessels may be torn by excessive traction on the uterine body. To determine the source of bleeding, each ligature is inspected. To do this efficiently, the abdominal incision is lengthened. Erosion of the uterine vessels or infection around the uterine vessel ligatures can cause intermittent bleeding from the vagina 4 to 16 days after ovariohysterectomy. Recurrent estrus following ovariohysterectomy is caused by residual ovarian tissue.

The diagnosis and treatment of recurrent estrus require an exploratory laparotomy through a midline incision and removal of all remaining tissue. It may be easier to find residual ovarian tissue if the operation is performed during estrus.

Uterine stump pyometra can occur in dogs and cats after incomplete ovariohysterectomy. The source of progesterone may be from residual ovarian tissue or from exogenous progestational compounds. *Uterine stump inflammation and granuloma* can be caused by ligatures of nonabsorbable suture material, poor aseptic technique, or excessive remaining devitalized uterine body. *Fistulous tracts* can develop from inflammatory response to ligature material. The tract extends from the ligature around the ovarian pedicle or uterine body through the muscle planes to the skin. Dissection of the fistulous tracts is of little value. A midline exploratory laparotomy is performed, and all pedicles examined. Accidental *ligation of a ureter,* causing hydronephrosis or atrophy of the kidney, is prevented by careful identification of uterine horns and body before ligating the uterine body. *Urinary incontinence* following ovariohysterectomy can be caused by adhesions or granulomas of the uterine stump that interfere with urinary bladder sphincter function.

Estrogen-responsive incontinence can occur in older spayed bitches. The recommended therapy is either oral administration of diethylstilbestrol (0.1 to 1.0 mg/day for 3 to 5 days, followed by a maintenance dose of 1.0 mg/week) or parenteral administration of estradiol cypionate (0.1 to 1.0 mg at intervals of weeks to months, as needed).

Body weight gains of 26 to 38 per cent have been reported after ovariohysterectomy. Inactivity and increased food intake contribute to weight gain. Ovariectomy may produce a *eunuchoid syndrome* in working dogs (i.e., decreased aggression, interest in working, and stamina).

CHAPTER 94

Vagina, Vestibule, and Vulva
(pages 1308–1316)

Congenital Anomalies (pp. 1308–1316)

Congenital abnormalities of the vagina probably occur commonly in bitches but are only occasionally associated with clinical disease. They result from abnormal development of the paramesonephric ducts (müllerian ducts) or urogenital sinus.

Acquired Abnormalities
Vaginal Edema (Formerly "Vaginal Hyperplasia")

During the follicular phase of the estrous cycle, the vaginal and vestibular mucosa normally becomes edematous and thickened. Exaggeration of this estrogenic response occasionally results in excessive mucosal folding of the vaginal floor cranial to the urethral tubercle. This redundant mucosa begins to protrude through the vulvar labia as a fleshy red mass. Vaginal edema is most frequently seen during the first estrous period and usually regresses spontaneously during the luteal phase. Recurrence is common during succeeding estrous periods.

Megestrol acetate (2 mg/kg PO daily for 7 days) can be given in early proestrus in an attempt to prevent the development of vaginal edema in bitches with a predisposition. Gonadotropin-releasing hormone (GnRH) has also been used to treat vaginal edema in bitches (50 µg GnRH IV once).

Temporary relief can be provided by application of K-Y Jelly or normal saline to minimize drying of the exposed mucosa. In addition to interfering with coitus, the edematous tissue is aesthetically displeasing to many owners, and surgical resection becomes the treatment of choice.

Surgical Treatment. Episiotomy exposes the caudal vaginal floor and allows delineation of the prolapsed tissue margins. Redundant vaginal tissue is amputated by making a transverse elliptical incision around its base.

Vaginal Prolapse

Vaginal prolapse is less common than vaginal edema in dogs and can be either partial or complete. In contrast to partial vaginal prolapse, the cervix is exteriorized with complete prolapses. In either case, a doughnut-shaped eversion of the complete vaginal circumference (including the urethral tubercle) protrudes through the vulvar labia. Brachycephalic breeds such as boxers and Boston terriers appear predisposed to vaginal prolapse. Both vaginal prolapse and vaginal edema must be differentiated from tumors arising from the vaginal and vestibular wall (leiomyomas, fibromas, polyps).

Treatment. With mild prolapse, no treatment may be necessary, because spontaneous regression occurs during diestrus. More severe prolapses require protection of exposed tissues until estrus passes. Attempts to replace the vaginal mucosa usually require general anesthesia. Episiotomy provides additional exposure for easier reduction.

Severe acute or long-standing vaginal prolapse may be attended by hemorrhage, infection, or necrosis of the prolapsed tissue. Affected animals may become hypotensive or septic and are treated accordingly. Surgical resection of the devitalized tissue is necessary to prevent further sepsis and self-mutilation and to restore the vaginal lumen.

A bitch with a vaginal prolapse during late pregnancy will probably have difficulty with parturition. Therefore, surgical resection of the prolapsed tissue at the time it occurs is preferred to waiting until parturition is evident.

THE VULVA (pp. 1314–1315)

Vulvar Stenosis (p. 1314)

Anovulvar Cleft (Vulvovestibular Cleft) (pp. 1314–1315)

Atresia of the Vulva (p. 1315)

Clitoral Hypertrophy (p. 1315)

Acquired Vulvar Abnormalities (p. 1315)

CHAPTER 95

Normal and Abnormal Parturition (pages 1316–1322)

PHYSIOLOGY OF PARTURITION (pp. 1316–1317)
Fetal Factors Contributing to Parturition

The fetus is important in initiating parturition; normal fetal adrenal-pituitary-hypothalamic axis is necessary for eutocia in many animals.

Maternal Factors Contributing to Parturition

A decrease in the progesterone/estrogen ratio at the myometrium is accepted as important for initiating normal parturition. As progesterone declines (or estradiol increases) in the serum, oxytocin initiates and maintains uterine contractions. Relaxin, a polypeptide hormone and homologue of insulin, has an important role in remodeling the reproductive tract for parturition. Corticoids are elevated in the serum before whelping, but their contribution to lowering concentrations of serum progesterone and initiating labor is unclear.

HEMATOLOGICAL CHANGES DURING PREGNANCY (p. 1317)

The packed cell volume declines in pregnant bitches, with an observed anemia (packed cell volume < 40 per cent) reportedly occurring between 7 and 9 weeks after estrus.

SIGNS OF IMPENDING PARTURITION (p. 1317)

The rectal temperature drops to less than 99°F (37.22°C) approximately 8 to 24 hours before parturition and 10 to 14 hours after concentrations of progesterone in the serum decline to less than 2 ng/ml.

For several days before parturition, a bitch becomes restless, seeks seclusion, and may not eat. Mammary turgidity and secretion of milk may be seen 1 to 2 weeks and nesting behavior 12 to 24 hours before parturition.

STAGES OF NORMAL PARTURITION (pp. 1317–1318)

Stage 1

The first stage of labor is characterized by subclinical uterine contractions and dilation of the cervix.

Stage 2

During the second stage of labor, each fetus passes through the birth canal and is expelled. Although the average duration of this stage is 6 to 12 hours, it may continue for 24 hours. A bitch usually lies down during the second stage of labor. Stage 2 can be inhibited if she is disturbed or distressed.

Although puppies are usually delivered every one-half to 1 hour until whelping is finished, the interval between puppies can be variable, with up to 4 hours between eutocic births.

Stage 3

The third stage of parturition involves expulsion of the fetal membranes and involution of the uterus. Fetal membranes usually pass 5 to 15 minutes after birth of each pup.

A thick greenish discharge (lochia) accompanies normal placental separation and may be observed in all three stages of labor.

Uterine Involution

Uterine involution may continue for a period of several weeks after whelping, with complete endometrial recovery occurring by 3 months postpartum. Although subinvolution of placental sites is fairly common in young females, retention of the whole placenta is unusual at any age.

ABNORMAL PARTURITION (pp. 1318–1320)

Taking a thorough history is important in establishing whether dystocia is present. Gestation lengths, when based on single breeding dates, can range from 59 to 71 days. Nevertheless, a pregnancy longer than 68 days is considered suspect for dystocia.

Fetal heartbeats are difficult to hear through the abdominal wall in most females. Real-time ultrasonographic equipment can accurately evaluate the heart rate and viability of individual fetuses. Survey radiographs of the abdomen can also be used to evaluate fetal viability; radiographic changes denoting fetal death usually do not occur until puppies have been dead for several hours. Survey radiographs are probably most valuable in determining the number of fetuses yet to be delivered. Late decelerations of the fetal heart rate are an early sign of fetal hypoxia, and a decline in fetal blood pH is a late and advanced sign of fetal distress due to hypoxia.

Criteria for Dystocia

The following criteria for determining the presence of dystocia are guidelines and are not absolute:

1. Signs of toxicity in a pregnant bitch.
2. Strong and frequent abdominal straining with failure to produce a puppy within 30 minutes.
3. Weak straining that fails to produce a puppy within 2 hours.
4. More than 4 hours since the birth of the last puppy.
5. Prolonged gestation.
6. Retained puppy visible at vulva.
7. The presence of normal and abnormal discharge at the vulva.

TYPES OF DYSTOCIA AND BREED INCIDENCE
(pp. 1320–1321)

Both maternal and fetal factors can contribute to abnormal parturition, with most episodes of dystocia rarely being caused by a single morphological or physiological problem.

The most common factors leading to dystocia are an oversize fetus (single puppy or puppy of a breed predisposed to large head or shoulder widths); developmental defects (fetal monsters, ascites, anasarca, hydrocephalus or hydropic conditions, hypothalamic-pituitary-adrenal axis abnormalities); and faulty presentations, positions, or postures at birth.

UTERINE INERTIA (p. 1321)

Uterine inertia is failure of the uterus to expel a fetus normally and is a common cause of canine dystocia. Uterine inertia is either primary or secondary.

Primary inertia is complete if no signs of second-stage labor occur. In secondary uterine inertia, the uterine muscles become exhausted after prolonged contraction against an obstructing fetus or following efforts to expel a large litter or an oversized puppy. In both types of inertia, the uterine musculature fails to respond to the administration of oxytocin and the bitch fails to strain when pressure is applied *per vaginam* to the pelvic canal (lack of the Ferguson reflex).

NONSURGICAL TREATMENT OF DYSTOCIA (p. 1321)

Whether to use medical or surgical treatment to alleviate dystocia depends on the duration and cause of the dystocia.

Ecbolics are administered only with *nonobstructive* dystocias and when uterine inertia is not complete (pups produced but not for 2 to 3 hours). The most commonly used ecbolic is oxytocin, which can be given intramuscularly or subcutaneously at 0.2 units/5 kg every 30 minutes. If a bitch fails to respond to therapy during the first hour or delivers only a single puppy every 2 or 3 hours, surgical intervention should be considered.

Calcium solutions are frequently given with dystocias, because calcium is required for myometrial contractions. However, because most bitches presented for dystocia have normal concentrations of calcium in the serum, it is probably safer to use a balanced electrolyte solution (lactated Ringer's solution) without additional calcium unless she is showing clinical signs of hypocalcemia (prepartum eclampsia).

OBSTETRICAL MANAGEMENT OF DYSTOCIA: VAGINAL DELIVERY BY DIGITAL AND FORCEPS MANIPULATION
(pp. 1321–1322)

The indications for assisted deliver *per vaginam* are (1) to correct abnormal fetal positions (breast-head, lateral head deviation); (2) to relieve obstruction due to slight fetal oversize (assuming secondary uterine inertia has not occurred); (3) to extract the last remaining fetus in secondary uterine inertia; or (4) to relieve obstruction by extracting a dead fetus. If the obstructed fetus is beyond digital reach, vaginal delivery of the fetus is discouraged.

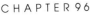

CHAPTER 96

Cesarean Section (pages 1322–1325)

TREATMENT OF DYSTOCIA (pp. 1322–1323)

When the decision for surgery is made, the dam has often endured hours of intensive labor. Abnormalities can include physical exhaustion, dehydration, acid-base disorders, hypotension, hypocalcemia, or hypoglycemia. Before anesthetic induction, physiological abnormalities are stabilized or corrected to minimize risks to the dam and fetuses. Intravenous fluids (balanced electrolyte solution with dextrose if indicated, given at minimum of 10 ml/kg/hr), corticosteroids, antibiotics, and calcium gluconate are administered as needed.

ANESTHESIA (see Chapter 173)

Regional anesthesia advantages include minimal depression of the fetuses and dam, immobilization of the hindquarters, and reasonable visceral analgesia. Disadvantages are regional vasodilation, often resulting in hypotension, fetal hypoxia, and exacerbation of surgical bleeding.

General anesthesia advantages are complete analgesia and immobilization. Disadvantages are depression of the fetuses and dam.

SURGICAL TECHNIQUE (pp. 1323–1324)

CARE OF NEONATES AND DAM (pp. 1324–1325)

Neonatal resuscitation is instituted immediately by attendants. Neonates are introduced to the dam after both have completely recovered from the effects of anesthesia.

COMPLICATIONS (p. 1325)

Potential postoperative complications include hemorrhage, hypovolemia and hypotension, and peritonitis due to exposure to uterine fluids. In animals in which uterine viability is questionable, ovariohysterectomy (with prior owner approval) is performed concurrently with cesarean section.

CHAPTER 97

Testes and Epididymides
(pages 1325–1336)

ANATOMY (pp. 1325–1326)

PHYSIOLOGY (pp. 1326–1328)

DISORDERS (pp. 1328–1335)

Anorchism and Monorchism

Diagnosis of these conditions is made after careful palpation of the scrotum and inguinal region and exploratory celiotomy.

Testicular Hypoplasia

Testicular hypoplasia may be present unilaterally or bilaterally. Treatment is orchidectomy.

Cryptorchidism

Cryptorchidism, the most common congenital testicular defect, is a failure of one or both testes to descend into the scrotum at the usual time. The usual time of testicular descent is at birth, although descent may occur normally at any time up to 6 months of age.

Cryptorchidism may be a hereditary condition involving a single recessive autosomal gene. Long-term exposure to normal body temperatures results in degeneration of the germinal epithelium and loss of exocrine function. Because the interstitial cells and Sertoli cells continue to function, endocrine function of the ectopic testis is nearly normal.

Ectopic testes, particularly intra-abdominal testes, are more susceptible to torsion and neoplasia than descended testes. Cryptorchid dogs have a risk of testicular tumors 13.6 times that of normal dogs. Signs of feminization have also been more commonly observed with Sertoli cell tumors of cryptorchid testes than scrotal testes.

Diagnosis of cryptorchidism, particularly in a young pup, may be difficult. A final diagnosis of cryptorchidism should not be made until the dog is approximately 6 months of age. Medical and surgical attempts to move ectopic testes into the scrotum have been largely unsuccessful in dogs. Orchiopexy is not condoned in veterinary medicine because of the heritable nature of cryptorchidism. Although the incidence of testicular neoplasia in dogs is unknown, the higher risk of neoplasia in cryptorchid testes may justify prophylactic removal of undescended testes. The high incidence of multiple tumors of more than one histological type in the same or opposite testis justifies bilateral orchidectomy. Another advantage of early bilateral orchidectomy in a unilaterally cryptorchid dog is that it decreases the possibility of perpetuating the defect.

Orchitis

Clinical signs of acute orchitis include testicular pain, tenseness, and scrotal edema. Acute orchitis is usually suppurative, with the formation of one or more abscesses in the testis and epididymis. Systemic signs of infection, including leukocytosis, pyrexia, and listlessness, may be present.

Severely traumatized or abscessed testes are surgically removed. Removal of chronically inflamed testes is justified to prevent continuing episodes of acute inflammation. Antibacterial drugs, local hypothermia, and possibly anti-inflammatory drugs are used to treat less severe orchitis. The prognosis for maintaining fertility is guarded, because orchitis is quite resistant to antibiotic or chemotherapeutic treatment. Orchidectomy is usually the treatment of choice, particularly if the patient is not a valuable breeding dog.

Testicular Trauma

Testes may be injured by either blunt trauma or penetrating wounds. Any trauma to the testis, epididymis, or spermatic cord is potentially dangerous because it is frequently accompanied by hemorrhage.

Medical treatment is indicated for minor testicular trauma. Local hypothermia, possibly supportive bandaging, and antibiotics and corticosteroids are often used. Analgesics and diuretics may also be indicated. Fluid accumulations are aseptically aspirated. If blood refills the scrotum, surgical exploration is considered for hemostasis.

Severe testicular trauma often requires unilateral or bilateral orchidectomy, possibly with scrotal ablation. Indications for orchidectomy following trauma include persistent pain, swelling, or local hyperthermia.

Testicular Tumors

Testicular tumors are the second most frequently reported tumors in male dogs. The three common neoplasms are seminoma, interstitial cell tumor, and Sertoli cell tumor, each with about equal frequency.

Orchidectomy
Orchidectomy in Dogs

Canine orchidectomy can be performed by either open or closed methods. Both methods use a midline prescrotal skin incision. In the open method, an incision is made through the parietal vaginal tunic covering the spermatic cord at the point where ligatures are to be placed. The components of the spermatic cord are double ligated using a transfixation ligation. In the closed method, the intact spermatic cord and vaginal tunics are double ligated using two transfixation ligatures.

Orchidectomy in Cats

Feline orchidectomy is usually performed by making a separate longitudinal scrotal incision over each testis. Occlusion of the components of the spermatic cord can be accomplished by ligation, overhand or figure-eight knot in the spermatic cord, or square knot of the ductus deferens to the testicular vessels.

Complications

Complications following orchidectomy include scrotal bruising and swelling, hemorrhage, and infection. Hemorrhage after orchidectomy may be serious, particularly if it occurs within the abdomen.

Scrotal Ablation

Scrotal ablation is recommended at the time of orchidectomy whenever trauma to the scrotum is severe and suggests ischemia. Ablation of the scrotum may be preferred at orchidectomy in old dogs with pendulous scrotums to avoid postoperative problems such as scrotal irritation and edema.

Epididymides

Aplasia and Occlusion of the Epididymis

Bilateral epididymal aplasia results in obstruction to flow of spermatozoa and infertility. Spermatoceles and spermatic granulomas develop immediately proximal to the obstructed segment.

Epididymitis

Epididymitis usually accompanies orchitis. Epididymitis can result from an ascending infection of the genital tract, canine distemper virus, or a hematogenous infection. Hematogenous infection, particularly *Brucella canis*, can result in epididymitis without orchitis. Treatment of acute suppurative epididymitis is orchidectomy.

CHAPTER 98

Penis, Prepuce, and Scrotum
(pages 1336–1348)

ANATOMY (pp. 1336–1340)

PHYSIOLOGY (pp. 1340–1341)

Penis

Erection is essential for the penis to function during copulation in all species except dogs. Enlargement of the bulbus glandis in dogs is an important part of the "tie" that occurs during copulation. The cornified spines of a cat's penis are proposed to stimulate ovulation.

Prepuce

At birth, the epithelial surfaces of the prepuce and penis adhere. Separation of the prepuce from the penis is under androgenic influence and usually occurs at puberty.

Scrotum

The scrotum functions in thermoregulation of the testes.

DISORDERS (pp. 1341–1348)

Penis

Hypospadias

Hypospadias, the most common developmental anomaly of the male external genitalia, is most frequently encountered in Boston terriers. Failure of fusion of the urogenital folds and incomplete formation of the penile urethra are noted. The external urethral orifice can be located anywhere on the ventral aspect of the penis from the normal opening to the perineal region, with glandular, penile, scrotal, and perineal hypospadias occurring.

Deformity of the Os Penis (p. 1341)

Penile Wounds

The most common clinical sign of penile wounds is hemorrhage. Penile wounds may occur during mating, dog fights, and fence jumping or from automobile or gunshot accidents.

Minor injuries of the penis can be cleaned and treated with a topical antibiotic ointment. Arterial bleeding is controlled by ligation, and cavernous bleeding is controlled by suturing the tunica albuginea with fine absorbable material. A transected urethra is sutured with fine absorbable material and catheterized. Severe wounds may require partial penile amputation and a scrotal urethrostomy.

Fracture of the Os Penis (p. 1342)

Balanoposthitis

Infections of the penis and prepuce are fairly common, constituting 20 per cent of canine penile and preputial lesions in one study. A copious yellow or blood-tinged preputial discharge suggests balanoposthitis or prostatic disease. Balanoposthitis may be seen after penile injury or accompanying phimosis, preputial foreign bodies, or neoplasia. Treatment is elimination of the primary cause. The prognosis following treatment is guarded, because balanoposthitis tends to recur.

Strangulation of the Penis

Malicious application of a rubber band around the penis or constriction by a ring of preputial hairs can cause strangulation of the penis. The dog usually seems to be in pain and may frequently lick the prepuce. Dysuria can also be noted. The penile mucosa becomes swollen with a necrotic circle, or the entire penis distal to the constriction may be necrotic.

This condition must be distinguished from paraphimosis because the treatment differs. When damage to the penis is minor, removal of the cause and topical application of an antibiotic ointment result in prompt healing.

Partial amputation of the penis is indicated when the distal portion is gangrenous or when the urethra is severely damaged. Shortening the prepuce may be necessary when a large part of the glans penis has been removed.

Penile Tumors

Tumors of the canine penis are not uncommon. There are almost no reports of genital neoplasia in male cats. Tumors of the penis in dogs include transmissible venereal tumor, papilloma, and squamous cell carcinoma. Transmissible venereal tumors respond to many modes of treatment, including radiation therapy, chemotherapy, and surgery. Tumors of the distal portion may require partial penile amputation.

Tumors involving most of the penis may require more extensive penile amputation and perineal urethrostomy. Bilateral orchidectomy and scrotal ablation may also be necessary.

Persistent Penile Frenulum

Persistence of the penile frenulum occurs in cocker spaniels, miniature poodles, mixed-breed dogs, and Pekingeses. Pain may be evident during sexual excitement or when an attempt is made to retract the prepuce.

Surgical severing of the minimally vascular connective tissue is readily performed after administration of a short-acting anesthetic. The prognosis is favorable after surgery.

Paraphimosis

In paraphimosis, the penis protrudes from the preputial sheath and cannot be replaced to its normal position. The exteriorized glans becomes congested and discolored owing to the constricting band of retracted prepuce. Necrosis of the exposed penis and urethral obstruction can occur quickly.

Lubricants, hyperosmolar solutions, and local heat or cold may be adequate to reduce the size of the penis and permit replacement. Temporary or permanent surgical enlargement of the preputial orifice may be necessary. Recurrence is common.

Prolapse of the Urethra

Prolapse of the urethra occurs uncommonly in male dogs. This condition is mainly encountered in young English bulldogs, although it has been reported in a Boston terrier. Swelling, hemorrhage, and drying of the prolapsed tissue occur relatively early, and self-inflicted trauma perpetuates the inflammation. Diagnosis is made by finding a small red pea-shaped mass at the end of the penis. Treatment is surgical, because spontaneous recovery does not occur. The prognosis after surgical repair is favorable, and prolapse usually does not recur.

Prepuce
Phimosis

Phimosis is the inability to protrude the penis beyond the preputial orifice. Clinical signs depend on the cause (congenital or acquired) and the size of the preputial orifice. Congenital phimosis is usually accompanied by a distended prepuce and inability to urinate normally. Preputial retention of urine results in balanoposthitis, and the infected area may ulcerate. Acquired phimosis results from scarring after preputial trauma or neoplasia. Surgical enlargement of the preputial orifice and correction of the primary condition result in successful treatment.

Abnormalities of the Prepuce

The prepuce may be hypoplastic or absent or may fail to fuse normally. Clinical signs of congenital preputial abnormalities usually are due to exposure of the distal part of the penis. Failure of preputial fusion usually accompanies hypospadias and underdevelopment or absence of the penis.

Surgical management of congenital preputial abnormalities other than phimosis is difficult. Failure of preputial fusion is usually treated by removal of the open prepuce, partial penile amputation, and scrotal or perineal urethrostomy. Orchidectomy, scrotal ablation, and perineal urethrostomy may be necessary if the preputial defect is severe.

Preputial Foreign Bodies (pp. 1346–1347)
Preputial Wounds

Wounds may be inflicted during mating or by trauma caused by barbed wire, motor accidents, and gun pellets. Wounds that penetrate into the preputial cavity or are near the preputial orifice are most likely to require surgical management.

Preputial Tumors

Mast cell tumors are the most frequently reported tumors of the external genitalia. Transmissible venereal tumors, melanomas, and perianal gland tumors have also been reported.

Scrotum
Scrotal Injury

Scrotal injury is uncommon despite the exposed location of the scrotum. Minor abrasions and lacerations may be initially undetected because of the paucity of clinical signs. Significant wounds are likely to become infected if treatment is delayed. Trauma to the parietal vaginal tunic of the testis can result in infection within the cavity of the vaginal tunic and even orchitis.

Infection of the Scrotal Skin

The exposed location and delicacy of the scrotal skin make it relatively susceptible to irritants. A disinfectant such as iodine is frequently the cause of scrotal irritation and subsequent infection, particularly in surgical procedures and in kennels.

Varicosities of the Scrotal Blood Vessels

Varicose dilation of scrotal veins occurs in older dogs. The varicosities are seen as flattened and irregular thickenings of the scrotal skin. Trauma leads to ulceration and repeated episodes of profuse bleeding.

Treatment consists of either stimulating thrombosis of the varicose vessels with styptics or surgically removing the involved scrotal skin and blood vessels.

Chronic Hyperplasia of the Scrotum

Hyperplasia of the scrotum is common in older dogs. The ventral part of the scrotum is thickened, wrinkled, and usually heavily pigmented. Scrotal hyperplasia usually is not clinically significant unless secondary infection occurs.

Scrotal Neoplasms

Many cutaneous neoplasms involve the scrotum. Mastocytomas are commonly reported.

CHAPTER 99

The Prostate (pages 1349–1367)

ANATOMY AND PHYSIOLOGY (pp. 1349–1351)
Anatomy

The prostate gland is the only accessory sex organ in male dogs. Although cats have a prostate gland, prostatic disease is rare. The gland lies within the abdomen after birth until degeneration of the urachal remnant occurs around 2 months of age, after which it assumes a position in the pelvic cavity. With advancing age, the prostate continues to increase in size by hyperplasia, and it moves cranially. By 4 years of age, approximately half of the gland is located in the abdomen, and by 10 years, it may be completely abdominal.

Histology

The prostate has epithelial and stromal (smooth muscle, fibroblasts, and collagen) components. The epithelial cells predominate, with the stroma occupying 10 per cent of the organ. The architecture of the prostate is characterized by compound tubuloalveoli that drain into the urethra.

Physiology

Secretions

Although prostatic secretions provide a vehicle for spermatozoa, they may not be essential for fertility. This fluid becomes part of the semen during the third phase of ejaculation, after the contributions of the urethral mucous glands and the testes have been expressed. Active secretion induced by ejaculation produces a product that is high in protein, slightly acidic, and isotonic.

Benign Prostatic Hyperplasia

As a dog ages, the prostate undergoes spontaneous enlargement, commonly referred to as *benign prostatic hyperplasia*. Clinically, it can sufficiently enlarge the prostate to cause obstruction of the colon and rectum, and under severe conditions, urethral obstruction can also occur.

Two distinct histotypes, glandular hyperplasia and complex hyperplasia, have been described. The glandular form may be an antecedent of the complex form. Glandular hyperplasia begins at 1 to 2 years of age and its prevalence peaks at 5.1 to 6 years.

The second histotype, complex hyperplasia, generally develops later, with the first evidence of complex benign prostatic hyperplasia appearing at 2 to 3 years of age. This histotype increases with age and affects 70 per cent of dogs between 8 and 9 years old. Cystic, dilated alveoli filled with eosinophilic material are a characteristic feature and can give the surface of the prostate an irregular contour.

That hormones may be involved in the induction or maintenance of benign prostatic hyperplasia has long been recognized, because dogs castrated early in life do not develop the problem. If dogs with preexisting benign prostatic hyperplasia are castrated, the hyperplasia regresses but is restored if exogenous testosterone is administered.

To induce hyperplasia in castrated dogs, estradiol-17β had to be coadministered with dihydrotestosterone or androstanediol.

RADIOGRAPHY AND ULTRASONOGRAPHY
(pp. 1351–1353)

Prostatic Radiography

The position of the prostate depends on bladder distension and the age and conformation of the dog, as well as pathological prostatic enlargement. An immature or involuted prostate in a castrated dog may be too small to be apparent on radiographs. In some instances, administration of contrast material is necessary to identify the bladder and to outline the border of the prostatic urethra.

Prostatic Ultrasonography

Ultrasonography is more informative and sensitive than radiology for detecting intraparenchymal prostatic disease, but neither is specific for investigating the underlying cause. Ultrasonography is useful in guiding a biopsy needle into diseased areas to help establish a final diagnosis. A 10- or a 7.5-MHz transducer or both are recommended for most dogs because they provide clear resolution of the prostatic parenchyma. The entire prostate is evaluated. The urinary tract, testicles, periprostatic tissue, and medial iliac lymph nodes are also examined.

The prostate is evaluated for size, shape, symmetry, echogenicity, and cavitational areas. Ultrasonography may differentiate prostatomegaly attributable to cysts, abscesses, cystic hyperplasia, neoplasm, and paraprostatic cysts and abscesses. The sonographic appearance of these disease processes overlaps.

An immature prostate encircles the urethra, is small, has indistinguishable or faintly distinct lobes, and has a homogeneous hypoechoic appearance. A fully developed prostate has a uniform homogeneous echoic pattern throughout both lobes. The urethra may be traced from the trigone of the urinary bladder through the prostate gland.

Cystic hyperplasia, which frequently accompanies benign prostatic hyperplasia, is recognized by small hypoechoic to anechoic areas in the parenchyma. Clinical history, physical examination, and laboratory findings are important in differentiating cystic hyperplasia from prostatitis or small abscesses because they have a similar ultrasonographic appearance. Large cavitary areas (> 1 cm) are more likely abscesses, cysts, or hemacysts. Acute prostatitis has a varying sonographic pattern. Tumors of the prostate are often hyperechoic and contain mineralization. Early tumors may have a hypoechoic appearance.

PROSTATE DISORDERS (pp. 1353–1361)

Clinical Disorders

Diseases of the prostate can produce clinical signs from weight loss and lethargy to septic shock with cardiovascular collapse. Male dogs that demonstrate tenesmus, penile discharge, hematuria, pyuria, stranguria, urinary incontinence, caudal abdominal pain, an acute abdomen, or ambulatory difficulty due to pelvic cavity discomfort are evaluated for prostatic disease.

Diagnostic Techniques

A complete anamnesis should be obtained. Physical examination includes careful abdominal and rectal palpation. If urinary retention or obstruction is suspected, catheterizing the urethra allows determination of urethral lumen patency and measurement of residual urine volume. Minimum data base includes a complete blood count, biochemistry profile, *Brucella canis* titer, urinalysis, and caudal abdominal radiographs.

Prostatic fluid may be obtained for cytological study and culture by ejaculation, prostatic wash, or fine-needle aspiration. Prostatic tissue may be obtained for histopathological examination and culture by percutaneous techniques or during laparotomy. Fine-needle aspiration of the prostate can be performed percutaneously via a perineal or prepubic approach. Percutaneous biopsy is performed with an actuated biopsy cutting needle via an abdominal or perineal approach. Whenever possible, a laparotomy for biopsy is preferred

Benign Prostatic Hyperplasia and Cystic Hyperplasia

Clinical signs of constipation, tenesmus, hemorrhagic urethral discharge, or urine retention may be noted. Dyschezia is much more common than dysuria. Rectal palpation reveals a symmetrically enlarged, nonpainful prostate of normal spongy consistency. Urinalysis or prostatic fluid analysis may show hemorrhage, especially with cystic hyperplasia. The recommended treatment is castration. Permanent involution of the prostate and relief of clinical signs occur in 2 or 3 weeks. Medical therapy for constipation and urine retention may be indicated until the prostate shrinks.

Suppurative Prostatitis and Prostatic Abscesses

The proximity of the prostate to the urethra, with its normal bacterial flora, predisposes the prostate to infection. Additionally, *Brucella canis* or other bacterial infection can ascend from the testicles during orchitis. As multiple foci of purulent material coalesce, large abscesses form. Prostatic abscesses can rupture into the peritoneal cavity or retroperitoneal space.

Clinical Signs and Diagnosis. Acute prostatitis typically causes lethargy, anorexia, and fever. Urine retention and constipation may occur. A purulent or bloody urethral discharge is frequently noted. Caudal abdominal or pelvic pain may cause abnormal posture or gait. The prostate is enlarged and usually asymmetrical, and it often has fluctuating areas of purulent material. If an abscess ruptures, acute peritonitis causes overt septic shock with cardiovascular collapse.

Treatment. Antibiotic therapy is based on culture and sensitivity testing of prostatic fluid. Trimethoprim-sulfadiazine or chloramphenicol is recommended initially until the sensitivity is determined. With chronic infection, aminoglycosides may be indicated for resistant bacteria. Antibiotic therapy is continued for 3 weeks. Castration is indicated for suppurative prostatitis to decrease the size and activity of the prostate and the chance of recurrence. Surgery is indicated to drain or excise large prostatic abscesses. Surgical techniques include drainage of parenchymal abscesses with gravity or suction drains and prostatectomy. Large prostatic abscesses may be marsupialized or resected during prostatectomy.

Prostatic Cysts and Paraprostatic Cysts

Oversecretion by glandular tissue with functional obstruction of the ducts causes fluid retention with cyst formation. The cysts may occur as multiple cavitary areas within the gland or as large fluid-filled structures extending into the abdominal cavity or pelvic canal.

Paraprostatic cysts may originate from the blind-ended uterus masculinus, an embryonic structure formed from the müllerian duct system. These cysts have no direct communication with the prostatic parenchyma and can become quite large. A large amount of pale yellow to orange fluid is contained within the cyst.

Clinical Signs and Diagnosis. Patients with prostatic or paraprostatic cysts may have vague clinical signs related to the large caudal abdominal mass. Inappetance, dysuria, constipation, and tenesmus are common. Incontinence, dysuria, or retention may be more common with cysts than with other prostatic diseases; pelvic pain may result in ambulatory difficulties.

Treatment. The goal of surgical therapy is to remove, reduce, or drain the cyst. Castration decreases the secretory activity of the prostate. Cyst resection may be coupled with partial or complete prostatectomy. Semipermanent drainage is achieved by marsupialization or temporarily by Penrose or suction drainage.

Prostatic Neoplasia (see also Chapter 159)

Adenocarcinoma and transitional cell carcinoma are the most common types of prostatic neoplasia in dogs. Older dogs typically are affected.
   Clinical Signs and Diagnosis. Prostatic carcinoma may be focal or disseminated throughout the gland; metastasis is common. Differentiating prostatic carcinoma from suppurative prostatitis may be difficult without biopsy.
   Treatment. Successful treatment of prostatic carcinoma is difficult because of its aggressive biological behavior. If the diagnosis is made before detectable metastasis, prostatectomy is recommended.

Prostatic Trauma (p. 1356)

Surgical Procedures and Complications

General Considerations and Surgical Approach

The prostate gland is usually approached by caudal laparotomy. It may also be approached from the perineum, usually as part of surgical repair of perineal hernia. As for any operation on the urogenital tract, preparations are made for aseptic urethral catheterization at any point in the procedure. If further caudal exposure is necessary, pubic osteotomy is indicated. Pubic osteotomy exposes the cranial portion of the pelvic canal.
   Drainage Techniques. Gravity or suction drains can be quickly placed in septic patients that cannot withstand more time-consuming resection techniques. In most drainage techniques, a stab incision is made into one prostate lobe, and suction is used to remove any purulent material. If leakage is severe, abdominal drains or open abdomen drainage after surgery is considered. Gravity drainage with various configurations of Penrose drains has been described. When gravity drains are used, preventing ascending infection by covering drain exit sites with a sterile dressing is a difficult but important postoperative goal. Drains are removed as soon as possible to decrease the risk of nosocomial infections and urethrocutaneous fistula.
   Because of the difficulty in maintaining clean drain exit sites and the inability to accurately quantitate discharge from gravity drains, I use closed-system suction drains. Regardless of the technique chosen for drainage of the infected prostate, aggressive antibiotic, fluid, electrolyte, and supportive therapy is indicated. If infection recurs after surgical drainage, castration, and proper antibiotic therapy, partial or complete prostatectomy is indicated.
   Cyst Resection. Discrete paraprostatic cysts or true prostatic cysts that have a narrow attachment to the prostate gland may be amenable to local resection. When paraprostatic cysts adhere to the prostate or when prostatic cysts narrow to a manageable stalk at the prostate, partial prostatectomy may be possible.
   Marsupialization. Marsupialization is used for prostatic or paraprostatic cysts. Abscesses within the parenchyma cannot be treated with this technique. A permanent stoma is created into the cyst for drainage. For marsupialization, the cyst must be mobilized to the ventral abdominal wall, and the capsule of the cyst must be strong enough to hold sutures without tearing. Drainage decreases over several weeks, and the stoma contracts and closes. Marsupialization may have major postoperative complications.

Prostatectomy. Complete prostatectomy is performed during laparotomy. A pubic osteotomy is occasionally necessary for better exposure.

Dogs that have undergone prostatectomy for prostatic disease are usually incontinent. Until this complication can be avoided or treated effectively, prostatectomy is reserved for severe prostatic trauma or prostatic neoplasia or is used in dogs in which minimizing recurrence of prostatic disease is more important than urinary continence.

Partial prostatectomy reduces glandular parenchyma without causing permanent incontinence. An intracapsular technique that removes 80 per cent of the parenchyma has been described in normal dogs.

In a different partial prostatectomy technique, all tissue is removed by electroscalpel, except for the prostatic urethra surrounded by a thin rim of glandular tissue around the urethra. The results of a similar technique using the neodymium:yttrium-aluminum-garnet laser for cutting and hemostasis have been reported. Two configurations of partial prostatectomy were used, depending on the location of the prostatic disease as determined by ultrasonography and visual observation. The role of partial prostatectomy in the treatment of prostatic abscesses will become better defined as more data accumulate.

TREATMENT OF CANINE ABSCESSED PROSTATE
(pp. 1361–1366)

Complications of surgical treatment of abscessed prostates are common. Sepsis and shock occurred in 32 to 64 per cent of dogs undergoing surgery. Hypoproteinemia occurred in 59 per cent of dogs, hypokalemia in 59 per cent, hypoglycemia in 59 per cent, anemia in 46 per cent, and peripheral edema in 43 to 69 per cent. Less frequent complications included polyuria/polydipsia, diarrhea, wound infection, ventricular arrhythmias, and hemorrhage.

Mortality rates for dogs with prostatic abscesses are high. An overall mortality rate of 51 per cent for 23 dogs with abscesses was reported in 1978, whereas 21 per cent of 89 dogs that survived surgical drainage for an abscessed prostate died within 1 week of surgery. Sepsis and associated shock were the most common causes of death. All the listed complications, including death, should be anticipated in a dog with a life-threatening septic process. A plan for recognizing and treating sepsis is necessary.

History and physical examination findings suggesting sepsis can be vague (Table 99–1). In a septic patient, several intravenous lines (in-

TABLE 99–1. LABORATORY RESULTS COMPATIBLE WITH SEPSIS

Complete Blood Count	Serum Biochemistry
Neutrophilia or neutropenia	Hyper- or hypoglycemia
Increased band neutrophils	Increased alkaline phosphatase
Degenerative left shift	Hypoalbuminemia
Toxic changes in neutrophils	Increased alanine aminotransferase
Monocytosis	Bilirubinemia
Decreased platelet count	

Clotting Tests	Acid-Base
Prolonged prothrombin and activated partial thromboplastin times	Metabolic acidosis with respiratory compensation
Increased fibrin degradation products	

cluding one central line) are placed to supply fluids, administer drugs, and withdraw blood samples. An indwelling urinary catheter is placed to monitor urine output. Systemic antibiotic therapy is initiated, not to treat the abscess but to avert potential dissemination of infection. Intravenous antibiotics are usually required because of shock and gastrointestinal failure.

A combination of amikacin (7 to 10 mg/kg IV every 8 hours) and ampicillin (20 to 40 mg/kg IV every 8 hours) is recommended if renal function is normal. If renal function is compromised, cefoxitin (20 mg/kg IV every 8 hours) is safe and usually effective. If oral antibiotics can be used, enrofloxacin (5 to 8 mg/kg PO every 12 hours) is recommended.

The choice of cardiovascular support therapy before surgery depends on the presence of shock. Once fluid administration has been initiated, the need for metabolic therapy is assessed. Antiendotoxin therapy is chosen carefully. Corticosteroids are effective when used before shock or within the first hour of onset. The clotting status of septic dogs can range from hypercoagulable to disseminated intravascular coagulation. During surgery, anesthetic management of patients with prostatic abscess is similar to that of any patient in critical condition.

Prostate fluid samples are submitted for Gram staining, cytological evaluation, aerobic and anaerobic cultures, and sensitivity testing. Urine is submitted for aerobic culture and sensitivity studies. Patients that are in obvious septic shock at the onset of surgery or that develop shock after surgery are carefully monitored for multiple organ failure.

Urinary System (pages 1368–1495)

CHAPTER 100

Anatomy of the Urinary Tract
(pages 1368–1383)

DEVELOPMENT OF THE URINARY SYSTEM (pp. 1368–1372)

Normal Development

Kidneys and Ureters

Kidneys are compound tubular glands composed of uriniferous tubules. They arise in the embryo in a mesodermal plate called the *nephrotome*, which lies between the somatic and splanchnic mesoderm. From the nephrotome, three classes of organs develop sequentially. The first to form is the pronephros. This is the functional kidney of primitive vertebrates such as cyclostomes and the provisional kidney of larval fishes and amphibians. The mesonephros is the permanent kidney of fishes and amphibians. The metanephric kidney, the third class in the sequence, is the functional kidney of reptiles, birds, and mammals. Secretory units, or nephrons, consist of the Bowman capsule, proximal and distal convoluted tubules, and the loop of Henle.

The drainage duct system of the metanephros is derived from a bud growing off the mesonephric duct close to the cloaca. This bud pushes into the metanephrogenic mesoderm and, by a process of repeated dichotomous branching and absorption, differentiates into ureter, pelvis, calyces, papillary ducts, and straight collecting tubules.

Abnormal Development

Renal Agenesis. This can occur if the mesonephric ducts fail to develop or if no ureteric bud forms.

Supernumerary Kidneys. If two ureteric buds grow from the same mesonephric duct, supernumerary kidneys will result.

Renal Hypoplasia. This is a deficiency in the total nephron population. *Dysplasia* refers to the presence of abnormal nephrons.

Ureteral Ectopia. If the ureter buds off the mesonephric duct too far cranially, then with growth and absorption the metanephric duct (ureter) might not open separately into the bladder.

Ureterocele. A ureterocele is a cystic dilatation of the intravesicular portion of the ureter.

Faulty Differentiation of the Cloaca. This can result in incomplete separation of the rectum and urogenital sinus.

GROSS ANATOMY OF THE URINARY SYSTEM
(pp. 1372–1383)

The characteristic features of the kidneys of dogs and cats are summarized in Table 100–1.

Arterial Circulation. Multiple renal arteries have been observed

TABLE 100–1. CHARACTERISTIC FEATURES OF THE KIDNEYS

Feature	Dog	Cat
Type	Unipyramidal (fused pyramids)	Unipyramidal (single pyramid)
Weight per kidney (g)	50 to 60	7.5 to 15
Color	Brownish red to reddish blue	Red to yellowish red
Kidney mass as a percentage of body weight	0.6	0.6 to 1.0
Total nephrons per kidney	415,000	190,000
Kidney length in proportion to length of lumbar vertebra (L2)	2.9	2.7
Kidney width in proportion to length of L2	1.6	1.7
Ventral displacement in proportion to length of L2	L 0.7 R 0.3	0.7 0.7

in the left kidney in 13 per cent of dogs but are uncommon in cats. Most dogs have a single renal artery to the right kidney.

Ureters

The ureters are retroperitoneal urine conduits that pursue a relatively tortuous route to the bladder.

Bladder

The bladder is a urine reservoir that varies in form, size, and position, depending on the volume of urine it contains.

Urethra

The urethra is the canal that extends from the neck of the bladder to the urethral meatus. It conveys urine from the bladder to the external environment. In males, the urethra also carries seminal secretions.

CHAPTER 101
Physiology of the Urinary Tract (pages 1384–1395)

OVERVIEW OF RENAL FUNCTION (p. 1384)

The primary function of the kidneys is regulation of the composition of extracellular fluid. Thus the kidneys indirectly control the composition of intracellular fluid as well. These functions are accomplished through filtration, reabsorption, secretion, and hormone production.

STRUCTURAL ORGANIZATION OF THE KIDNEYS
(p. 1384)

Renal function is the sum of the function of individual nephrons, approximately 190,000 per kidney in cats and 415,000 to 580,000 per kidney in dogs.

RENAL CIRCULATION (p. 1384)

The kidneys receive approximately 20 to 25 per cent of cardiac output, despite the fact that they account for less than 1 per cent of total body weight. Normal renal blood flow in dogs is approximately 4 ml/minute/g of kidney weight. Approximately 90 per cent of renal blood flow traverses the cortex, 10 per cent perfuses the outer medulla, and 1 to 2 per cent reaches the inner medulla and papilla.

GLOMERULAR FILTRATION (pp. 1385–1386)

Formation of glomerular filtrate, which is the central function of the kidneys, occurs as a result of Starling forces in the glomerular capillary bed. The filtrate formed is most accurately termed *glomerular ultrafiltrate*. The Starling forces under consideration are the colloid (protein) osmotic and hydrostatic pressure gradients.

MECHANISMS CONTROLLING RENAL BLOOD FLOW AND GLOMERULAR FILTRATION (pp. 1386–1387)

The driving force for glomerular filtration rate, glomerular capillary hydrostatic pressure, is controlled through the relative resistance of the afferent and efferent arterioles. Most vasoactive compounds affecting renal blood flow and glomerular filtration rate act by altering the relative or absolute tone of these arterioles.

A central concept of renal hemodynamics is that renal blood flow and glomerular filtration rate tend to remain constant despite variations in systemic arterial pressure between 75 and 160 mm Hg. This capacity is referred to as *autoregulation,* and because it occurs in a denervated, isolated-perfused kidney, it is an intrinsic property of the kidney.

RENAL SOLUTE HANDLING (pp. 1387–1390)

Although in excess of 100 l of glomerular filtrate is formed daily in the average dog, less than 1 per cent of this ultimately remains in the urine. Because of the large quantity of electrolytes, water, amino acids, and glucose in the filtrate, tubular modification is essential for the maintenance of homeostasis. The reabsorptive process is arranged axially along the nephron, with most reabsorption occurring in an isosmotic manner without regard to body needs via high-capacity, low-affinity transport systems in the early portions of the tubule. As fluid progresses along the length of the tubule, reabsorption occurs in accordance with body needs through low-capacity, high-affinity transport processes. For some solutes, such as glucose and amino acids, this entire process occurs within the proximal tubule, and all filtered solute is normally removed from the tubular fluid. For other solutes, such as sodium and potassium, the bulk of filtered solute is reabsorbed in a poorly regulated fashion in the proximal tubule, and the amount of solute finally to appear in the urine is adjusted according to body needs in the distal tubule and collecting duct.

Glucose

At normal plasma concentrations, reabsorption of glucose is complete as the filtrate passes through the first 20 per cent of the proximal tubule. The plasma glucose concentration at which glucosuria first occurs is referred to as the *renal threshold for glucosuria*, which is approximately 180 to 200 mg/100 ml in dogs and 290 mg/100 ml in cats.

Amino Acids

Amino acid reabsorption is nearly complete (> 99 per cent) in the proximal tubule. One exception is felinine, which is normally present in the urine of cats. The functional significance of this sulfur-containing amino acid is unknown.

Sodium

Sodium is the principal extracellular cation, and its concentration and total body content are important determinants of extracellular fluid composition. The concentration of sodium in plasma is a main determinant of plasma osmolality. Body sodium content determines extracellular fluid volume and influences systemic arterial pressure. Although sodium reabsorption occurs along the length of the tubule, most filtered sodium is reabsorbed in the proximal tubule. In both the proximal tubule and the loop of Henle, sodium reabsorption occurs without regard to body needs. In the distal tubule and collecting duct, aldosterone enhances sodium reabsorption in accordance with needs.

Chloride

Chloride transport in the proximal tubules occurs by secondary active transport and passive transport through intercellular spaces.

Potassium

Potassium is predominantly an intracellular ion. A high intracellular potassium concentration is required for optimal cellular functions and for maintenance of the transmembrane potential. Plasma potassium concentration does not provide a reliable method to assess whole-body potassium homeostasis. Cats with normal or diseased kidneys are predisposed to urinary losses of potassium and subsequent development of a polymyopathy secondary to potassium depletion. The relative contributions of inadequate dietary potassium intake versus enhanced urinary potassium losses have not been determined.

Phosphate

The kidneys are the main organs responsible for phosphate homeostasis. Phosphate is freely filtered and reabsorbed in the proximal tubule by a sodium-dependent mechanism, which is inhibited by parathyroid hormone.

Calcium

The most important mechanism for maintenance of homeostasis of calcium is gastrointestinal absorption, which is influenced by vitamin D. Although only ionized calcium is physiologically active, calcium exists in plasma in protein-bound, chelated, or ionized forms. Only chelated and ionized forms are freely filtered by the kidneys and account for approximately 50 per cent of total calcium in normal animals.

Magnesium

Plasma magnesium concentration is regulated by the kidneys. Most magnesium in plasma is freely filtered, and about 25 per cent of this is reabsorbed in the proximal tubules.

ACID-BASE BALANCE (pp. 1390–1392)

Acid-base homeostasis is controlled by the kidneys and lungs. The CO_2/HCO_3^- buffer system has an integral role in maintenance of acid-base balance by both kidneys and lungs via the following reactions:

$$H_2O + CO_2 \xrightleftharpoons[\text{anhydrase}]{\text{carbonic}} H_2CO_3 \xrightleftharpoons{} HCO_3^- + H^+$$

Although the lungs can bring about an acute change in body acid-base status by altering carbon dioxide pressure, the kidneys provide long-term control of body acid-base status through the related processes of bicarbonate reabsorption and proton excretion.

Bicarbonate Reabsorption

Bicarbonate freely passes the glomerular filtration barrier and must normally be reabsorbed to maintain acid-base homeostasis. Bicarbonate is reabsorbed by proton secretion into the proximal tubular lumen. Unlike most electrolytes, bicarbonate has several mechanisms contributing to control of its reabsorption in the proximal tubules.

Proton Excretion

Although the addition of alkalinizing agents (e.g., sodium bicarbonate, potassium citrate, or calcium carbonate) or the ingestion of a cereal-based diet may have a net alkalinizing effect, cats and dogs ingesting a meat-based diet must usually generate acidic urine to maintain acid-base balance. Proton secretion by the distal tubules and collecting ducts is responsible for the final adjustment of urine pH and the maintenance of total-body acid-base balance.

The final urine pH is a product of distal tubular proton excretion and the net secretion of hydrogen ions and can be quantitated as the sum of urinary content of ammonium and titratable acid.

Factors Affecting Tubular Reabsorption

Although the uptake of solutes and water from the lumen depends on cellular transport mechanisms, the transit of solutes and water from the interstitium into the peritubular capillaries depends on Starling forces. Hence, peritubular physical forces—specifically interstitial colloid osmotic and hydrostatic pressures—greatly affect renal handling of solutes and water. Consequently, any process that causes fluid to accumulate in the interstitium lowers interstitial colloid osmotic pressure and raises interstitial hydrostatic pressure, both changes that hinder fluid movement out of the tubule.

An important property of the kidneys is the presence of glomerulo-tubular balance, which allows that for most solutes, the rate of transport reflects the rate of filtration. Thus, elevations of glomerular filtration rate lead to increases in filtered load, which are met with increases in absolute reabsorption. As a consequence, transient changes in glomerular filtration rate do not cause wide fluctuations in urinary content of solutes or in concentrations of solutes within the extracellular fluid.

Many hormones have direct effects on tubular reabsorptive processes.

WATER REABSORPTION: THE URINE-CONCENTRATING MECHANISM (pp. 1392–1393)

The kidneys are responsible for maintaining water homeostasis. This includes the ability to conserve or excrete water, depending on body needs. In a normal 20-kg dog, the daily glomerular filtration rate exceeds 100 l, and even polyuric animals must reclaim the majority of filtrate. As with most filtered substances, water reabsorption occurs primarily in the proximal portions of the nephrons. As a consequence of water reabsorption in the proximal tubules and the loop of Henle, approximately 10 per cent of the filtered load of water reaches the final portion of distal tubules, regardless of body needs.

As the tubular fluid reaches the terminal portion of the distal tubules and the collecting ducts, water could be passively reabsorbed along the osmotic gradient provided by medullary hypertonicity. In the absence of antidiuretic hormone, the collecting duct epithelium is impermeable to water, resulting in formation of dilute urine. Water movement from collecting duct to interstitium is promoted by antidiuretic hormone, resulting in the production of concentrated urine.

ASSESSMENT OF RENAL FUNCTION (pp. 1393–1394)

Renal function is assessed by analysis of urine, measurement of serum concentrations of creatinine (SCr) and blood urea nitrogen (BUN), or specialized tests to assess glomerular filtration rate, renal blood flow, or renal solute handling.

Serum Creatinine and Blood Urea Nitrogen

Because of wide variability and the effects of nonrenal factors, measurement of SCr and BUN is generally worthwhile only for clinical detection of marked impairment of renal function (glomerular filtration rate). Normal BUN and SCr values may be noted in dogs and cats with as little as 25 per cent of normal glomerular filtration rate.

Measurement of Renal Clearance

The standard measure of renal function is the clearance procedure in which a timed, total collection of urine is used with the standard clearance formula:

$$C = UvUc/Pc$$

where C = clearance (milliliters per minute), Uv = urine flow rate (milliliters per minute), Uc = concentration of solute in urine, and Pc = concentration of solute in plasma. Inulin, a fructose polymer that is freely filtered, not metabolized, and neither reabsorbed nor secreted, is the standard compound for measurement of glomerular filtration rate (inulin clearance). A timed collection of urine in a metabolism cage (24 hours) is used to measure endogenous creatinine clearance. This method is useful clinically. Exogenous infusion/injection of creatinine for short-term measurement of clearance (20 to 60 minutes) minimizes the contribution of noncreatinine chromogens, providing a reliable method for measuring glomerular filtration rate in dogs.

MICTURITION (p. 1394)

The entire process of urine storage and voiding is referred to as *micturition*. A lesion of the bladder, urethra, or any component of the neural pathway may lead to a disorder of the storage or voiding phase of micturition.

CHAPTER 102

Pathophysiology and Therapeutics of Urinary Tract Disorders (pages 1396–1415)

RENAL INSUFFICIENCY AND RENAL FAILURE
(pp. 1396–1403)

This section deals with reduced renal function in three characterized syndromes: urinary tract obstruction, acute renal failure, and chronic renal failure.

Renal insufficiency is defined as reduction in renal function in the absence of dramatic clinical signs. The term *renal failure* refers to more significant loss of renal function with dramatic clinical signs. Renal failure is associated with a group of metabolic abnormalities termed *uremia*.

Urinary Tract Obstruction

Urinary tract obstruction is generally divided into two forms, acute and chronic. When acute obstruction is complete and bilateral, it threatens life. Death results within 65 to 70 hours if the obstruction is not relieved. Chronic urinary tract obstruction is commonly unilateral or incomplete and may remain unrecognized for long periods.

Causes

The most common mechanical cause of obstruction is urinary calculi (Chapters 108 and 110). The most common cause of functional obstruction is neurogenic or atonic bladder (see the later section on urine incontinence).

Clinical Signs and Laboratory Findings

The clinical signs of acute complete obstruction are straining on urination, increased frequency of attempts to urinate, dysuria with oliguria or anuria, and abdominal pain. Table 102–1 outlines the clinical and laboratory data commonly used to identify urinary tract obstruction and distinguish it from acute or chronic renal failure. Physical findings associated with chronic obstruction are more discrete, and affected animals may require special diagnostic tests including radiography.

TABLE 102–1. CLINICAL AND LABORATORY DATA BASE

Finding	Urinary Tract Obstruction	Acute Renal Failure	Chronic Renal Failure
Azotemia	X	X	X
Uremic symptoms		X	X
Urinary retention	X		
Edema/ascites		X	X
Anuria/oliguria	X	X	
Tender bladder	X		
Distended bladder after voiding	X		
Gross polyuria			X
Blood chemistry			
↑ Urea nitrogen/creatinine	X	X	X
↑ or ↓ sodium			
↑ potassium	X	X	
↑ chloride or ↓ carbon dioxide		X	X
↑ phosphorus	X	X	X
↑ or ↓ calcium			X
Blood count anemia			X
Urinalysis			
proteinuria		X	X
glycosuria	X	X	
casts		X	X

Pathophysiology

Dramatic changes in renal function occur during the first 24 hours of complete bilateral obstruction. After relief of obstruction, sodium and water excretion in the urine markedly increases despite a severe reduction in glomerular filtration rate (GFR), a natriuretic state referred to as postobstructive diuresis.

Urine-concentrating capacity is the first function lost after any form of urinary tract obstruction. Loss of the ability to excrete acid occurs when urine is not excreted. After 24 hours of complete ureteral obstruction in dogs, renal blood flow decreases to approximately 50 per cent of normal. During acute bilateral urinary tract obstruction, GFR is markedly reduced and is approximately 20 per cent of normal immediately after relief of 24 hours of obstruction. During acute bilateral obstruction, plasma potassium concentration increases. After relief of obstruction, potassium loss in the urine increases.

Urethral obstruction (complete or partial) can cause overdistension of the bladder, resulting in loss of tight junctions within the bladder wall. Impaired detrusor function may improve in response to drug therapy, but the owner should be informed that this may be permanent.

Treatment

The site of blockage must be determined and the obstruction removed as soon as possible. Severe acidosis, hyperkalemia, and azotemia may preclude immediate surgery. Animals with azotemia, hypothermia, and dehydration should be hospitalized for intensive treatment.

Expansion of the extracellular fluid volume may partially correct the reduced GFR associated with obstruction. Based on the severity of clinical signs or on specific measurement of the severity of acidosis, sodium bicarbonate should be administered intravenously. Although potassium-containing solutions are contraindicated initially because of hyperkalemia, reduced potassium intake combined with increased urinary potassium loss tends to cause hypokalemia during recovery.

Complications of obstruction, such as renal failure, anemia, calculi, and infection, require specific management before or after surgery. All animals that have had recurrent obstruction with or without infection require careful long-term surveillance.

Acute Renal Failure

Acute renal failure is defined as recent loss of renal function owing to potentially reversible damage of the renal parenchyma. It may be difficult to distinguish from chronic renal failure.

Causes

Reduced renal hemodynamics represent a major predisposing factor to acute renal failure. Reduced renal perfusion, hypotension, hypovolemia, and sudden circulatory collapse are the most common initiating factors. Various nephrotoxins may also cause acute renal failure, including heavy metals, organic compounds, antimicrobial agents, pigments, acute infectious agents, and hypercalcemia.

Clinical Signs and Laboratory Findings

Animals with acute renal failure are generally depressed, hypovolemic, and hypothermic and have acute and severe gastrointestinal signs. Kidneys are usually normal in size or enlarged. Oliguria with concentrated urine suggests acute rather than chronic renal failure. Laboratory studies should include a complete blood count; BUN, serum creatinine, sodium, potassium, phosphorus, and calcium determinations; acid-base evaluation; and urinalysis (see Table 102–1).

Radiographic studies to confirm acute failure are of limited practical value. A wedge biopsy or even a percutaneous needle biopsy may be contraindicated owing to the dangers of anesthesia and bleeding tendencies associated with renal failure.

Pathophysiology

Acute renal failure occurs in four stages: (1) onset, (2) oliguric or maintenance stage, (3) diuretic stage, and (4) recovery.

No single event or sequence of events uniformly represents the pathophysiological sequence. After an ischemic or nephrotoxic insult, alterations in renal hemodynamics, cellular injury to the glomerulus, arteriolar vasoconstriction, tubular ischemia, tubular leakage, intratubular obstruction, and decreased glomerular permeability occur. The exact sequence of these events is unclear.

Treatment

Surgery is seldom indicated in the treatment of acute renal failure. The first priority is correction of renal hemodynamic disorders and alleviation of biochemical abnormalities until renal repair can take place. Diuretic agents have been advocated in the treatment of oliguric acute renal failure when volume replacement alone fails to initiate urine production.

After surgery, trauma, or nephrotoxic exposure resulting in oliguria, mannitol administration may be of considerable benefit in protecting renal function. Infusion of 0.25 to 0.5 g/kg given with fluid replacement to dogs is beneficial. If diuresis results, a maintenance infusion of 5 to 10 per cent mannitol in normal saline or a balanced electrolyte solution can be continued to promote diuresis for 12 to 24 hours. If diuresis does not occur within 1 hour of the first dose, additional doses should not be given. Repeated bicarbonate administration every 6 to 12 hours may be necessary for several days to combat acidosis. Peritoneal dialysis and hemodialysis may be considered and applied for 3 to 14 days until it is clear whether renal function will return and be adequate to support the animal.

Chronic Renal Failure

In chronic renal failure, GFR has been reduced for a long interval, and there is little likelihood of rapid deterioration or hope of significant improvement.

Causes

The causes of chronic failure are usually not surgical diseases and cannot be corrected by surgical intervention.

Clinical Signs and Laboratory Findings

The common clinical and laboratory findings seen with chronic failure are outlined in Table 102–1. Evidence of chronicity includes stable azotemia and stable reduced GFR for more than 3 months and a gradual decline of function over years. Most animals have some degree of polyuria, anorexia, or osteodystrophy or small kidneys observed on routine x-ray films. In conjunction with signs of renal disease, nonresponsive anemia suggests chronic rather than acute failure.

Chronic renal failure in dogs and cats can also result in systemic hypertension. Chronic failure may also include the coexistence of acute renal failure, which may obscure the duration of disease.

Metabolic Abnormalities in Uremia

As chronic failure progresses, a number of complex alterations in renal function occur to maintain metabolic balance until the later stages of renal failure. The pattern of metabolic abnormalities in uremia is irregular. Therefore, during the early course of chronic failure, the presenting signs may be highly variable and confusing.

A typical animal with progressive chronic failure may pass through four stages.

Stage 1. During this stage there is only a reduction in renal reserve. Until at least 50 per cent of normal nephrons have been lost, there is no evidence of chemical abnormalities or azotemia. The excretory and regulatory functions of the kidneys are preserved in this stage, and clinical signs are absent. This stage is commonly missed in clinical evaluation unless renal clearance studies are performed.

Stage 2. This stage may be termed *renal insufficiency*. Manifestations include mild azotemia, impaired ability to concentrate urine, nocturia, and polyuria. Anorexia may occur intermittently, but body weight and physical appearance are relatively normal. A mild anemia may be present. The animal is in a precarious state, which may be revealed by reduced fluid intake, vomiting, or diarrhea leading to more pronounced azotemia.

Stage 3. This stage is associated with persistent and frank renal failure with anemia, hyperphosphatemia, isosthenuria, and marked polyuria. Intermittent anorexia, weakness, listlessness, and intermittent vomiting with debilitation occur.

Stage 4. The final stage is uremia, when all the consequences of metabolic abnormalities become obvious. Clinical signs are more advanced than in stage 3 and include severe gastrointestinal disturbances, nervous signs, and severe anemia.

The major metabolic abnormalities of uremia are listed in Table 102–2.

Uremia is associated with various endocrine abnormalities, including excessive production of hormones, inadequate production of hormones, reduced metabolic or renal clearance of hormones, and abnormal metabolism of hormones. In some cases, as with parathyroid hormone, clinical disturbances have been identified, and the role of the hormone has been clarified.

The anemia of chronic renal failure may be a major limiting factor in survival of these animals. The pathogenesis of anemia includes deficiency of erythropoietin. Renal osteodystrophy is a major metabolic abnormality with widespread secondary effects. The pathogenesis of renal osteodystrophy involves three main abnormalities: malabsorption of calcium, altered vitamin D metabolism, and hyperparathyroidism. Several toxic effects have been attributed to excessive parathyroid hormone, and this substance may now be considered a uremic toxin.

METABOLIC CONSEQUENCES AND ALTERED RENAL FUNCTION AFTER URINARY DIVERSION (pp. 1403–1404)

Urinary diversion procedures include ureteroileostomy, ureterosigmoidostomy, trigonal-colonic anastomosis, transureteroureterostomy, and cutaneous end ureterostomy. The objectives of urinary diversion are to provide for adequate urinary drainage, to preserve renal function, and to minimize secondary effects of diversion. Untoward consequences are not expected when a technically competent transureteroureterostomy is performed. Problems associated with the use of bowel as a urinary conduit include ascending infection resulting in pyelonephritis and reduced renal function, electrolyte imbalances secondary to absorption of urinary solutes, and stenosis at the site of intestinal anastomosis causing impaired ureteral function, leakage of urine, or progressive hydronephrosis. The problems of cutaneous end ureterostomy in domestic animals have not been studied because this procedure is considered impractical in domestic animals. Infection of the upper urinary tract is a major concern when using any urinary diversion technique.

Abnormal levels of plasma electrolytes and other solutes are less likely with urine diversion into the colon than with diversion into the small intestine. Electrolytes are more readily absorbed from the small intestine than from the colon. However, ureterocolonic anastomosis in

TABLE 102–2. METABOLIC DISTURBANCES OF UREMIA

Uremic toxins
Cellular function and composition
Biochemical disturbances
Nitrogen metabolism
Fat metabolism
Endocrine alterations
Gastrointestinal changes
Fluid, electrolyte, and acid-base changes
Hematological abnormalities
Renal osteodystrophy
Neurological changes
Cardiovascular abnormalities

dogs has been accompanied by uremia due to dehydration, ureteral obstruction, renal dysfunction or absorption of urea, and metabolic acidosis and hyperchloremia.

Problems associated with urinary diversion are usually obvious within a few days of surgery. The metabolic complications must be distinguished from deterioration of renal function, which is monitored by long-term surveillance.

PATHOPHYSIOLOGY AND PHARMACOLOGICAL MANAGEMENT OF URINARY INCONTINENCE
(pp. 1404–1409)

Urinary incontinence is the failure of voluntary control of the urinary bladder and urethral sphincters, resulting in inability to control urination. This disorder is more common in dogs than in cats and in females than in males.

Pathophysiology of Urinary Incontinence

Urinary incontinence and urinary outflow obstruction can occur secondary to neurological lesions, hormonal imbalances, congenital abnormalities, and diseases of the bladder, urethra, or prostate gland.

Neurological Causes of Urinary Incontinence
Upper Motor Neuron Lesions

Lesions from the pons-L7 spinal cord segments may result in detrusor areflexia, with hyperreflexia and increased tone of the external urethral sphincter. Thus, there is loss of voluntary control of urination, and manual expression of the bladder is difficult.

Abnormalities of the cerebellum or partial long tract lesions may result in detrusor hyperreflexia with little or no residual urine. In these cases, urination is frequent and inappropriate. Partial long tract lesions may also result in detrusor urethral dyssynergia or reflex dyssynergia, a condition in which bladder contraction and urethral relaxation are not synchronous.

Lower Motor Neuron Lesions

Injuries of the sacral spinal cord or nerve roots or branches may result in detrusor areflexia with or without sphincter areflexia. Atony of the detrusor muscle results in overdistension, which, if prolonged, may cause separation of the tight junctions and increased bladder capacity with large amounts of residual urine.

Non-Neurological Causes of Urinary Incontinence
Congenital Abnormalities

The most common congenital abnormality resulting in urinary incontinence is ectopic ureter (see Chapter 106). Surgery may correct the urinary incontinence, depending on the location of the ectopic ureters.

Other congenital abnormalities that may result in urinary incontinence include patent urachus, urethrorectal fistulas, and urethrovaginal fistulas. In patients with patent urachus, urine is voided through the umbilicus, and surgical correction is warranted.

Hormone-Responsive Urinary Incontinence

Estrogen-responsive incontinence in female dogs is an uncommon and poorly understood sequela to ovariohysterectomy. It develops in dogs after a variable period of time following surgery. The reported mean age of dogs in which this type of incontinence has been recognized is 8.3 years. Hormone-responsive incontinence has also been reported in a castrated male dog.

Incontinence Due to Cystitis, Urethritis, or Prostatic Disease

An inflamed or irritated bladder may become hyperactive or unstable, resulting in a syndrome called *urge incontinence*, which is characterized by detrusor contractions that cannot be voluntarily inhibited. Chronic cystitis, urethritis, or prostatic disease can also cause urethral incompetence resulting in urinary incontinence.

Paradoxical Incontinence Due to Mechanical Obstruction of the Urethra

Bladder Position and Urethral Length

Caudal displacement of the bladder (pelvic bladder) in female dogs has been variously reported to be a cause of urinary incontinence or an incidental finding.

Idiopathic Urinary Incontinence

Diagnosis

An accurate history, recorded chronologically, is important in the diagnosis of the cause of urinary incontinence. Observation of the animal's urination, attempted urination, or lack of urination can provide important clues to the dysfunction. Measuring residual urine may provide additional information. Normally, residual urine volume should be less than 10 ml. The presence of voluntary control of urination is important in the diagnosis of urinary incontinence.

In addition to observation of urination, a complete physical and neurological examination is essential to the correct diagnosis of disorders of continence. Palpation and careful manual expression of the bladder provide information about bladder and urethral tone. If the physical examination reveals dribbling of urine and an easily expressed bladder, the urethral sphincter mechanism is inefficient. Difficulty in expressing the bladder in a dog with signs of bladder-urethral incoordination is further evidence that dyssynergia exists. Increased urethral tone due to sympathetic discharge can occur in animals with cauda equina lesions such as intervertebral disc protrusion, lumbosacral instability, or cauda equina tumors.

In all continence disorders, thorough examination must be performed for urinary tract infection or mechanical obstruction to urination. If functional obstruction is suspected but mechanical obstruction cannot be ruled out on the basis of physical and neurological examination, further examination of the urethra and bladder should be initiated. Other diagnostic tests that are usually available through referral centers and that may be necessary in making a definitive diagnosis include the electromyogram (EMG), the cystometrogram (CMG), and the urethral pressure profile (UPP).

Treatment (p. 1407)

Micturition disorders that are responsive to specific drug therapy are listed. Doses should begin at the low end of the range given and are increased gradually until the desired response is seen or the maximum dose is reached. The duration of the therapeutic trial at maximum dose depends on the individual drug but in general should be 1 to 2 weeks. If no response to the chosen drug is noted within this time period, the drug can be considered ineffective and discontinued.

Hormone-Responsive Urinary Incontinence (p. 1407)

Recommended drugs and dosages, mode of action, and potential side effects are given.

Urethral Incompetence

Phenylpropanolamine is an alpha stimulant that is effective in increasing urethral pressure and resistance to urine leakage when given orally.

Urge Incontinence

Oxybutynin and flavoxate are antispasmodic drugs with little or no anticholinergic action and fewer potential side effects than propantheline. Imipramine pamoate is a tricyclic antidepressant that has been used successfully in humans to treat detrusor instability and facilitate urine storage. Empronium bromide is an anticholinergic drug with antimuscarinic and antinicotinic actions. In one study, only 7 of 21 female dogs with urinary incontinence responded favorably to treatment with empronium bromide.

Functional Urethral Obstruction

Sympathetically induced urethral obstruction can be treated effectively with the alpha-adrenergic blocking agents phenoxybenzamine or prazosin hydrochloride. Somatically induced urethral obstruction can be treated with diazepam or dantrolene.

Detrusor Atony and Detrusor Atony with Functional Urethral Obstruction

Bethanechol is a cholinergic agent that has been used successfully to stimulate detrusor contraction in neurogenic and non-neurogenic hypotonic bladder dysfunction. Because bethanechol stimulates the parasympathetic receptors of smooth muscle, it may cause increased urethral resistance, and its efficacy in improving bladder emptying depends on its effect on the detrusor exceeding its effect on the urethra.

Surgical Treatment of Urinary Incontinence

URINE SPRAYING AND MARKING IN CATS
(pp. 1409–1419)

Even though male cats are castrated to prevent urine spraying and female cats spray urine infrequently, this behavior remains a clinical problem in feline practice. Alternative therapeutic approaches include behavioral control, administration of progestins and, as a last resort, neurosurgical or bilateral ischiocavernosus myectomy techniques. None of the therapeutic approaches currently used are 100 per cent effective.

Normal Urine Spraying and Urine Marking Behavior

Territorial Marking

By creating a recognizable olfactory field in the home envionment, it is believed that the cat may feel more self-assured and confident, especially in regard to agonistic encounters with other cats.

Sexually Dimorphic Aspects

Spraying is a behavior normally associated with tomcats, and the onset is related to sexual maturation. Like fighting, roaming, and sexual behavior, urine spraying is sexually dimorphic behavior that occurs less frequently in females than males.

Differential Diagnosis of Problem Spraying

When urine is found 1 to 2 feet above the ground on vertical objects, it is a result of spraying. In both urine spraying and marking, certain objects are usually selected and repeatedly hit.

Inappropriate Urination
Urinary Disorders

The presence of a urinary disorder is usually evident from the medical history.

Androgenic Steroids

An occasional cause of spraying may be administration of androgenic steroids to stimulate metabolism, increase muscle tone, or treat certain skin conditions.

Incidence of Urine Spraying
Effects of Postpubertal Castration

Castration of tomcats after puberty, even after spraying has begun, is quite effective in eliminating or markedly reducing spraying.

Effects of Prepubertal Castration

It is not unusual to find that male or female cats, neutered at 6 months of age, begin spraying as late as 3 or 4 years of age. The onset of spraying is often related to the introduction of new cats into a household with other cats, changing households, or altering a major aspect of the cat's life-style, such as making an outdoor cat an indoor cat.

A survey including 136 male and 124 female cats revealed that prepubertal castration is not likely to be more effective in preventing objectionable spraying than postpubertal castration is in eliminating the behavior once it has started.

Therapy for Problem Spraying
Predisposing and Causal Factors

When treating urine spraying and marking, it is a good idea to determine why the cat started spraying and continues to spray.

Behavioral Approaches and Management

A remote punishment, such as upside-down mouse traps near the soiled areas, may be effective. Ambushing a cat with a squirt gun or water sprayer when it is beginning to spray is another technique. It is important that remote punishment be delivered without the cat knowing that the owner is involved in the punishment process. In this way the animal makes the association between the target areas and the punishment rather than between the owner and the punishment.

Progestin Therapy

Synthetic progestins are related to the hormone progesterone; the progestins suppress malelike behavior, such as spraying, even when the behavior occurs in females. The long-acting progestins effective in correcting spraying include the commercially available medroxyprogesterone (MPA; Depo-Provera) and megestrol acetate (MA; Ovaban). MPA is given as an injection and MA orally.

Because MPA and MA seem to be about equally effective in the initial treatment of spraying but MA results in more depression and appetite stimulation than MPA, it is recommended that injectable MPA be used in most cases for initial treatment. The use of an injectable drug also eliminates the need for a client to follow a complex dosage regimen.

Bilateral Ischiocavernosus Myectomy

The exact cause of the beneficial effect is unknown, but it is postulated that the surgery prevents the cat from holding the penis at the preferred position to spray urine.

Olfactory Tractotomy

Olfactory tractotomy has been successfully used to eliminate spraying in cats that do not respond to progestin treatment. The rationale for the operation is that spraying is usually initiated by a cat's smelling the target area. The olfactory tracts and caudal parts of the olfactory bulbs are approached dorsally through the frontal sinus.

Transient anorexia occurs in about half of the patients, but one can usually stimulate a cat to start eating by placing chicken or turkey baby food in its mouth or smearing the food on its lips. Individual responses to the operation vary. Our clinical evaluation of the effectiveness of this operation is 50 per cent for male cats and 80 to 90 per cent for female cats.

CHAPTER 103

Principles of Urinary Tract Surgery (pages 1415–1428)

PATIENT EVALUATION (pp. 1415–1420)

The physical examination narrows the examiner's focus and, with the history, supplies most of the information needed to make a diagnosis.

Radiography

The presence of urinary tract disease or injury may be suggested by plain radiographs. The observation of calculi is diagnostic, but contrast studies are frequently required to confirm the presence, location, and extent of urinary tract disease.

Excretory Urography

If the renal blood supply is intact and the kidneys are capable of concentrating and excreting contrast material, excretory urography (intravenous pyelography) outlines the kidneys and ureters and provides information about the junction of the ureters and the trigone of the bladder. The location of injury to the kidneys or ureters can often be identified precisely. Rapid intravenous administration of aqueous organic iodide (880 mg/kg) is recommended. Many contrast media can be used.

Renal Angiography

Renal angiography is infrequently done. Options include selective or nonselective renal angiography.

Retrograde Urethrocystography

The integrity of the urethra and bladder is best assessed by retrograde positive-contrast urethrocystography. Negative-contrast or double-contrast studies may identify intraluminal calculi, masses, or blood clots.

Ultrasonography

The contour and size of the kidneys are easily determined, and mass or cystic lesions of the kidneys are readily detected and biopsy performed. Ultrasonography is efficacious in evaluating the bladder.

Abdominoparacentesis

If fluid is present in the abdomen or if intra-abdominal urinary tract trauma is suspected, abdominoparacentesis and diagnostic peritoneal lavage (if necessary) should be performed. The concentration of creatinine or urea in the fluid retrieved from the abdomen is compared with that in peripheral blood.

SURGICAL PRINCIPLES (pp. 1420–1422)
Surgical Instruments

A gentle touch with delicate, high-quality equipment and minimal handling of the tissues minimizes edema. A scalpel causes minimal tissue trauma. An electroscalpel is a useful tool for incising the bladder and urethra and for hemostasis by coagulation of small vessels.

Grasping instruments with strong jaws and large teeth are not required for operating on delicate urinary tract tissues. Hemostats are never used for temporary vascular occlusion because they crush vessels and promote clotting and stricture. Polypropylene catheters with rounded, sealed ends and a side hole in a range of sizes from 3 to 8 French can be used for catheterizing the urethra or ureters of cats and dogs. Some type of suction apparatus is useful to aspirate urine and flushing solutions.

Suture Materials

The choice of suture material depends on the normal strength of the tissues, the rate at which the wound recovers strength, the strength of the suture material, the rate at which the suture material loses strength in tissues, and interactions that occur between sutures and tissues. The bladder, along with the proximal colon, is one of the weakest organs in the body; however, tissues regain nearly 100 per cent of pre-wounded strength in 14 to 21 days. Sutures should be at least as strong as the tissue through which they are placed. Nonabsorbable sutures are not used in the urinary tract, because they provide a nidus for formation of urinary calculi.

Splinting (Stenting) in Urethral and Ureteral Surgery

Urinary epithelium is damaged by indwelling urethral catheters. If primary intention healing is sought, splinting catheters are avoided because of (1) interference with healing and (2) risk of ascending infection. Urine leakage at the urethral anastomosis can delay healing; if this is considered a possibility, urine can be diverted during healing by placing a Foley catheter in the bladder and exteriorizing it in the antepubic position. If sound microsurgical techniques are used for ureteral anastomosis in dogs, splinting catheters are not required.

ALTERED RENAL FUNCTION DUE TO ANESTHESIA, SURGERY, AND DRUGS (pp. 1422–1423)

Indirect Effects of Anesthesia

Circulation. Renal blood flow is decreased owing to renal vasoconstriction and systemic hypotension.

Sympathetic Nervous System. In response to moderate stress, efferent arteriolar constriction occurs. Thus, although renal blood flow has decreased, glomerular filtration rate remains constant.

Endocrine Effects. These are significant and are closely related to circulatory changes.

Direct Effects of Anesthesia

Immediate effects are masked by the indirect effects outlined previously. Delayed effects are related to direct nephrotoxicity as a result of anesthetic agents containing fluorinated hydrocarbons, principally methoxyflurane. Affected patients are unable to concentrate urine, resulting in high-output renal insufficiency. Light anesthesia and an adequate fluid regimen with a balanced electrolyte solution ensure that patients have only minimal and transient depression of renal function.

Antimicrobial Agents

The kidneys are a major excretory pathway for many antibiotics. Nephrons are exposed to high concentrations by glomerular filtration, tubular reabsorption, and secretion. The relative nephrotoxicity of various antimicrobials is listed.

Analgesic Nephropathy

Inhibition of prostaglandin synthesis by nonsteroidal anti-inflammatory agents has little effect on renal blood flow or glomerular filtration rates in normal animals but profoundly diminishes these indices in animals subjected to hemorrhage, salt depletion, general anesthesia, biliary cirrhosis, or heart failure.

Radiographic Contrast Agents

If an iodinated contrast agent is injected through a catheter that is obstructing arterial blood flow, organ damage results.

URINARY TRACT INFECTION (pp. 1423–1426)

Most urinary tract pathogens originate in the gut or on the skin. Organisms ascend from the urethral orifice, and most are mechanically cleared by normal voiding. Urine may be collected by free catch, catheterization, or cystocentesis for analysis and microbial culturing. Quantitative urine cultures may be performed to determine if an infection is present. Contamination of the urine can occur from the urethra, prepuce, or vagina when a clean-catch or catheterized specimen is obtained.

Use of open indwelling urethral catheters for temporary urine diversion has to be weighed against the known risk of infection. Organisms can enter around or through the lumen of the catheter, and most patients with previously sterile urine have bacteriuria within 24 hours of catheter placement. Closed catheter drainage systems with nonreturn valves prevent catheter-associated urinary tract infection for short periods. The prevalence of urinary tract infections in cats is less than in dogs, possibly because of superior antibacterial qualities of cat urine.

Antibiotic, Antibacterial, and Analgesic Therapy

Antibiotics

Penicillins. As a group, the penicillins are generally active against gram-positive organisms. Penicillin G and ampicillin, when given orally, reach urine concentrations 100 times greater than serum concentrations and can be effective against gram-negative as well as gram-positive organisms.

Aminoglycosides. Streptomycin at the recommended dose is bactericidal against many gram-negative organisms. Neomycin is not recommended for parenteral use because of the risk of nephrotoxicity and ototoxicity. Gentamicin is bactericidal and has a broad spectrum of activity. Ototoxicity, renal toxicity, and neuromuscular blockade with the risk of respiratory paralysis can occur with this drug. Tobramycin is like gentamicin.

Cephalosporins. Cephadroxil and cephalexin are effective in the treatment of urinary tract infection due to *Escherichia coli* and *Klebsiella pneumoniae*, respectively.

Tetracyclines. These antibiotics have a broad spectrum of activity and are bacteriostatic at usual concentrations. Oxytetracycline is more freely excreted in the urine than chlortetracycline.

Chloramphenicol. This antibiotic is effective in treating urinary tract infections in dogs, including *Proteus* spp. and *Pseudomonas* spp. infections.

Fluoroquinolones. The fluoroquinolones are bactericidal and are effective against many gram-positive and gram-negative bacteria. Enrofloxacin is approved for veterinary use.

Polymyxins. These drugs are decidedly nephrotoxic and are only used if other, less toxic drugs are unavailable.

Antibacterials

Sulfonamides. These drugs are bacteriostatic, with a gram-positive spectrum of activity.

Enhanced Sulfonamides. When a sulfonamide is combined with trimethoprim, another bacteriostatic drug, the combination is bactericidal and has a broad spectrum of activity.

Nitrofurans.

Methenamine and Its Salts. Methenamine is excreted in the urine, where, in the pH range of 5 to 6, it breaks down to form ammonia and formaldehyde. Bacterial resistance to methenamine has not been demonstrated; therefore, it can be used with its acid salts for long-term therapy.

CHAPTER 104

Kidneys (pages 1428–1442)

CONGENITAL ABNORMALITIES (pp. 1428–1430)

ACQUIRED ABNORMALITIES (pp. 1430–1440)

Trauma

Automobiles inflict most injuries to the urinary tracts of dogs and cats. The most common injury is rupture of the urinary bladder, followed by rupture of the kidney, urethra, and ureter. Renal parenchymal damage as a result of blunt trauma can vary from minor subcapsular bleeding with hematuria to a shattered kidney from which death due to exsanguination, hemorrhagic shock, or acute renal failure may occur.

The objectives of treatment of renal trauma are to control hemorrhage, excise devitalized tissue, and repair injured structures. Parenchymal tears can be packed with a topical hemostatic agent such as gelatin sponge or polymerized methylcellulose. If the damage is confined to one pole, partial nephrectomy may be considered. If the kidney is shattered, it is removed, provided the other kidney is present and functioning satisfactorily.

Nephrectomy

Partial Nephrectomy

Idiopathic Hematuria

Nephrolithiasis

Calculi may form anywhere along a dog's urinary tract, but the kidneys are involved in only 4 per cent. Calculi are occasionally found in the kidneys of cats.

Nephrotomy

Nephrotomy temporarily decreases renal function by 20 to 50 per cent. If calculi are present in both kidneys, a choice of one operation or two operations spaced a few weeks apart must be made.

When bisection nephrotomy is performed, a longitudinal sagittal incision is made with a scalpel through the convex lateral surface of the kidney. Alternatively, an intersegmental nephrotomy can be performed by dividing the kidney along an avascular plane between the terminal branches of the renal artery identified by intra-arterial injection of dye.

Pyelolithotomy

If renal calculi have resulted in dilation of the proximal ureter and renal pelvis, they may be removed through an incision made into these structures (pyelolithotomy). If the renal pelvis and proximal ureter are not dilated, this technique is not attempted. Use of this technique in cats has not been reported.

Alternative Methods for Removing Renoliths
Hydronephrosis

Hydronephrosis is progressive dilation of the renal pelvis and progressive atrophy of the renal parenchyma, most often due to ureteral obstruction. Dogs are more often affected than cats. When urine outflow obstruction affects both kidneys, the animal dies before pressure atrophy can cause much reduction in renal mass. When the obstruction is unilateral, the degree of hydronephrosis can reach such proportions that the renal parenchyma is only a shell. Urine production continues after the lower urinary tract is obstructed, because the obstruction is not complete. Urine is reabsorbed through the renal vein and the renal hilar lymphatics. If the obstruction is relieved within 1 week, the renal damage is totally reversible.

If hydronephrosis is advanced and the kidney is only a fluid-filled sac, the prognosis is hopeless, and the remains of the kidney are removed. If some kidney function is evident on excretory urography and if the cause of the urine obstruction can be identified and corrected, it is vital to try to save that kidney, particularly if the other kidney is also damaged. Nephrostomy drainage of urine immediately relieves intrarenal pressure. Drainage can be maintained until the cause of the obstruction has been corrected.

Purulent Nephritis

Bacterial infection by the hematogenous route is a common complication of obstructive uropathy. Renal injury also predisposes the kidney to blood-borne infection. Purulent nephritis also can occur as an ascending infection from the lower urinary tract, particularly in the presence of vesicoureteral reflux.

Kidney Worm

Dioctophyma renale, the giant kidney worm, is found sporadically in dogs and wild fish-eating carnivores, particularly mink. Cats are resistant to this parasite.

Acute Renal Failure

Acute renal failure is characterized by the rapid onset of oliguria or anuria, reduced renal blood flow, reduced glomerular filtration rate, and sudden azotemia. Acute renal failure is potentially reversible, but some renal tubular damage has invariably occurred. Recovery depends on the extent of renal injury and the capacity of the remaining nephrons to regain normal function.

Two major predisposing factors that contribute to acute renal failure are decreased renal blood flow and exposure of the kidneys to nephrotoxic agents such as heavy metals, organic compounds, and antimicrobial drugs. Decreased renal perfusion can be the result of hemorrhage, trauma, prolonged anesthesia, extensive surgery, or impaired cardiac function. Any of these inciting factors may be present in various proportions in all surgery.

If surgery must be performed on animals with renal disease, consideration is given to fluid balance, serum concentrations of electrolytes (hyperkalemia often occurs in acute renal failure, and hyponatremia in chronic failure), and the pH of peripheral blood (metabolic acidosis accompanies the impaired ability to excrete hydrogen ions).

Needle Biopsy

It is possible to obtain a sample of kidney tissue without opening the abdomen by using the blind percutaneous, keyhole, or percutaneous approach guided by ultrasonography. The kidneys can also be sampled under direct observation during laparoscopy. Before biopsy, the benefits must be weighed against the risks. Absolute contraindications to needle biopsy are hemorrhagic tendencies, inexperienced diagnosticians, and damaged equipment. Complications observed after keyhole kidney biopsy in dogs and cats have included gross and microscopic hematuria, fatal hemorrhage, and hydronephrosis.

Two types of needles are currently in use, the modified pediatric Franklin-Silverman biopsy needle* and the Vim Tru-Cut biopsy needle.† The Tru-Cut needle is disposable, sharp, and easy to use. It can be cleaned and resterilized with ethylene oxide.

Wedge Biopsy

A larger sample of renal tissue can be obtained during nephrotomy. A wedge of tissue 2 to 5 mm thick can be removed from the exposed parenchyma by making a scalpel incision parallel to the nephrotomy incision.

Dialysis

The metabolic waste products that accumulate during acute renal failure and contribute to the signs of uremia can be eliminated by dialysis. Two techniques of dialysis are available, hemodialysis and peritoneal dialysis. Fluid and solute in the extracellular fluid are exchanged across a semipermeable membrane. This membrane is cellulose in hemodialysis and the peritoneum in peritoneal dialysis. Hemodialysis is more efficient, but it requires special equipment and trained staff because the blood has to be removed from the body, circulated through an artificial kidney, and returned to the body.

Peritoneal dialysis is quite feasible in dogs and cats. The dialysate contains at least 1.5 per cent glucose‡ to prevent rapid water absorption from the peritoneum due to the hyperosmotic state of uremic plasma. Hyperosmotic dialysis solutions with 4.25 and 7 per cent glucose are also available, and their use effectively reduces plasma volume in edematous patients.

---

*Mueller Company, Chicago, IL.
†Travenol Laboratories, Deerfield, IL
‡Dianeal, Travenol Laboratories, Deerfield, IL.

The major difficulty with peritoneal dialysis has been removing the bulk of the fluid instilled. This problem has largely been overcome by the development of two efficient silicone rubber peritoneal dialysis cannulas. The recommended volume of dialysis fluid to infuse is 30 to 40 ml/kg. It remains in the abdominal cavity (dwell) for 30 minutes. A cycle of infusion, dwell, and recovery takes about 1 hour. Six to eight exchanges can be completed in 24 hours. Complications of peritoneal dialysis include peritonitis, hypoproteinemia, malnutrition, hydrothorax, and signs associated with renal failure.

Chronic Renal Failure

Chronic renal failure is the result of progressive nephron loss, regardless of etiology, eventually leading to uremia when the process has reached its end-stage.

Renal Transplantation
Renal Autotransplantation

In renal autotransplantation, the kidney is removed from its orthotopic position and transferred to a heterotopic position, such as the iliac fossa. This procedure could be an alternative to nephrectomy if a damaged distal ureter were too short to be reimplanted into the bladder.

CHAPTER 105

Ureters (pages 1443–1450)

CONGENITAL ABNORMALITIES (pp. 1443–1444)
Ectopic Ureters

Failure of the ureters to open into the bladder in the normal location has been reported in dogs, cats, horses, cattle, poultry, and humans. Ureteral ectopia is due to abnormal differentiation of the mesonephric and metanephric ducts. The ureters open into the uterus, neck of the bladder, urethra, or vagina rather than the normal location in the trigone of the bladder. Although the condition has been reported in both male and female dogs and cats, it is more common in dogs than cats and occurs more frequently in females of both species.

The most common complaint of owners of animals with ectopic ureter(s) is urinary incontinence. Many of these animals void a small to nearly normal quantity of urine at appropriate intervals. The perineal area (females) or tip of the prepuce (males) is constantly damp from the uncontrolled flow of urine. Surgical treatment (see Chapter 106) frequently corrects incontinence associated with ectopic ureter in cats, but as many as 50 to 60 per cent of dogs treated surgically for ectopic ureter may have some degree of incontinence (positional, exertional, nocturnal, or other) after surgery.

Ureterocele

A ureterocele is a cystic dilation of the intravesicular, submucosal segment of the distal ureter. This disorder is rare in dogs and has not been described in cats. Ureteroceles may cause pain, stranguria, pollakiuria, or hematuria. Stranguria is the result of the physical presence of the dilated distal ureter, which applies pressure on the neck of the bladder. Preoperatively, the diagnosis of ureterocele is most often made by excretory urography. If the associated kidney is still functional, the affected ureter can be severed and reimplanted into the bladder (see Chapter 106).

VESICOURETERAL REFLUX (pp. 1444–1445)

Retrograde flow of urine from the bladder into the ureter and renal pelves is prevented by the valvelike effect of the bladder wall on the intravesicular portion of the ureter. In sedated or lightly anesthetized animals, vesicoureteral reflux was a relatively common occurrence (50 per cent of dogs and 40 per cent of cats) during manual compression of the bladder and distension of the bladder with radiographic contrast material. Vesicoureteral reflux may also occur in association with cystitis, obstruction of the bladder neck or urethra, or neurogenic bladder disease.

ACQUIRED ABNORMALITIES (pp. 1445–1449)
Ureteral Injury—Accidental

Ureteral disruption may be the result of accidental or iatrogenic injury or it may be a sequel to ureteral obstruction. Because of their position ventral to the lumbar musculature, the ureters are injured much less frequently than other abdominal organs as a result of blunt trauma.

Ureteral Injury—Iatrogenic

Iatrogenic injuries of the ureter occur most commonly during ovariohysterectomy.

If a ligature or clamp has been applied to the ureter, the ultimate degree of injury may be difficult to assess initially. It has been recommended that crush injuries not be treated immediately but instead be evaluated at regular intervals by excretory urography and treated if abnormalities persist. If a ligature is removed from the ureter within 1 week of application, normal function of the ureter and kidney may be regained. Obstruction of the ureter for 4 weeks or longer results in total loss of function of the associated kidney.

Diagnosis of Ureteral Trauma

Radiography.
Excretory Urography. Excretory urography usually allows the presence and location of ureteral disruption to be precisely determined.
Renal Angiography. Renal angiography is described in Chapter 103.
Antegrade Ureterography. A catheter is passed through the renal parenchyma into the pelvis or ureter, and contrast material is injected.

Management of Ureteral Trauma

When the ureters have been injured, four treatment options exist: ureteronephrectomy, placement of a ureteral catheter, ureteral anastomosis, or reimplantation of the ureter into the bladder (neoureterocystostomy—see Chapter 106). A common solution to ureteral trauma in veterinary medicine is to perform ureteronephrectomy.

Reimplantation of a ureter after it has avulsed from the renal pelvis is technically difficult. Ureteral anastomosis is difficult in small patients and is associated with an extremely high rate of postoperative obstruction in cats. In most dogs, no more than 3 to 5 cm of ureter can be resected without creating tension on the anastomosis.

Compensation for Loss of Ureteral Length

If a segment of ureter is permanently damaged, the surgeon can reduce the distance between the kidney and the bladder to facilitate reimplantation of the ureter or attempt to replace the ureter. The kidney can be freed of its retroperitoneal attachments and displaced caudally. The bladder may also be drawn cranially and sutured to the fascia of the sublumbar musculature (psoas hitch).

The most successful techniques for replacing the ureter have used autogenous tissues. Bladder flaps, pedicle grafts of the intestine or bladder mucosa, or free grafts of buccal mucosa all have been used successfully, clinically in man or experimentally in animals.

Ureteral Obstruction

Ureteral obstruction may be the result of trauma, intraluminal objects or structures, intramural mass lesions, or extramural compression. Intraluminal obstruction of the ureters by calculi in cats and dogs are rare. Extramural causes of compression, apart from tumors, include intrapelvic cysts, which are developmental abnormalities, and uterine stump granulomas, which occur as sequelae of ovariohysterectomy.

Treatment

Experimental studies in dogs have shown that if ureteral obstruction is relieved within 10 weeks of its occurrence, the dilated segment returns to its normal size and shape. If the ureter does not regain its normal diameter or if the dilation is not related to obstruction, ureteral plication can be tried.

Ureterotomy. Because of the nonspecific signs associated with ureteral calculi in dogs and cats, the diagnosis may be delayed. The prolonged presence of calculi within the ureter may result in necrosis of the ureteral wall. If there is no radiographic evidence within 24 hours that a stone has moved, ureterotomy is indicated.

CHAPTER 106

Urinary Bladder (pages 1450–1462)

ANATOMY (pp. 1450–1451)

The bladder is a hollow muscular organ that receives urine from the kidneys via both ureters and stores the urine until expulsion through the urethra.

PHYSIOLOGY (p. 1451)

In the storage phase of micturition, the bladder acts as a flaccid, low-pressure reservoir for urine and the urethra acts as a high-pressure valve preventing passage of urine. Sympathetic innervation via the hypogastric nerve dominates this phase of micturition while parasympathetic activity is inhibited.

Parasympathetic input begins to dominate the emptying phase, which is initiated by smooth-muscle (detrusor) depolarization and contraction. As the detrusor muscle contracts, the bladder neck opens. Simultaneously, the sympathetically innervated urethral smooth muscle and the somatically innervated urethral striated muscle relax.

Non-neurogenic causes of urinary incontinence include ovariohysterectomy, ectopic ureters, and chronic disease of the bladder, urethra, or prostate. Central or peripheral lesions anywhere in the normal neural pathway of micturition may cause dysuria or incontinence.

DIAGNOSIS OF BLADDER DISEASE (pp. 1451–1452)
Physical Examination

Findings noted on palpation include size, pain, wall thickness, calculi, and intraluminal or intramural masses.

Urinalysis/Microbiology

It is recommended that all nonelective surgical patients have a urinalysis performed as part of a preoperative data base. In general, urine obtained by cystocentesis is most easily interpreted because contamination with cells and bacteria from the distal urethra is avoided. Cystocentesis is easily and safely performed in small animals by using a 22-gauge or smaller needle and syringe. Specific components of the urinalysis that may assist in diagnosis of bladder disease include microscopic examination of urine sediment and urine culture. Cytological evaluation of urine sediment is especially important if bladder neoplasia is suspected. Samples obtained by cystocentesis are sterile in normal dogs and cats.

Radiology/Ultrasonography

Radiographic examination of the bladder is begun with survey radiographs, but contrast radiographs are often required to demonstrate most diseases. Ultrasonography is a useful aid to radiography in evaluating the bladder, especially when space-occupying masses are present.

Cystoscopy

Cystoscopy as a diagnostic technique was previously limited to the use of rigid endoscopes in females. With the advent of flexible fiber-optic instruments, the bladders of large male dogs can be examined without the need for surgical intervention.

Cystometrogram/Urethral Pressure Profile

Urodynamic studies provide functional data that may give a diagnosis and prognosis and aid in treatment of a micturition disorder. Urodynamic studies measure pressure, volume, and flow relationships within the bladder and urethra during various phases of micturition. Cystometry and urethral pressure profilometry evaluate bladder and urethral function in incontinent dogs.

The urethral pressure profile assesses nonvoiding urethral pressure measured from the bladder to the external urethral meatus and is plotted against that distance. The urethral pressure profile may localize areas of increased urethral resistance (obstruction) or decreased urethral resistance (incompetence).

CONGENITAL SURGICAL DISEASES (pp. 1452–1455)

Ectopic Ureters (see also Chapter 105)

Ectopic ureter is a congenital anomaly in which one or both ureters terminate and drain at a site other than the bladder. In dogs, approximately 70 to 80 per cent are unilateral, whereas cats more frequently have bilateral involvement.

Most animals with ectopic ureters are females, and they exhibit some urinary incontinence at the time of birth or weaning. A tentative diagnosis of ectopic ureter may be confirmed by radiography, vaginoscopy, or exploratory laparotomy. The method of choice for confirming the diagnosis of ectopic ureter is excretory urography, which provides information about the renal pelvis and ureter size and may identify the site of termination of the ureters.

Urinary tract infection is found in many animals with ectopic ureters and may cause pyelonephritis in both the affected and contralateral kidneys if not properly treated. The prognosis for urinary continence after surgery is guarded and depends on several factors. Bilateral ectopia is accompanied by cystic hypoplasia, thereby reducing bladder storage volume after surgery. The incidence of ectopic ureter and concurrent urethral sphincter incompetence is unknown. Similarly, the cause of continued incontinence after correction of ectopic ureter in some animals is unknown.

The choice of surgical technique for correcting ectopic ureter depends on whether the condition is unilateral or bilateral, the type of ectopic ureter, and functional status of the kidneys. Nephrectomy-ureterectomy is selected only when severe hydronephrosis or pyelonephritis and unilateral ectopic ureter are present.

Ectopic ureters may be intramural or extramural. In either case, a thorough exploration of the urinary tract precedes a ventral cystotomy. If an ectopic ureter is extramural, it is ligated and transected, preserving the maximum length of ureter available, and ureteroneocystostomy is performed. The goal of implantation is to salvage the affected ureter and kidney and prevent vesicoureteral reflux of urine into the ureter. Complications of all methods of implantation or neoureterostomy include hydroureter and hydronephrosis and continued incontinence.

ACQUIRED SURGICAL DISEASE (pp. 1455–1459)

Bladder Rupture

Bladder rupture may be caused by blunt or penetrating abdominal trauma or improper catheterization. Spontaneous rupture is uncommon but may occur secondary to prolonged urethral obstruction or necrosis. Urine leakage into the peritoneal cavity results in uremia, dehydration, hypovolemia, and death if undiagnosed or untreated.

Clinical signs of urinary tract trauma can be vague. Hematuria, dysuria, abdominal pain, lack of a palpable bladder, fluid accumulation within the abdomen, and abdominal and perineal bruising are early signs.

Radiographic examination of the abdomen is indicated if urinary tract trauma is suspected. Radiographic signs that suggest urinary tract injury include nonvisualization or asymmetry of the kidneys, enlargement of the retroperitoneal space, loss of normal intra-abdominal contrast, and reduced size or absence of the bladder. Positive-contrast cystography is the method of choice to evaluate bladder integrity.

Surgical repair is the definitive treatment for most rents in the bladder. In the preoperative period, urinary diversion can be accomplished by inserting an indwelling urinary catheter into the bladder and connecting the catheter to a closed collection system. A peritoneal dialysis catheter may be placed directly into the abdomen to divert urine that has accumulated within the peritoneal cavity.

Cystostomy

Antepubic urinary diversion by temporary cystostomy provides urinary drainage that may allow stabilization of an ill patient before definitive urological surgery. It may also serve to divert urine from a urethra that has been traumatized or surgically repaired. Either of two methods of cystostomy provide satisfactory urine diversion. The first method requires a 6 to 12 French Foley catheter. A second method of urine diversion is by percutaneous placement of a Stamey catheter.

Cystic Calculi

The most common surgical procedure performed on the bladder in companion animals is cystotomy for removal of uroliths. Magnesium ammonium phosphate (struvite) is the main component of approximately 60 to 70 per cent of all calculi in dogs. These stones are commonly associated with urinary tract infection but may also form in sterile urine. In decreasing incidence, the other types of calculi found in dogs are calcium oxalate, urate, cystine, silicate, and calcium phosphate. The composition of calculi may be reasonably determined without surgery based on urinalysis and identification of crystals within the urine and bacterial culture and sensitivity tests. If the calculi are magnesium ammonium phosphate, dietary and appropriate antibiotic therapy may result in stone dissolution. Diagnostic radiographs are indicated in the clinical evaluation of any patient with cystic calculi.

Surgical removal of cystic calculi is indicated for stones other than magnesium ammonium phosphate or stones that are causing or may cause urinary tract obstruction. The incision site for cystotomy and removal of uroliths is made in the most avascular and convenient area of the bladder. A second consideration is avoidance of the trigonal area and the ureteral orifices.

Palpation of the bladder neck and passage of a catheter through the urethra are indicated to ensure that the bladder neck or urethra is not blocked by calculi. Repeated flushing and aspiration are indicated to remove all discrete calculi and small particles of sand. Thorough medical management by dietary therapy, induced diuresis, or appropriate antimicrobial therapy is indicated to minimize the incidence of calculi recurrence, which ranges from 12 to 25 per cent.

Neoplasia

Bladder neoplasia accounts for less than 1 per cent of all canine neoplasia, and the prevalence is even lower in cats. Malignant neoplasms are more common than benign tumors in both dogs and cats. Transitional cell carcinoma is the most commonly diagnosed tumor in dogs and cats, followed by squamous cell carcinoma and adenocarcinoma. Fibromas, leiomyomas, and papillomas are the most common benign tumors of the bladder.

Patients with bladder neoplasia usually show clinical signs of hematuria, stranguria, and pollakiuria. Contrast radiography is often necessary to detect bladder masses as well as to assess the remainder of the urinary tract.

Surgical therapy for bladder neoplasia consists of partial cystectomy if the location of the mass allows complete excision of the tumor while sparing the urethral and ureteral orifices (trigone). If the trigone is preserved, 75 per cent of the bladder may be resected, with return to near-normal function over a period of weeks.

Transitional cell carcinoma frequently involves the trigone of the bladder, making partial cystectomy a poor treatment option. Urinary diversion consisting of total cystectomy and ureteral transplantation into the gastrointestinal tract may be considered as a treatment option. The ideal goals of treatment are cure or palliation of the disease and maintenance of urinary continence.

URINARY INCONTINENCE (pp. 1459–1461)

Urinary incontinence is a complex problem with multiple causes. A complete medical and neurological evaluation is necessary before considering surgical treatment of urinary incontinence. Several surgical techniques have been described for managing incontinence caused by bladder neck and proximal urethral dysfunction. All of the procedures described provide a mechanical means of increasing urethral resistance to urine flow. There are insufficient data on clinical cases to document the success of any procedure.

Cystourethroplasty

The creation of a bladder neck sling using autogenous fascia has been described. A sling urethroplasty technique using seromuscular urethral flaps has also been described. Three female dogs with sphincter incontinence were treated by suturing Dacron-impregnated Silastic strips around the urethra.

CHAPTER 107
Surgical Diseases of
the Urethra (pages 1462–1473)

CONGENITAL OR HEREDITARY LESIONS AFFECTING THE URETHRA (pp. 1462–1463)

Urethral anomalies are uncommon.

Hypospadias

Hypospadias is due to failure of fusion of the urogenital folds and incomplete formation of the penile urethra. In dogs, hypospadias is usually associated with failure of fusion of the prepuce and underdevelopment or absence of the penis. Corrective surgery, if performed, includes identifying and preserving the urethral opening, excising the urethral groove and remnants of the prepuce and penis, and castration.

Urethrorectal Fistula

Urethrorectal fistula is a developmental anomaly of the fetal cloaca in which a communication between the urethra and rectum persists. In dogs, urethrorectal fistulas have been reported in both sexes. Urine passes simultaneously through the urethra and anus. Surgical correction is performed via ventral pubic symphysiotomy.

ACQUIRED NONTRAUMATIC LESIONS AFFECTING THE URETHRA (pp. 1463–1469)

Urethritis

Urethritis is generally associated with other inflammatory diseases of the urogenital tract, such as cystitis, prostatitis, or vaginitis.

Urethral Prolapse

Urethral prolapse has been reported in young male dogs of the brachycephalic breeds. Diagnosis is based on observing the protruding mucosa.

Urethral Obstruction

Urethral Calculi

Urethral calculi are the most common cause of urethral obstruction in male dogs. Less-organized debris causes obstruction in male cats. Urethral obstruction due to calculi may be complete or incomplete and most often occurs just behind the os penis. Diagnosis is based on an inability to pass a urethral catheter and radiological demonstration of the presence of stones.

Urethral calculi that cannot be moved by either catheterization or hydropulsion to the exterior or into the bladder require urethral surgery.

Urethrotomy/Cystotomy

With a urethral catheter in place to the obstruction, a longitudinal incision is made over the calculus (or catheter tip), and the stone is carefully removed. The catheter is advanced, and any remaining calculi are flushed into the bladder with a stream of saline. These calculi and any other cystic calculi are removed via cystotomy. The major complication associated with urethrotomy is urethral stricture formation.

Urethrostomy

Creation of a permanent opening into the urethra can be used for (1) calculi that cannot be removed by flushing, (2) animals that cannot be kept free of calculi medically, (3) strictures of the urethra resulting from one or more episodes of prior urethral surgery or trauma, and (4) severe penile trauma when penile amputation is required.

Canine Urethrostomy. In dogs, urethrostomy can be performed in four locations: prescrotal, scrotal, perineal, and prepubic. The location selected is based on the site of obstruction and the surgeon's preference. If a choice exists and if the patient can be castrated, scrotal urethrostomy is recommended.

Feline Urethrostomy. There are many techniques for urethrostomy in male cats, but I prefer perineal urethrostomy using the Wilson and Harrison technique.

Urethral Prostheses in Cats. Prosthetic conduits manufactured from steel and Teflon, silicone rubber and Dacron velour, and silicone rubber alone have been advocated as treatments for urethral stricture and urethral obstruction in cats.

A correctly performed perineal urethrostomy remains the surgical method of choice for treating cats with recurrent urethral obstruction.

Neoplasia

Neoplastic processes can involve the urethra, producing partial or complete obstruction. Tumors of the urinary tract are uncommon in cats. In dogs, primary urethral tumors are uncommon but are most likely to occur in females.

TRAUMATIC LESIONS AFFECTING THE URETHRA
(pp. 1469–14711)

Traumatic lesions of the urethra include contusion, laceration, rupture, and obstruction. The causes of traumatic urethral injuries are many, but the overall incidence is low.

Clinical Signs

Clinical signs associated with urethral trauma may be masked by other problems or may be absent. The usual clinical signs include dysuria, anuria, hematuria, pain, fluid in the abdomen, and swelling and discoloration of the skin in the perineal area. Clinical signs vary, depending on the severity of the lesion. If the urethra is ruptured, urine leakage produces cellulitis that leads to fistula formation. If the urethra is obstructed, signs of uremia occur.

Diagnosis

Diagnosis is based on a high level of suspicion (abdominal or pelvic trauma), clinical signs, and positive-contrast urethrography. Negative-contrast studies with room air are contraindicated because of the potential for development of air emboli.

Treatment

Treatment of urethral trauma takes advantage of the remarkable regenerative ability of the urethral mucosa. The entire length of the urethra will regenerate from a longitudinal strip of mucosa if an intraurethral catheter is maintained for 3 weeks. After complete transection, however, the urethral muscle and mucosa retract. Primary repair to prevent the almost inevitable stenosis or delayed repair to excise it is essential in most cases of complete urethral transection.

Lacerations

Lacerations that permit extravasation of urine into the surrounding tissues are explored and sutured with 3-0 or 4-0 polyglactin 910 or polyglycolic acid suture material, and the urine is diverted with an intraurethral catheter for 3 to 5 days. If gross infection is present, primary closure is delayed.

Intrapelvic Partial Urethral Rupture

Incomplete rupture of the intrapelvic urethra without impingement by fracture fragments may be treated by diverting urine through the largest urinary catheter that can be comfortably passed and maintained in place for 7 to 21 days (depending on the size of the urethral tear).

Complete Urethral Rupture

When possible, primary suture repair is the best treatment for complete rupture of the urethra. Urethral anastomosis over an indwelling catheter produces less stricture formation than suturing without an indwelling catheter. With severe trauma to the urethra and periurethral tissue, accumulation of blood, urine, and devitalized tissue may preclude primary suturing. In these cases, an indwelling catheter and delayed urethral repair are indicated.

Urethral Obstruction

Urethral obstruction generally necessitates some temporary measures to decompress the bladder as well as fluid and electrolyte therapy to correct metabolic abnormalities before definitive treatment. Cystocentesis and urinary diversion through catheters, either urethral or prepubic, are helpful lifesaving techniques. If the obstruction is associated with pubic fractures, exploration, reduction, and stabilization of the fracture are required. If the urethra is traumatized, it is treated as previously described.

Urethral Strictures

Urethral obstruction may be due to stenosis or stricture following urethral trauma or urethral surgery. Extrapelvic urethral strictures are best managed by urethrostomy as discussed earlier. Intrapelvic urethral strictures of 1 cm or less are best treated by resection and anastomosis. Larger defects require heroic measures.

PREPUBIC URETHROSTOMY (pp. 1471–1472)

Prepubic urethrostomy results in the creation of a urethrostomy opening on the ventral surface of the abdomen cranial to the pubis and should be considered when an insufficient length of normal urethra is available to perform urethrostomy in one of the more commonly used sites. This technique has been used with considerable success in dogs and cats of both sexes.

Although the urethra is usually shortened significantly, urinary continence will be maintained if the sphincter mechanism and innervation are preserved. Urine scalding of the skin surrounding the urethrostomy opening has not been a significant problem. Animals may be predisposed to bacterial cystitis after prepubic urethrostomy. I have seen urethral obstruction after prepubic urethrostomy owing to stricture of the urethrostomy opening, and urethral obstruction could occur owing to compression of the urethra as it passes across the abdominal wall or owing to kinking of the urethra as a result of severe shortening of the urethra or selection of an inappropriate site for the urethrostomy opening.

Potential complications limit application to cases of prepubic urethrostomy in which standard techniques for urethrostomy are unsatisfactory.

Feline Urological Syndrome

(pages 1473–1487)

Feline urological syndrome (FUS) is defined as idiopathic lower urinary tract disease characterized by dysuria and hematuria with or without urethral obstruction. Urethral obstruction is common in affected male cats and rare in affected females. When present, urethral obstruction in males usually occurs in the penile urethra. This definition excludes urolithiasis, which is characterized by organized concretions in the urinary tract. It implies that a reasonable diagnostic effort has been made to rule out other documented causes of lower urinary tract disease.

The obstructing material typically is unorganized and composed of crystalline and matrix components. The primary crystalloid is struvite (magnesium ammonium phosphate hexahydrate). The origin, composition, and significance of the matrix component are unknown.

EPIDEMIOLOGY (pp. 1474–1475)

PATHOGENESIS (pp. 1475–1480)

The lack of consensus about etiology and results of several epidemiological studies suggest that FUS is a multifactorial disorder.

Infectious Agents

Bacteria

Most cats with lower urinary tract disease do not have bacterial urinary tract infections. Thus, bacterial urinary tract infection is not a primary factor in FUS. Bacterial urinary tract infection can be a complicating factor after urethral manipulation, use of indwelling urinary catheters, antibiotic therapy, and perineal urethrostomy.

Viruses

Attempts to demonstrate viruses in naturally occurring FUS have been unsuccessful.

Struvite Crystalluria

The urethral plugs in cats with FUS typically contain struvite. Struvite crystals have been observed in the urine of normal cats and those with FUS. Struvite solubility is reduced in alkaline urine, and struvite crystals were common in urine with pH greater than 6.8. Many cats with FUS have acidic urine at presentation, and the amount of struvite crystalluria does not correlate with the occurrence of FUS. These observations do not preclude a role for struvite crystalluria in FUS, because urinalysis in cats examined for FUS may not reflect the status of their urine between episodes.

Diet

The moisture content, mineral composition, nutrient content and digestibility, and caloric density of the diet may be important in the etiology of FUS.

Moisture Content

Cats fed dry food drink more water than cats fed canned food but much of this water contributes to fecal moisture so that urine volume is lower and urine specific gravity higher in cats fed dry food. The urine concentration of all solutes, including potentially calculogenic crystalloids, depends on urine volume. Urine volume is influenced by the water and nutrient content of the diet, by drinking, and by water excretion via feces and the respiratory tract.

Cats fed canned food and meat diets had higher urine volumes and slightly lower urine specific gravity values than cats fed dry food. In this study, the ratio of total water to dry matter intake (TH$_2$O/DM) was higher in cats fed canned (3.7) than dry diets (2.0 to 2.4).

A high-fat, high-calorie diet may prevent FUS.

The effect of water intake and urine volume on the development of FUS is incompletely understood. It is recommended that canned food be fed to cats with FUS to increase TH$_2$O/DM and decrease urine specific gravity.

Mineral Content (pp. 1476–1478)

Ash refers to all noncombustible components of a diet and thus includes most of the mineral content without regard to the specific elements present. Ash does not cause FUS. Although some components of ash may be important in the pathogenesis of FUS, the term *ash* itself is of no value.

Dietary minerals that have been examined for their effects on the development of FUS include sodium, magnesium, calcium, and phosphorus. Addition of sodium chloride to the diet increases total water intake in cats. The diet may be supplemented with salt to increase water consumption in cats, but it is unclear whether it prevents recurrence of FUS.

Studies suggest that the amount of magnesium found in commercial diets is safe if urine pH is maintained near 6. In contrast, if urine pH is too high, even normal amounts of dietary magnesium may cause increased risk of FUS.

The quantity of magnesium required to saturate urine with struvite at alkaline pH is very small. As pH decreases below 6.4, the amount of magnesium required to saturate the urine with struvite increases exponentially. Conversely, as urine pH increases above 6.9, the amount of struvite that forms in the urine increases markedly. When urine pH is alkaline, the amount of struvite formed in urine is proportional to the dietary magnesium concentration. At urine pH values less than 6.1, struvite does not form regardless of the magnesium concentration of the diet. Thus, the tendency of struvite to form is a function of urine pH. The magnesium content of the diet only becomes important when urine pH is greater than 6.1.

Nutrient Content and Digestibility

Constituents of foodstuffs exert major effects on urine pH. Urine volume was greatest and urinary magnesium excretion least in cats fed highly digestible diets regardless of whether a dry or canned food was fed.

Feeding Patterns

An *ad libitum* feeding pattern attenuates postprandial alkalinization of the urine.

Urine Acidification (pp. 1478–1480)

Changing urine hydrogen ion concentration tenfold (1 pH unit) inhibits struvite precipitation six times more effectively than a tenfold change in the concentrations of magnesium, ammonium, or phosphate. A tenfold change in urine magnesium, ammonium, or phosphate concentration is greater than that likely to occur when diets formulated especially to decrease the risk of FUS are substituted for normal diets. The range of urine hydrogen ion concentration that may be produced by dietary manipulation is much greater, at least one-thousandfold (3 pH units).

Acidification of the urine is not without potential toxicity. When fed experimentally to cats at a dosage of 0.5 to 1.0 g/kg/day (2.8 to 5.5 per cent of diet dry matter), *dl*-methionine caused hemolytic anemia, methemoglobinemia, and Heinz body formation. Ammonium chloride also is potentially toxic. Some cats given 1 g/day of ammonium chloride developed anorexia, vomiting, and diarrhea.

Additional concerns about chronic acidification are its potentially detrimental effects on renal function and bone development. Dietary potassium content also may be important because chronic metabolic acidosis can cause potassium depletion, which can contribute to renal dysfunction.

We recommend that cats with FUS be fed a canned food that is high in digestible energy (greater than 4 Kcal/g dry matter) and contains less than 0.2 per cent magnesium. If a cat is meal-fed, its urine pH is monitored 4 hours after feeding to be sure that it is 6.0 to 6.5. If the urine pH is higher, ammonium chloride is administered with the food.

PATHOPHYSIOLOGY OF OBSTRUCTION (p. 1480)

Bilateral ureteral obstruction causes acute renal failure and anuria. The postobstructive diuresis that follows relief of obstruction is incompletely understood.

DIAGNOSIS (pp. 1480–1482)

Anamnesis

Cats without urethral obstruction are presented for evaluation of *stranguria, pollakiuria,* and *hematuria.* Cats with urethral obstruction make frequent unsuccessful attempts to urinate. Pain is evidenced in some cats by reluctance to move, a hunched-up posture, and a guttural cry. When complete urethral obstruction has been present for more than 48 hours, signs of postrenal uremia such as anorexia, muscle weakness, lethargy, and vomiting occur. Cats die after 72 to 144 hours of complete urethral obstruction.

Physical Findings

An affected cat without obstruction is not systemically ill and has a small, firm, painful bladder. When a cat has been obstructed for more than 36 to 48 hours, the bladder is firm, distended, and painful, and there is evidence of dehydration (e.g., reduced skin turgor). The distal portion of the penis is examined for discoloration and for the presence of a urethral plug that could be dislodged manually.

Laboratory Findings

In cats without urethral obstruction, the complete blood count and serum biochemical determinations usually are normal. The hallmark of FUS on routine urinalysis is hematuria without pyuria. Results of urine culture usually are negative in cats when samples are taken before urethral manipulation and catheterization. Struvite crystals may be observed in the urine sediment. Their presence is not diagnostic, because they can be observed in the urine of normal cats.

Cats with urethral obstruction may have leukocytosis with a normal distribution of leukocytes or a stress pattern. Increased hematocrit and total plasma protein concentration reflect hemoconcentration. Azotemia, hyperphosphatemia, hypocalcemia, hypermagnesemia, mild hyponatremia, metabolic acidosis with inadequate respiratory compensation, hyperproteinemia, hyperglycemia, and hyperkalemia may occur.

After relief of obstruction, cats that survived had polyuria, but nonsurvivors were oliguric.

Radiographic Findings (p. 1481)

Pathological Findings

Lesions are limited to the urinary tract and consist primarily of erosion, hemorrhage, edema, and inflammation in the bladder.

TREATMENT (pp. 1482–1484)

Uncomplicated Obstruction (<24 to 48 Hours)

Consideration must first be given to relief of urethral obstruction. Adequate restraint can be achieved with ketamine (1 to 2 mg/kg IV) or sodium thiamylal (4 to 10 mg/kg IV).

The distal portion of the penis is examined, and an attempt is made to manually dislodge obstructive material. If the obstruction is not located at the tip of the penis, the next step is aseptic passage of a well-lubricated polypropylene urinary catheter (e.g., open-end tomcat catheter) and irrigation of the urethra. The urethra is flushed retrograde with 0.9 per cent saline or lactated Ringer's solution at room temperature. The catheter can be lubricated with lidocaine gel.

If hydropulsion is successful, the urethra and bladder are irrigated until the returning fluid is free of blood and crystalline debris. If hydropulsion fails, cystocentesis is used to decompress the bladder, and retrograde flushing is attempted again.

Indwelling urinary catheterization is considered if marked urethral trauma occurs during catheterization, an insufficient urine stream is observed, hematuria is severe, or the bladder fails to return to normal size after relief of obstruction. After the catheter is removed, urine is cultured and antibiotic treatment instituted if indicated.

Subcutaneous administration of a balanced electrolyte solution such as lactated Ringer's solution at approximately 1.5 to 2 times maintenance (0 to 80 ml/kg/day) promotes diuresis and prevents early recurrence. No benefit was observed with subcutaneous fluid therapy of nonobstructed cats with FUS. The bladder is palpated periodically to detect recurrence of obstruction or bladder hypotony.

The use of antibiotics after relief of obstruction is controversial. Urinary acidifiers are not used in cats that have been obstructed recently and have metabolic acidosis. Anti-inflammatory drugs such as glucocorticoids and dimethylsulfoxide (DMSO) are controversial.

Complicated Obstruction (>24 to 48 Hours)

The major therapeutic goals are to correct hyperkalemia, acid-base imbalance, dehydration, and azotemia with appropriate fluid therapy and to relieve obstruction. Initially, blood is drawn for laboratory evaluation. An intravenous catheter is placed, and a crystalloid solution (0.45 per cent sodium chloride with 2.5 per cent dextrose solution) given. Rehydration is established during the first 4 to 6 hours of hospitalization by rapid intravenous fluid administration.

An electrocardiogram is obtained. If severe hyperkalemia is suspected, sodium bicarbonate may be administered intravenously. Some clinicians have advocated administration of 0.5 to 1.0 units/kg regular insulin intravenously and 2 g of glucose per unit of insulin to translocate potassium intracellularly, but this therapy is controversial.

Relief of urethral obstruction is performed as described for uncomplicated obstruction. Anesthesia is dangerous in severely depressed or moribund cats and is not used except when necessary to prevent undue urethral trauma. An indwelling urinary catheter is placed, and urine output monitored. This approach is recommended because ensuing postobstructive diuresis can be marked, and dehydration occurs if urinary fluid losses are not replaced.

After normal hydration is restored and hyperkalemia resolved, a balanced electrolyte solution is administered to provide insensible needs (approximately 20 ml/kg/day) plus a volume equal to the daily urine output. Urinary acidifiers and nephrotoxic antibiotics (e.g., aminoglycosides) are avoided. Hypokalemia occurs frequently during postobstructive diuresis and may be treated with supplemental potassium chloride.

Unobstructed Cat

There is no evidence that antibiotics are useful in initial treatment of FUS. It is important that clinical studies be properly controlled before concluding that a particular treatment is beneficial, because FUS without obstruction is a self-limiting disorder.

No commercial cat foods cause FUS, nor do any specific foods prevent recurrence of naturally occurring FUS. Cats fed *ad libitum* have less variable urine pH values than cats that are fed meals. Urinary acidifiers may not be needed, because some foods promote acidic urine.

Owners are informed of the high recurrence rate of FUS (approximately 40 per cent) and are instructed to observe their cat's urination carefully to detect obstruction early.

COMPLICATIONS OF FELINE UROLOGICAL SYNDROME
(pp. 1484–1485)

Increased Outlet Resistance

Increased outlet resistance is suspected when manual compression of the bladder results in a weak urine stream. It is first necessary to rule out and treat early recurrence of intraluminal obstruction caused by additional crystalline, mucoid, or inflammatory debris. If intraluminal obstruction is not present, extraluminal obstruction caused by edema, inflammation, and hemorrhage is considered. If such changes are likely, an anti-inflammatory dose of glucocorticoids (e.g., 0.5 to 1.0 mg/kg prednisolone) may be beneficial if a cat is not azotemic and does not have bacterial urinary tract infection or an indwelling urinary catheter.

Another extraluminal cause of obstruction is urethral spasm. Treatment of functional outlet resistance can be attempted with alpha-adrenergic blocking drugs such as phenoxybenzamine or acepromazine.

Detrusor Hypotony

Affected cats have large, flaccid bladders that can be expressed manually without excessive force. Detrusor hypotony can be treated with bethanechol (1.25 to 2.5 mg PO TID) for a few days.

Bacterial Urinary Tract Infection

Bacterial urinary tract infection occurs in 40 to 60 per cent of cats with recurrent urethral obstruction and is a serious complication of indwelling urethral catheterization.

PREVENTION OF FELINE UROLOGICAL SYNDROME (p. 1485)

No studies of specific dietary alterations or drug treatments have been shown to prevent recurrence of naturally occurring FUS in cats. Conservative recommendations are suggested for unobstructed cats.

CHAPTER 109
Medical Treatment of Canine Uroliths (pages 1488–1495)

The majority of uroliths in dogs are found in the bladder or urethra, and only 5 to 10 per cent are located in the kidneys or ureters. Uroliths are most frequently observed in dogs between 3 and 7 years old.

ETIOLOGY AND PATHOGENESIS (pp. 1488–1490)

Conditions that contribute to crystallization of crystalloids and urolith formation include a sufficiently high concentration of crystalloids in the urine, adequate time within the urinary tract (urinary retention of crystalloids), a favorable urine pH for crystallization to occur, a nucleation center or nidus on which crystallization may occur, and decreased concentrations of crystallization inhibitors in the urine. High dietary intake of minerals and protein and the ability of dogs to produce highly concentrated urine contribute to urine supersaturation with crystalloid substances. In some cases, decreased tubular reabsorption of crystalloids (e.g., calcium, cystine, and uric acid) or increased production of crystalloids secondary to bacterial infection also contributes to urine supersaturation.

Struvite or *magnesium ammonium phosphate* uroliths are the most common uroliths in dogs. Urinary tract infection is an important factor predisposing to the formation of struvite uroliths, and *Staphylococcus aureus* and *Proteus* spp. are commonly associated pathogens. These organisms contain urease and are capable of splitting urea to ammonia and carbon dioxide. Hydroxyl and ammonium ions are formed from hydrolysis of ammonia, which reduces hydrogen ion concentrations in urine and results in increased urine pH. Alkaline urine decreases struvite solubility and facilitates crystal formation. Because of the close association with urinary tract infection, struvite uroliths are more frequent in female dogs; 80 to 97 per cent of uroliths in female dogs are struvite.

Calcium oxalate uroliths are the most common type in hum. incidence of calcium oxalate uroliths in dogs is increasing. Fac. involved in the pathogenesis of calcium oxalate urolithiasis in dogs are not well understood, but increased concentrations of calcium in the urine may contribute to their formation.

Most *urate* uroliths are composed of *ammonium acid urate*; 100 per cent uric acid and sodium urate uroliths are rare in comparison. Uric acid is derived from the metabolic degradation of endogenous purine ribonucleotides and dietary nucleic acids. Decreased production of allantoin in Dalmatians results in increased urinary excretion of uric acid.

The cause of silicate uroliths is unknown.

Cystine uroliths occur in dogs with cystinuria, an inherited disorder of renal tubular transport involving cystine and, in some cases, other amino acids (tubular reabsorption of cystine, the immediate precursor of cystine, and lysine may also be decreased). Not all dogs with cystinuria develop cystine uroliths; cystinuria is therefore a predisposing rather than a primary causative factor.

CLINICAL SIGNS AND DIAGNOSIS (pp. 1490–1491)

Clinical signs associated with urolithiasis depend on the number, type, and location of the stones within the urinary tract. Most uroliths are located in the urinary bladder, and clinical signs of cystitis (hematuria, pollakiuria, and stranguria/dysuria) are frequently observed. In male dogs, smaller uroliths may pass into the urethra, causing partial or complete obstruction with signs of bladder distension and postrenal azotemia (depression, anorexia, and vomiting). Uroliths frequently lodge within a male's urethra at the caudal end of the os penis.

Uroliths within the bladder and urethra can often be palpated via the abdomen or rectum; however, a thickened, irritated bladder wall may obscure small uroliths. Ultrasonography or plain or contrast radiographs of the urinary tract are often necessary to confirm a diagnosis of urolithiasis.

Urinalysis findings in dogs with urolithiasis often suggest urinary tract inflammation (hematuria, pyuria, increased numbers of epithelial cells, and proteinuria). Bacterial culture and antibiotic sensitivity testing of the urine are performed in all cases of urolithiasis to identify and properly treat any concurrent urinary tract infection.

The patient's signalment along with laboratory and radiographic findings are often helpful in determining urolith type; however, a quantitative urolith analysis is performed if uroliths are passed or removed surgically.

MEDICAL MANAGEMENT (pp. 1491–1494)

General principles of treatment include relief of any urethral obstruction and decompression of the bladder, if necessary. This can usually be accomplished by passage of a small-bore catheter, cystocentesis, dislodgment of urethral calculi by hydropulsion, or emergency urethrotomy. Fluid therapy is initiated to restore fluid and electrolyte balance if postrenal azotemia exists. Hyperkalemia is a potentially life-threatening electrolyte disturbance that may occur with postrenal azotemia due to urethral obstruction or of rupture of the urinary bladder or urethra.

Medical dissolution of struvite, urate, and cystine uroliths is effective. The choice between surgical removal of uroliths and medical dissolution is not always clear.

General preventive measures that should be used with surgery or medical treatment of uroliths include induction of diuresis and eradication of urinary tract infections. Diuresis lowers urine specific gravity and the urinary concentration of crystalloids. Daily addition of 0.5 to 1.0 g of salt (1 tsp = 3.5 g of sodium chloride) to the diet is usually recommended, although there are exceptions to this recommendation.

Struvite uroliths can usually be dissolved by feeding a calculolytic diet. Hill's Prescription Diet Canine s/d is severely restricted in protein, calcium, phosphorus, and magnesium. It has a high salt content and results in acidic urine.

In addition to decreasing the concentration of crystalloids in the urine, elimination of any bacterial urinary tract infection is an essential part of the medical treatment of struvite urolithiasis. Antibiotics are selected by urine culture and sensitivity testing, and in severe or persistent urinary tract infections caused by urease-producing bacteria, the urease inhibitor acetohydroxamic acid may be added to the treatment regimen.

Measures to prevent struvite urolith recurrence include prevention and control of urinary tract infections, maintenance of acidic urine, and decreased dietary intake of calculogenic crystalloids. Medical treatment for dissolution of oxalate urolithiasis has not been developed. Medical dissolution of urate urolithiasis that is not associated with hepatic insufficiency (e.g., portosystemic shunts) includes a diet low in protein and nucleic acids, alkalization of the urine, xanthine oxidase inhibition, and elimination of urinary tract infections. Guidelines for medical dissolution of silicate uroliths are unavailable. Recommendations for medical dissolution and prevention of cystine uroliths include reduction of dietary protein and methionine, alkalization of urine, and administration of thiol-containing drugs.

Endocrine System (pages 1496–1544)

CHAPTER 110

Hypophysectomy (pages 1496–1510)

Canine hyperadrenocorticism (Cushing's syndrome) was recognized in 1939, marking the beginning of a long Dutch predominance in exploring the pathophysiology and treatment options. Hypophysectomy was investigated in 28 dogs with spontaneous pituitary-dependent hyperadrenocorticism (PDH; Cushing's disease*) and reported as a valuable alternative to adrenalectomy or medical therapy. Few other reports describe hypophysectomy in other centers. This lack of widespread clinical experience is in sharp contrast to the wealth of information on experimental hypophysectomy in dogs and cats, which has a history dating back to the past century.

EXPERIMENTAL HYPOPHYSECTOMY (pp. 1496–1497)

Experimental Hypophysectomy in Veterinary Medicine

Veterinary surgeons have just begun to conduct trials to improve clinical hypophysectomy techniques. The stimulus for these efforts lies in the still unsatisfactory safety record of hypophysectomies, in the difficulty in accurately approaching and exposing the pituitary in dogs of various sizes and with diverse skull shapes, and in the uncertainty of achieving and assessing completeness of hypophysectomy.

INDICATIONS FOR HYPOPHYSECTOMY AND DIAGNOSTIC REQUIREMENTS (pp. 1497–1500)

Large-scale studies have been performed only in dogs. Clinical experience sufficient to recommend hypophysectomy in cats is lacking.

The presence of any primary tumor in the pituitary gland represents a potential indication for hypophysectomy. In general, only pituitary microadenomas (sellar tumors) and functional adenohypophyseal hyperplasia† are amenable to surgical treatment by hypophysectomy.

In dogs, more than 60 per cent of all neoplastic disorders of the pituitary are endocrinologically active. Adenomas producing excess adrenocorticotropic hormone (ACTH) and eliciting Cushing's disease are the most frequent pituitary disorder in dogs. Approximately two-thirds of all canine adenohypophyseal tumors are microadenomas (<1

---

*Cushing's syndrome is referred to as *Cushing's disease* when caused by a pituitary source, either a tumor or hyperplasia.

†The term *functional pituitary hyperplasia* is sporadically used in the literature. Clinically and by computed tomography (CT) scan, functional pituitary microadenomas and functional pituitary hyperplasia cannot be differentiated. The distinction is of pathophysiological importance only and at present has no impact on therapeutic strategies.

cm diameter), the remainder being macroadenomas*; pituitary carcinomas account for less than 3 per cent of all pituitary neoplasms. Thus, nearly 70 per cent of all dogs with PDH have surgically resectable, hyperactive corticotrophs and are definite candidates for hypophysectomy. In dogs with functional macroadenomas (<30 per cent of the dogs with PDH), the benefit/risk evaluation for hypophysectomy has to be considered. In dogs with concomitant signs of Cushing's disease and neurological deficits, the advantage of partial tumor ablation might outweigh the surgical risk. From the diagnostic viewpoint, CT scanning of the sella turcica area is required to differentiate hypophyseal macro- and microadenomas.

If ACTH stimulation tests or low-dose and high-dose dexamethasone suppression tests or plasma endogenous ACTH measurements or metyrapone suppression tests suggest PDH, pituitary CT scan should be performed. If a CT scan of the sella region cannot be obtained, ultrasonographic assessment of bilateral adrenal enlargement might suffice to justify hypophysectomy; there is a 30 per cent chance of encountering a pituitary macroadenoma (which potentially is nonresectable) and less than 3 per cent probability of a pituitary carcinoma.

In veterinary medicine, indications for hypophysectomy have only been established for PDH. Growth hormone supplementation after hypophysectomy is not essential in adult animals. Diabetes insipidus is transient after hypophysectomy. Hypophysectomy renders most animals of both sexes infertile, and the gonads undergo varying degrees of atrophy.

TRANS-SPHENOIDAL HYPOPHYSECTOMY (NIEBAUER)
(pp. 1500–1508)

Surgical Anatomy

The canine sella turcica is a shallow depression on the dorsal surface of the sphenoid bone. To reach the sella via the trans-sphenoidal route, the soft palate is transected, the mucoperiosteal cover of the sphenoid bone reflected, the sphenoid bone trephined, and the dura mater incised. Reliable landmarks to consistently pinpoint the sellar center for sphenoid bone trephination are absent. Thus, in the surgical technique described, the use of additional points of reference in the form of radiographic markers combined with a cranial sinus venogram is described.

The cavernous sinus system is located within the extradural space on the interior surface of the sphenoid bone in immediate proximity to the pituitary gland. These sinuses are the most vulnerable vascular structures during hypophysectomy, and severe, potentially fatal hemorrhage occurs when they are inadvertently lacerated.

INSTRUMENTATION

Anesthesia

There are no specific requirements for general anesthesia. Manipulation or drugs significantly increasing intracranial pressure are avoided.

---

*The definition of macroadenoma is controversial. Any pituitary neoplasm visible without optical devices during surgery or on necropsy can be regarded as macroadenoma. Some authors define macroadenomas in dogs as lesions >5 mm, others of >1 cm in diameter. The size of the individual animal and the size of its pituitary gland might also affect these distinctions. From a surgical standpoint, we regard any dog with confirmed PDH and a negative contrast-enhanced CT scan as having a microadenoma and any animal with Cushing's disease and a pituitary mass lesion, visible on CT image, as having a macroadenoma (or carcinoma).

Preparation for Surgery

Trans-sphenoidal hypophysectomy is a contaminated surgical procedure.

Angularis Oculi Vein Catheterization

The area of the angularis oculi vein (unilaterally) is shaved and routinely prepared for a cutdown procedure, which is preferably performed before positioning the animal for the trans-sphenoidal surgery. Radiographic markers are placed on the same side as the catheter (discussed later).

Surgical Procedure (pp. 1504–1507)

Part 1: Approach to the Sphenoid Bone, Placement of Radiographic Markers

Part 2: Venous Sinus Angiography

Part 3: Sphenoid Ostectomy, Hypophysectomy, Closure

Surgical Aftercare

Immediately after surgery, vasopressin (Pitressin) is given (approximately 0.2 IU/kg IM) every other day and continued for 1 to 2 weeks as necessary. Corticosteroid and thyroid hormone supplementation is initiated shortly after recovery from anesthesia.

Antibiotic therapy is continued for at least 1 week after surgery.

Long-term Endocrine Supplementation

Corticosteroids (prednisone, 0.2 mg/kg) and thyroid hormone* (0.02 mg/kg) are given daily, preferably in the morning.

Complications

Severe complications are rare and depend to some degree on the experience of the surgeon. Such complications include severe hemorrhage and iatrogenic damage to the hypothalamus or adjacent central nervous structures. Should either of these complications occur, the damage becomes apparent immediately or during recovery from anesthesia. Survival of such dogs is questionable. Another major potential complication is dehiscence of the palate incision (usually on the second to fourth day after surgery).

Assessment of Completeness of Hypophysectomy

In successfully treated dogs, signs of Cushing's disease begin to diminish shortly after surgery. If signs persist or if recovery is unsatisfactory, endocrine screening tests are repeated.

ALTERNATIVE SURGICAL APPROACHES: INTRACRANIAL AND PARAPHARYNGEAL ROUTES (p. 1508)

Intracranial Transtemporal Approach

The intracranial transtemporal approach to the dog's pituitary has been fully explored experimentally and is indicated for attempted resection of macroadenomas and suprasellar or parasellar pituitary tumors.

*Synthetic L-thyroxine (levothyroxine sodium), peroral form, Soloxine, Daniels Pharmaceutical, St. Petersburg, FL; injectable form, Synthroid, Flint Laboratories, Morton Grove, IL.

Parapharyngeal Approach

The parapharyngeal approach was developed experimentally in dogs and reported once. Visibility is limited, and the surgical exposure is inferior to the oropharyngeal approach.

PROGNOSIS (pp. 1508–1509)

Dogs with pituitary microadenomas or sellar lesions (confirmed by CT scan) are definite candidates for hypophysectomy, and their prognosis is excellent.

The size of the sellar lesion, completeness of hypophysectomy, and histological diagnosis are of equal prognostic importance. Accurate assessment of each of these factors is generally the exception rather than the rule. Therefore, in all cases except those with microadenomas and subsequent complete hypophysectomy, the prognosis is guarded.

CHAPTER 111

Adrenalectomy (pages 1510–1514)

Adrenalectomy is a challenging surgical procedure performed on animals that are usually at high risk. Hyperadrenocorticism due to a unilateral adrenal tumor and bilateral hyperplasia are the most common indications for surgery. Pheochromocytoma, a less common but equally devastating tumor, is another indication for adrenalectomy.

ANATOMY (pp. 1510–1511)

The paired adrenal glands are retroperitoneal, located cranial and medial to the cranial pole of each kidney.

PREOPERATIVE CONSIDERATIONS (p. 1511)

Efforts are made to correct metabolic derangements such as hyperglycemia and fluid and electrolyte imbalances. Hyperalimentation is considered in patients that are malnourished and hypoproteinemic.

SURGICAL TREATMENT (pp. 1511–1514)

Monitoring of patients during adrenalectomy is extremely important. Adrenalectomy for hyperadrenocorticism causes a precipitous decline in serum cortisol concentrations. Glucocorticoid replacement is necessary to avoid severe adrenocortical insufficiency. Dexamethasone (0.1 to 0.2 mg/kg) or prednisolone sodium succinate (1.0 to 2.0 mg/kg) is given intravenously immediately after anesthetic induction and repeated immediately after surgery.

Surgical Technique

The ventral midline approach allows exposure of both adrenal glands and other abdominal organs, such as the liver, through one incision. The retroperitoneal (flank) approach provides adequate exposure of either the right or left gland.

Ventral Midline Approach (pp. 1511–1513)

Retroperitoneal Approach (p. 1513)

Postoperative Care and Complications

Hemorrhage, fluid and electrolyte imbalances, pancreatitis secondary to iatrogenic trauma, wound infection or pneumonia due to impaired immune system function, and poor wound healing are potential problems. Adrenal insufficiency develops after either bilateral gland removal or unilateral removal for adrenal neoplasia. Glucocorticoids are administered postoperatively. Mineralocorticoid therapy is also necessary after removal of both adrenal glands. Dogs are re-evaluated every 3 to 6 months to check for evidence of recurrence of the adrenal tumor or other associated problems. Adrenalectomy for adrenal tumors in cats has also been reported, although much less frequently than in dogs. The ventral approach is preferred for adrenalectomy in cats.

CHAPTER 112

The Thyroid (pages 1514–1523)

ANATOMY (p. 1514)

In dogs and cats, the thyroid gland consists of two distinct lobes adjacent to the first five to eight tracheal rings. Two parathyroid glands are associated with each of the two thyroid lobes. The thyroid gland is highly vascular. Ectopic thyroid tissue is present in most dogs and cats. This accessory thyroid parenchyma is found mainly in the cervical region but can also be located within the thorax. Carcinoma or adenoma can arise from ectopic thyroid tissue in both dogs and cats.

THYROID PHYSIOLOGY (p. 1515)

CANINE AND FELINE HYPOTHYROIDISM (pp. 1515–1517)

Etiology of Hypothyroidism

Abnormally low circulating levels of thyroid hormone are the most common thyroid disorder in dogs. Hypothyroidism results from inadequate production and secretion of thyroid hormone. The specific defect most commonly originates in the thyroid gland; rarely, the defect is present in the hypothalamus or pituitary gland. Thyroid dysfunction is termed *primary hypothyroidism,* whereas pituitary and hypothalamic causes are called *secondary* and *tertiary hypothyroidism,* respectively.

Naturally occurring adult primary hypothyroidism is most common in dogs. Sporadic reports describe histological changes in the mature feline thyroid gland that are consistent with primary thyroid dysfunction, but naturally occurring clinical cases have not been identified.

Clinical Signs of Hypothyroidism

The major difficulty in diagnosing hypothyroidism is the nonspecific and variable clinical signs in affected animals. Adult-onset hypothyroidism most frequently afflicts middle-aged medium to large dogs, with no predilection for a particular sex. The golden retriever, Irish setter, Doberman pinscher, dachshund, and cocker spaniel are at increased risk. Because thyroid hormone's main role is generation of energy throughout the body, many of the clinical signs in hypothyroid animals are manifestations of decreased metabolic rate, which creates lethargy, exercise intolerance, and generalized weight gain.

Dermatological alterations include alopecia, dry haircoat, thickening of the skin, and hyperpigmentation. The hypothyroid state can inhibit myocardial function to the point of producing bradycardia and a weak apex beat. One of the more important consequences of hypothyroidism is the potential relationship between low thyroid function and von Willebrand's disease. Thyroid insufficiency should be considered as having a possible role in canine infertility; both males and females should be evaluated.

Diagnosis of Hypothyroidism

The major hematological finding is a normocytic normochromic anemia. Primary biochemical abnormalities are elevations in serum cholesterol and triglyceride concentrations. The most frequently used laboratory tests to diagnose hypothyroidism are serum T_4 concentration and the thyrotropin thyroid-stimulating hormone (TSH) response test. The TSH response test is the dynamic test most suitable for general veterinary practice, and its application has been described in detail.

Therapy

Synthetic thyroxine is the most effective drug. The recommended replacement dosage range for T_4 in dogs is 0.02 to 0.04 mg/kg/day.

FELINE HYPERTHYROIDISM (pp. 1517–1522)

Feline hyperthyroidism is one of the more commonly diagnosed endocrine diseases. It is a systemic disorder that results from sustained high circulating levels of T_4 and T_3. The origin of the excessive thyroid hormones is usually adenomatous hyperplasia in one (30 per cent) or both (70 per cent) thyroid glands. Most hyperthyroid cats are middle-aged to old; no breed or sex predilection is noted. The clinical signs in these cats involve many organ systems. Cardiac involvement and an increase in metabolic rate are often the most profound clinical signs.

The key to diagnosing this disease on physical examination is gentle, deliberate ventral cervical palpation. Normal thyroid glands are not palpable in cats. In approximately 90 per cent of hyperthyroid cats, the enlarged thyroid glands can be palpated. Because these are usually elderly sick cats, a complete hemogram and biochemical profile are indicated. The simplest method of diagnosing hyperthyroidism is by determining resting serum concentrations of T_4 or T_3. In most laboratories, the normal range for T_4 is 1 to 4 µg/100 ml, whereas the normal range for T_3 is 10 to 100 µg/100 ml.

Because high levels of circulating thyroid hormone can lead to hypertrophic changes within the myocardium, a thoracic radiograph is obtained in all suspected cases of feline hyperthyroidism.

Thyroid scanning (imaging) is helpful in treating hyperthyroid cats; this relies on an increased uptake of radioiodine by the overly active thyroid gland. The goal of thyroid imaging is to determine the extent of the primary disease process and to detect distant metastases.

Antithyroid drugs inhibit the formation of thyroid hormone and maintain levels of circulating T_3/T_4 at low to normal values; hyperplastic thyroid tissue persists. Methimazole (Tapazole) and propylthiouracil are two antithyroid drugs used to treat hyperthyroid cats. The disadvantages of antithyroid medication are that (1) the abnormal thyroid tissue persists, and this benign disease is never cured, (2) daily medication must be given for the life of the cat, and (3) these drugs can potentially produce mild to serious side effects. Methimazole is as effective as and safer than propylthiouracil and therefore is the antithyroid drug of choice.

Another effective nonsurgical treatment for feline hyperthyroidism is radioactive iodine. ^{131}I is a radioactive isotope that is taken up by the thyroid gland after being given intravenously and is concentrated in the hyperplastic cells. These cells are destroyed by the emission of beta particles. The disadvantages are that cats must be isolated in a hospital environment for 1 to 2 weeks, possibly leading to anorexia and depression.

In our opinion, radioactive iodine is the best treatment for feline hyperthyroidism when all factors are collectively considered. If nuclear medicine facilities are unavailable, surgical thyroidectomy is then recommended. Long-term antithyroid drug treatment should only be recommended for cats in which hospitalization, anesthesia, and surgery carry a substantial risk.

Before thyroidectomy, a complete blood count, serum chemistry profile, and, when available, a thyroid scan are performed using intravenous ^{99m}TC as pertechnetate. Most cats are treated preoperatively with methimazole until euthyroidism is achieved, usually 2 to 4 weeks after the onset of drug therapy. Once hyperthyroidism has been reversed, the risks associated with anesthesia are markedly diminished.

Surgical Techniques

Surgical treatment of feline hyperthyroidism is accomplished via extracapsular or intracapsular thyroidectomy. In the extracapsular technique, the entire thyroid gland and capsule are removed without opening the capsule. In the intracapsular technique, the capsule is opened and the thyroid gland is gently teased away from the capsule and removed. In the initial description of the intracapsular technique, the thyroid capsule was left in place and not removed. The modified intracapsular technique involves removal of the thyroid capsule after the gland has been removed.

Postoperative Complications

There are several potential complications after thyroidectomy, including hypocalcemia, laryngeal paralysis, hyperthyroid recurrence, and hypothyroidism. Hypocalcemia occurs after inadvertent removal of all four parathyroid glands during bilateral thyroidectomy or as a result of damage to the blood supply of the external parathyroid glands. Laryngeal paralysis becomes clinically significant when bilateral recurrent laryngeal nerve damage occurs during bilateral thyroidectomy.

Recurrence of hyperthyroidism after bilateral thyroidectomy can be caused by adenomatous changes in ectopic thyroid tissue or more commonly hypertrophy of thyroid remnant cells left behind at the initial site of thyroidectomy.

CANINE THYROID TUMORS (p. 1522)

Most feline thyroid tumors are benign; in dogs, most thyroid tumors are malignant carcinomas. Most of these carcinomas are nonfunctional, with only about 15 per cent producing excessive levels of thyroid hormones. Most canine thyroid tumors have an abundant blood supply and are locally invasive. These tumors are surgically approached with caution because they are often difficult to resect completely.

CHAPTER 113

Parathyroid Glands (pages 1523–1536)

The parathyroid glands regulate the concentration of calcium in the circulation through the actions of parathyroid hormone (PTH). PTH stimulates reabsorption of calcium by the kidneys, mobilization of calcium from bone, and, indirectly, absorption of calcium through the intestine by regulation of vitamin D hydroxylation in the kidneys.

ANATOMY AND VASCULAR SUPPLY (p. 1523)

Dogs and cats have four parathyroid glands. Two parathyroid glands are closely associated with each thyroid gland. Most of the parenchyma is composed of a single cell type called the *chief cell*. The vascular supply of the parathyroid glands is derived from branches of the thyroid arteries and veins.

EMBRYOLOGY (p. 1523)

PARATHYROID HORMONE (pp. 1523–1527)

Secretion

The parathyroid glands store a small quantity of PTH secretory granules in the chief cells. PTH is rapidly synthesized and released in response to decreases in serum calcium concentration.

Physiological Effects

The main function of the parathyroid glands is regulation of the serum calcium concentration.

Parathyroid Hormone and Vitamin D Metabolism

Several effects of PTH on calcium homeostasis are mediated by vitamin D. PTH controls 1-hydroxylation of 25-hydroxyvitamin D_3, which occurs in the mitochondria of the proximal tubules of the kidneys. The end product of renal hydroxylation, 1,25-dihydroxyvitamin D_3 $[1,25(OH)_2D_3]$, is the most metabolically active form of vitamin D. It is 100 times more potent than 25-hydroxyvitamin D_3 in promoting bone calcium resorption activity and functions three times faster in promoting calcium absorption through the intestine. Feedback inhibition of PTH secretion by the parathyroid glands is provided by $1,25(OH)_2D_3$.

Parathyroid Hormone and Intestinal Calcium Absorption

Effects of PTH on intestinal calcium absorption are mediated through vitamin D. Ingested calcium is absorbed from the gut by two different processes. The first process occurs mainly in the proximal jejunum, is transcellular, and is vitamin D dependent. The second process by which calcium is absorbed occurs throughout the small intestine and functions independently of vitamin D.

Renal Effects of Parathyroid Hormone

PTH has three effects on the the kidneys: It (1) potentiates the renal reabsorption of calcium, (2) increases renal excretion of phosphate, and (3) potentiates the 1-hydroxylation of vitamin D. Renal reabsorption of calcium occurs at several sites in the kidneys, with most (50 to 60 per cent) of the reabsorption occurring in the proximal convoluted tubule. The major site of PTH effect on renal reabsorption of calcium is in the distal convoluted tubule.

Although PTH increases renal reabsorption of calcium, it decreases the reabsorption of phosphorus. This is a homeostatic mechanism that preserves calcium but prevents the calcium-phosphorus solubility product from exceeding saturation limits, thus preventing precipitation of calcium phosphate salts in the soft tissues of the body.

Parathyroid Hormone and Bone

PTH acts on bone to stimulate the release of calcium and phosphorus from bone mineral stores. Bone minerals are released into the circulation by two mechanisms, osteoclastic bone resorption and osteocyte-mediated release of calcium and phosphorus from an exchangeable pool of bone minerals. PTH causes increased metabolic activity in osteoblasts and increased intracellular levels of second messengers such as cyclic adenosine monophosphate, calcium, diacylglycerol, and inositol triphosphate.

Osteoclasts do not have PTH or $1,25(OH)_2D_3$ receptors. Activation of osteoclasts occurs through the action of an osteoclast-stimulating factor released by osteoblasts in response to PTH. The greatest effect of PTH on acute release of calcium from bone is not the result of an increase in osteoclast activity but an augmentation of calcium release from the exchangeable pool of calcium in bone.

CALCITONIN (p. 1527)

Calcitonin is a 32-amino-acid polypeptide hormone synthesized and secreted by the parafollicular C cells of the thyroid gland. Calcitonin reduces serum calcium concentrations to the normal range by antagonizing some of the actions of PTH.

PARATHYROID NEOPLASIA (pp. 1527–1528)

The most common parathyroid neoplasm in dogs is functional parathyroid adenoma. Some solitary parathyroid tumors are histologically classified as hyperplasia because of the difficulty in differentiating hyperplastic from adenomatous change. Parathyroid neoplasia is rare in cats. Parathyroid adenomas are usually unilateral and affect only one thyroid-associated parathyroid gland. Clinical signs associated with functional parathyroid neoplasms (primary hyperparathyroidism) are related to hypercalcemia caused by excessive secretion of PTH.

The clinical signs of primary hyperparathyroidism are often subtle and most commonly include polyuria/polydipsia, lethargy, inappetence, and weakness. Less commonly reported clinical signs include vomiting, stiff gait, pathological fractures, facial deformity, loose teeth, and urolithiasis.

Hyperparathyroidism produces hypercalciuria, which may predispose to urolithiasis. Chronic administration of exogenous PTH produces calcium phosphate uroliths in dogs. Increased PTH secretion causes proliferation of osteoblasts and osteoclasts and stimulates bone remodeling sites. The result is augmented bone turnover, with osteoclasia in excess of bone synthesis. The radiographic and histological picture of hyperparathyroidism is bone resorption and replacement of resorbed bone by fibrous connective tissue (osteitis fibrosa). The skull, maxilla, and mandible are most commonly affected.

Clinical Pathological Changes of Primary Hyperparathyroidism

No consistent abnormalities in the hemogram of dogs with functional parathyroid neoplasms have been reported. Urinalysis may reveal calcium phosphate or calcium oxalate crystals associated with hypercalciuria.

The most consistent hematological abnormalities associated with primary hyperparathyroidism are hypercalcemia with normo- or hypophosphatemia. In dogs, serum calcium concentrations may be affected by the concentration of serum albumin or protein. Approximately 50 per cent of serum calcium is protein bound, so elevations of serum albumin or protein may elevate total serum calcium measurement. Some dogs with primary hyperparathyroidism may have elevations of serum alkaline phosphatase concentration, attributed to increased bone resorption.

DIFFERENTIAL DIAGNOSIS OF HYPERCALCEMIA
(pp. 1528–1531)

Hypercalcemia of Malignancy

Nonparathyroid malignancy is the most common cause of hypercalcemia in dogs but is infrequent in cats. Hypercalcemia may be caused by direct destruction of bone by the tumor or tumor metastases. Findings now support the concept that hypercalcemia of malignancy is most often caused by the action of humoral factors produced by nonparathyroid neoplasms. The most commonly reported neoplasms causing hypercalcemia in dogs are lymphosarcoma, adenocarcinoma of the apocrine glands of the anal sacs, and multiple myeloma.

Hypercalcemia Associated with Renal Failure

Renal failure is usually associated with increased secretion of PTH and hyperplasia of the parathyroid glands. Despite the presence of increased circulating levels of PTH, hypercalcemia is not common during chronic renal failure. Most dogs and cats with renal failure have normal or low serum calcium concentrations. The factor that makes some chronic renal failure patients with secondary hyperparathyroidism hypercalcemic whereas most are normocalcemic or hypocalcemic is unknown.

Animals with secondary renal hyperparathyroidism may suffer from pathological fractures, loose teeth, and soft mandibles, as do animals with primary hyperparathyroidism.

Hypoadrenocorticism

Approximately 30 to 45 per cent of dogs and 15 per cent of cats with hypoadrenocorticism are hypercalcemic. The cause of the hypercalcemia is unknown; it may be related to elevated serum protein concentration due to dehydration. Hypocalciuria is present in hypoadrenocorticoid patients even though hypercalcemia is present. The hypocalciuria may be due to increased renal reabsorption of calcium.

Hypervitaminosis D

Excessive intake of vitamin D causes hypercalcemia and hyperphosphatemia. The most common causes of hypervitaminosis D in dogs and cats are excessive administration of vitamin D-containing dietary supplements, excessive vitamin D therapy for hypocalcemia, ingestion of vitamin D-containing rodenticides, and ingestion of ovine and bovine liver.

Hypercalcemia and Inflammation

Hypercalcemia is an infrequent complication of blastomycosis in dogs. The hypercalcemia is not associated with bone destruction; indeed, few hypercalcemic patients with granulomatous disease have evidence of bone involvement. The hypercalcemia may be due to endogenous production of $1,25(OH)_2D_3$ by macrophages in granulation tissue associated with fungal infection.

EVALUATION OF HYPERCALCEMIC PATIENTS
(pp. 1531–1532)

The differential diagnosis of hypercalcemia in small animals includes primary hyperparathyroidism, secondary renal hyperparathyroidism, hypercalcemia of malignancy, hypervitaminosis D, granulomatous disease, hypoadrenocorticism, and hyperproteinemia.

To diagnose hypercalcemia, elevated calcium levels must be present on more than one occasion.

A physical examination is performed initially. Serum chemistry profile may enable differentiation of other causes of hypercalcemia.

Hyperkalemia with hyponatremia may suggest hypoadrenocorticism. Hypercalcemia with hyperphosphatemia and normal renal function is compatible with vitamin D toxicity. Hyperphosphatemia and uremia may signal hypercalcemia associated with renal failure. An elevated serum globulin concentration (monoclonal gammopathy) is present in dogs with multiple myeloma. Thoracic and abdominal radiographs are also helpful in determining the cause of hypercalcemia.

The chief diagnostic dilemma is in distinguishing between hypercalcemia of malignancy due to occult, nonparathyroid neoplasia and hypercalcemia due to primary hyperparathyroidism. PTH radioimmunoassay has been validated for dogs and cats. Many PTH assays are commercially available; however, it is essential to select an assay that has been validated for the specific species of animal in question. The PTH assay validated for dogs measures intact PTH.* If primary hyperparathyroidism is suspected on the basis of history, physical examination, and hematological findings, PTH assay is the next step.

SURGICAL TREATMENT OF HYPERPARATHYROIDISM
(pp. 1532–1534)

Surgical excision of neoplastic parathyroid glands is the treatment of choice for primary hyperparathyroidism.

Preoperative Treatment

Animals with primary hyperparathyroidism usually have mild symptoms and require little preoperative treatment. Because increased serum calcium levels can potentially cause cardiac conduction abnormalities, an electrocardiogram is performed. Animals with primary hyperparathyroidism should be well hydrated. Hypercalcemic damage to renal tubular cells is magnified if glomerular filtration is decreased.

Patients in a hypercalcemic crisis with severe weakness, vomiting, depression, dehydration, and uremia require emergency management consisting of rapid rehydration with isotonic saline solution. Once the

---

*The validated canine PTH assay is currently available at the endocrinology laboratory, Michigan State University School of Veterinary Medicine.

animal is hydrated, furosemide may be administered in high doses (5 mg/kg initially, then 5 mg/kg/hr until the calcium level is lowered) to enhance calciuresis. It is important to maintain hydration during diuretic therapy, or calcium reabsorption in the proximal tubules occurs along with sodium reabsorption. If saline and furosemide diuresis are unsuccessful in lowering calcium concentrations, corticosteroid administration (prednisone, 2 mg/kg) may reduce serum calcium concentration. Calcitonin is effective for rapidly reducing serum calcium concentrations.

Cimetidine, an H_2-receptor blocker, lowers serum calcium and PTH levels in humans with hyperparathyroidism associated with parathyroid neoplasia. Bisphosphonates have been used to treat hypercalcemia in man, and one report described bisphosphonate use for treatment of hypercalcemia in a dog.

Preoperative Localization of Parathyroid Tumors

It is desirable to identify parathyroid neoplasms before surgery, not only to plan the surgical approach but also to confirm the diagnosis.

Surgical localization of parathyroid tissue may be enhanced with methylene blue. Methylene blue is selectively taken up by the parathyroid glands by an unknown mechanism. Methylene blue can cause fatal Heinz body anemia in cats, so the use of methylene blue infusion for identification of parathyroid tissue is not without risk.

Parathyroidectomy

Surgical excision of adenomatous or hyperplastic parathyroid glands is the treatment of choice for primary hyperparathyroidism in dogs and cats. All parathyroid neoplasms reported have involved only one parathyroid gland. The unaffected glands are of normal size or slightly smaller owing to suppression from elevated PTH concentrations.

If there is any question about the completeness of excision or if the internal parathyroid gland is to be excised, partial or unilateral thyroidectomy is indicated. If none of the parathyroid glands are enlarged, there are two possible explanations. The animal may have some other cause of hyperparathyroidism or a neoplasm involving ectopic parathyroid tissue. If all four parathyroid glands are enlarged, the most likely diagnosis is parathyroid hyperplasia.

Postoperative Treatment

The most common complication after surgical removal of a parathyroid tumor is postoperative hypocalcemia. The major cause of postoperative hypocalcemia is suppression of the remaining parathyroid glands due to negative feedback from chronically elevated PTH concentrations. The suppressed glands require 2 to 3 weeks to begin secreting PTH.

Postoperative hypocalcemia is treated with a combination of vitamin D and calcium supplementation. Severe hypocalcemia is treated with intravenous administration of 15 mg/kg of 10 per cent calcium gluconate (100 mg/ml). The vitamin D supplement most commonly used in dogs and cats is dihydrotachysterol. Starting dihydrotachysterol and oral calcium therapy immediately after surgery may reduce the incidence of postoperative hypocalcemia. The dose is gradually tapered during a 4- to 8-week period, while serum calcium concentration is monitored.

Prognosis

The majority of parathyroid tumors are benign and are cured by complete excision. Most bony lesions caused by chronic hyperparathyroidism resolve after parathyroidectomy. Mild renal disease caused by hypercalcemia often improves after parathyroidectomy.

CHAPTER 114

Surgical Diseases of the Endocrine Pancreas (pages 1536–1544)

Surgical diseases of the endocrine pancreas are uncommon in animals and generally are limited to diseases of the islet cells. Cells of the endocrine system and autonomic nervous system are referred to as *APUD* cells because a major cytochemical characteristic of these cells is the capability of *a*mine *p*recursor *u*ptake and *d*ecarboxylation. Tumors arising from APUD cells are called *apudomas*. Pancreatic beta-cell carcinoma (insulinoma) is the most commonly observed apudoma in veterinary medicine.

PANCREATIC BETA-CELL CARCINOMA (pp. 1536–1542)

Pancreatic beta-cell carcinomas are also referred to as *insulinomas* and islet cell adenocarcinomas. Insulinomas are most commonly observed in middle-aged to older dogs. A breed predisposition exists for boxers, German shepherds, standard poodles, Irish setters, and collies.

Pathology and Pathophysiology

Insulin-secreting tumors result in hyperinsulinemia and hypoglycemia. Neurological signs predominate in hypoglycemic animals because glucose is the primary energy source used by the central nervous system (CNS). Clinical signs are related to the rate of development of hypoglycemia rather than the degree of hypoglycemia.

Insulinomas are malignant, slow-growing tumors in animals. Early metastasis to the liver, regional lymph nodes, and spleen is common, and the recurrence rate approaches 100 per cent. Demonstration of hypoglycemia in an animal with episodic weakness does not confirm a diagnosis of insulinoma. Numerous disorders such as hypoadrenocorticism, hepatic lipidosis, hepatic glycogen storage diseases, hepatic cirrhosis, inanition, cachexia, portosystemic shunt, pregnancy toxemia, and hunting dog hypoglycemia may result in hypoglycemia and signs of neuroglycopenia.

Diagnosis

A tentative diagnosis of insulinoma is based on demonstration of the Whipple triad: (1) neurological signs associated with hypoglycemia, (2) fasting blood glucose concentration of 40 mg/100 ml or less at the time the animal is symptomatic, and (3) relief of neurological symptoms by feeding or parenteral administration of glucose. The Whipple triad is characteristic of hypoglycemia regardless of etiology and is not specific for insulinoma.

History

Characteristic clinical signs are slowly progressive and episodic and include weakness, depression, disorientation, incoordination, bizarre behavior, seizures or seizure-like activity, and collapse. Clinical signs may be triggered by excitement, stress, exercise, fasting, or eating.

Clinical Findings

Physical examination findings generally are nonspecific and subtle.

Radiology

Ultrasonography often is beneficial in identifying liver metastases and may be helpful in delineating the primary pancreatic mass.

Laboratory Evaluations

Nonfasting blood glucose concentrations frequently are quite low.

Fasting Blood Glucose

Demonstration of a profoundly low blood glucose concentration after a fast suggests an insulinoma but is not confirmatory.

Plasma Insulin

Plasma insulin concentration is reported in micro-units/milliliter (μunits/ml) of immunoreactive insulin (IRI).

Animals with insulinoma have persistently elevated IRI levels because hypoglycemia fails to have the normal suppressive effect on insulin secretion if the insulin arises from autonomous neoplastic cells.

Amended Glucose/Insulin Ratio

Several glucose/insulin ratios have been suggested. The amended glucose/insulin ratio (AGIR) is the most reliable. The AGIR is not used as a sole criterion for diagnosis of insulinoma, because the ability of this test to consistently distinguish between hypoglycemic animals with and without insulinoma has been questioned.

Glucagon Tolerance Test

Provocative tests for insulin secretion are rarely necessary to make a diagnosis of insulinoma in animals.

Preoperative Treatment

Important considerations in the preoperative period are protection from hypoglycemia and clinical signs of neuroglycopenia and maintenance of fluid and electrolyte balance. Frequent assessment of the blood glucose concentration is imperative and easily accomplished with commercially available reagent strips. Serum electrolytes are assessed during dextrose infusion, and potassium supplementation is provided as needed. Food and water are withheld for 12 hours before surgery. Five per cent dextrose solution is administered intravenously during the preoperative fast and surgery. Multiple blood glucose analyses are performed during this time.

Surgical Therapy

Surgical exploration may be necessary to definitively diagnose a pancreatic beta-cell carcinoma. The therapeutic and prognostic value of an exploratory laparotomy justifies surgery when the diagnosis has previously been established. Surgical therapy is considered palliative owing to the almost 100 per cent incidence of recurrence. A thorough visual and *gentle* digital inspection of the pancreas is necessary.

The goal of surgery is to reduce the tumor mass by removing as much obvious tumor as possible, including metastases to the liver and regional lymph nodes. Reduction in tumor mass frequently results in remission or reduction of clinical signs and improved response to medical therapy. Euthanasia during surgery should not be recommended regardless of the findings because most dogs can be treated medically for several months.

Pancreatic or extrapancreatic nodules occasionally cannot be positively identified as beta-cell carcinoma. Intravenous methylene blue infusion is beneficial in differentiating metastatic nodules from nonmetastatic nodules in dogs.

Postoperative Management

Maintenance of normoglycemia and management of iatrogenic pancreatitis are primary considerations in the immediate postoperative period. Frequent blood glucose analyses are essential, and 24-hour monitoring of patients is ideal. Animals may be hypo-, hyper-, or euglycemic after surgical excision of an insulinoma. All dogs that undergo partial pancreatectomy for insulinoma excision are treated for pancreatitis for 24 to 48 hours after surgery.

Medical Therapy for Insulinoma

Animals that are euglycemic and symptom free after surgery usually remain so for several months, occasionally for 1 year or longer. Medical therapy is not recommended as long as an animal remains euglycemic. Medical therapy of malignant insulinoma consists of dietary, hormonal, and antineoplastic regimens. Each therapeutic method, starting with dietary control, is continued until hypoglycemic signs recur. At that time, another treatment regimen begins without discontinuing the first.

Diet

Feeding three to six small meals per day provides a continuous supply of glucose and avoids the sudden excessive insulin secretion commonly generated by large meals.

Antihormonal Drugs

Glucocorticoids.
Diazoxide. Diazoxide is a benzothiadiazide diuretic with potent hyperglycemic properties.

Antineoplastic Drugs

Streptozotocin. Streptozotocin is extremely nephrotoxic, and its use in animals with recurrent insulinoma cannot be recommended at this time.
Somatostatin.

Prognosis

The long-term prognosis for dogs with insulinoma is poor. The recurrence rate is nearly 100 per cent. Appropriate and timely surgical intervention and adjunctive medical therapy typically result in survival for 12 to 15 months, although 2-year survival has been reported.

GASTRINOMA (pp. 1542–1544)

In 1955, Zollinger and Ellison described a syndrome in humans of gastric acid hypersecretion, gastrointestinal ulcerations, and a non–beta-cell pancreatic tumor and postulated that an ulcerogenic humoral factor of pancreatic islet origin was responsible. It was later discovered that the pancreatic tumor consisted of cells that secreted large quantities of gastrin. The syndrome, termed the *Zollinger-Ellison syndrome*, was first described in dogs by Jones in 1976.

Pathology and Pathophysiology

Zollinger-Ellison syndrome is rare in man and exceedingly rare in animals. The few case reports of gastrinoma in the veterinary literature suggest the condition is more common in middle-aged to older dogs.The disease is insidious in onset, and metastasis to the liver and regional lymph nodes occurs in more than 50 per cent by the time the diagnosis is made.

Diagnosis

The diagnosis of gastrinoma is based on demonstration of hypergastrinemia and an elevated rate of gastric acid secretion in any animal with typical clinical signs of upper gastrointestinal ulcer disease.

History

Animals with gastrinoma typically have a 1- to 2-month history of anorexia, weight loss, intermittent diarrhea, depression, vomiting, and hematemesis that is partially responsive or nonresponsive to conservative therapy.

Clinical Findings

Clinical findings are nonspecific and may include weight loss, dehydration, melena, hematemesis, and rarely signs of generalized peritonitis from a perforated ulcer.

Radiology

An upper gastrointestinal series may be helpful in establishing a diagnosis based on findings of thickened gastric mucosa, prominent gastric rugal folds, and hypermotility of the small intestine.

Laboratory Evaluations

Hypoproteinemia is a consistent finding in animals with gastrinoma. Hypokalemia, hypochloremia, and metabolic alkalosis occur.

Endoscopy (pp. 1542–1543)

Serum Gastrin Level

Demonstration of hyperchlorhydria in conjunction with increased serum gastrin concentration is the most reliable nonsurgical means for establishing a diagnosis of gastrinoma in animals. Provocative tests using oral protein loading, intravenously administered secretin, or intravenously administered calcium gluconate are indicated when basal serum gastrin levels are nondiagnostic. Hypergastrinemia is not pathognomonic for gastrinoma.

Basal Gastric Acid Secretion

Dogs do not constantly secrete hydrochloric acid; therefore, basal gastric acid secretion values are almost zero in normal dogs.

Medical Therapy

Medical therapy of gastrinoma involves inhibition of gastrin-stimulated gastric acid secretion with H_2 antagonists such as cimetidine and ranitidine and treatment of ulcer disease. Sucralfate, a sulfated disaccharide that coats ulcerated surfaces in the stomach and duodenum, may be used in animals with gastric or duodenal ulcers.

Surgical Therapy

Surgery is the best therapeutic alternative for animals with gastrinoma. Exploratory celiotomy is the most advantageous method for establishing a diagnosis and allows complete excision or debulking of the tumor mass and evaluation for metastasis. Extensive metastatic disease is often present; however, reducing the tumor mass may enhance the success of medical therapy postoperatively.

Prognosis

The prognosis is poor, and long-term survival is unlikely.

Ear (pages 1545–1576)

CHAPTER 115

The Pinna (pages 1545–1559)

ANATOMY (p. 1545)

INJURIES (pp. 1545–1548)

Aural Hematoma

Aural or auricular hematoma is the most common physical injury of the pinna. It is usually self-inflicted by scratching and head shaking. The hematoma is lined by cartilage on both sides, suggesting fracture or splitting of the cartilage as an etiological factor. With chronicity, fibrosis and contraction thicken and deform the ear. The therapeutic objectives for an auricular hematoma are to identify the source of irritation, evacuate the hematoma, maintain tissue apposition, reduce fibrin deposition, and prevent recurrence.

Conservative Therapy

Needle aspiration may evacuate the hematoma and restore tissue apposition if used soon after hematoma formation. A pressure bandage is applied after aspiration. Recurrence is common with needle aspiration as the only treatment.

Incision

Large, severe, or chronic (thick-walled) hematomas are treated by incision to remove the fibrin and by suturing to reappose the tissue. Longitudinal contracture is less likely to cause deformity with S-shaped incisions. The fibrin clot is thoroughly curetted, and the cavity copiously irrigated. Loosely tied mattress sutures are placed through the ear, parallel to the major vessels.

Lacerations

The ears are commonly injured during fights. Regardless of severity, the therapeutic objectives are cleaning, débridement, apposition of tissues, protection, and prevention of secondary infection.

Skin Wound

Suturing is mandatory when a two- or three-sided flap has been formed.

Skin and Cartilage Wound

For best results, the skin is sutured by using a vertical mattress pattern with the deeper bite aligning cartilage and the superficial bite aligning skin.

520

Perforating Wound

The most serious lacerations are those in which the full thickness of the ear is lacerated through a helical border. Such lacerations should be sutured soon after injury.

LOSS OF TISSUE (pp. 1548–1549)
Inflammatory Lesions

Defects of the pinna can be caused by minor trauma (fissures), ear tip dermatitis, or avulsions. The primary objective is to treat the cause of head shaking.

Avulsive Injuries
Partial Amputation

Ears with shallow auricular defects can be cosmetically improved by partial amputation of the auricle.

Pedicle Flaps

A larger auricular margin defect can be reconstructed by transposing a pedicle flap from the lateral cervicobuccal region. Both the concave and convex epithelial surfaces are replaced.

SOLAR AND COLD INJURIES (pp. 1549–1552)
Actinic Keratosis of White Feline Ears

The initial lesions are a mild sunburn, causing alopecia. During a period of years, the cartilage and overlying skin begin to deform. The lesion is preneoplastic and may lead to squamous cell carcinoma. The therapeutic objectives are to decrease the ear's exposure to direct sunlight and to amputate progressive ulcerative lesions.

NEOPLASIA OF THE EXTERNAL EAR (p. 1552)
Staging and Diagnosis

Neoplasms arising from the external ear originate from the skin, adnexa, or connective tissue. Neoplasms commonly associated with the external ear include ceruminous gland or sebaceous adenoma or adenocarcinoma, papilloma, squamous cell carcinoma, histiocytoma, mast cell tumor, basal cell carcinoma, and melanosarcoma.

Ceruminous gland tumors are the only tumors unique to the pinna. They remain small but recur readily after incomplete excision.

Neoplasms that arise in the central portion of the pinna are more common on the convex surface.

COSMETIC OTOPLASTY* (pp. 1552–1559)

Cosmetic otoplasty is performed on the ears of certain breeds to meet breed specifications. There are no medical reasons for these techniques to be performed.

---

*Editor's note: This technique is not considered ethical and is illegal in some areas. Local details should be sought.

Standards of Ear Trimming

Regardless of the trimming standard, all ears cannot be trimmed alike. Variations are justified depending on the sex of the animal and conformation of the breed. Females generally are trimmed to have a finer ear than males.

General Considerations

Trimming the ears of a puppy that is in poor condition is delayed until the puppy's general health improves. Puppies are vaccinated before having their ears trimmed.

Surgical Technique

Instruments such as ear-trimming forms are often not satisfactory because placement is difficult and they usually fail to provide the trim desired. Finely serrated cartilage scissors are essential for the final trimming of the cartilage.

Postoperative Care

Many ears fail to stand because of improper aftercare. The ears must be pulled above the head, stretched when taped or braced to obtain proper ear carriage, and examined closely for exudates, odors, and malpositioning.

Rolled Gauze Sponge and Tape

Cardboard Tube

Styrofoam Cups

Complications

The most severe problem, at least in the owner's eyes, is failure of the ears to stand.

Corrective Ear Surgery

If discovered early, faulty ear carriage may be corrected by proper taping procedures, particularly in dogs younger than 6 months. Numerous techniques have been used to correct faulty ear carriage; most result in only slight improvement.

Conservative Treatment

The ear is rolled opposite to the way it is breaking. Tape is left on the ear for 5 days, and the ear is observed for 1 day to see if improvement has occurred.

Surgical Correction

Medial Deviation.
Lateral Deviation.

External Ear Canal (pages 1560–1567)

OTITIS EXTERNA (pp. 1560–1567)

Otitis externa is the most common ear disease in veterinary practice. In dogs, miniature poodles, cocker spaniels, and fox terriers have the highest incidence, and Himalayan and Persian cats may also be at risk. Pendulous and hair-filled ears predispose to otitis. Differences in the number and distribution of adnexal structures and overall skin disease may provide better explanations for the breed association.

Etiology

The causes of otitis externa are numerous, and it is most often a multifactorial disease. The anatomy of the ear and the presence of hair in the canal may predispose to infection. Bacterial pathogens include *Staphylococcus*, *Streptococcus*, *Pseudomonas*, *Proteus*, *Escherichia coli*, and *Corynebacterium*. Although otitis may be caused by a single species of bacteria, a combination of organisms are more commonly isolated. Small numbers of gram-positive organisms are cultured from normal ears. Gram-negative bacteria are usually found only in diseased ears. *Staphylococcus* is the most common organism isolated, with *Proteus* the most common gram-negative organism in dogs and *Pasteurella* the most common gram-negative organism in cats.

Malassezia canis is the most common yeast isolated from otitis cases and can be found alone or in combination with bacteria. *Candida* can also be found in diseased ears.

Otodectes cyanotis is a mite that commonly causes otitis in cats and occasionally in dogs. Other parasites leading to otitis include fleas, spinous ear ticks, *Demodex*, chiggers, and *Cheyletiella*. Irritation due to foreign bodies may produce otitis by creating an environment favorable to opportunistic bacteria and fungi. In certain regions, grass awns (foxtails) are found within the ear canal.

Atopy, food allergy, and contact sensitivities may predispose or cause otitis. The ear canal is often affected by diseases that cause generalized skin disorders. These diseases may be seasonal or related to diet and topical medications. Metabolic diseases including hypothyroidism and seborrhea may cause severe otitis. The appearance can be that of an oily film or large, soft flakes within the ear canal. Finally, immune-mediated diseases, such as lupus, pemphigus vulgaris, and pemphigus foliaceus may be manifested as otitis externa.

Pathophysiology

Once the disease begins, its progression is quite similar despite the original etiology.

The inflammatory response with otitis results in damage to the superficial protective stratum corneum of the canal. Hyperplasia and hypertrophy of sebaceous and ceruminous glands occur, along with a diffuse cellular infiltration of macrophages, mast cells, lymphocytes, plasma cells, neutrophils, and eosinophils. Moisture, debris, foreign bodies, hair, and glandular secretions are trapped because of the shape of the canal. Retained wax is broken down by the lipolytic action of microorganisms. Erosions and ulcerations occur within the canal, resulting in serum exudates and necrotic debris, which form additional culture media for bacterial proliferation.

523

Metabolic disorders are associated with increased secretion of free fatty acids. Allergic reactions result in mast cell degranulation and release of lymphokines. Parasites elicit both allergic and mechanical irritation in the canal. Long-standing otitis results in significant hyperplasia of the dermis and epidermis and stenosis of the lumen of the canal. Fibroplasia of the dermis in chronic cases can result in total occlusion of the external auditory meatus. This chronic inflammatory response may give rise to polyps in cats. The tympanic membrane opacifies, scleroses, ulcerates, and eventually ruptures, predisposing to otitis media.

Clinical Signs

Initial clinical signs may be pruritus, manifested by scratching, rubbing the ears, and shaking the head. As the disease evolves, the animal becomes head shy and exhibits pain when examined. Aural exudate becomes prominent, varying from dry, brown exudate of *Otodectes cyanotis* to a purulent, smelly exudate of bacterial infection. (Eventually the external acoustic meatus becomes completely obstructed with proliferative granulation tissue). Infection and ulceration may erode through the wall of the ear canal and result in a para-aural abscess and fistula. In one study, 80 per cent of dogs with end-stage ear disease had one or more dermatological problems, including seborrhea, pyoderma, atopy, or hypothyroidism. Some animals have neurological signs such as facial nerve paralysis, vestibular signs, and head tilt. Severe infection may extend to the temporomandibular joint or surrounding tissues, resulting in pain when opening the mouth. Chronic infection causes calcification of the ear cartilages.

Diagnosis

Definitive diagnosis necessitates a thorough examination of the ear, which usually requires sedation or anesthesia, cytological study and culture of the aural exudate, allergy testing, endocrine evaluation, and determination of immune diseases. Although present in high numbers, microorganisms may be opportunistic and disguise the primary systemic cause.

Radiography is of value in some cases to determine the extent of disease. Cartilage calcification may extend to the osseous bulla. Changes in the bulla suggesting severe otitis externa with extension to the middle ear include osseous bulla thickening, lysis, or periosteal reaction and radiodense tympanic cavity.

Examination and Medical Therapy

A ceruminolytic agent applied to the ears a few hours before the examination softens debris and exudate. Samples are collected for culture and cytological study before adding chemicals to the ear canal. The canal is gently irrigated with warm water or saline to remove exudate and debris. The addition of 0.5 per cent chlorhexidine or 1:100 povidone-iodine to the lavage solution is beneficial for antimicrobial effect but may be toxic to the middle ear if the tympanic membrane is ruptured.

After the canal is cleaned and dried, specific antimicrobials and anti-inflammatory and drying agents are applied. Definitive treatment depends on the total evaluation of the patient for systemic disease and the results of the ear culture, antimicrobial susceptibility, and cytological study.

Surgical Therapy

Lateral Wall Resection (Zepp procedure)

Lateral wall resection is indicated when (1) otitis externa has not responded favorably to proper medical management, (2) otitis externa has recurred despite proper medical management, or (3) exposure is needed for biopsy or to remove benign polyps of the canal. (In the first two instances, it is important that irreversible hyperplastic disease has not occurred.)

Lateral wall resection permits drainage of the ear canal and provides ventilation to reduce moisture, humidity, and temperature, all of which favor infection. Surgery improves conditions for treatment but often is not a cure. Proper topical and systemic management must be continued.

Complications. Failure of lateral wall resection is often related to failure to recognize and treat underlying systemic disease, irreversible changes in the ear canal, failure to drain the horizontal canal properly, strictures of the horizontal canal, presence of concurrent otitis media, failure to perform lateral wall resection correctly, or undue postponement of resection.

Vertical Canal Ablation

Vertical canal ablation is used to salvage a functional horizontal canal when the vertical canal is severely diseased. The procedure combines the advantages of lateral wall resection (drainage, ventilation, and preservation of hearing) with total ear canal ablation (total removal of severely diseased tissue). Vertical canal ablation has certain advantages over lateral wall resection including (1) total removal of vertical canal tissue, (2) less postoperative exudate, (3) less postoperative pain, (4) less incised cartilage, resulting in better healing, and (5) improved cosmetic effect. Indications for vertical canal ablation are irreversible hyperplastic otitis, severe trauma, or neoplasia limited to the vertical canal.

Complications. Vertical canal ablation has fewer complications than lateral wall resection. Postoperative stenosis of the horizontal canal may occur but is less likely if the baffle plate is used. Others have reported extremely high success rates with this procedure and its various modifications. If there is doubt that lateral wall resection will result in a cure, then vertical canal ablation or total canal ablation is recommended.

Total Ear Canal Ablation

Total ear canal ablation is a procedure for removal of both vertical and horizontal ear canals. Indications for surgery include (1) chronic end-stage proliferative otitis with obstruction of both vertical and horizontal canals, (2) persistent otitis following lateral wall resection or vertical canal ablation, (3) neoplasia involving the vertical and horizontal canals, (4) collapsed or stenotic horizontal ear canal with or without ossified cartilages, (5) severe trauma to the vertical and horizontal canal, (6) congenital anomalies of the ear canal, (7) para-aural abscessation, and (8) unremitting otitis media. The most common indication is chronic end-stage otitis, encountered in cocker spaniels.

Total ear canal ablation may be contraindicated when otitis media is present because of a lack of drainage pathway of the middle ear. Most animals with end-stage disease have extension of the disease into the middle ear through perforated tympanic membranes but can be successfully managed with total ear canal ablation combined with bulla osteotomy and drainage.

Complications. Postoperative complications of total ear canal ablation are numerous and frequent. Most frequently encountered are facial nerve paralysis or neuropraxia, wound drainage or dehiscence, cellulitis and infection, hemorrhage, vestibular disease, hypoglossal nerve dysfunction, deafness, and fistula formation. The overall complication rate is 29 to 82 per cent. Most complications can be prevented by proper surgical technique or are temporary and can be resolved with postoperative care.

Postoperative abscessation or fistulation (which may occur up to 1 year or more after surgery) are due to failure to completely remove all infected cartilage and epithelium of the external ear canal or failure to thoroughly remove all debris and infected tissues from the osseous bulla. Correction requires reoperation and thorough débridement of the remaining tissues.

NEOPLASMS OF THE EXTERNAL EAR CANAL (p. 1567)

Neoplasms of the ear canal are most common in cats and usually are ceruminous gland carcinoma. Squamous cell carcinoma has also been reported. Neoplasms in dogs include malignant melanoma, squamous cell carcinoma, and ceruminous adenocarcinoma. The majority of the tumors are malignant, and 50 per cent are metastatic at the time of diagnosis in the cat. Metastases are most frequent to the local nodes and lungs. The clinical presentation resembles otitis that is usually unilateral. Careful examination and biopsy are required for diagnosis. Lateral wall resection may be required for adequate exposure. Although favorable results have been reported in dogs after surgical treatment by total ear canal ablation, other reports describe surgery alone as usually unsuccessful. Radiation following surgery may improve the prognosis, but adequate confirmatory studies are not available.

Inflammatory polyps of cats are the most common benign lesions. These growths may arise from the epithelial lining of the ear canal or middle ear. The clinical signs mimic otitis externa but may also cause signs of otitis media or pharyngeal obstruction when the polyp extends to the middle ear or pharynx (see Chapter 117). The polyps can often be removed by traction through the external meatus.

CHAPTER 117
Middle Ear (pages 1568–1576)

Otitis media frequently afflicts dogs. In one survey of 100 patients with otitis externa, 16 per cent with acute otitis externa had concurrent otitis media and 50 per cent with chronic otitis externa had concurrent otitis media. The most common cause of otitis media is otitis externa; thus, middle ear disease should always be suspected in dogs with chronic or recurrent external ear disease. Other less common causes of otitis media include foreign bodies, trauma, neoplasia, or blood-borne pathogens.

ETIOLOGY AND PATHOGENESIS (p. 1569)

The common pathogens cultured from the middle ear include *Staphylococcus* spp., *Streptococcus* spp., *Pseudomonas* spp., *Escherichia coli*, and *Proteus mirabilis*.

Inflammation of the middle ear can be initiated via three routes: across the tympanic membrane, through the eustachian tube, or by hematogenous spread. Extension of otitis externa across the tympanic membrane is the most common route.

Any organism capable of eroding or ulcerating the epithelial tissue and tympanic membrane can cause severe pathological changes in the tympanic cavity. Such changes include swelling and occlusion of the eustachian tube, erosion of the mucosal lining of the tympanic cavity, metaplasia of the epithelium of the middle ear to hypersecretory stratified squamous epithelium with variable keratinization, degenerative or proliferative changes of the osseous tympanic bulla, and accumulation of inflammatory debris in the tympanic cavity.

CLINICAL SIGNS (p. 1569)

Patients with otitis media generally have signs of otitis externa. These include discharge from the external ear canal, pawing or rubbing the affected ear, shaking the head, or pain when the head is touched. Some animals may have so much pain that they hold their head tilted because of discomfort rather than because of abnormal vestibular function. Because the facial and sympathetic nerves pass near the middle ear, a facial nerve palsy or Horner's syndrome may occur on the same side as the otitis media. If middle ear infection is chronic or severe enough to cause otitis interna, signs of abnormal vestibular function (head tilt, nystagmus, and ataxia) may occur. Nystagmus frequently disappears after the first week, and ataxia may disappear or be rapidly compensated for, but the head tilt generally remains.

PHYSICAL FINDINGS (pp. 1569–1570)

A thorough history and physical examination are performed to rule out systemic disorders (i.e., immune-mediated diseases, generalized seborrhea, atopy, and hypothyroidism) that may be contributing to the etiology of the middle ear disease. Patients should also be examined for the presence of facial palsy, Horner's syndrome, exposure keratitis, and vestibular signs. The temporomandibular joints and base of the ear are palpated for swelling or pain. A careful oral and pharyngeal examination is performed to rule out an abscess or mass associated with the eustachian tube. Proper cleaning of the external ear canal facilitates otoscopic examination of the tympanic membrane. Careful examination of the external ear canal, particularly the tympanic membrane, is helpful in early diagnosis of otitis media. The normal tympanic membrane is slightly concave, translucent, pearl gray, and glistening. Alteration in its color, tension, or integrity indicates pathological change in the middle ear.

RADIOGRAPHY (p. 1570)

Radiographic examination of the osseous bulla may be helpful in establishing a diagnosis of otitis media. Lateral, ventrodorsal, open-mouth, and lateral oblique projections allow adequate observation of the osseous bulla. Radiographic changes in the interior of the bulla compatible with otitis media include the presence of a fluid or bone density. Fluid density may be caused by purulent exudates, granulation tissue, neoplasia, or cellular debris. In patients with chronic otitis media, the tympanic cavity may occasionally be replaced with bone. Although radiographic changes are helpful in establishing a diagnosis of otitis media, these changes may occur late. If the clinical signs and physical findings are compatible with otitis media, with normal radiographs, a presumptive diagnosis of acute otitis media can be made.

TREATMENT OF OTITIS MEDIA (pp. 1570–1574)

The goals of treating patients with otitis media are to gain access to the tympanic cavity; remove inflammatory, infected, or foreign debris; perform culture and susceptibility testing; and provide an avenue for adequate ventilation and drainage.

Medical Treatment: Myringotomy

If the tympanic membrane is intact but discolored and bulging, it is incised (myringotomy) to obtain samples for culture and susceptibility testing and cytological study and to provide drainage from the middle ear cavity. Myringotomy also relieves pain and pressure and provides for lavage and instillation of medication.

The disadvantages of myringotomy include poor exposure of the tympanic cavity, poor postoperative drainage, exposure of the middle ear to the external ear canal (particularly in patients with otitis externa), and damage to the delicate middle ear structures. If medical treatment proves ineffective or a neoplasm, inflammatory mass, or foreign body is found, surgical drainage is indicated.

Surgical Treatment

Numerous surgical techniques are used for treatment of otitis media, but only two provide adequate exposure and drainage of the tympanic cavity: lateral bulla osteotomy and ventral bulla osteotomy.

Lateral Bulla Osteotomy

Lateral bulla osteotomy may be performed as a separate procedure or in combination with other procedures involving the external ear canal. Many patients with otitis media have concurrent signs of otitis externa and may benefit from combined lateral ear resection and bulla osteotomy. Patients frequently have otitis media *and* severe obstructive otitis externa or otitis media *and* a previously unsuccessful lateral ear resection. In either case, a total ear canal ablation and lateral bulla osteotomy can be performed.

A high rate of complications has been reported with total ear canal ablation and lateral bulla osteotomy and is attributed to two main factors: technical difficulty in performing the two procedures and bacterial contamination of the surgical site from contaminated tissues. Complications include facial palsy, wound infection, fistula tract formation, various degrees of hearing loss, and vestibular damage. The overall long-term success rate of total ear canal ablation and lateral bulla osteotomy is 90 to 95 per cent.

Ventral Bulla Osteotomy

Ventral bulla osteotomy may be performed alone or in combination with other procedures involving the external ear canal. This technique has the advantage of providing improved exposure and more consistent ventral drainage of the tympanic bulla than the lateral bulla osteotomy. With bilateral otitis media, both bullae can be approached without repositioning. The major disadvantages of this technique are the technical difficulty of performing the procedure and repositioning of patients that require concurrent external ear canal surgery (i.e., lateral ear resection or total ear canal ablation).

Results. Results following ventral bulla osteotomy alone are excellent in 90 per cent of reported cases. This is most likely due to excellent exposure of the tympanic cavity, allowing careful examination of its contents and adequate ventral drainage.

Patients with end-stage otitis externa and otitis media can be helped by a combination of total ear canal ablation and ventral bulla osteotomy. The complications encountered with total ear canal ablation and ventral bulla osteotomy are comparable to those with total ear canal ablation and lateral bulla osteotomy.

NEOPLASMS OF THE MIDDLE EAR (p. 1574)

Inflammatory Polyps of the Middle Ear in Cats (p. 1574)

Musculoskeletal System
(pages 1577–2026)

CHAPTER 118

Gait Analysis and Orthopedic Examination
(pages 1577–1586)

THE DIAGNOSIS OF CANINE LAMENESS (p. 1577)

Lameness is defined as interference in normal locomotion of an animal, usually involving the propulsion mechanism of one or more limbs. It is often assumed that lameness originates in the skeletal system, but when the cause cannot be found there, attention is directed to other systems, such as the muscular system or neurological system or to referred pain from internal organs.

Lameness is caused by an animal's attempting to minimize pain, which usually occurs during the contact phase, but protraction can sometimes cause pain and interference with the swing phase.

QUANTIFICATION OF LAMENESS (p. 1578)

Although a 1–5 method is used by some clinicians, especially equine veterinarians, the 1–10 method is more useful, for subtle lameness:

Degrees of Lameness
  0: Sound
  1: Occasionally shifts weight
  2: Mild lameness at a slow trot, none while walking
  3: Mild lameness while walking
  4: Obvious lameness while walking, but places the foot when standing
  5: Degrees of severity
  6: Degrees of severity
  7: Degrees of severity
  8: Degrees of severity
  9: Places toe when standing, carries limb when trotting
  10: Unable to put the foot on the ground

ORIGIN OF LAMENESS (pp. 1578–1579)

HISTORY (p. 1579)

One wishes to know the duration of the problem, whether the onset was sudden or gradual, whether an accident preceded the lameness, and whether the lameness only appears at certain times.

It is also necessary to know the progress of the lameness; has it evolved to its present state, or is it of an intermittent nature? Does the lameness abate for some time and return unexpectedly? Is the animal more lame at certain times of the day or in certain kinds of weather?

Is it particularly lame after exercise or does it "warm out" of the lameness? Is the lameness always in one limb, or does it move around (shifting lameness), producing lameness in different limbs at different times? It is also essential to know if the animal has previously been treated for the condition and if it is currently receiving medication.

Certain breeds have congenital abnormalities that predispose to lameness. The valgus and plantigrade stance of the forelimbs of a basset hound predispose to radiocarpal problems. The bowed limbs of a Pekingese predispose to degenerative arthritis of the elbows.

EXAMINATION FOR LAMENESS (pp. 1579–1580)

It is tempting to place the patient on a table and start to palpate. Palpation in the initial stage of investigation is contraindicated. Before seeing an animal move, it is essential to observe it when it is still. One should preferably see it rise, because difficulty in rising may show signs pertaining to the particular area involved. *During the time the history is being taken, the animal is watched because many salient features may emerge when it believes it is not being observed: weight shifting from one limb to another, easing of a joint, and loading one limb more than the other.* If the lameness is not obvious at a slow walk, the animal is induced to trot.

In cases of hindlimb lameness, the stride length is shortened, and animals carry their head lower to minimize, via a cantilever effect, the amount of weight that is carried on the hindlimb(s). When lame in the hips, a dog shifts weightbearing to the forelimbs and the pelvis is tilted more vertically than normal. If the lameness is unilateral, the pelvis is tilted sideways, and an oscillating motion is seen during locomotion. The oscillation is toward the sound side. When viewed from the rear, particularly if a dog is lame in both hips, the pelvis swivels from side to side. This maneuver minimizes hip motion and instead uses lateral bending of the spine to achieve forward movement.

With lameness in a forelimb, an animal lifts its head when the unsound limb bears weight and drops its head with weightbearing on the sound limb.

SPECIFIC TESTS FOR THE EXAMINATION OF LAMENESS (p. 1580)

Inspection

Once an animal has been observed in locomotion, it is stood quietly in front of the observer or, if it is small, on the table, and the body inspected. Observe whether or not the musculature is diminished in any part of the body. Note particularly the muscles of the shoulders and the thighs. Their state may be evaluated by standing over the patient and comparing one side with the other.

Palpation

Light palpation is used to search for puffiness of an area, particularly a joint; swelling, whether fluctuating or tense; and an increase in local temperature.

Deep palpation of the bones must be carefully performed because the observer may inadvertently put pressure on either a nerve or muscle, causing discomfort. In a condition such as panosteitis, lesions may be present in more than one bone. The stoicism of some animals and the sensitivity of others can be extremely misleading.

Shoulder

In the shoulder joint, the compression test is particularly helpful. With the joint held in its normal position, the head of the humerus is compressed into the glenoid cavity in three different ways: with slight abduction, with slight adduction, and in a rotational movement during compression. When this is being carried out, the area of the scapular tuberosity and the bicipital bursa is examined at the same time for specific point pain.

Muscular conditions causing lameness include infraspinatus contracture, dorsal displacement of the scapula, avulsion of the origin of the biceps brachii, medial displacement of the tendon of origin of the biceps brachii, and partial or complete avulsion of the triceps tendon. In the acute stages, the limb is nonweightbearing, and there is usually displacement of the scapula according to the muscles involved. Loss of musculature and fibrous contraction of the remaining muscle tissue occur with chronicity, impairing joint function. One should ascertain the neurological status of the limb, because acute trauma may have caused brachial plexus damage or damage to peripheral nerves such as the suprascapular nerve.

When the biceps brachii muscle is involved, the lameness may not be greater than a grade 3 or 4 but is variable. Pain may be elicited on flexion and extension of the shoulder joint, and cranial displacement of the humerus may be detectable. Rupture of the transverse humeral ligament permits displacement of the biceps tendon of origin, usually in a medial direction. The animal becomes acutely lame, but this lameness may subside after a few days, becoming exacerbated after prolonged exercise. The displacement may be determined by palpating the area, noting a sensation of the tendon popping in and out of the groove when the leg is flexed and extended, particularly if internal rotation of the scapula and external rotation of the humerus are performed.

Elbow Joints

Lameness in the elbow is similar to that in the shoulder. Elbow lameness is characterized by reduced joint motion during ambulation.

Most elbow lameness arises from problems within the joint rather than the surrounding ligaments and tendons. The joint is examined in flexion and extension to search for any decrease in the range of motion. At the same time, capsular distension or soft-tissue swelling can be palpated.

Antebrachium

The radius is a common site for panosteitis, and it is relatively easy to palpate. Confirmation of the diagnosis requires radiography. Panosteitis may cause a shifting lameness, and the signs may disappear from one area and reappear elsewhere.

Fractures of the styloid process of the ulna or radius may be acute and cause severe lameness. With minimal displacement and a fibrous tissue connection, they can be extremely difficult to diagnose. Radiographs may be helpful, but the fracture may not be visible. The area is carefully palpated, and if pain is produced, radiographs are taken at various angles to demonstrate the fracture.

Carpus

When a dog is lame in the carpus, weight is not put on the main footpad, and the animal tends to ''toe'' as it walks. This is particularly apparent when the animal trots.

Carpal bone injuries are common in racing animals. Hyperextension of the carpus is usually caused by jumping from heights. Lameness from traumatic radiocarpal luxation is extremely acute, and the area does not bear weight. Over time, a plantigrade stance develops and diagnosis is not difficult. Stress radiographs are necessary to differentiate radiocarpal, intercarpal, or carpometacarpal subluxation.

Phalanges

Diagnosis of lameness due to a problem in the toes is not usually difficult because of the localized effect that occurs. Sesamoid bones should be carefully palpated to detect pain. Radiographs are necessary to confirm fragmentation.

Hip Joint

Hip dysplasia is one of the most common causes of hindlimb lameness. Dogs with hip dysplasia often demonstrate a typical gait pattern (Table 118–1). Marked subluxation is occasionally associated with an audible clicking sound as a dog walks, caused by the femoral head snapping in and out of the acetabulum.

Stifle Joint

The stifle joint is a common site of lameness in the hindlimb. The signs caused by this lameness are characteristic. In an attempt not to use the joint, greater use is made of the hip joint in the swing phase to permit the animal to cover the necessary distance.

"Dipping" of the hip results on the sound side. In severe cases, the carriage of the head is also affected, and it too dips when the opposite forelimb is in the contact phase. In milder cases, discomfort in the stifle joint causes the animal to move the limb continually to ease the load. If the lameness is severe, the animal puts only its toe on the ground.

Hock Joint

The tarsal joint is a complicated group of joints collectively known as the *hock*. Diagnosis of lameness in the hock is not difficult in severe cases but may be elusive in subtle conditions such as mild osteochondrosis of the talus.

Lesions of the Spine
Cervical Spine

Lesions high in the cervical spine, such as in the atlanto-occipital area, may produce anesthesia caudal to the lesion or more commonly may

TABLE 118–1. HIP DYSPLASIA GAIT PATTERNS

Upright hindlimb
Stiff hindlimb—reaches forward
Low head carriage
Weight carried on hind toe and not the whole foot
Lateral bending of lumbar spine associated with lateral rotation of the pelvis, which is greater on the side that is more painful
Decreased protraction (swing phase)

produce exquisite pain. This causes the animal to walk with its head extremely depressed and to take very short steps. Great care should be used in examining such a patient because the lesion may be exacerbated and become irreversible.

Lesions farther down the spine, C3–C7, may produce the classic gait of a "wobbler."

Lesions in the Lumbar Spine

Animals with a lesion in the lumbar area have difficulty in rising and show marked shortening of steps. Chronic lumbosacral pain may be due to nerve entrapment. The pain may be intermittent but is usually progressive. Manipulation of the area, particularly dorsal flexion of the lumbosacral junction, can increase the discomfort and may aid in localizing the pain. A condition termed *cauda equina syndrome* may manifest itself by signs that include difficulty in rising, urinary or fecal incontinence, perineal hyperalgesia or analgesia, paresis of the tail, paresthesia, self-mutilation of the tail and perineal area, and a decrease in the lumbosacral spinal reflexes. It is important to distinguish cauda equina syndrome from hip dysplasia; early cases bear some similarity in that the animal is reluctant to rise and to walk upstairs. The two conditions may be differentiated by dorsal flexion of the spine. Unfortunately, radiographs that are positive for hip dysplasia may not rule out involvement of the lumbosacral spine because the diseases may exist concurrently.

CHAPTER 119
Connective Tissues of the Musculoskeletal System
(pages 1587–1595)

Connective tissues serve many functions in the body: They hold it together, organize its compartments, and provide cohesion and internal support. Differing in form and function, the connective tissues, skin, tendons, ligaments, cartilage, bones, teeth, lungs, spleen, capsules and sheaths of muscles, synovium, blood vessels, lungs, and so forth have several common features. All consist of cells, fibers, and nonstructured (amorphous) ground substances; all are derived primarily from mesenchyme; and all show the characteristic presence of banded fibers (collagen) under the light microscope. Variations in the density and arrangement of the collagen fibers relative to the cells that produce them determine the functions of the connective tissues.

Tissues that provide tensile strength (i.e., the ability to withstand stress) contain long, parallel bundles of fibers. The ability of ligaments and tendons to stretch depends on the presence of both collagen and another protein—rubbery, expansible elastin.

In cartilage, the collagen fibrils are spaced farther apart, with a more random orientation to provide mechanical strength and resilience while giving the tissue flexibility. Hyaline cartilage is a semitransparent cartilage found at the bone/joint surface, on the ventral ends of ribs, and in the respiratory system. It is extremely flexible owing to the presence of high-molecular-weight macromolecules known as *proteoglycans*. Elastic cartilage, such as that found in the external ear, has even greater elasticity and opacity than hyaline cartilage. Fibrocartilage, found in the intervertebral discs and in close association with joints, contains denser collagen fibers and proteoglycans similar but not identical to those in hyaline cartilage.

The "synovial system," consisting of articular cartilage, synovial membrane, and synovial fluid, contains various tissue types crucial to the functioning of the joints. The synovial cells (fibroblasts and chondrocytes) within the synovial membrane secrete and synthesize hyaluronic acid, a heteropolymer of N-acetylglucosamine and glucuronic acid. The presence of large (3 mg/ml) quantities of the highly charged hyaluronic acid in the synovial fluid allows it to provide lubrication and nutrition to the joints.

Bones and teeth are mineralized connective tissues that differ from the other connective tissues because they contain calcium phosphate mineral crystals (hydroxyapatite), which are deposited in an oriented fashion on the collagen fibers. The calcium phosphate mineral crystals make the tissue strong and rigid, providing the capacity for locomotion and protection. These crystals also provide a storage site for mineral deposition and are important in controlling mineral ion homeostasis.

Collagen

The major fibrous component synthesized by connective tissue cells is collagen.

At least 13 different types of collagens have been identified. These collagens vary in size, structure, and the ability to form aggregates. However, all contain (to variable extents) three tightly coiled polypeptide chains known as *alpha chains*. The alpha chains are twisted about one another in a triple-helix configuration. Most of the connective tissue collagens form supermolecular aggregates (fibrils and fibers).

The most abundant class of connective tissue collagen is type I. It is found in skin, bones, tendons, and ligaments. Type I collagen consists of two identical alpha chains and one alpha chain of different amino acid composition. Type II collagen is the principal collagen of cartilage, the nucleus pulposus, and vitreous humor.

Elastin

The other fibrous component of the connective tissue matrix is elastin. This rubber-like component of elastic ligaments, blood vessels, skin, and lungs accounts for only a small amount of the matrix in nonextensible tissues and a major proportion of the matrix of deformable tissues. Skeletal ligaments contain less elastin and more collagen than the specialized ligaments. In contrast to the highly oriented, regularly arranged collagen fibrils, elastin generally occurs in a compacted nonstructured (amorphous) form that is rubbery and soft and can be extended to double its length.

Proteoglycans

The high-molecular-weight proteoglycans, with their component acidic glycosaminoglycans, provide resilience and flexibility to the connective tissue matrix. Although proteoglycan structure differs among the connective tissues, all proteoglycans consist of a protein core to which glycosaminoglycans are covalently attached.

Matrix Proteins

Improved methods for isolating and characterizing proteins from the connective tissue matrix have led to the identification of numerous noncollagenous matrix proteins in the connective tissues. These proteins, which include glycoproteins, phosphoproteins, gamma-carboxylated proteins, and proteolipids, are less abundant than collagen but are believed to have important roles in their component tissues.

Glycoproteins, as distinct from proteoglycans, are protein compounds that contain no large repeating sugar units and therefore tend to have a high protein/sugar ratio. Among the less abundant but important connective and related tissue glycoproteins are fibronectin, laminin (basement membranes), osteopontin (bone sialoprotein), and chondronectin (cartilage). Each of these proteins functions *in vitro* to regulate cell adhesion, motility, or alignment.

ANATOMY AND PHYSIOLOGY OF SPECIALIZED CONNECTIVE TISSUES (pp. 1592–1594)

Bone

Bone consists of several functionally distinct regions. At the articulating surfaces is articular cartilage. Surrounding the entire bone is a membranous structure, the periosteum. Lining the area enclosing the cartilage (capsule) of the joints and also lining tendon sheaths, providing nutrition and lubrication to the articular cartilage while serving as a protective barrier, are the synovial membranes. Below the articular cartilage, in the epiphysis, lies the secondary center of ossification, and below that, in growing animals, the physis, or growth plate. Woven lamellar cancellous bone lies below the physis in a metaphysis, and the compact cortical bone surrounds a marrow cavity in the diaphyseal region.

Three principal cell types are found in all bones: osteoblasts, osteoclasts, and osteocytes. The osteoblasts are the bone cells responsible for synthesizing the matrix. Once encased in mineral, these osteocytes do not die but rather communicate via long processes with other mineral-encased cells and with unencased cells. Osteoclasts, the large multinucleated cells with ruffled borders that lie on the surface of the mineralized matrix, are directly responsible for removing the mineral and matrix (bone resorption). In healthy bone, the activities of the osteoclasts and osteoblasts are coupled (via protein factors released from the bone); thus resorption stimulates new bone formation.

The component of the extracellular bone matrix that distinguishes it from other connective tissue matrices and enables it to perform its unique functions is the mineral. The mineral found in bone is an analog of the naturally occurring mineral hydroxyapatite. Bone mineral is in equilibrium with body fluids, and demineralization of bone (resorption) occurs when the intake of minerals (calcium, magnesium, phosphorus) necessary for bone formation is inadequate (as in vitamin D-deficiency rickets) or when loss of mineral ions is excessive (as in hyperparathyroidism). Regulation of the serum concentration of minerals (homeostasis), via control of bone formation and resorption, is principally controlled by three substances: parathyroid hormone, calcitonin, and vitamin D.

Muscle

Fibrous proteins are found intracellularly as well as in the extracellular matrix. Motion of single cells and whole tissues, as well as motion of organelles within the cells, depends on these intracellular proteins, called the *cytoskeletal proteins* because of their location (cytoplasmic) and structure (insoluble and fibrous). The cytoskeletal proteins are those fibrous elements that hold the cell intact, maintain its shape, and provide it with contractible, locomotive, and adhesive properties.

In the muscle cell, bundles of thick filaments, held in place by intermediate filaments, interact with thin filaments (actin), contracting and producing mechanical work. The contractile proteins of the muscle cells produce work in the form of motion, sustenance of weight, balance, propulsion of blood, regulation of temperature, secretion, and excretion.

The Contractile Process (p. 1594)

CHAPTER 120
Fracture Biology and Biomechanics (pages 1595–1603)

Long bones are subjected to physiological and nonphysiological forces. Nonphysiological forces occur in unusual situations such as automobile accidents, gunshot injuries, or falls. They can be transmitted to bone directly and may easily exceed the ultimate strength of bone, giving rise to a fracture. Physiological forces are generated by weightbearing, muscle contraction, and associated physical activity. They are transmitted to the bone through the joint surfaces and muscle contraction. Physiological forces are uniaxial (tension or compression) and can give rise to torsional and bending moments. Physiological forces do not commonly exceed the ultimate strength of bone and are not responsible for bone fractures except in unusual cases.

A bending moment occurs when a force causes an object to bend about an axis, and a torsional moment occurs when a force causes an object to rotate about an axis. A bending or torsional moment is the product of a force times the moment arm (lever arm) over which it acts. The moment arm is equal to the perpendicular distance from the line of action of the force to the point where the moment acts (e.g., when the front foot strikes the ground, a primarily vertical ground reaction force is produced). The perpendicular distance from the line of action of the ground reaction force to the carpal joint is the moment arm. The product of the ground reaction force and the moment arm is the bending moment that causes the foot to bend cranially about the carpal joint. The moment of the ground reaction force acting at the carpal joint is balanced by muscle contraction to maintain equilibrium. Because of relatively short moment arms (lever arms), muscles must exert considerable force to maintain equilibrium.

The sum of the physiological forces is transmitted to the bones via the joint surfaces and causes axial compression, axial tension, bending moments, and torsional moments on the column of bone. The percentage of the joint load transmitted as axial compression or bending is determined by the point and direction of force application at the articular surface relative to the column of bone, the normal curvature of the bone, and limb position. If the force is applied eccentric (off center) to the bony column, both compression and bending occur; a force applied concentric (in line) with the bony column produces compression. Bones loaded more eccentrically (femur, humerus) are subject to greater bending; bones loaded more concentrically carry a greater compressive force. A second factor that determines the amount of bending versus axial compressive force is the normal curvature of the bone. Although the radius and tibia are loaded through a joint surface that is more in line with the longitudinal axis of the bony column and are subject to compressive loading, the normal curvature of these bones results in significant bending loads. In fact, *in vivo* strain analysis has shown that 85 to 89 per cent of the predominant physiological internal stress in most bones is derived from bending.

Torsion arises from the twisting of the body when the foot is firmly planted on the ground. Muscle forces also contribute significantly to torsion because their points of attachment are peripheral to the axis of rotation of the bone.

The four primary physiological forces are (1) axial compression, (2) axial tension, (3) bending, and (4) torsion. Each of these alone or in combination results in a complex pattern of internal stresses and strains within the bone. The normal stresses and strains are associated with tension and compression at a cross-sectional surface, whereas shear stress and strain are directed obliquely or parallel to cross-sectional surfaces of the bone. When a fracture occurs, these internal stresses and strains are present at the fracture line. Internal shear stress and tensile stress damage fragile tissues crossing the fracture gap. Internal stresses and strains can be neutralized with stabilizing devices.

When a significant component of the joint force is transmitted eccentrically to the column of bone, bending occurs. It may result from the joint surface being eccentric to the column of bone (e.g., proximal femur) or from the normal curvature of the bone (e.g., radius). When a structure such as bone undergoes bending, internal tensile stress is produced on the convex surface and internal compressive stress is produced on the concave surface. The surface experiencing tension is referred to as the *tension band surface*, whereas the surface experiencing primary compressive stress is referred to as the *compression surface*. It is important to know the tension band surface of each long bone to resist tension and prevent fracture gap widening. The tension band surface of the femur is the craniolateral surface. It is the craniolateral surface of the tibia, the craniolateral surface of the humerus, the cranial surface of the radius, and the caudal surface of the ulna.

Although it is convenient to categorize these physiological forces and subsequent internal stresses, clinically the bones experience combined axial compression, axial tension, bending, and torsional loading.

After a fracture, the morphological features of repair tissue depend on a number of factors; two of these are the vascular and mechanical environment at the fracture site. When healing of a fracture occurs, the principal components of the normal afferent vascular system (nutrient artery, metaphyseal and periosteal arteries) are enhanced. In addition, the area receives a temporary new blood supply that is entirely distinct from normal. This is termed the *extraosseous blood supply of healing bone* and is derived from the surrounding soft tissues. Gentle reflection of soft tissues during open reduction of a fracture is vital for preservation of early nutrient supply to the pluripotential cells near the fracture site.

Biomechanically, the interfragmentary strain theory proposes that pluripotential cells are responsive to local deformation within the fracture gap. Different tissue cells are able to withstand specified levels of deformation (stretching) beyond which they are unable to survive. Granulation tissue can withstand 100 per cent deformation before failure. Cartilage and fibrous tissue tolerate 10 per cent deformation, and bone tolerates 2 per cent deformation before failure. Interfragmentary deformation is eventually reduced to the point where bone survives and unites the fragment ends. Surgical implants alter the local environment by providing stability to reduce interfragmentary deformation.

Bony union can occur by two different repair mechanisms: (1) direct healing (osteonal reconstruction) and (2) indirect healing (intermediate callus formation). The effectiveness of the implant in providing stability, coupled with the biological environment at the fracture surface, determines whether bony union occurs directly or indirectly.

The method of bone healing is determined by the stability given by the implant and by biological factors. Different implants are able to prevent compression, bending, and rotation to different degrees. For example, intramedullary pins resist bending only. Rotation and compression are not adequately prevented in most cases. When properly applied to a simple fracture, bone plates and screws act with the bone to form a composite that exhibits strength and stiffness resembling normal bone. As the fracture becomes more fragmented, the plate and bone cannot act as a functional composite, markedly reducing the strength and stiffness of the osteosynthesis. External fixators can be assembled to provide strength and stiffness similar to bone plates and screws. In addition, a surgeon has the flexibility to destabilize the osteosynthesis as healing progresses. All implants, when used properly, can result in direct healing (primary or secondary osteonal reconstruction of the cortex).

Some of the biological factors that are important include the age and size of the patient, type and location of the fracture, whether the fracture is stabilized through closed or open reduction, the presence of multiple fractures, high-velocity versus low-velocity injury, and whether the injury is an open or closed fracture. Clinical factors include a patient's and a client's compliance, postoperative limb function desired, available equipment, and experience of the surgeon. The method of fixation is chosen by evaluating the radiograph to determine the areas of tensile and shear deformation, knowledge of the stabilization properties and principles of application for each implant, and consideration of the biological and clinical factors described.

CHAPTER 121

Emergency Management of Fractures (pages 1603–1610)

INITIAL MANAGEMENT (p. 1603)

Traumatic musculoskeletal injury is a common problem in companion animal practice. A rapid but careful initial physical examination should be conducted to assess the patient. Priorities are establishing a patent airway, securing hemostasis, and providing circulatory support. After a patient is stabilized, re-examination, including assessment of the thoracic and abdominal cavities, is completed. Fluid or free air within the thorax, detected by radiography, may require further diagnostics and therapeutic intervention.

Orthopedic injuries have been divided into three groups in an effort to establish priorities for treatment. In the first group are those injuries requiring immediate intervention. These include fractures with the potential for injury to the central nervous system, such as depressed skull fractures and spinal fractures/luxations. Also included in group I are open fractures.

Injuries in group II include luxations, intra-articular fractures, and physeal fractures. Treatment of these injuries may be safely delayed for 1 to 2 days. Definitive treatment of group III injuries, which include closed long-bone shaft fractures, nonarticular pelvic fractures, scapular fractures, and metacarpal/tarsal fractures, may also be delayed.

CLOSED FRACTURES (pp. 1603–1608)

Closed fractures below the elbow or stifle may benefit from temporary external support. Closed fractures of the humerus and femur can be initially treated with cage rest or by use of a spica splint, which immobilizes the shoulder or coxofemoral joint.

OPEN FRACTURES (pp. 1608–1610)

Classification

Open fractures have arbitrarily been divided into three separate grades, based on severity of the injury.

A grade I open fracture typically has a small external wound that may be difficult to identify unless the limb is carefully examined. The break in the skin is caused by the bone penetrating to the outside.

The skin wound in a grade II open fracture results from external trauma. More damage to the soft tissues has occurred than with a grade I fracture. Some low-velocity gunshot injuries could be included in this category.

Grade III is the most severe open fracture. The frequent high degree of comminution of these fractures reflects the severity of the injury to the soft tissues. Examples of grade III open fractures are gunshot injuries from weapons with high muzzle velocities and shearing injuries of the distal extremities.

Pathophysiology

Treatment

Ideally, a sterile bandage is placed over the wound. Because most clients do not have access to bandaging materials, a clean cloth is used to cover the wound. Compression may be used to control hemorrhage.

When the animal arrives at the hospital, a sterile dressing is applied to the wound. Careful assessment of the neurological and vascular status of the limb is extremely important. Because open fractures are contaminated, administration of an antibiotic is appropriate. Gram-positive isolates commonly found are the coagulase-positive *Staphylococcus* spp. and *Streptococcus* spp. Gram-negative organisms are *Escherichia coli, Proteus* spp., *Pasteurella* spp., and *Pseudomonas* spp. Mixed infections also may be found. Intravenous administration of a broad-spectrum antibiotic that achieves therapeutic levels in both bone and soft tissue, such as a cephalosporin, should be considered.

Radiographic evaluation of the fracture includes a minimum of two views, lateral to medial and cranial to caudal, and includes the joints above and below the fracture.

Adequate débridement of the wound is critical in the treatment of open fractures. In an effort to convert a contaminated wound to a clean one, adherence to aseptic technique cannot be overemphasized. Cap, mask, and gloves should be worn and sterile instruments used. After surgical preparation of the limb, copious lavage of the wound is performed. Lavage can be accomplished with a 35-ml syringe and an 18-gauge needle. A satisfactory solution for lavage is sterile isotonic saline either with or without 0.05 per cent chlorhexidine.

Culture and sensitivity testing are performed. A prospective study in man concluded that infection was correlated with the organisms in the wound at the end of débridement, not at the beginning. In light of these findings, culture and sensitivity test results should be obtained when the débridement is finished.

Guidelines for débriding bone are as follows: Small pieces that have no soft-tissue attachment may be removed. If a piece of bone with no soft-tissue attachment is integral to the reconstruction of the fracture, an attempt is made to salvage it. Bone fragments with soft-tissue attachments are left in the fracture site whether or not they are incorporated into the fracture repair.

Fracture Fixation

Definitive stabilization of the fracture is carried out as soon as possible. Stabilization improves blood supply to the tissues, facilitates healing, and promotes resistance to infection. Coaptation devices are rarely used except as temporary support or on stable fractures with easily managed soft-tissue wounds.

Intramedullary pins may be used in grade I and II open fractures if adequate stabilization is achieved. Rigid fixation is provided by bone plates and screws. Their use is indicated in grades I and II. The extensive soft-tissue dissection required for their placement makes plates less attractive as an option for grade III fractures.

In many grade III open fractures, external fixators are ideal. The pins may be placed away from the fracture site and the traumatized soft tissue, preserving blood supply and aiding wound care.

Well-débrided, clean grade I and II fractures are candidates for primary closure. Grade III open fractures are rarely closed primarily. Delayed closure or second intention healing is the method of choice. If large cortical bone defects are present, the use of a delayed cancellous bone auto graft, after the wound is covered with granulation tissue, helps speed union of the fracture.

CHAPTER 122

Methods of Internal Fracture Fixation (pages 1610–1640)

General Principles (pp. 1610–1631)

CHOICE OF FIXATION (pp. 1610–1612)

The method of fracture repair is based on the type and location of the fracture, the size and age of the animal, the number of bones or limbs involved, and concurrent soft-tissue disease. Other factors to consider include the animal's behavior and environment, the owner's cooperation during the convalescent period, and the animal's expected level of performance after bone union. Cost, surgical expertise, and the availability of equipment and technical assistance must be considered. It is better to provide the optimum in fixation or to offer referral to a specialist than to compromise the principles of fracture repair.

Fractures in small or medium-sized animals may be adequately stabilized with intramedullary pins. If one considers other factors, this type of fixation may not be adequate. A small animal that is 12 years of age and housed outdoors without restriction of activity may require the more stable fixation provided by a bone plate. A plate may be indicated when a disease process such as a fracture, dislocation, or even arthritis is present in another limb. The resulting early return to full function of the fractured limb enables the animal to walk sooner and allows the application of an Ehmer sling or similar device to another limb.

The type and location of a fracture may dictate using one implant over another. For instance, it is technically easier to apply a bone plate to a pelvic fracture than to attempt fixation with alternative methods. Conversely, some fractures do not readily lend themselves to bone plate application. Metaphyseal and epiphyseal fractures may not leave enough bone length to allow adequate plate fixation.

A fracture associated with extensive soft-tissue damage may require stabilization with an external skeletal fixator. Application of an external skeletal fixator stabilizes the bone until the soft tissues heal, at which time additional fixation may be undertaken, if necessary.

FRACTURE FORCES (pp. 1612–1614)

For most purposes in clinical orthopedics, it is sufficient to consider four basic forces. These are rotational, bending, and shearing forces and fragment apposition. A fixation device, whether it involves external or internal stabilization, must neutralize inherent forces acting on that particular fracture to prevent motion at the fracture site. If fracture forces are neutralized, soft-tissue structures are preserved, vascular integrity is maintained, and infection is prevented, optimal conditions have been established for fracture healing.

Rotational force is present in all fractures. Rotation is most often a problem in transverse or slightly oblique long-bone fractures that do not interdigitate. Rotation at the fracture site may cause delayed union or nonunion and can result in rotational deformities of the limb distal to the fracture site.

Bending results from eccentric axial loading, the presence of a cortical defect on the compression side, or both. The common tendency is to use inadequate fixation where *bending forces* predominate. A common error in fracture fixation is application of an external coaptation device as secondary support for a femoral or humeral fracture. These devices seldom provide additional support for the implants and may be detrimental because the top of a cast or the bar of a Schroeder-Thomas splint can act as a fulcrum to enhance bending forces.

Shearing force is most commonly associated with an oblique fracture. Shearing force causes the two bone ends to slide relative to each other in a direction parallel to their plane of contact. Shearing forces can have devastating effects on a fracture; every effort is made to neutralize the impact of shear on the fracture site (Table 122–1).

The ability of a single intramedullary pin to counteract horizontal or angular shearing force depends on the size of the pin in relation to the medullary cavity. If the pin is smaller than the medullary cavity, shearing may occur, resulting in horizontal movement or over-riding of fracture segments. Because most bones are not perfect cylinders, the pin rarely fills the medullary cavity of both fracture segments. Either supplemental fixation or an alternative means of repair is required to neutralize the shearing forces.

The ability of an intramedullary pin to resist bending force is directly proportional to its diameter as well as to the ratio of the pin diameter to the medullary diameter. It may be necessary to add supplemental fixation such as an external fixation device to resist the bending forces. Rotation is not effectively counteracted by a single intramedullary pin, regardless of its size. Rotational forces may be counteracted

TABLE 122–1. ABILITY OF VARIOUS IMPLANTS TO NEUTRALIZE
FRACTURE FORCES

Implant	Rotational Force	Bending Force	Shearing Force	Fragment Apposition
Single intramedullary pin	−	+	−	−
Multiple intramedullary pins	+	+	−	−
Bone plate	+	+	+	+
External fixator	+	+	+	−
Cerclage wire	(+)	(+)	(+)	+
Lag screw	(+)	(+)	(+)	+

+, neutralization achieved; −, neutralization not achieved; (+), neutralization achieved but devices must be protected by another implant to minimize failure.

by interlocking of fragments and by compression caused by internal and external loading forces.

Multiple pins provide additional fixation in the cancellous bone of the distal end of the bone and emerge from separate points in the proximal end of the bone. The use of multiple intramedullary pins is called *stack pinning.*

Properly applied, bone plates provide the most stable form of fracture fixation. They neutralize rotational, shearing, and bending forces and maintain apposition of multiple fragments.

Lag screws and cerclage wire are effective in achieving fragment apposition, but their ability to maintain reduction under clinical loading conditions is poor. Their primary function is to maintain fragment apposition to facilitate application of the primary implant.

Wire is effective in neutralizing the tension or distracting force that occurs at an apophysis such as the tibial tubercle, olecranon process, or trochanter major. A tension band device consisting of two parallel pins and a figure-eight wire is used to repair fractures or osteotomies of these apophyses.

SURGICAL CONSIDERATIONS (pp. 1614–1615)

THEORY AND TECHNIQUE OF INTRAMEDULLARY PINNING (pp. 1615–1623)

Equipment

Round Steinmann pins are available in various sizes. The most commonly used pins are 9 and 12 inches in length and 1/16 to 1/4 inch in diameter. Smaller pins, called Kirschner wires, are available in diameters of 0.028, 0.035, 0.045, and 0.062 inch. Intramedullary pins are available with chisel, trocar, and threaded trocar points. Nonthreaded trocar points are the most commonly used for intramedullary pinning because of their ability to penetrate cortical bone. Threaded trocar-point intramedullary pins are more difficult to insert and offer no advantage over nonthreaded points.

A pin chuck is required to insert the pins into the bone, and a pin cutter is necessary to cut them to the proper length. Auxiliary fixation devices such as cerclage wire and external fixator components should be available.

Principles of Intramedullary Pinning

Pins can be placed by the closed or open technique. The closed method avoids surgical exposure and is applicable to stable fractures of palpable long bones. An open approach may expedite fracture repair and cause less soft-tissue damage.

Angular stability, or resistance to bending, is achieved by stable anchorage of the pin in the cortical or cancellous bone of the proximal and distal ends of the bone. Because of the natural curvature of most long bones and variations in cross-sectional diameter, the pin rarely fills the medullary canal. Therefore, bending and horizontal shearing forces may cause motion at the fracture site. Filling the medullary canal at the fracture site may be undesirable, because the pin interferes with medullary blood supply. It also complicates application of a secondary fixation device, such as an external fixator. A good compromise is to select a pin diameter that occupies approximately 60 to 70 per cent of the medullary cavity.

Intramedullary pinning techniques are restricted to small and medium-sized animals. The large and giant breeds have such a large medullary cavity that standard round pins are unable to maintain adequate alignment and stability. The size and weight of these large animals generate forces that cannot be counteracted by Steinmann pins; therefore, plate and screw fixation is generally required.

Technique of Application

After exposure, the pin may be inserted into the bone via either a normograde or retrograde technique. With the normograde technique, the pin is started into the bone from an external landmark and advanced to the fracture site. With the retrograde method, the pin is started from the fracture site and advanced up the marrow cavity through the cortex and out of the skin.

Once the pin has been placed in the proximal fragment, the bone is anatomically reduced with the aid of bone forceps and held in reduction while an assistant seats the pin into the distal fracture segment. If the pin is seated without anatomical reduction, adjustments in alignment may be difficult, because the pin may have a different axial alignment in each of the two fracture segments. A comminuted fracture is reconstructed first to a two-piece fracture; then the two remaining pieces are reduced.

Once the pin is seated in the distal fracture segment, the reconstructed bone is stressed to evaluate stability. Adjacent joints are also flexed and extended to determine if the pin is interfering with normal joint motion. If any malalignment or instability is present, the fragments are correctly aligned and additional fixation applied. Two common techniques are to add additional intramedullary pins or a two- or four-pin unilateral external fixator.

Surgical Anatomy and Landmarks for Pin Placement

Femur

The femoral shaft is exposed from a lateral approach centered over the fracture site. Adductor muscle attachment to any major fragments is left intact to promote rapid incorporation of these fragments.

Pin insertion in the femur is from the proximal end. The pin is inserted through the skin and underlying soft tissues, sliding along the medial surface of the trochanter major into the trochanteric fossa. At this point, the pin is inserted into the medullary cavity and down to the fracture site. During retrograde pin insertion, the hip is held in slight extension and the leg is adducted to minimize soft-tissue penetration and avoid the sciatic nerve as the pin emerges from the bone proximally.

Because of the cranial bowing of the canine femur, the intramedullary pin engages the cranial cortex near the patella. If an attempt is made to seat the pin the remaining distance, the pin may inadvertently enter the stifle joint. To avoid this, the distal fracture segment is angled slightly cranial to direct the pin caudally in the distal segment. The caudal angulation allows the pin to be seated into the cancellous bone of the femoral condyles.

If the animal suddenly stops using the limb and shows signs of unusual pain or a proprioceptive deficit, entrapment of the sciatic nerve is suspected. If exploration of the pin is undertaken for nerve impingement, the leg is prepared for surgery in a normal walking position. A hanging leg preparation may result in additional nerve damage.

Tibia

The entire shaft of the tibia can be exposed from a medial approach. The incision is centered over the fracture site and extended proximally and distally according to the extent of the fracture. The pin must never be passed retrograde from the fracture site because it will emerge in the stifle joint, resulting in extensive destruction of articular cartilage, cruciate ligaments, and menisci, as well as permanent disability. The proper point of pin insertion is on the medial side of the tibial tubercle, halfway between the attachment of the patellar tendon and the cranial edge of the medial femoral condyle. Because of the curvature of the tibia, it is necessary for the pin to curve as it passes down the medullary canal. Too large a pin may engage the cortex and leave the bone rather than bending and following the medullary cavity. If a large pin is required, it is helpful to insert a smaller pin first, then remove it and pass the larger pin through the established guide hole.

The base of the medial malleolus is the landmark for distal pin placement. Once the pin is properly seated, the proximal end is cut off short enough so that its end does not damage the articular cartilage of the femoral condyles during extension of the joint. One successful method is to seat the pin to the desired point and then retract it 5 to 7 mm and cut it off close to the tibia. At this time, the distal aspect of the limb is held firmly to provide counterpressure while the pin is driven the remaining 5 to 7 mm with a mallet and center punch device.

Humerus

Careful consideration must be given to selecting the appropriate surgical approach for a fracture of the humerus. The proximal aspect of the shaft is approached through a lateral skin incision. The distal portion of the shaft can be approached either medially or laterally. If it is necessary to extensively reconstruct the condylar region of the humerus, an osteotomy of the olecranon process is performed to expose the intercondylar region of the joint and the caudal surface of the distal aspect of the humerus.

Pins can be inserted into the humerus by either the normograde or the retrograde method. The landmark for normograde insertion is the cranial crest of the proximal aspect of the greater tubercle. If the retrograde method is chosen, care must be taken to avoid entering the shoulder joint. The pin is started at the medial cortex of the proximal fracture segment and aimed laterally as it passes up the medullary cavity. This angle directs the pin toward the greater tubercle and also positions it near the medial cortex at the fracture site. The medial location is advantageous, because the pin must be directed down into the medial aspect of the distal humeral condyle to avoid the elbow joint and gain the best anchorage. The pin is directed medially because the medial portion of the condyle is larger and in direct axial alignment with the shaft.

A unilateral external fixator can be applied to the lateral aspect of the humerus for secondary fixation. In fractures of the distal portion of the humerus, it is often desirable to insert a cross pin from the lateral epicondyle proximally into the medial cortex of the shaft for additional fixation.

Radius and Ulna

Because of the anatomical configuration of the radius, it is impossible to pass an intramedullary pin retrograde from the fracture site without the pin entering the adjacent joints. A pin can be inserted into the radius with a normograde technique. Simple fractures of the radius and ulna in small and medium-sized dogs are frequently managed with external casts. Fractures of the distal portion of the radius and ulna in toy breeds are prone to nonunion. Unilateral external fixators are recommended in all but very young animals. If plate fixation is used in these toy breeds, a plate is chosen that is not too stiff. The veterinary cuttable plate* is useful for distal radius fractures in toy breeds. If the plate does not allow loading of the bone, nonunion may result. Oblique and comminuted fractures of the radius in large dogs are best stabilized with bone plates or unilateral or bilateral external fixators rather than with intramedullary pins.

Advantages and Disadvantages of Intramedullary Pinning

Pins are less costly to purchase, are less time-consuming to use, require less exposure, and are easier to implant and remove than bone plates. These advantages must be considered along with the disadvantages of less stable fixation, slower return to function, secondary bone union, and more involved aftercare. These are generalizations that do not apply to all individuals or situations. With experience, bone plate application may be as fast as pin fixation, even with a simple fracture. After bone plate fixation, return to function is almost immediate, few follow-up examinations are required, and the chance of a successful outcome is greater.

Postoperative Management

THEORY AND TECHNIQUE OF RUSH PINNING
(pp. 1623–1624)

THEORY AND TECHNIQUE OF BONE PLATING
(pp. 1624–1631)

Specialized training and equipment are required to apply bone plates properly. A complete set of instruments, a full range of implants, and knowledge of their use are necessary before fracture repair is attempted. A plate may be used on any fracture when there is enough bone length on each side of the fracture site to adequately attach the plate.

Interfragmentary Compression

Compression of fractures increases fracture stability through frictional impact loading and narrowing the gap between fragments, providing optimum conditions for direct bone union. Fracture compression can

---

*Synthes USA, Paoli, PA.

be achieved through interfragmentary compression with lag screws or axial compression with a plate.

Cancellous screws have relatively thin core diameters and wide threads. The cancellous screw is used in soft cancellous bone of the metaphysis and epiphysis. To achieve interfragmentary compression with a cancellous screw, it is important that only the smooth shank be within the near fragment and that the entire threaded portion be within the far fragment. If threads are present on both sides of the fracture, the threads maintain the fracture gap and compression cannot occur. Only the first few millimeters of the hole are tapped to facilitate starting the screw. As the screw is advanced into the cancellous bone, the trabeculae are tightly compressed, resulting in greater holding power.

To achieve evenly distributed interfragmentary compression, the screw is centered in the middle of both fragments. If the screws are placed eccentrically, they produce shear instead of pure compression, resulting in loss of reduction. To achieve interfragmentary compression of a butterfly fragment, the screw is inserted to bisect the angle subtended between a line perpendicular to the long axis of the bone and one perpendicular to the fracture plane. The primary function of a lag screw is to provide fragment apposition through interfragmentary compression. The resulting fracture alignment and stability must be protected against the forces acting on the fracture with a bone plate. Such a plate is called a *neutralization plate.*

Principles of Bone Plate Application

There are three types of plates: straight, special, and angled. Straight plates are used for the diaphysis, special plates for the epiphysis and metaphysis, and angled plates for the proximal and distal regions of the femur. In the AO system, plates are available in 2.0-mm, 2.7-mm, 3.5-mm, and 4.5-mm sizes, denoting the screw size used with each plate. The 3.5-mm and 4.5-mm plates are available in narrow and broad widths.

The dynamic compression plate is an improvement over the original round-hole plate. The special geometry of its oval screw holes has increased the potential uses of the plate. The dynamic compression plate does not require a tension device for axial compression and can be used to compress fractures without additional surgical exposure.

A plate's ability to provide rigid fixation is directly proportional to its distance from the fulcrum of the bending moment. At least six cortices should be firmly engaged by screws on either side of the fracture. Plates are contoured to the original shape and curvature of the particular bone. They must be bent and twisted to fit the bone properly, requiring a bending press or bending irons.

A plate can serve various functions, depending on the manner in which it is used. It may act as a tension band plate if it is placed on the tension side of a weightbearing bone such as the lateral femur. It may act as a neutralization plate if it is used to protect a comminuted area that has been reconstructed with lag screws. It may also function as a buttress plate if it is used to bridge a diaphyseal defect. With a tension band, tensile forces are counteracted and converted into compressive forces. If a plate is applied to the lateral side of the femur and a portion of the medial cortex is absent, the requirements of the tension band plate have not been met because the bone cannot absorb compression.

The tension band side of weightbearing bones may change, depending on the phase of stride. The tension band side of a fractured bone (e.g., humerus) may vary, depending on the location of the fracture within the bone. These factors, as well as the difficulty of the surgical approach, are considered when deciding where the plate is to be applied to the bone. Plates are usually applied to the medial aspect of the tibia, because the lateral approach is more difficult. The femur is usually plated on the lateral side rather than on the craniolateral aspect so that the plate will not interfere with gliding of the quadriceps muscle. The humerus may be plated caudally, medially, cranially, or laterally, depending on the fracture location and the surgeon's preference. The radius is usually plated cranially, and the proximal aspect of the ulna may be plated caudally, laterally, or medially.

Neutralization plates are used to stabilize comminuted fractures in which the butterfly fragments have been reconstructed with lag screws. First, the comminuted fracture is reduced and fixed with lag screws, and then a carefully contoured plate is applied to the two main fragments. When a plate is applied as a neutralization plate, it must be prebent to prevent gaps from forming in the cortices opposite the plate.

In animals, a buttress plate is primarily used to bridge a diaphyseal defect filled with cancellous bone graft while the graft is being incorporated. Its function is to prevent the fracture from collapsing until the diaphyseal defect can be filled with new bone.

Postoperative Treatment

Achieving stable internal fixation is only one aspect of fracture management. The postoperative and convalescent care is important to allow healing of the fracture before failure of the implant and to promote early function of the injured limb. After stable fracture fixation with a bone plate, the affected limb can be placed in a light support wrap, which helps prevent postoperative swelling and reduce any swelling present before the fracture repair. The animal is encouraged to use the limb as soon as possible to maintain muscle tone and gliding function of muscles and tendons and to prevent fibrous adhesions from forming, thus preventing fracture disease.

Stress Protection and Implant Removal

Plate removal is advised after bone union, not only because of possible corrosion but also because bone under a plate never becomes physiologically or biomechanically normal. Cortical osteopenia occurs in the bone directly underneath the plate. The explanation for the osteopenia appears related to interference with periosteal blood flow under the plate. Also, the rigid plate prevents the bone from responding to normal physiological stimuli because of the difference in the modulus of elasticity between the bone and the implant. If a plate is too stiff, thinning of the underlying cortices may result. Because this response, known as *stress protection*, is partially the result of improper implant selection, it is important not to "overplate" a fracture.

There are some exceptions to the rule of implant removal. Plates are usually not removed from healed pelvic fractures, because stress protection of this bone seldom occurs. Plates are seldom removed from humeral fractures if there is no evidence of stress protection. The approach is difficult, and the likelihood of damaging major nerves is increased because they are more difficult to identify in the scar tissue that forms after fracture repair. Single screws in the metaphysis or epiphysis need not be removed. Plates are often not removed from old animals.

Long bones must be protected from excessive stress after implant removal. An animal's activity must be restricted for 8 to 12 weeks after plate removal to prevent refracture of the bone.

Cerclage Wiring and Tension Band Fixation (pp. 1631–1640)

Virtually every small animal general practice equipped to perform basic internal fixation of fresh fractures should have the minimal equipment and implants needed to apply the basic forms of wire fixation—namely full-cerclage, hemicerclage, and tension band fixation.

MATERIALS (pp. 1632–1633)

INSTRUMENTS FOR WIRE APPLICATION (pp. 1633–1634)

INFLUENCE OF WIRE IMPLANTS ON BONE HEALING (pp. 1634–1635)

After fracture, loss of the medullary blood vessels results in a transient shift in blood supply to the cortex from a medullary- to extraosseus-derived, centripetal blood flow to the healing callus. With adequate stabilization, rapid restoration of the medullary vessels occurs within the first few weeks, and a centrifugal blood flow pattern to the cortex is re-established. At this point, the dominant blood supply to the endosteal, intercortical uniting, and periosteal callus is once again derived from the medullary arteries. Tight application of small-diameter wire implants to the periosteal surface of the cortex does not impair or alter this pattern of blood supply to the healing fracture.

Wide bands applied tightly to the cortex (e.g., Parham-Martin bands) are reputed to interfere with the extraosseus arterial blood supply to the cortex and venous drainage from the periosteal surface and thus result in detrimental cortical avascularity. Most investigators discourage the use of these bands in fracture repair.

GENERAL INDICATIONS (p.1635)

In general, wire is best able to maintain fragment apposition in long oblique fracture planes, thus reducing shear and rotational forces. Additional stabilization in the form of intramedullary pins, bone plates, or external skeletal fixation is necessary to decrease the bending forces acting on the wire implant.

FULL-CERCLAGE WIRES (pp. 1635–1638)

Indications

Full cerclage implies the use of wire loops that completely encircle the diaphysis of the bone. They are best suited for uniform, cylindrical long bones such as the femur, tibia, and humerus, where they are commonly used in combination with intramedullary pins. Full-cerclage wires are often used around long oblique and spiral fractures of the diaphysis, where they serve to counteract shear, rotational, and angular forces and provide compression across the fracture line.

Full-cerclage wire may be used around longitudinal undisplaced fissure fractures in the main fracture segments before attempting reduction or application of intramedullary devices to prevent further distraction or propagation of these fissures into complete fractures.

Principles of Application

Wires must be applied tightly and directly against the periosteum. In areas of muscular or fascial attachments, a wire passer may be used to place the wire directly against the bone with minimal soft-tissue dissection while avoiding entrapment of tissues beneath the wire.

Orthopedic wire in sizes 0.64 and 0.8 mm (22 and 20 gauge) is generally used for fractures in cats and small dogs. Fractures in medium-sized and larger dogs are usually repaired using 0.8-mm (20-gauge) and 1.0- to 1.25-mm (18- to 16-gauge) diameter wire, respectively.

Wire cerclage is placed perpendicular to the long axis of the bone. If placed obliquely to the bone shaft, the previously tight wire may shift to a position perpendicular to the bone's long axis, resulting in a loose wire.

In general, a minimum of two cerclage wires is used for repair of oblique or spiral fractures. If a single wire is used, it may serve as a fulcrum for motion of the fracture segments, with subsequent loss of fixation or delayed union. Full-cerclage fixation is only considered for oblique fractures whose length is at least two times the diameter of the bone shaft. Wire removal after uncomplicated fracture healing is not performed.

INTERFRAGMENTARY WIRES (pp. 1638–1639)

Cerclage wire placed through holes in the cortex, partially around the bone shaft, and across a fracture line is referred to as an *interfragmentary wire*. These wires may be placed in a number of configurations including figure-eight, horizontal mattress, or simple interrupted patterns across transverse fractures of the diaphysis to neutralize rotational forces that are not controlled by intramedullary devices. Interfragmentary wiring, or hemicerclage, is also commonly used as a method of reduction and fixation of fractures of the scapula, mandible, maxilla, and occasionally the pelvis. The wire provides reduction and compression across the fracture site. Interfragmentary wires are commonly used in combination with other implants such as bone plates, screws, or intramedullary pins.

TENSION BAND WIRES (pp. 1639–1640)

The engineering principle of the tension band may be used in the repair of certain fractures and osteotomies to convert tensile and distractive forces into compressive forces across the fracture line. The principles of the tension band wire can be applied to any fracture or osteotomy in which the pull of muscles, tendons, or ligaments results in distraction of a bone fragment away from the parent bone. When the tension band wire is applied to the tension surface of the fracture, it exerts a tensile force equal in magnitude and 180° opposite to the distracting force created by the muscle, tendon, or ligament. The force vector generated by these two opposing forces results in compression across the fracture.

Tension band repair is indicated for the following fractures and osteotomies: greater trochanter of the femur, tibial tuberosity, medial and lateral malleoli of the tibia/fibula, tuber calcis, tuber ischii, supraglenoid tubercle, scapular acromion, greater tubercle of the humerus, olecranon, patella, and various avulsions or osteotomies of collateral ligaments.

Principles of Application

COMPLICATIONS (p. 1640)

Inappropriate choice of fracture for cerclage application, too few cerclage wires, undersized wires, loosely applied wires, and inadequate ancillary fixation may contribute to fixation failure and nonunion. Failure should not be blamed on the inadequacies of the wire implants but instead on the poor judgment of the surgeon.

CHAPTER 123

External Skeletal Fixation
(pages 1641–1661)

General Principles (pp. 1641–1656)

External skeletal fixation is a means of stabilizing fractures or joints using percutaneous fixation pins that penetrate the bone cortices internally and are connected together externally to form an external frame. It is particularly useful in those open or highly comminuted fractures with poor circulation that require prolonged fixation.

FIXATOR NOMENCLATURE AND CHARACTERISTICS
(pp. 1641–1644)

Nomenclature of the external fixation device is based on components used and their geometric arrangement.

Simple Fixators

The simplest fixators consist of relatively rigid fixation pins attached to longitudinal connecting bars or frames. Fixation pins that pass through one side of the limb and both bone cortices are called *half pins*. They can be connected together to form a type I (half-pin) splint. Type I configurations can be used on the humerus or femur to avoid interfering with the body wall. They can also be positioned to avoid soft-tissue injuries on the lower limbs. This type I single connecting bar configuration provides adequate stability for treating most relatively stable simple fractures in small animals. For large animals or less stable fractures, a second connecting bar can be added to the same fixation pins, creating a double connecting bar configuration that nearly doubles the splint's resistance to compressive forces. Two single connecting bar splints can be applied parallel to and at 60° to 90° of axial rotation to each other. The ends of the connecting bars are joined to form a triangular cross section. The resulting biplanar type I configuration is more resistant to craniocaudal bending forces than even full-pin uniplanar splints. It can be applied to very proximal or distal fractures because its biplanar design allows an adequate number of fixation pins to obtain good stability.

Fixation pins that pass through both sides of the limb and the bone are called *full pins*. The pins can be connected together to form a type II (full-pin) splint. Type II configurations are very resistant to compressive forces. They can be used on relatively unstable fractures. To avoid interference with the body wall, they are limited to use below the elbow or the stifle.

A type I and a type II splint can be combined to form a type III (trilateral) frame. Type III configurations are the most rigid of currently used configurations and are roughly ten times more resistant to axial compression than type I splints. Consequently, they are used for highly unstable or infected fractures, nonunions, and arthrodesis when prolonged rigid fixation is needed.

Circular Fixation

Circular (ring) fixators use small-diameter flexible Kirschner wires instead of rigid fixation pins. These wires are driven through the bone fragments at perpendicular angles and attached under tension to rigid rings. The rings are then connected together with three adjustable longitudinal rods. In addition to fracture fixation, they have great application potential for limb lengthening and deformity correction.

EXTERNAL FIXATION DEVICES AND EQUIPMENT
(pp. 1645)

The most common external skeletal fixation device is manufactured by Kirschner Medical Company. Three sizes are useful for small animal application. The small apparatus is appropriate for use on cats, dogs up to approximately 8 to 10 kg, some exotic pets, and raptors. The medium apparatus is the most commonly used and is appropriate for most dogs. The large apparatus has been redesigned based on the human tibial frame. It is useful on large dogs and other larger animals. We prefer to use a low-speed power drill for pin insertion. A variable-speed 3/8-inch electric drill with a cord works well but requires gas sterilization. Extended chucks and drill shrouds that can be autoclaved are available for rechargeable drills and can be obtained at moderate cost. A nut wrench (both open ended and spin tite are useful) and pin cutter are needed for application of a Kirschner apparatus.

Another form of external fixation that was originally described for use in treating human mandibular fractures and is being increasingly used for veterinary patients replaces the connecting bar and clamps with a column of methyl methacrylate. This is commonly known as an *acrylic-pin splint*. The strength and stiffness of these splints directly depend on the diameter of the acrylic column.

PRINCIPLES OF APPLICATION (pp. 1645–1647)

One of the most important advantages of external skeletal fixation is that it can be applied with little additional damage to vascularity and the healing process. Closed reduction of the fracture minimizes such damage. Closed reduction may not provide adequate fracture reduction or alignment, particularly with complex fractures or fractures located proximal to the elbow or stifle joint. Delayed union, nonunion, or malunion can result. I prefer a limited open approach for better fracture alignment and reduction. A limited open approach also allows placement of autogenous cancellous bone graft into fracture defects.

External fixation is only as effective as the pin contact with bone. Because premature loosening of fixation pins is the most common cause of postoperative problems and even fixation failure, attention to pin design and application is essential. Both clinically and experimentally, threaded pins offer a firm grip on bone and increase stiffness of the fixator. Threaded pins used in veterinary medicine are manufactured by cutting threads into the shaft, resulting in a decreased core diameter. Consequently, these pins have a tendency to break or bend at the junction of the threaded and nonthreaded shaft. A new half-pin design (sold by Kirschner as the Ellis pin), which is threaded only far enough to engage the far cortex, offers five to seven times the resistance to pullout of nonthreaded pins while maintaining all of their resistance to bending and is about twice the cost of nonthreaded pins. Alternatively, pins with enhanced threads "raised" over a constant shaft diameter (Turner half pins and Bonnell full pins) have excellent pullout resistance and bending strength. They are expensive (at least five times the cost of nonthreaded pins owing to the complicated manufacturing process) and often require predrilling a pilot hole. Consequently, I often use one of these raised-thread pins in each fragment, with the balance nonthreaded or Ellis pins to reduce costs.

Before pins are placed, the fracture is approximately reduced so excessive skin tension does not develop against the pins when final reduction is achieved. When pins are inserted, they are placed through small separate skin incisions. When possible, the fixation pins should not penetrate large muscle masses and areas of extensive soft-tissue motion because this is a common cause of poor postoperative limb use and serum drainage from the pin tract. Even when applying a half-pin splint, the pins are driven so the tip completely penetrates the far cortex.

If nonthreaded pins are used, they are placed at a divergent angle to each other to maintain a mechanical grip on bone. An angle of 30° to 40° between the outermost pins placed in each fragment offers the best compromise between pin strength and bone grip.

A minimum of three and preferably four pins on each side of a fracture is preferable. These pins are best spread over the length of the fractured bone to distribute the disruptive forces and maintain maximum fixator strength.

GENERAL PROCEDURE FOR FIXATOR APPLICATION
(pp. 1647–1650)

TECHNIQUE FOR ACRYLIC-PIN SPLINT APPLICATION
(pp. 1650–1651)

ORIENTATION OF EXTERNAL FIXATORS ON SPECIFIC LONG BONES (p. 1651)

INDICATIONS FOR CLINICAL USE OF EXTERNAL FIXATION (pp. 1651–1654)

Adjuncts to Other Internal Fixation

External skeletal fixation can be effective in controlling axial rotation and, to some degree, axial collapse of the fracture site when used with intramedullary pins. This supplementary fixation can usually be removed in 3 to 5 weeks, when the callus becomes sufficiently organized to control rotation.

Comminuted Fractures

Severely comminuted fractures may be treated with external fixation when more exacting reconstruction is impossible. External fixation requires minimal bone for fixation and can span large defects. A closed reduction or limited open reduction with massive cancellous bone autograft is necessary. Overall joint alignment but not necessarily perfect fracture reduction is sought. A relatively rigid configuration is initially applied to neutralize disruptive forces. Dynamization after early fracture healing has occurred (6 to 10 weeks) is considered to enhance callus hypertrophy and remodeling.

Open, Gunshot, and Infected Fractures

External fixation has the advantage of not invading the fracture site and spreading contamination or infection. External fixation is particularly useful for stabilizing severe open-wound fractures because it supports the fracture and soft-tissue vascularity while preserving access to the traumatized area for continued treatment. Gunshot fractures often combine the problems of severe comminution and bone loss with significant contamination and severe soft-tissue vascular damage. Moderate débridement followed by rigid external fixation, cancellous bone autografting, and packing the wound open is indicated.

Mandibular Fractures

External fixation has the advantage of being able to avoid the placement of implants in open wounds and infected alveolar sockets. An acrylic-pin splint works well, particularly for bilateral mandibular fractures.

Nonunions

Treatment requires open reduction, removal of unstable hardware, decortication of avascular bone, opening of the medullary canal, and packing with cancellous bone graft to stimulate vascular proliferation and callus production. External fixation can be used to provide necessary stabilization while allowing the bone-stimulating stress of weightbearing.

Transarticular Stabilization

External fixation is ideal for cases of ligamentous rupture associated with adjacent soft-tissue injury. The ligament may be repaired or replaced with a prosthesis and protected by the external fixator while treatment of the open wound continues.

Transarticular external fixation may be used to help protect articular or periarticular fractures from weightbearing forces. Because of their metaphyseal location, such fractures heal quickly, so the transarticular portion of the fixator can usually be removed after 4 to 8 weeks. External fixation may also be used for arthrodesis of certain joints. It is especially useful in cases with severe soft-tissue damage or infection, when the use of internal fixation would be less desirable.

Growth Deformities

External fixation is a very effective means of treating growth deformities, particularly of the radius and ulna. A distraction splint can be used in the dynamic treatment of a progressive growth deformity. The circular fixators (Ilizarov) have potential here.

POSTOPERATIVE MANAGEMENT OF EXTERNAL FIXATION (pp. 1654–1655)

POTENTIAL COMPLICATIONS AND THEIR MANAGEMENT (p. 1655)

The most common complication of fracture repair with external skeletal fixation is drainage around the fixation pins. This is often caused by excessive skin and soft-tissue movement or tension against the pins. Careful placement of the pins through nondisplaced soft tissue and avoiding large muscle masses minimize this problem.

Loosening of the fixation pin at the pin–bone interface commonly results in drainage and infection of the pin tract. Once a pin becomes loose, the only effective treatment is removal. The drainage usually resolves rapidly. Aside from the nuisance of drainage, loosening of pins may decrease leg use. If too many pins loosen too quickly, stability may be lost and nonunion develops. The use of three or four threaded pins per fragment prevents most pin loosening and subsequent drainage or infection.

The Ilizarov External Ring Fixator: Principles, Techniques, and Uses
(pp. 1656–1661)

CHAPTER 124
External Coaptation (pages 1661–1676)

PRINCIPLES OF AN ORTHOPEDIC BANDAGE (p. 1661)

A well-padded bandage is almost always comfortable to the animal wearing it and provides sufficient support for stabilization of many orthopedic conditions during healing. If a fracture is present, too much padding within a splint or cast may allow movement of bone fragments at a fracture site and be detrimental to healing. Too little padding in a splint or cast may also cause complications. If a rigid cast with minimal padding is applied to a heavily traumatized limb and soft-tissue inflammation is not properly anticipated, poor vascular supply may develop and lead to pressure ulceration of the skin and underlying structures.

The four primary functions of a bandage are protection, absorption of draining material, compression of soft tissue, and stabilization. Protection of the soft tissue is necessary to prevent external contamination with bacteria if an open wound is present. Absorptive qualities of a bandage limit accumulation of exudates and decrease wound infection. Compression of soft tissue by the bandage further helps to limit the development of exudates within "dead space" and reduces fluid accumulations (hematoma, seroma, edema) that may affect healing.

PRINCIPLES OF EXTERNAL COAPTATION (pp. 1661–1662)

Internal fixation of a fracture may best be described as "bone splinting." External coaptation is thought of as "limb splinting." An external splint depends on compressive or tensile properties of soft tissue in the affected limb to augment stability at a fracture site, whereas internal fixation depends less on soft tissue to provide stability.

Fracture Forces

Different methods of external coaptation vary in their ability to counteract fracture forces and stabilize an injury. Bending and rotational forces are adequately neutralized in most fractures by a cast, as long as the joints above and below the injury are immobilized. Compressive or shear forces are difficult to neutralize with a cast. Distraction forces at a fracture site, such as those in olecranon fractures or fractures of the greater trochanter of the femur, are caused by muscle tension and are poorly neutralized by external coaptation.

GUIDELINES FOR COAPTATION (pp. 1662–1663)

Basic Guidelines

Fracture Reduction

Minimally displaced stable fractures are best suited to healing by external coaptation. Reduction of fracture fragments does not improve after a cast or splint has been applied and so must be achieved before application. Further loss of reduction may develop after anesthesia recovery when the animal is awake and bearing weight. Radiography must be used to ensure that fracture reduction remains adequate for healing. If sufficient fracture reduction cannot be maintained by closed methods, surgical intervention for reduction and fixation must be considered. Cortical positioning of fracture ends should have at least 50 per cent contact to expect fracture healing.

Fracture Alignment

Fracture fragments are positioned so that the approximate anatomical relationship of the joint above and below the injury is maintained. Failure to align bone fragments with respect to the joints of the limb may result in rotational or angular malunion severe enough to cause functional gait abnormality and lameness from secondary degenerative joint disease.

Standing Position

Splints, bandages, and casts are applied so that the limb is maintained in a neutral standing position. Stiffness of joints commonly develops secondary to trauma, surgery, and immobilization of a limb. If a joint has been positioned in a standing position for coaptation, the animal will bear weight on the limb while the splint is in place and after splint removal.

Joint Above and Below

A basic principle in external coaptation is that the joints above and below a fracture must be immobilized. Consequently conventional splints and casts are adequate for fractures below the elbow or stifle but not above. Use of a conventional cast or splint as treatment for a femoral or humeral fracture is contraindicated.

BANDAGES, SPLINTS, SLINGS, AND CASTS
(pp. 1664–1676)

Robert Jones Bandage

The bulk and mild compression of a Robert Jones bandage provide support and reduce swelling. Tissue heals with less tension at sutured margins, and the animal's comfort is usually dramatically improved. Well padded with bulk cotton and compressed with successive layers of elastic gauze and tape, a Robert Jones bandage provides excellent temporary support for an injured extremity before or after surgical intervention. A Robert Jones bandage extends from the toes to mid-humerus or femur and so may be used to provide temporary support of fractures or dislocations at or below the elbow and stifle joints. Adequate immobilization of a fracture is achieved to prevent worsening of fracture displacement and further injury to the soft tissues by sharp bone fragments. Immobilization by a Robert Jones bandage is inadequate as primary stabilization for a fracture.

The Robert Jones bandage is a safe bandage, and few complications occur with its use. Clients must be advised to observe the toes for swelling or abrasion. The bandage is kept dry by covering it with plastic sheeting if the animal is to be walked during wet conditions. A wet bandage rapidly causes acute moist dermatitis that is difficult to treat without bandage removal. With proper care, a Robert Jones bandage is easily maintained by a pet owner for several weeks.

Light or Modified Robert Jones Bandage

A light or modified Robert Jones bandage is applied in similar fashion to the Robert Jones bandage, except that much less cotton padding is used. Cast padding may be substituted for roll cotton. Less immobilization of the limb is achieved because the reduced padding is more flexible. This bandage is indicated whenever a lightly compressing support wrap is needed to reduce soft-tissue edema, but not in circumstances requiring rigid stability.

Reinforced Robert Jones Bandage

A light Robert Jones bandage is frequently reinforced with rigid material to enhance immobilization of the joints. The improved stability and the reduced bulk of a reinforced Robert Jones bandage make it an excellent choice for temporary stabilization of a fracture before surgery or as adjunctive external coaptation for a tenuous internal repair.

Spica Splint

A spica splint envelopes the affected limb and torso of an animal to immobilize the shoulder or hip joint in addition to the more distal joints of the extremity. Because the shoulder or hip joint is immobilized in a spica, this splint may be used as temporary preoperative support of humeral and femoral fractures. Most femoral and humeral fractures are usually too displaced to use the spica splint as primary fixation. A greenstick fracture of the humerus or femur occasionally is seen in a young puppy or kitten. It may then be appropriate to use a spica splint as primary fixation.

Schroeder-Thomas Splint

Aluminum splint rod and bandage material are used in a Schroeder-Thomas splint to provide traction at a fracture site and immobilization of the joints in a limb. This splint has been widely used in the past for small animals, but its indications have become progressively fewer. The Schroeder-Thomas splint may be used as primary fixation for selected minimally displaced midshaft fractures of the radius, ulna, and tibia. Because the Schroeder-Thomas splint does not adequately immobilize the shoulder or hip joint, it is not used to stabilize fractures of the humerus or femur.

Velpeau Sling

A Velpeau sling maintains the carpus, elbow, and shoulder joints in a flexed position and prevents weightbearing on the forelimb. A Velpeau sling immobilizes the shoulder joint and is used as primary or adjunctive stabilization for shoulder luxations, bicipital bursitis, minimally displaced fractures of the scapula and proximal humerus, and conditions of the distal forelimb if nonweightbearing is desired.

Care is taken in application of the sling not to compress the animal's thorax or to compress the flexed carpus and paw with gauze and elastic tape.

Ehmer Sling

An Ehmer sling is used to prevent weightbearing on a pelvic limb and to maintain a limited degree of internal rotation of the hip and abduction of the limb. It is commonly used as primary coaptation after closed reduction for craniodorsal coxofemoral luxation. Internal rotation of the hip rotates the femoral head beneath the dorsal rim of the acetabulum to help prevent reluxation of that joint. Unfortunately, internal rotation of the hip joint is not rigidly fixed with this sling, and reluxation of the joint can and does occur. An Ehmer sling is also commonly used as adjunct stabilization for coxofemoral luxations after surgical correction and to prevent weightbearing after internal repair of acetabular and femoral fractures.

Pelvic Limb Sling

A pelvic limb sling (Robinson sling) prevents weightbearing on the hindlimb but allows relatively free movement of the joints. It is only rarely used as primary stabilization of an injury but serves as an excellent adjunct to surgical repair. The sling may be used to prevent stress on healing fractures of the femur and tibia and is also used after coxofemoral and stifle joint operations.

Carpal Flexion Bandage

A carpal flexion bandage prevents weightbearing on the forelimb and firmly flexes the carpus to relieve tension from the flexor tendons. It is most commonly used to shield stress from tendon repairs after traumatic laceration and to prevent weightbearing for other orthopedic repairs of the forelimb.

Caution is required when using this bandage in the presence of generalized carpal soft-tissue injury. If the carpus is maintained in an extreme flexed position for too long, adhesions that are strong enough to prevent extension of the carpus may form.

Hobbles

Hobbles are circumferential tape strips constructed to allow weightbearing on the hindlimbs and walking but prevent abduction of the limbs at different levels. Tarsal hobbles are placed just above the tarsus and provide mild support and assistance in walking to animals recovering from pelvic trauma.

Full Leg Cast

A cast is a limb splint constructed with light padding and casting tape applied circumferentially to rigidly enclose an extremity. The stability achieved is adequate fixation for healing of many fractures and joint conditions. A full leg cast encloses the limb from the toes to the midshaft humerus in the forelimb or midshaft femur in the hindlimb. The shoulder and hip joints are not immobilized in the conventional full leg cast, effectively limiting the use of casts for fractures below the level of the elbow or stifle joint. Casts are most effective in treating minimally displaced stable fractures of the radius, ulna, tibia, and fibula in young, fast-healing animals.

Cast Materials (p. 1674)

Method of Application

Modifications of Casts

Half Cast. A half cast is shorter than a full leg cast and does not extend above the elbow or stifle. Also called a *walking cast*, a half cast is indicated in minimally displaced fractures of the metacarpus and metatarsus and to immobilize various carpal and tarsal conditions.

Walking Bar. A walking bar may be applied to any cast by contouring aluminum splint rod to the end of the cast and taping it in place.

Bivalved Cast. Changing a cast frequently to examine the limb is usually contraindicated. Excessive movement at the fracture may cause loss of fracture reduction and delay healing. If a major wound is present, bivalving the cast allows frequent cast changes without the added expense of new casting tape at each change. If bivalving a cast is anticipated, the stockinette and tape stirrups are not incorporated into the casting tape but taped to the outer surface of the cast.

CHAPTER 125

Delayed Union, Nonunion, and Malunion (pages 1676–1685)

Most delayed union, nonunion, and malunion complications are directly related to conservative treatment or nontreatment of fractures, orthopedic infections, technical errors in fracture fixation, and errors in clinical judgement.

DELAYED UNION (pp. 1676–1680)

A delayed union is a fracture that has not healed in the expected time when compared with other similar fractures (type, location) treated similarly in comparable patients. A delayed union infers that the fracture healing process is continuing but at a less than optimal rate.

Pathophysiology and Pathology

Histological Characteristics

Delayed union is characterized by abundant periosteal and endosteal callus and vigorous intracortical remodeling.

Clinical Signs and Diagnosis

A delayed union may be described as a fracture that is relatively stable, will likely end in clinical union, but is healing at a less than optimal rate. A delayed union may also be described as a fracture that is grossly unstable and will likely end in nonunion (i.e., the healing process ceases).

A comparison of sequential radiographs taken at 4- to 6-week intervals should show progression of healing. Radiographic characteristics of ongoing fracture healing include limited bone resorption at the fracture site, periosteal new bone formation somewhat proximal and distal to the fracture site, periosteal and endosteal bridging callus, and bridging callus mineralization. The medullary cavity remains open at the fracture site throughout the healing process.

Noninfected Delayed Unions

Surgical intervention is indicated for delayed unions in which the main fracture fragments are significantly malaligned and cannot be adequately realigned by closed reduction. Gentle use of a fracture distractor and incision of the tissues within the fracture site permit distraction and alignment of the fragments. Fibrous or cartilaginous tissue within the fracture gap need not be excised if adequate reduction and rigid stabilization with compression can be achieved. Dynamic compression bone plating, bone plating using a compression jig, and a rigid external fixator configuration in a compression mode are options.

Surgical intervention is also indicated in adequately aligned delayed unions in which skeletal implants have loosened, significant instability is present at the fracture site, and conservative treatment may end in nonunion.

Delayed unions involving aligned main fracture fragments may be treated conservatively if skeletal implants have remained firmly attached to the bone fragments, instability at the fracture site is minimal, no obvious signs of osteomyelitis are present, and a united fracture in 8 to 12 additional weeks is highly probable.

Infected Delayed Unions

Fracture healing has been shown to progress to union in the presence of infection if fracture fragments are rigidly immobilized.

Surgical treatment is indicated in infected delayed unions that radiographically demonstrate unstable implants and large sequestra. Deep culture and sensitivity testing, débridement of necrotic soft tissues, sequestrectomy, and rigid skeletal fixation with interfragmentary compression are indicated. The fracture site may then be treated as an open wound and grafted with autogenous cancellous bone after resolution of the osteomyelitis. Delayed unions that radiographically demonstrate mild osteomyelitis but no evidence of bone sequestra, draining fistula, or implant loosening may be treated conservatively.

NONUNION (pp. 1680–1682)

A nonunion is an ununited fracture usually characterized by a pseudoarthrosis at the fracture site. Without surgical intervention, eventual union is highly doubtful because the fracture healing process has ceased.

Pathophysiology and Pathology

Classification

Nonunions may or may not be capable of a biological response and have been classified accordingly as viable (hypervascular) or nonviable (avascular).

Nonviable nonunions are subclassified as dystrophic, necrotic, defect, or atrophic. *Dystrophic nonunions* are characterized by an intermediate fragment that has healed to only one main fragment. The poorly vascularized intermediate fragment is incapable of stimulating a sufficient osteogenic response to bridge the gap with the second major fragment. *Necrotic nonunions* are associated with comminuted fractures in which major fragments are avascular or poorly vascularized and eventually die. The necrotic fragments do not become incorporated in the fracture callus. *Defect nonunions* result from the loss of a significant section of bone at the fracture site. *Atrophic nonunions* are sequelae to the other three types of nonviable nonunions. Significant bone resorption at the fragment ends, loss of all vascularity and osteogenic activity, and osteoporosis characterize these nonunions.

Clinical Signs and Diagnosis

The clinical signs of nonunion differ from delayed union. Motion at the fracture site is usually greater, and movement of the main fracture fragments is often painless or only mildly uncomfortable. Partial weightbearing on the affected limb is not unusual; however, limb deformity and muscle atrophy are present.

Radiographic characteristics of nonunion may include a variable amount of nonbridging periosteal and endosteal callus, interfragmentary radiolucency, sclerosis and smoothing of the ends of the fracture fragments, mineralized tissue sealing over the medullary cavity, and (particularly in older nonunions) a pseudarthrosis.

Clinical Treatment

Noninfected Nonunions

A reasonable chance of achieving relief of discomfort, improved limb function, and correction of limb deformity should accompany any chosen treatment. Nontreatment may be the preferred choice in an older sedentary animal with a minimally displaced chronic nonunion that has formed a relatively stable, functional, and painless pseudarthrosis.

Restoring fragment stability by rigid internal or external skeletal fixation, reducing the fracture gap by fragment alignment and compression of interfragmentary tissues, and stimulating vascularity and osteogenesis by the use of débridement, bone grafting, and decortication all are important in encouraging fracture healing in all nonunions. With hypertrophic viable nonunions, removal of interfragmentary tissue (nonmineralized fibrocartilage) is not necessary. Only enough periosteal callus is removed to create a flat cortical surface for secure plate fixation. Although oligotrophic nonunions are capable of a biological response, in addition to the previously mentioned procedures, débridement of the fragment ends and packing the fracture gap with generous amounts of autogenous cancellous bone improve the chance of union.

All nonviable nonunions benefit from débridement of the ends of the fracture fragments, opening the medullary cavity if necessary, and packing the fracture site with autogenous cancellous bone. Necrotic nonunions require removal of all avascular bone fragments. Defect nonunions or large defects created by the removal of necrotic fragments often require large volumes of autogenous cancellous bone or autogenous corticocancellous bone (ilial wing, rib chips) to fill the defect, as well as the use of strong buttress plates.

Infected Nonunions

As with infected delayed unions, deep cultures are taken before antimicrobial therapy, and all necrotic bone and soft tissue at the fracture site are débrided. Depending on the severity of the infection, the fracture gap may be packed with autogenous cancellous bone and closed immediately, or the site may be treated as an open wound followed by cancellous bone grafting after granulation tissue has covered the exposed bone. After union, skeletal implants are removed to resolve residual osteomyelitis.

MALUNION (pp. 1682–1684)

A malunion is a fracture that has healed in an abnormal position, usually causing various degrees of functional impairment of the limb. Limb shortening, angulation, or rotation may cause improper balance or abnormal gait; uneven distribution of weight across the joint may cause degenerative arthritis, and movement of an adjacent joint may be restricted.

Pathophysiology and Pathology
Clinical Treatment

Surgical treatment of malunion is indicated if, by performing the surgical procedure, significant functional improvement can be expected. Correction of a deformity resulting from malunion for cosmetic reasons alone is rarely justified. Because of the normal angulation in major joints of the forelimb and hindlimb of small animals, increasing joint extension can often compensate for over-riding malunions that have caused mild to moderate limb shortening. Dogs can compensate for up to 20 per cent of femoral shortening by decreasing the standing angle of the contralateral stifle.

Malunions that cause significant disability require osteotomy, gentle distraction of the soft tissues, débridement of the fracture ends and opening of the medullary cavities, alignment of the main fragments, and application of rigid fixation. Gaps created at the osteotomy site during realignment are filled with autogenous cancellous bone. Angular malunions with varus or valgus deformity (mediolateral displacement) require opening or closing wedge osteotomy to prevent subsequent degenerative arthrosis from unequal forces on articular cartilage. Transverse or dome osteotomy may be performed for correction of moderate to severe rotational malunions.

CHAPTER 126
Orthopedic Infections
(pages 1685–1694)

Wound infections in orthopedic surgery usually result from contamination of open fractures or from open fracture repair, resulting in osteomyelitis and soft-tissue infection. Osteomyelitis is inflammation of bone and its marrow contents. The majority of infections are caused by bacteria; fungi are occasionally involved, and parasites and viruses rarely. Chronic osteomyelitis may result from sequestra or contamination of implants. Young dogs may develop osteomyelitis from hematogenously delivered bacteria. Septic arthritis can occur as a postoperative complication, by wounds or hematogenous contamination.

Prophylactic Use of Antibiotics

Prophylactic therapy is considered in all clean orthopedic procedures involving implantation of foreign materials and in arthroscopy. The timing of administration and choice of antibiotic are important. Maximum tissue concentration of the antibiotic is necessary during the vulnerable period between skin incision and closure. Antibiotics administered 3 hours or more before contamination may select for resistant organisms. Single-dose intravenous prophylaxis 20 minutes before the incision is the present practice in human orthopedics. Antibiotic administration later than 3 to 5 hours after contamination is ineffective.

Coagulase-positive and coagulase-negative *Staphylococcus* spp. are the most common pathogens associated with orthopedic procedures. Cefazolin, a first-generation cephalosporin, is a bactericidal drug that is effective against staphylococcal organisms. It has a relatively long half-life (1.8 hours) and achieves excellent penetration into bone (25 per cent of blood levels when given intravenously).

ACUTE HEMATOGENOUS OSTEOMYELITIS (pp. 1686–1687)
Clinical Findings

In dogs, acute hematogenous osteomyelitis most often affects neonates or young individuals. The source of infection may be the umbilicus; however, older, immature dogs may develop the disease after umbilical closure. The history often includes focal infection or more generalized disease. Clinical signs include fever, malaise, and nonweightbearing lameness. Morbidity ranges from lameness to severe debilitation. Physical examination findings include soft-tissue swelling over the involved bone; it may fluctuate if purulent exudate has extended through the periosteum.

Pathophysiology
Diagnosis

A tentative diagnosis of acute hematogenous osteomyelitis is based on a history of prior infection and physical findings. The white blood cell count is usually elevated. Radiographs demonstrate only soft-tissue swelling for the first 2 to 3 weeks; thereafter, areas of lysis and new bone production involving the metaphysis become apparent. Fine-needle aspiration of fluctuant areas may yield positive cultures if samples are obtained before antibiotic administration. Gram-positive organisms such as *Staphylococcus* or *Streptococcus* spp. are most likely.

Treatment

A broad-spectrum bactericidal antimicrobial, such as a cephalosporin, is administered intravenously for 3 to 5 days, until culture and sensitivity test results are available. If the bacteria cannot be identified, continued administration of the antibiotic is based on the animal's clinical response. A favorable initial response permits an oral antibiotic, which should be continued for 4 weeks.

Palpable abscesses are drained and débrided, and culture specimens obtained before copious lavage. If débridement is adequate, closure over a drain can be considered. If the adequacy of débridement is in doubt, the wound is left open. Extension of infection into a joint is a surgical emergency.

OSTEOMYELITIS FROM EXOGENOUS SOURCES
(pp. 1687–1689)
Acute Osteomyelitis
Clinical Findings

Acute osteomyelitis is usually a complication of open fracture repair, and clinical signs are generally apparent after 5 to 7 days. Animals are febrile and often have leukocytosis. Surgical wounds are edematous, red, and warm. The animal may not bear weight on the limb, and the surgical site is painful.

Pathophysiology
Diagnosis

A history of recent fracture repair and evidence of wound infection (swelling, heat, drainage) suggest acute osteomyelitis. Radiographs demonstrate proliferative new bone and occasionally gas in soft tissues. Sequestra may be suspected, but they generally do not become visible radiographically for several weeks or months. Fine-needle aspirates from the fracture site or exudate from draining tracts are submitted for culture and sensitivity testing.

Treatment

Aggressive early intervention is necessary to prevent the development of chronic osteomyelitis. The fracture must be stable; if implants are not providing stabilization, they must be removed. External fixation devices are often indicated to provide stabilization and minimize soft-tissue damage. Broad-spectrum bactericidal antibiotics (e.g., cefazolin) are administered intravenously. Antibiotic protocols are modified depending on culture results and clinical response.

In most cases, the surgical wound is opened for débridement, lavage, and drainage. If débridement is thorough and the tissues appear healthy, the wound is closed over a drain. Low-vacuum closed suction systems minimize ascending contamination and provide effective drainage. Drainage systems are cared for aseptically and removed when fluid accumulation has subsided, usually in 3 to 5 days. Open wound management with delayed closure may be necessary in severely infected wounds.

Chronic Osteomyelitis

Chronic osteomyelitis usually results from inadequate treatment of acute osteomyelitis; it may also develop from cryptic infections associated with metallic prostheses.

Clinical Findings

Moderate to severe atrophy is present in the affected limb, and a draining tract is usually present. The drainage generally subsides with administration of antibiotics but invariably returns when the medication is discontinued. Pain at the fracture site and the amount of weight-bearing are variable and depend on whether or not the fracture has united.

Diagnosis

The history and physical findings are sufficient to make a tentative diagnosis. Radiographic signs include new bone production with areas of lysis, extensive remodeling, and often the presence of a sequestrum. Cultures from draining tracts are usually polymicrobic and do not necessarily include the causative organisms.

Treatment

Chronic osteomyelitis is a surgical disease, with antimicrobial chemotherapy an integral part of the treatment regimen. Aggressive débridement of necrotic tissue includes sclerotic bone that may be occluding the medullary cavity. Stabilization of the fracture is essential, if it has not already united. With significant soft-tissue infection, external fixators are preferred because they can be applied with minimal disruption of blood supply. If the soft tissues are healthy and the surgical procedure has consisted primarily of sequestrectomy and débridement of the fistulous tract, plate fixation may be considered. Intramedullary pins are contraindicated because they do not provide adequate stability and may permit extension of the infection throughout the medullary cavity. All implants are ultimately removed, if possible, because they harbor organisms and potentially contribute to fracture-associated sarcoma.

FUNGAL OSTEOMYELITIS (pp. 1689–1690)

SEPTIC ARTHRITIS (pp. 1690–1691)

Septic arthritis is a potentially devastating bacterial infection secondary to joint contamination from hematogenous or exogenous routes. The latter are most common and include injuries, surgical procedures, and intra-articular injections. Potential sources of hematogenously derived bacteria are the respiratory or digestive tracts, umbilicus, and endocardium.

Clinical Findings

Septic arthritis is usually monoarticular. The joint is swollen, painful, and warm, and rectal temperature is often elevated. The limb either does not bear weight or is markedly lame.

Pathophysiology

Diagnosis

A tentative diagnosis is based on clinical findings. Definitive diagnosis is based on evaluation of joint fluid obtained via arthrocentesis. Abnormal findings include increased numbers of polymorphonuclear leukocytes ($40,000/mm^3$ to $100,000/mm^3$ or greater), bacteria, and increased turbidity or purulent appearance. Direct culture of synovial fluid is commonly negative, so synovial fluid samples are immediately placed into blood culture medium to facilitate growth and culture.

Early radiographic signs are related to effusion and soft-tissue swelling. With progression of sepsis, radiographic signs include bone lysis, joint surface irregularity, and subluxation.

Treatment

Therapy is directed at minimizing cartilage destruction. Antimicrobial chemotherapy begins immediately after arthrocentesis for cytological study and culture. Intravenous administration of a broad-spectrum bactericidal drug such as a cephalosporin is indicated pending culture and sensitivity test results. Antibiotics are continued for a minimum of 4 weeks.

Joint lavage is essential to remove cellular and enzymatic constituents. In young animals, decompression is particularly important to reduce pressure and preserve epiphyseal vascularity. Needle aspiration and lavage do not adequately remove deleterious materials from the joint and may cause iatrogenic cartilage damage. Arthrotomy, surgical débridement, and copious lavage are indicated for (1) postoperative joint infections, (2) septic joints untreated for 72 hours or more, (3) joints that have not responded to 72 hours of conservative treatment, and (4) penetrating wounds involving a joint. The joint is lavaged with large volumes of isotonic solution to remove fibrin clots, purulent exudate, and foreign material. The use of antibiotic and antiseptic solutions for lavage is controversial. Antiseptic solutions may cause chemical synovitis. Each case must be considered individually, and for infections caused by extremely resistant organisms, the potential advantages of antibiotics or antiseptics in the lavage solution may outweigh the hazards.

Parenteral antibiotics, daily aseptic bandage changes, and hospitalization are recommended during the first postoperative week. Daily wound inspection allows assessment of the infection, lavage of blood clots and exudate, and passive range of motion exercises to facilitate drainage.

INFECTION ASSOCIATED WITH PROSTHETIC IMPLANTS
(pp. 1691–1693)

CHAPTER 127
Bone Grafting (pages 1694–1703)

A properly applied bone graft is often the critical factor differentiating a successful fracture repair from a nonunion or the possibility of a limb salvage procedure from the need for an amputation. The most commonly used bone graft is the fresh cancellous autograft, which has the advantages of histocompatibility, live cells, and excellent osteogenic and inductive potential. If the graft must provide mechanical stability or fill large defects, cortical bone is preferable.

BONE GRAFT TERMINOLOGY (p. 1694)

The term *graft* implies the transfer of living tissue, whereas *implant* refers to nonviable material placed in the body. Implants also can be nonbiological materials, such as metal or ceramic, in addition to dead bone (e.g., frozen or freeze-dried cortical bone). A graft moved from one site to another within the same individual is an *autograft*, described by the adjectives *autologous, autogenous,* or *autochthonous.* An *allograft* (adjective: *allogeneic*) is tissue transferred between two genetically different individuals of the same species. A *xenograft* is tissue of one species implanted into a member of a different species (adjective: *xenogeneic*).

FUNCTIONS OF BONE GRAFTS (pp. 1694–1695)

Osteogenesis

Osteogenesis refers to bone formation with no indication of cellular origin. When new bone is formed on or about a graft, it may be either of graft origin (i.e., from cells that survived the transfer and are capable of forming bone) or from cells of host origin. Surface cells on cortical and cancellous grafts that are properly handled can survive and produce new bone. This early bone formed by viable graft cells is often critical in callus formation during the first to 4 to 8 weeks after surgery. Cancellous bone, with its very large surface area covered by quiescent lining cells or active osteoblasts, has potential for more graft-origin new bone formation than does cortical bone. Host mesenchymal cells may be recruited to form bone and cartilage by the process of osteoinduction.

Mechanical Support

When placed in large defects resulting from trauma or *en bloc* resection of neoplastic bone and stabilized with internal fixation, bone grafts and implants act as weightbearing space fillers or struts and as scaffolds for the ingrowth of new host bone. The three-dimensional process of ingrowth of sprouting capillaries, perivascular tissue, and osteoprogenitor cells from the recipient bed into the structure of an implant or graft is termed *osteoconduction*. Osteoconduction may result from osteoinduction (e.g., in a fresh cortical autograft) or may occur without active participation of the implant, as with porous ceramic or mineral apatite implants.

FACTORS AFFECTING INCORPORATION OF BONE GRAFTS AND IMPLANTS (p. 1695)

INCORPORATION OF BONE GRAFTS/IMPLANTS
(pp. 1695–1699)

Incorporation is a partnership between the recipient site and the bone graft. The graft provides a small but critically important population of cells (if it is fresh), bioactive bone-inducing factors present in the matrix such as bone morphogenetic protein (osteoinduction), and a suitable structural shape to support new host bone formation (osteoconduction). The host provides the inflammatory response and ensuing fibrovascular stroma, which eventually revascularize the graft. Anything that interferes with the ingrowth of vessels or the availability of osteoprogenitor cells adversely influences the bone graft.

Summary

Fresh autologous cancellous bone is incorporated the most rapidly of any graft; it contributes to osteogenesis both by survival of graft cells and by induction of new bone formation at the graft site. Fresh autogenous cortical bone is incorporated more slowly because of its dense structure. Fresh allogeneic bone is subject to attack by the immune system of the recipient; thus, its course of incorporation is less predictable but is certainly slower and less complete than that of autografts. Preserved alloimplants are useful when they retain some osteoinductive capacity while being minimally immunogenic. Preserved alloimplants are not very biologically acceptable and are poorly incorporated.

INDICATIONS FOR BONE GRAFTS AND IMPLANTS
(pp. 1699–1700)

If rapid formation of large amounts of new bone is required (e.g., for an arthrodesis or for defects in a reconstructed comminuted fracture), cancellous autografts are clearly superior to allografts of any kind. When the graft functions primarily as a weightbearing strut and can be stabilized with internal fixation for a relatively long period, allogeneic material is an acceptable alternative to autologous bone.

In general, the two principal indications for bone grafts are to enhance healing and to replace bone lost through trauma or surgical resection. These indications are not mutually exclusive; in a severely comminuted fracture, both characteristics may be desirable.

Enhancement of Healing in Comminuted or Retarded Fractures

All comminuted fractures benefit from a graft of autologous cancellous bone because they frequently have avascular fragments that are resorbed. Additionally, it is not always possible to achieve stable internal fixation. Thus, early and vigorous production of new bone originating from and stimulated by fresh autologous cancellous bone is helpful. Even simple fractures of bones known to be slow to heal (e.g., the distal radius in small dogs) benefit from the osteogenesis provided by a cancellous autograft.

Arthrodesis

When an arthrodesis is performed, it is of utmost importance to achieve a stable bony union of the joint surfaces as quickly as possible. The usefulness of autogenous cancellous and corticocancellous bone has been confirmed.

Nonunions

Although the majority of nonunions following fractures of long bones in dogs are proliferative and are adequately treated by rigid internal fixation with compression if possible, avascular and infected nonunions profit greatly from internal fixation augmented by an autologous cancellous bone graft.

Cancellous autografts may also be used to advantage in the treatment of infected nonunions. The nonunion site is débrided, sequestra are removed, and open irrigation drainage with an appropriate antibiotic solution is performed if possible.

Contaminated and Infected Fractures: Osteomyelitis

Bone Loss

Relatively large segments of bone may be lost through trauma or surgical excision of tumors, cysts, or shattered fracture fragments. When the defect is not segmental and when the bone retains sufficient mechanical strength for weightbearing, the defect may be packed with autogenous cancellous bone. Large segmental defects require internal or external fixation and a cortical graft.

HARVESTING AND HANDLING OF GRAFTS AND IMPLANTS (pp. 1701–1702)

A key consideration is the selection of a donor site with a large population of surface cells. The most commonly selected sites in dogs are the proximal tibia and humerus for fresh cancellous bone and the iliac crest or rib for fresh corticocancellous bone. Once an appropriate site has been selected, the surgeon must harvest the graft with minimal trauma.

Once the donor bone has been removed, numerous precautions must be taken to prevent the death of surface cells. Exposing the graft to air for 30 minutes kills a significant number of cells. Immersion in saline inhibits osteogenesis, and exposing the grafts to antibiotic powders is absolutely contraindicated. Irrigation of the recipient bed before graft placement with dilute solutions of bacitracin (25 to 50 units/ml) and polymyxin B sulfate (25 to 50 μg/ml) is permissible. The use of antibiotic solutions after graft implantation is controversial and is probably best avoided. The optimal technique is to harvest the graft immediately before use and to transfer the graft directly into the recipient bed. If this is not possible because of risk of contamination of the donor site with bacteria or tumor cells, it is best to wrap the graft in a moistened blood-soaked sponge. The graft can be placed in a metal bowl, covered with additional saline-soaked sponges, and held for 3 to 4 hours if necessary.

Attention must also be paid to the recipient bed. Asepsis, hemostasis, and atraumatic technique are crucial. Additionally, several key steps are taken to promote effective diffusion of nutrients. First, prevent the interposition of dead space, hematoma, or necrotic tissue between the graft and the bed. Second, place cancellous portions of the graft next to cancellous portions of the bed. Third, do not pack the graft so tightly that diffusion is impossible. Fourth, the importance of stable fixation of the grafted area has already been mentioned but cannot be overemphasized.

Bone Graft Collection (pp. 1701–1702)

CHAPTER 128

Scapula (pages 1703–1710)

Because of the scapula's location, trauma sufficient to produce a scapular fracture can easily produce concomitant injury. It is important to assess each patient for cervical and rib fractures, shoulder luxations, thoracic trauma (pneumothorax and pulmonary injury), brachial plexus trauma, and suprascapular nerve trauma.

Fractures of the scapula are classified according to their location: (1) fractures of the body and spine, including the acromion process; (2) fractures of the neck; and (3) fractures involving the glenoid cavity, including fractures of the supraglenoid tuberosity.

FRACTURES OF THE SCAPULAR BODY (pp. 1703–1705)

Because of protection afforded by the thorax and lateral supporting musculature, fractures of the scapular body are often displaced minimally. These fractures are best treated by restricting activity for 3 to 4 weeks and applying scapular support bandages or Velpeau slings. The prognosis for full function is excellent. Open reduction and internal fixation are indicated for scapular body fractures exhibiting severe instability or displacement or when the displacement is cosmetically unacceptable.

FRACTURES OF THE ACROMION (pp. 1705–1706)

Affected animals generally have a weightbearing lameness with pain on palpation of the acromial process. The acromion serves as the origin of the acromial head of the deltoid muscle; therefore, constant muscle pull distracts the fragment, and internal fixation is recommended. If fixation is secure, postoperative bandages or slings are not necessary, and the prognosis for full recovery is excellent.

FRACTURES OF THE SCAPULAR NECK, GLENOID, AND SUPRAGLENOID TUBEROSITY (pp. 1707–1709)

Fractures in this area frequently are severely displaced and may involve the articular surface of the glenoid. Patients are presented with a nonweightbearing lameness, and pain and crepitus are palpable on manipulation of the shoulder joint. Because these fractures usually are severely displaced and are in close proximity to the shoulder joint, open reduction and internal fixation are indicated to prevent exuberant callus formation and possibly limited shoulder function. Articular involvement is also an indication for anatomical reduction and rigid fixation.

Fractures involving the articular surface can be particularly challenging, and the principles of anatomical reduction with rigid internal compression fixation must be followed. Avulsion fractures of the supraglenoid tuberosity are displaced by the pull of the biceps brachii muscle. After exposure and anatomical reduction, these fractures are stabilized with a lag screw or a pin and tension band. If stable fixation has been achieved, early limited weightbearing or passive range-of-motion exercises are encouraged. If necessary, a scapular support bandage may be applied for 10 to 14 days.

SCAPULAR DISLOCATION (p. 1709)

The ventral serratus muscle is a large muscle mass that covers the caudal half of the lateral thoracic wall and inserts on the proximal medial aspect of the scapula. It is the major muscular support for the scapula and thoracic limb. Rupture of this muscle can occur secondary to trauma. The resulting clinical signs are dramatic, with marked upward displacement of the scapula. If the distal limb is adducted, the proximal part of the scapula displaces laterally. Affected animals generally are not in pain but do have a characteristic gait abnormality.

Surgical repair is usually necessary for a functional and cosmetic result. Closed reduction and a tight Velpeau sling have been reported as a successful treatment for acute dislocations in cats. Primary wire support is also an effective method of repair.

CHAPTER 129

Luxation of the Scapulohumeral Joint

(pages 1710–1716)

Scapulohumeral luxation is unusual in dogs and very rare in cats. The majority of luxations are either medial or lateral; cranial and caudal types have been reported but occur much less often. The cause is often traumatic disruption of the supporting elements of the joint; however, congenital medial luxation in small dogs has been associated with capsular laxity and insufficiency of the glenoid cavity.

SURGICAL ANATOMY (p. 1710)

LATERAL SCAPULOHUMERAL LUXATION (pp. 1710–1711)

Lateral luxation of the scapulohumeral joint is a traumatic injury occurring most often in large dogs. Lateral luxation is attended by rupture of both the lateral joint capsule with its glenohumeral ligament and the tendon of the infraspinatus.

Clinical Findings and Diagnosis

The affected limb is carried in flexion, and the foot may be internally rotated. Pain and crepitation are noted on manipulation of the shoulder, and the greater tubercle of the humerus can be palpated lateral to its normal position. A complete neurological examination is essential to detect possible injury to the brachial plexus. Radiographs of the shoulder are necessary to confirm the diagnosis and to detect fractures or excessive wearing of the glenoid rim. If the luxation is intermittent, stress radiographs, with the limb held in adduction, may be required to demonstrate the instability.

Treatment

If the injury has occurred within the previous 5 to 7 days, closed reduction and splintage are often successful. If the joint tends to reluxate easily, the prognosis for successful closed reduction is guarded. If the reduction is stable, the limb is immobilized using a spica splint for 10 to 14 days.

More chronic injuries (> 1 week) or very unstable joints require surgical reduction and stabilization.

MEDIAL SCAPULOHUMERAL LUXATION (pp. 1711–1715)

Medial luxation can occur in any size dog, but is more common in small breeds. In large dogs, traumatic disruption of the subscapularis muscle and medial joint capsule is the cause of the instability. In small dogs and toy breeds, congenital or developmental laxity results in medial instability, and the condition is often bilateral. In some dogs, a malformed and hypoplastic glenoid cavity is present, and reduction is not possible.

Clinical Findings and Diagnosis

Acutely traumatized dogs carry the affected limb in flexion with the foot rotated outward. Pain is associated with extension of the shoulder, and the greater tubercle may be palpated medial to its normal position. Dogs with chronic luxations may not appear to be in pain. A thorough neurological examination is essential.

Small dogs with nontraumatic medial luxation may have intermittent or constant lameness. The joint may often be easily reduced and reluxated with manipulation and is not painful. Dogs with severe malformation of the glenoid usually do not bear weight and hold the affected limb in flexion.

Radiographic examination of dogs with traumatic luxations is important to verify the diagnosis and check for concurrent fractures, especially of the glenoid cavity. Radiographs of the shoulder in small dogs with chronic luxations may show considerable secondary degenerative changes, including erosion of the medial glenoid rim.

Treatment

Conservative care of acute traumatic medial luxations consists of closed reduction and placement of the limb in a Velpeau-type sling for 2 weeks. Unstable reductions and fractures involving the articular surfaces require surgical intervention.

Chronic luxations in small dogs may cause only intermittent lameness with minimal secondary degenerative changes. Decisions regarding surgical stabilization in these types of cases must be made on the basis of age, general health, and the severity of the disability. Nonweightbearing lameness associated with severe dysplasia of the glenoid cavity in small dogs requires arthrodesis or resection arthroplasty to restore limb use.

Prognosis

In evaluating medial translocation of the biceps tendon, one study reported satisfactory results in 11 of 12 dogs, another in 10 of 11 dogs.

Scapulohumeral arthrodesis provides good to excellent use of the limb in the majority of animals studied. Excision of the glenoid cavity provided excellent results in two of ten dogs and good results in the remaining eight dogs. Some reduction in range of motion, muscle atrophy, and slight climb shortening were noted in all limbs after surgery.

CRANIAL SCAPULOHUMERAL LUXATION (pp. 1715–1716)

CAUDAL SCAPULOHUMERAL LUXATION (p. 1716)

CHAPTER 130

Fractures of the Humerus
(pages 1716–1728)

Many humeral fractures occur within the shaft of the bone; thus the radial nerve may be injured when a humeral fracture occurs. Although the incidence of radial nerve injuries is low, the radial nerve is always checked when a humeral fracture is present. Other nerves of the brachial plexus may also be injured when a humeral fracture occurs, and thus a complete forelimb neurological evaluation is indicated with this type of injury. The location of the humerus in relation to the thoracic cavity makes it imperative that the chest be evaluated with auscultation and radiographs when humeral fractures occur.

FIXATION TECHNIQUES (pp. 1717–1724)

The circumstances under which a humeral fracture can be treated using an extended lateral splint (spica) or a Velpeau bandage occur very infrequently. They include minimally displaced nonarticular fractures in very young animals. External splintage of humeral fractures for more than 2 or 3 weeks may cause severe restriction of elbow motion and must be avoided. The difficulty in adequately splinting the humerus, the propensity for loss of elbow motion, and the unstable nature of most humeral fractures dictate the need for internal fixation in most of these fractures.

Intramedullary Pinning

Intramedullary pin fixation of the humerus may be performed either open or closed. Closed fracture fixation is limited to those cases that are neither complex nor greatly displaced. An animal with this fracture often is young, so rapid healing and good remodeling can be expected.

Open reduction is the most frequent manner in which humeral fractures are handled. Intramedullary pins may be introduced either retrograde or normograde with a hand chuck or power pin driver.

Generally, only one pin that is about two-thirds the diameter of the medullary canal at its narrowest point is used.

It is sometimes advantageous to place a second pin in the medullary canal. If two pins are to be used, the size of the first pin is reduced to not greater than half the diameter of the medullary canal. Stacked pins may be of the same or different sizes. When stacking two or more pins in the humerus, the pins may be placed either normograde or retrograde. Intramedullary pin fixation often needs some form of auxiliary support such as cerclage wire or external fixators to stabilize the fracture.

Plate Fixation

Bone plates, when applied to the humerus, as with any other bone, may have one of four functions: (1) neutralization, (2) buttress, (3) static compression, and (4) dynamic compression.

Bone plates can be placed on any surface of the humerus; therefore, position of the plate depends on the location of the fracture and the surgeon's preference. Cranial placement of the plate works well for very proximal fractures and can be used for fractures of the shaft that allow at least two and preferably three screws placed above and below the fracture line. The lateral surface of the humerus is used for fractures from the proximal third distally.

External Fixators

External fixators are placed on the lateral side of the bone to keep them from interfering with limb function and because anatomy prevents them from being placed medially. The type I fixator, which penetrates one skin level and two cortices of bone with the fixation pin, is the primary type of fixation used on the humerus. External fixators may be used as primary means of fracture fixation but more frequently are used as auxiliary fixation in combination with intramedullary pins.

PROXIMAL HUMERAL FRACTURES (pp. 1724–1725)

SHAFT FRACTURES (pp. 1725–1726)

Fractures of the shaft of the humerus are common owing to the tapering configuration of the bone, making this part relatively weaker than the proximal end.

Intramedullary pins, external fixators, and bone plates are the primary methods of fixation for humeral shaft fractures. Lag screws and orthopedic wires are auxiliary methods of fixation.

It is generally not possible to use intramedullary pins alone to repair humeral shaft fractures. Two-piece fractures that interdigitate and need no additional support are the exception. Because of the spiral configuration of the humeral shaft, two-piece fractures are often spiral or oblique. Shear and rotational forces thus must be neutralized.

With more complex fractures, the fragments are reduced and stabilized, when possible, with a combination of cerclage wires and intramedullary pins. An external fixator can be used in addition; a single pin above and below the fracture line is all that is needed to provide necessary stability.

Bone plates are an effective method of shaft fracture stabilization. By providing rigid internal fixation, they allow early ambulation. Most surgeons prefer to apply plates either cranially or laterally, but medial plate application is gaining acceptance.

SUPRACONDYLAR FRACTURES (pp. 1726–1727)

A patient's age often dictates the method of treatment used on supra-condylar fractures of the humerus. Bone plates, intramedullary pins, or external fixators can be used on adult animals, whereas animals with growth potential should be treated only with intramedullary pins. External fixators are rarely used to stabilize this fracture because of their relative inability to resist rotational forces. External fixators are usually used with intramedullary pins.

FRACTURES OF THE CONDYLE (pp. 1727–1728)

Fractures of the lateral portion of the humeral condyle are frequent in immature animals and occasional in adults. Adult cocker spaniels have a higher than expected incidence of these fractures. In immature dogs, this fracture is the most commonly encountered Salter IV fracture. Because the fracture is intra-articular, it is critical that anatomical reduction of the fracture be achieved.

An interfragmentary lag screw and an antirotation implant are used to stabilize fractures of the lateral portion of the humeral condyle. Stabilization of the proximal portion of the fracture segment eliminates rotation of the segment and provides added stability to the fracture repair. The antirotation implant may be either an additional lag screw if the proximal portion of the fragment is long enough or a small intramedullary pin.

Fractures involving only the medial condyle are uncommon. As with fractures of the lateral portion, they are repaired with lag screws and an antirotation implant. When both the medial and lateral portions of the condyle are involved, the fracture is referred to as a T or Y fracture, based on its configuration. These fractures usually occur in adult animals.

The first step in reducing these fractures is to use a lag screw to make the condylar segments one anatomically reconstructed piece. The fracture can then be treated like a supracondylar fracture using either intramedullary pins with or without external fixators or bone plates. The majority of intercondylar fractures can be adequately repaired with a single plate and axillary fixation. Plating provides the most rigid fixation, allowing early passive physical therapy and controlled weightbearing. This is important when dealing with elbow fractures because of that joint's tendency to stiffen when traumatized.

CHAPTER 131
Elbow Luxation (pages 1729–1736)

Elbow luxation can be congenital or can be acquired as a result of trauma. Because the elbow is inherently a very stable joint, acquired luxations are relatively uncommon. Congenital luxations are unusual in dogs and are unreported in cats.

SURGICAL ANATOMY (p. 1729)

TRAUMATIC ELBOW LUXATION (1729–1733)

The elbow joint is inherently stable owing to the configuration of the humeroulnar joint and the presence of periarticular ligamentous structures. Depending on the mechanism of injury, fracture-dislocations such as the Monteggia fracture may occur. When luxations do occur, the radius and ulna invariably luxate laterally, because of the restraining effect of the prominent medial epicondylar ridge of the humerus.

Complete luxation is associated with rupture or avulsion of the attachments of one or both collateral ligaments and the joint capsule. In more severe injuries, the origins of the flexor or extensor muscles may be ruptured or avulsed from the humeral condyle as well.

Diagnosis

In most cases of traumatic elbow luxation, the client describes a history of recent injury, with the dog having been hit by a car or involved in a dog fight.

Examination of the affected leg usually reveals (1) a nonweight-bearing lameness with the elbow in slight flexion, (2) abduction and external rotation of the antebrachium, (3) "widening" of the elbow with an indistinct lateral epicondyle but a distinct radial head laterally, (4) lateral position of the olecranon in relation to the humeral condyle, and (5) marked pain.

Radiographs are required to document the presence or absence of fractures and in chronic luxations to determine the degree of osteoarthrosis. Avulsion fractures of the attachment of the collateral ligaments are suspected when a separate bony density is present on the craniocaudal projection.

Treatment

In acute cases, every effort is made to achieve a closed reduction as soon as the animal can be safely anesthetized, because the results are generally quite satisfactory. Closed reduction is often difficult to achieve, however, because of the powerful muscle forces involved and the complex configuration of the elbow articulation. General anesthesia with sufficient muscle relaxation is essential, and suspending the limb from a drip stand for 5 minutes before attempted reduction is helpful. Neuromuscular blockade may also facilitate reduction.

If nonsurgical reduction is successful, the integrity of the collateral ligaments is evaluated to determine if further treatment is necessary. The elbow and carpus are flexed to 90°, and the antebrachium rotated. With an intact lateral collateral ligament, internal rotation is limited to 60°; with an intact medial ligament, external rotation should not exceed 40°. Manipulation of the extended elbow into varus and valgus is another test that is a simple and reliable means for assessing collateral stability. Collateral ligament injury is common with elbow luxations, and a judgement must be made after closed reduction about whether surgical reconstruction of the collateral ligaments is warranted. With marked varus or valgus instability, reconstruction is indicated. If, on the other hand, the postreduction instability is considered mild and the radiographs demonstrate only minimal subluxation, conservative treatment is indicated, especially if the animal is a companion and not an athletic or working dog.

Open Reduction and Stabilization. Open reduction is necessary when closed reduction is not possible or when luxation has recurred after a closed reduction. Chronic luxations are often impossible to reduce closed because of the associated fibrosis and muscle contracture. Surgical stabilization, including reconstruction of the collateral ligaments, is indicated if marked instability follows open reduction, particularly in cases in which closed reduction has failed and in chronic luxations that have a propensity for reluxation. If surgical exploration reveals that the joint surfaces are badly damaged, arthrodesis can be considered.

After surgical reduction and stabilization, joint stability is evaluated and postoperative radiographs are taken to evaluate anatomical alignment and placement of metallic implants. A soft padded bandage from midhumerus downward is applied for 24 to 48 hours to minimize postoperative swelling.

Aftercare (p. 1735)

Aftercare varies depending on the severity of injury, type of repair, and owner compliance.

Postoperative complications include reluxation, infection, decreased range of motion, and secondary osteoarthrosis. The prognosis after traumatic elbow luxation depends on the severity of cartilage and soft-tissue damage, duration before repair, degree of stabilization achieved, and owner compliance.

Lateral Rotation of the Ulna

Afflicted puppies are usually between 4 and 22 weeks old.

Affected puppies have a characteristic posture and gait. The elbow is held flexed, with the antebrachium markedly pronated. With bilateral involvement, the front legs may almost cross and the dog bears weight on the caudomedial aspect of the elbows and antebrachium. Palpation reveals prominent lateral displacement of the olecranon and triceps tendon, with moderate to severe muscle atrophy. Pain and crepitation are generally absent.

Significant radiographic findings include lateral displacement and cranial rotation of the proximal ulna, relatively normal position of the radial head, and narrowing of the radial neck.

Treatment

When discussing treatment options for congenital elbow luxation with a client, the possible hereditary etiology and the palliative nature of available treatments need to be clearly addressed. If a dog is able to ambulate reasonably well without pain, conservative management may be the best option. Surgical treatment provides good long-term clinical results if the procedure is performed when the dog is younger than 4 months. The surgical approach is determined primarily by the age of the dog at the time of diagnosis.

Caudolateral Luxation of the Radial Head

Diagnosis

Affected puppies show mild or no supination of the antebrachium, and the olecranon is in a normal position. A valgus deformity may be present at the carpus. The radial head is palpable on the lateral aspect of the elbow. Pain and crepitation are not present in young dogs, and the lameness is not nearly as severe as in dogs affected with lateral rotation of the ulna. Radiographs are necessary to document the abnormal position of the radial head and to evaluate the physes. The distal ulnar physis may appear abnormal, implying that retarded growth at this physis may have a role in this disease.

Treatment

If the condition is not severe, a conservative approach may be satisfactory. The dog is examined at 2- to 3-week intervals for evaluation of limb conformation and lameness, and radiographs are made to verify elbow joint congruity and continued growth, especially at the distal ulnar physis. In cases of complete luxation of the humeroradial joint, surgical reduction and stabilization are required.

CHAPTER 132

Fractures of the Radius and Ulna (pages 1736–1757)

Fractures of the radius and ulna represent a significant proportion (17 to 18 per cent) of all fractures in cats and dogs. The high incidence of delayed union and nonunion, carpal hyperextension and stiffness, and growth deformities reflects the potential complexity of treating these fractures.

FRACTURES OF THE OLECRANON (pp. 1736–1737)

Complete fractures of the olecranon result in severe proximal displacement of the fragment away from the ulna. Because external coaptation is unable to control the distractive pull of the triceps, open reduction and internal fixation are indicated.

Postoperative management depends on stability of the repair. A Robert Jones compressive bandage may be used for a few days to limit swelling. A traumatized elbow joint stiffens quickly if immobilized. Joint motion must be encouraged with either controlled walking or passive range-of-motion exercises. If a good tension band effect was achieved, additional support is not needed. If bony defects persist after surgery or if fixation is tenuous, a carpal flexion bandage is considered. This bandage allows active motion of the elbow while preventing weightbearing and can be left on for several weeks to allow early fracture healing.

PROXIMAL ULNAR FRACTURE WITH LUXATION OF THE RADIAL HEAD (pp. 1737–1739)

Proximal ulnar fracture with luxation of the radial head is known as the Monteggia lesion in the human literature. The ulnar fracture can occur anywhere from the trochlear notch to the midshaft of the ulna. The radial head usually displaces cranially and proximally. In small animals, the syndrome is thought to be caused by a severe blow to the caudal aspect of the ulna when the antebrachium is extended and bearing weight. A high incidence of concurrent radial head chip fractures (39 per cent) has been reported.

Treatment depends on the fracture configuration and the clinician's preference. Nonoperative closed reduction and external coaptation are not recommended because of the decreased elbow joint range of motion and delayed ulnar healing that commonly result. The syndrome can be divided into those cases in which the ulnar fracture is proximal and the annular ligament has ruptured and those cases in which the ulnar fracture is relatively distal and the ligament remains intact. In either situation, rapid swelling, muscle spasm, and fibrous proliferation necessitate early treatment.

If the annular ligament remains intact, as is often the case when the ulnar fracture occurs at the base or into the trochlear notch, the relationship of the radial head and the ulnar shaft remains normal. Reduction of the ulnar fracture occurs only with reduction of the radial head luxation. Stable fixation of the ulna fracture with pins and tension band wire or bone screws and plate stabilizes the radial head reduction.

If the annular ligament is ruptured, the radial head separates from the proximal ulnar shaft. This occurs when the ulnar fracture is distal to the annular ligament. Treatment requires not only reduction and stabilization of the fracture but also approximation and fixation of the normal radial and ulnar relationship.

FRACTURES OF THE RADIAL HEAD (pp. 1739–1740)

Fractures of the radial head are uncommon because the anatomy of the elbow joint predisposes to fractures of the lateral humeral condyle, sparing the radius. When fractures of the head occur, they usually involve the articular surface. Meticulous reduction and stable internal fixation are necessary to prevent secondary arthritis and joint stiffness.

The ideal method of radial head fixation is an intrafragmentary lag screw. Splitting of the fragment can be reduced by countersinking the screw head. A Steinmann pin or Kirschner wire may be needed to control rotation of the fragment around the screw. If screws are unavailable or are too large for fixation without splitting the fragment, stabilization can be achieved with multiple Kirschner wires placed at divergent angles.

If the fracture is chronic, with severe articular damage, or is not reconstructible owing to severe comminution, a salvage procedure may be necessary. Resection of the radial head has been described as treatment for lateral luxation of the radial head secondary to growth deformities in small dogs. This technique has also been cited as a potential method of treating radial head fractures. In larger, more athletic dogs, an elbow arthrodesis should be considered.

FRACTURE/SEPARATION OF THE PROXIMAL RADIAL PHYSIS (p. 1740)

FRACTURES OF EITHER THE RADIAL OR ULNAR SHAFTS (pp. 1740–1741)

Fractures of the radial or ulnar shafts with continuity of the other bone occur relatively often, particularly in young animals, with nonvehicular trauma such as horse kicks, bite wounds, and low-velocity gunshot injuries. Treatment with external coaptation in the form of a cast or splint is satisfactory in nearly all cases.

SHAFT FRACTURES OF BOTH THE RADIUS AND ULNA (pp. 1741–1745)

Fractures of both the radius and ulna are common. Selection of a fixation technique depends on a patient's age and size, axial stability of the fracture, concurrent musculoskeletal injuries, and the condition of associated soft tissues. An algorithm is presented to aid in this selection (Fig. 132–1).

FRACTURE SEPARATION OF THE DISTAL RADIAL PHYSIS (pp. 1745–1746)

Fracture separations of the distal radial physis, much like proximal physeal separations, can often be treated by closed reduction and

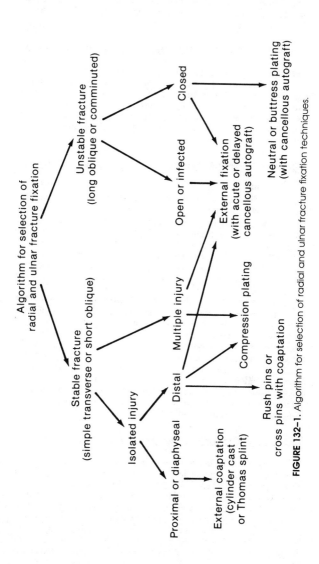

FIGURE 132–1. Algorithm for selection of radial and ulnar fracture fixation techniques.

Algorithm for selection of radial and ulnar fracture fixation

Stable fracture (simple transverse or short oblique)

Unstable fracture (long oblique or comminuted)

Isolated injury

Multiple injury

Closed

Open or infected

Proximal or diaphyseal

Distal

External coaptation (cylinder cast or Thomas splint)

Rush pins or cross pins with coaptation

Compression plating

External fixation (with acute or delayed cancellous autograft)

Neutral or buttress plating (with cancellous autograft)

579

external coaptation. If open reduction is needed, stabilization with small pins or Kirschner wires placed perpendicular to the physis is usually adequate. A caudal splint may be applied for 10 to 14 days to control rotation and limit use of the limb. As with proximal physeal injuries, the owner is advised of the possibility of premature physeal closure and secondary growth deformity.

FRACTURES OF THE DISTAL RADIUS AND ULNA (p. 1746)

Major fractures into the radial articular surface can be treated with an interfragmentary lag screw or multiple divergent Kirschner wires as described for radial head fractures. Avulsion fractures of either the radial or ulnar styloid processes result from pull on the corresponding collateral ligament. Consequently, these fractures must be accurately reduced and stabilized to regain normal antebrachial carpal joint stability.

GROWTH ABNORMALITIES OF THE ANTEBRACHIUM
(pp. 1746–1756)

Deformities of the foreleg can occur for various reasons. The two-bone system of the antebrachium is predisposed to deformity caused by continued growth of one bone after premature growth cessation of the other. Premature closure of the distal ulnar physis is a recessive inheritable trait in Skye terriers, and growth deformities have been seen with retardation of endochondral ossification in giant-breed dogs, possibly associated with osteochondrosis or nutritional deficiencies. The most common cause of premature growth cessation is trauma to one of the physeal plates.

Growth deformities of the canine antebrachium can result from injury to any one of three physes: distal ulnar, distal radial, or proximal radial. Angular deformities are seen more in the longer-limbed dogs, whereas shorter-limbed dogs develop more severe joint malarticulations. The age of the animal at the time of premature closure also affects the relative degree of deformity and joint malarticulation, perhaps because of the variation in stiffness of bone with age and the duration of altered growth until maturity. Growth deformities usually have a history of progressive limb angulation or lameness 3 to 4 weeks after forelimb trauma. Growth deformities in cats are quite uncommon; congenital agenesis of the radius has been reported.

Premature Closure of the Distal Ulnar Physis

The incidence of premature closure or fusion resulting in growth deformities is greatest in the distal ulnar growth plate of dogs. This may be due to the conical configuration of the distal ulnar physis.

Growth deformities that result from premature distal ulnar physeal closure are particularly severe because this physis contributes 75 to 85 per cent of ulnar longitudinal growth. Once the physis has fused, ulnar growth ceases and the ulna behaves like a retarding strap twisted around the radius. As the radius continues to grow, it bows away from the ulna. Three deformities of the radius result: lateral deviation (valgus), cranial bowing (curvus), and external rotation (supination). The radial head may also push the humeral condyles out of the trochlear notch of the ulna. Abnormal articulations resulting in irreversible degenerative osteoarthritis in the antebrachial carpal joint and the elbow are common sequelae. The appropriate treatment for antebrachial deformities due to premature ulnar closure depends on the patient's age and remaining growth potential.

Treatment of Distal Ulnar Physeal Closure in Immature Dogs

Animals that have a significant amount of radial growth potential remaining (usually less than 5 to 6 months of age) are treated with a technique that relieves the restraining effect of the ulna and allows the radius continued growth. Ulnar release permits lengthening of the limb and can result in partial correction of existing deformity.

The prognosis for adequate long-term function and completeness of spontaneous straightening obtained with segmental ulnar ostectomy depended on both the severity of the deformity and the remaining growth potential of the radius. Young puppies (median age of 5 months) with a valgus deformity of more than 25° and dogs near growth completion (median age of 6.5 months) with valgus deformities of more than 13° did not adequately respond to just a segmental ulnar ostectomy and required further definitive surgical treatment.

Definitive Correction of Ulnar Physeal Closure in Mature Dogs

If bone growth has ceased, definitive treatment is indicated. This treatment consists of two components if needed. The first is correction of the angular and rotational deformities. Whichever technique is used for angular deformity treatment, the correction is performed at the point of greatest curvature to provide the desired articular alignment with the best overall limb straightening.

Oblique osteotomies stabilized with external skeletal fixation result in some restoration of leg length, can be applied to short and irregular fragments, and allow significant adjustment of alignment during surgery.

Cuneiform wedge ostectomies provide a wide, flat surface for fragment contact, significantly contributing to fixation stability and bone healing. Although a wedge ostectomy does not increase the anatomical limb length, correction of the valgus deformity increases the functional length of the limb. The cuneiform ostectomy is a wedge with an angle in both the craniocaudal plane and the mediolateral plane. The angle of these wedges can be determined by drawing perpendicular lines to the long axis of the proximal and distal fragments.

The second component of treating a mature deformity is treatment of the humeroulnar subluxation by repositioning the elbow articular components. Because the affected limb is already shortened, lengthening of the ulna is more appropriate than shortening the radius.

Premature Radial Physeal Closure

Either the proximal or the distal radial physis can prematurely cease growing and cause antebrachial abnormalities. Premature closure of the proximal radial physis with continued ulnar growth results in malarticulation of the elbow joint, characterized by widening of the radial-to-humeral space and the humeral-to-anconeal joint space. Severe malformation of the articular components with secondary arthritis rapidly develops. The abnormalities that result from premature closure of the distal radial physis can be quite variable. If ulnar growth continues, the elbow malarticulation just described for proximal closures is common. If a complete symmetrical premature closure of the physis occurs, the limb may remain straight and develop a widened radial carpal joint space, or a caudal bow may develop in both the radius and ulna. More commonly, the physeal closure is asymmetrical, with bony bridging on one side of the physis and continued growth of the opposite. Premature closure of the medial side of the physis causes a varus angular deformity and occasionally inward rotation of the manus. Premature closure of the lateral side of the physis causes valgus angular deformity and external rotation, characteristic of premature distal ulnar physeal closure with which it is often concurrent.

Treatment of Radial Physeal Closure in Immature Dogs (pp. 1755–1756)

Synostosis of the Radius and Ulna in Growing Dogs

Synostosis of the radius and ulna is not a disease of the physeal growth plates but a restriction in the relative proximal movement of the ulnar shaft that normally occurs during growth. This movement reflects the virtually total contribution to ulnar length by the distal ulnar physis, while the contribution to radial length is nearly equal between the proximal and distal radial growth plates. When this movement is restricted, a relative overgrowth of the proximal radius occurs, with proximal displacement of the humeral condyles and trochlear notch deformation. Significant shortening, angular deformity, or antebrachial carpal joint alterations usually do not occur. The strong pull of the distal ulnar growth through the radioulnar ligament apparently stimulates additional growth from the distal radial physis.

Treatment of synostosis is removal of the restricting element and realignment of the elbow joint. Transfixing pins or screws are removed. Bridging callus can be resected, and the defect filled with an autogenous fat graft to prevent reformation. A dynamic proximal ulnar osteotomy is performed to treat the elbow malarticulation.

CHAPTER 133

Carpus and Digits (pages 1757–1769)

ANATOMY (pp. 1757–1759)

FRACTURES (pp. 1759–1764)

Radial Carpal Bone

Fractures of the radial carpal bone are rare. They occur most often in working dogs (e.g., sled dogs and field trial dogs) during heavy exertional activity. These fractures are usually the result of jumps or falls but may result from direct trauma.

Fractures of the radial carpal bone are usually chips or slabs involving the articular surfaces. Clinical signs depend on the severity of the fracture and degree of displacement. The lameness is severe initially but may subside in a few weeks. A dog may be sound when rested but lame after exercise.

Radiographs. The diagnosis requires a high index of suspicion, especially if the fracture is not displaced. High-quality radiographs are essential. Dorsopalmar, mediolateral, and oblique views are often required. Fractures of the radial carpal bone include chip fractures, dorsal slab fractures, body fractures, or avulsion fractures of the medial palmar prominence.

Treatment

Undisplaced or incomplete fractures may heal if the leg is coapted for 6 to 8 weeks. If the fragments are displaced, surgery is indicated. If the fragment is large, it may be reattached with a lag screw or K wires. Small chip fractures are excised if they cannot be reattached. The defect usually fills in with fibrocartilage. Carpal arthrodesis is indicated for comminuted radial carpal bone fractures and chronic radial carpal bone fractures with degenerative joint disease.

The main complication of radial carpal bone fracture is degenerative joint disease, the development and prognosis for which depend on the nature of the fracture, quality of repair, and length of time between injury and treatment. If the fracture lends itself to accurate reduction and rigid internal fixation, the prognosis is favorable. If the bone is eburnated or the fracture is chronic and arthritis is present, the prognosis is guarded or poor.

Accessory Carpal Bone

Fractures of the accessory carpal bone are uncommon except in racing greyhounds. Most accessory carpal bone fractures in greyhounds occur in the right leg. Racing in a counterclockwise direction is a contributing factor in these fractures. As a dog rounds the turns, all of the body weight is placed on the right front leg, and a fracture occurs. These fractures are classified as avulsion fractures. Other accessory carpal bone fractures usually result from a jump or fall.

In racing dogs, clinical signs are usually not apparent until the day after the injury. The dog shows a slight lameness, and swelling around the accessory carpal bone may be observed. The lameness and swelling usually subside with rest but return when the dog exercises again.

Slight hyperextension of the carpus may occur with distal ligamentous avulsion fractures. There may be decreased range of motion and pain on flexion of the joint. Conversely, normal range of motion exists with proximal tendinous avulsion fractures, along with increased soft-tissue swelling and pain on extension. An extended mediolateral radiograph distracts the fragments and enhances visibility of the fracture.

Treatment

Splints or casts rarely result in complete healing of avulsion fractures. Internal fixation of comminuted fractures is rarely feasible; these fractures are most often treated by casting the carpus in 20° of flexion.

The surgical treatment of accessory carpal bone avulsion fractures depends on the size of the fragment. If the fragment is too small to be reattached, it is excised. When the fragment is excised, successful healing depends on the ligaments becoming reattached to the bone by scar tissue. If such healing has insufficient strength, the accessory carpal bone becomes unstable and degenerative joint disease results. An animal may not return to racing with this treatment.

The prognosis for accessory carpal bone fractures depends on the type of fracture, method of treatment, and anticipated use of the dog. At one institution, less than 50 per cent of the greyhounds treated by excision of the fracture fragment won a race afterward. Repair of these fractures is a more rational approach to treatment, but there are insufficient data to support a definitive prognosis.

Ulnar and Numbered Carpal Bones (p. 1761)
Metacarpal Bone Fractures

Metacarpal bone fractures occur most commonly in young dogs or cats that have been stepped on or have had the foot trapped under a rigid object. Fractures may involve one or more metacarpal bones. Animals usually do not bear weight and are lame.

Animals with metacarpal fractures have soft-tissue swelling, pain, and crepitus over the fracture site. The skin is examined closely for penetrating wounds suggesting an open fracture. Varus or valgus deformities may be present if metacarpals II or V are fractured.

Treatment may be achieved with a cast or splint if only one or two metacarpal bones are fractured with mild displacement and if one of the main weightbearing bones (III or IV) is intact. The remaining intact bones act as internal splints to aid alignment.

Internal fixation is performed if more than two metacarpals are fractured, both metacarpals III and IV are fractured, severe displacement or comminution exists, articular surfaces are involved, or the base of metacarpal II or V is fractured. Pins and wires in a tension band or lag screws may be used to repair basilar fractures of metacarpals II and V.

Sesamoid Bones (p. 1763)

LIGAMENTOUS INJURIES (pp. 1764–1767)

Radial/Ulnar Collateral Ligaments

The radial collateral ligaments are more commonly injured than the ulnar collateral ligaments. Injuries of the ulnar collateral ligaments are reportedly less serious because they are not subject to as much tension. Most injuries to carpal ligaments result from jumps or falls, but some are due to vehicular trauma. The integrity of the collateral ligaments may be assessed by manipulating the carpus to place valgus and varus stresses on the carpus. This is done with the carpus in extension and flexion. Nonscreen or high-detail screen radiographs are necessary to confirm the diagnosis. Several views are often necessary. Widening of the joint space on the affected side may be seen on the stress views.

Primary repair of the radial collateral ligament may be possible in acute injuries. It is important to repair both the straight and oblique parts. Suture repair of the ligaments followed by appropriate splinting may be adequate, but reinforcing such a repair with synthetic material is advisable.

Palmar Ligaments and Palmar Fibrocartilage

Rupture of the palmar carpal ligaments and palmar fibrocartilage is commonly referred to as a *hyperextension injury* and is one of the more common carpal injuries. It is often thought that carpal hyperextension is the result of tendon injury, but tendons have only a minor role in supporting the palmar aspect of the carpus.

The affected carpus may be swollen. Manually extending the carpus (i.e., stressing the palmar ligaments) reveals the area of instability. Forcing a dog to stand on the leg produces the typical stance of carpal hyperextension. A stressed lateral view is the most helpful in determining the level of injury. One should try to determine what joint is involved to select the appropriate treatment. The distribution of joint involvement has been reported as antebrachiocarpal, 10 and 31 per cent; middle carpal, 50 and 22 per cent; and carpometacarpal, 40 and 47 per cent.

Splinting the carpus is usually not rewarding because randomly oriented scar tissue does not have sufficient strength to support the stress placed on the carpus.

Surgical treatment is usually more successful. Although panarthrodesis of the carpus can be used to treat all carpal hyperextension injuries, partial arthrodesis may be better for injuries involving the middle carpal and carpometacarpal joints and to maintain function of the antebrachiocarpal joint.

If hyperextension injury is at the antebrachiocarpal joint, panarthrodesis of the carpus is recommended. Although technically possible to fuse the antebrachiocarpal joint only, it is not recommended because the increased stress placed on the distal carpal joints predisposes them to injury. The prognosis after partial or complete carpal arthrodesis is favorable. Dogs compensate well for the loss of carpal motion.

FLEXOR TENDON LACERATIONS (p. 1767)

Severance of the digital flexor tendons is generally the result of laceration by sharp objects. Hemorrhage may be profuse, and the skin and other surrounding soft tissues are commonly traumatized. The superficial and deep digital flexor tendons insert on the proximal ends of the second and third phalanges, respectively.

In acute tendon laceration, the cut ends of the tendons may be visible. Laceration of the superficial digital flexor tendon may have little functional or physical consequence. However, complete severance of both the superficial and deep digital flexor tendons results in palmigrade positioning of one or more digits, especially during weight-bearing.

Acute lacerations of the flexor tendons with minimal contamination may be definitively repaired if surgery is performed within 4 to 6 hours. Older injuries or those that are severely contaminated or infected are treated by surgical débridement and proper open wound management until the tissues are healthy.

Complications include breakdown of the repair as a result of excessive tension on the anastomosis, infection, and adhesions of the tendons to surrounding soft tissues. The prognosis for acute injuries with minimal tension on the anastomosis is generally favorable but for massive injuries with excessive tension or chronic injuries is guarded to poor.

SHEARING INJURIES (pp. 1767–1768)

CARPAL LAXITY SYNDROME IN YOUNG DOGS (p. 1768)

CHAPTER 134

Pelvic Fractures (pages 1769–1786)

Approximately 25 per cent of all fractures involve the pelvis. The majority of pelvic fractures are multiple because of the boxlike configuration of the pelvis and the short, strong musculotendinous support of the osseous structures. Because of the tendency toward multiple fractures and the degree of trauma necessary to fracture the pelvis or cause a fracture-dislocation, adjacent soft tissue and surrounding organ systems must be carefully evaluated.

Injury to the genitourinary organs is suspected in a patient with pelvic fracture if the patient is unable to void or has hematuria or a bloody urethral discharge. Rupture of the urethra is more common in male dogs. Ureteral avulsion and urinary bladder rupture occur with equal frequency in males and females.

PHYSICAL EXAMINATION (pp. 1770–1771)

Patients that have sustained trauma of sufficient magnitude to fracture the pelvis are exposed to a high risk of associated injuries.

Extensive palpation and manipulation of the pelvis are unnecessary, because diagnostic radiographs are taken. A greater trochanter that is difficult to palpate and seems medially displaced, with crepitus, decreased rotation, and pain elicited by manipulation suggests an impacted acetabular fracture. Dorsal and cranial displacement of the greater trochanter is associated with a coexisting craniodorsal hip luxation, whereas dorsal displacement alone is more compatible with a femoral neck fracture, capital physeal separation, or a combination of femoral head or neck fracture and avulsion of the greater trochanter. Cranial displacement of the iliac crest occurs with sacroiliac separations and sacral fractures. Severe bruising and inability to palpate the ventral abdominal wall occur with rupture of the prepubic tendon or avulsion fracture of the pubis.

Finally, a rectal examination is gently performed. If this procedure is unusually painful for the animal, a sacral or coccygeal fracture is suspected. Blood on the examining finger is presumptive evidence of rectal injury. During rectal palpation of a male dog, the prostate is sought; if it is not palpable, a tear in the pelvic urethra may be assumed.

Evidence of genitourinary damage is confirmed by radiography. A retrograde urethrogram is obtained before catheterization of the bladder. If the urethra is lacerated or separated, catheterization may introduce infection into the pelvic hematoma, add to the trauma of the injured urethra, and fail to reveal an incomplete urethral injury. If the urethra is intact, a cystogram is performed, including a postevacuation film. Intravenous pyelography is used to evaluate the upper urinary tract.

Once the general examination is over, the animal is carefully raised to a standing position. Most of the weight on the rear limbs is borne by the examiner. Conscious proprioception is evaluated, but musculoskeletal pain may render the test useless. The most important criterion is the presence of pain in the distal extremity, acknowledged by cerebral recognition. Femoral and sciatic responses are checked. The absence of sensation in the lateral digits implies sciatic injury due to nerve root avulsion, sacroiliac luxation, acetabular fracture, or a proximal third femoral fracture. Anesthesia of the medial digit and inability to lock the stifle in extension are evidence of femoral nerve injury and possibly a lower lumbar fracture.

TREATMENT PLAN (pp. 1771–1783)

Conservative treatment is used for animals with little or no displacement of the fracture segments, an intact acetabulum, and essentially intact continuity of the pelvic ring. Conservatively treated pelvic fractures almost always heal. Unfortunately, many pelvic fractures are treated conservatively because of the tired old axiom that "the fractures will heal and your dog will be a functional pet." If one critically assesses these dogs months and years after injury, many are not functioning as well as expected. Patients *correctly selected* for conservative management of pelvic fractures generally do well.

A successful conservative regimen consists of confinement, comfortable quarters, restricted and supervised exercise, and attention to hydration, alimentation, urination, and defecation. A padded area with easy access to water and food is provided. Because of musculoskeletal pain due to the fracture, dogs lie continuously on the unaffected side and may develop decubital ulcers. Hydrotherapy helps relieve aches and pains from bruised muscles and healing areas.

An animal with a minimally displaced unilateral caudal acetabular fracture with an intact contralateral hemipelvis is a candidate for a nonweightbearing sling. A figure-eight (Ehmer) sling is not necessary, because a neutral position of the hip is preferred. The sling is maintained for 10 to 14 days, the toes are checked carefully for swelling during this time, and the dog is gradually returned to normal activity during the following 2 to 3 weeks.

Renal function is monitored and assisted if necessary. Water intake may be limited because of reluctance to move around, and urination may be difficult because of inability to posture and reluctance to break house training. For the same reasons, constipation may develop, necessitating enemas, laxatives, or suppositories.

Surgical Therapy

The criteria for prompt surgical intervention are (1) marked decrease in the size of the pelvic canal, (2) fracture of the acetabulum (displacement of articular surfaces), (3) instability of the hip (fracture of the ilium, ischium, and pubis on the same side; segmental or Malgaigne fracture), and (4) unilateral or bilateral instability, particularly if accompanied by coxofemoral dislocation or other limb fractures.

Early surgical treatment of pelvic fractures is encouraged. Concomitant pelvic stabilization may reduce damage to the lumbosacral plexus, diminish hemorrhage, and prevent further genitourinary trauma. Surgical repair is attempted as soon as feasible for the condition of the animal, preferably within 4 days of injury. Each additional day considerably increases the effort and iatrogenic trauma necessary for repair. After 8 or 9 days, reduction of major iliac shaft fractures in large dogs is almost impossible.

Iliac Fractures

Acetabular Fractures

Open reduction is indicated for acetabular fractures of the cranial and middle thirds of the articular surface. Most weightbearing occurs on the cranial two-thirds of the acetabulum. Cranial and medially displaced caudal third fractures are repaired because the caudal buttress of the acetabulum is usually in contact with the femoral head.

Minimally displaced fractures, especially of the caudal third of the dome, are treated by confining the dog for 3 or 4 weeks. Preferably, a nonweightbearing sling is used with confinement to minimize motion at the fracture site. The sling maintains the hip joint in a neutral position, and no attempt is made to internally rotate or flex the hip as with the Ehmer sling. Owners are advised that some degree of secondary degenerative joint disease will develop. In 15 dogs with nonsurgically treated caudal third acetabular fractures, evaluated from 6 to 67 months after injury, 13 dogs had radiographic evidence of moderate to severe osteoarthrosis. Twelve dogs had decreased range of motion or pain in the affected hip, and seven dogs were lame. Surgical repair of these fractures is difficult, and most surgeons treat them conservatively.

Open reduction and fixation of acetabular fractures pose a challenge. The prognosis depends on the type of fracture, the amount of damage to the weightbearing surface, the degree of persistent displacement or incongruity of the articular surface, and the presence or absence of other pelvic fractures. Whenever dislocation or instability of fracture segments is present, surgical repair is advised to decrease the severity and extent of the osteoarthritis that inevitably develops. Crepitus is usually felt when the hip is manipulated. Regardless of the plan, the priority sequence is the patient first, the limb second, and the fracture third. With concomitant limb injury, more important fractures may pre-empt definitive repair of the acetabular fracture. An attempt is always made to first repair the fracture that affords a patient the most benefit.

Acetabular fractures have been classified into four groups according to the course of the fracture line—cranial, central, caudal, and comminuted. Central transacetabular fractures occur most commonly, with comminuted transacetabular fractures second in frequency. In addition to standard views, an oblique lateral view with the upper unaffected limb abducted and pulled caudally prevents superimposition of structures and aids in defining comminuted acetabular fractures.

The principles and goals of articular surgery are anatomical reduction of the articular surfaces, rigid reduction, and early return to full function. These principles must be adhered to for successful results with repair of acetabular fractures.

Ischial Fractures

Isolated ischial fractures are uncommon and seldom need surgical repair. When ischial fractures accompany other pelvic fractures, stabilization and reduction of the major fragments usually result in acceptable reduction and stabilization of the ischial fracture. When the ischial fragment is large and isolated from the rest of the pelvis, the resulting instability justifies correction. Conservative therapy consists of confinement and a nonweightbearing sling in a neutral position.

Sacroiliac Joint Fracture-Luxation

Unilateral separation of the sacroiliac joint is much more common than bilateral luxation. Because of the geometry of the pelvis, unilateral displacement cannot occur without associated fractures or a pelvic symphyseal separation. Surgery is indicated for fractures with marked instability, pain, or bilateral instability.

After operation, a dog is in much less pain and can be rehabilitated more quickly. Exercise is limited for 4 to 6 weeks to decrease mechanical force on the screws and to permit a strong soft-tissue repair, because bone-to-bone union does not occur. Dogs are observed for sciatic nerve dysfunction after operation, because the sciatic nerve passes just ventral to the lateral aspect of the body of the sacrum. Sacral nerve injuries may be evidenced by abnormal urination or defecation.

Pubic Fractures and Pelvic Symphyseal Separation

Pubic fractures commonly accompany other pelvic fractures. Stabilization of the major segments usually provides adequate reduction and stability for the pubic fractures. Damage to the genitourinary system may result from pubic bone fracture or separation-displacement of the pelvic symphysis. Marked cranial displacement of the pubic brim suggests an avulsion fracture associated with the prepubic tendon. In these cases, the inguinal and groin area usually is severely bruised. Caudal ventral hernias are common with this particular injury.

COMPLICATIONS OF PELVIC FRACTURES (pp. 1783–1785)

Major complications may arise during conservative or surgical treatment of pelvic fractures. They stem from associated soft-tissue or multiorgan trauma. The importance of a thorough history and physical examination cannot be overemphasized. Serial monitoring of vital functions for several days is equally important. Traumatic myocarditis may not appear for 48 to 72 hours after trauma. Because of the strong muscular support of the pelvis, surgical intervention is needed within 2 to 4 days of injury. Reduction, especially in large dogs, becomes increasingly difficult with each passing day. Unfortunately, pulse deficits, a ruptured bladder, and occasionally a diaphragmatic hernia may not be diagnosed initially. Peripheral nerve injury is always a concern with craniomedial displacement of iliac bone fragments and cranial displacement of the ilium with sacroiliac fracture-dislocation. In one series, 11 per cent of dogs and cats with these injuries had peripheral nerve injury. Eighty-one per cent had good or excellent limb function 16 weeks after the peripheral nerve injury was sustained.

ADVANTAGES OF PELVIC FRACTURE REPAIR (p. 1785)

Dogs with repaired pelvic fractures convalesce and rehabilitate more rapidly and completely than those treated conservatively. Musculoskeletal function is better in surgically treated dogs. Clients are generally pleased with the results, and hospitalization and nursing care are less than required for conservative treatment. An important factor is the reduced morbidity from concomitant injuries and associated complications such as pressure sores, pulmonary problems in recumbent animals, and urine or fecal soilage.

CHAPTER 135
The Hip Joint (pages 1786–1805)

The hip is a ball-and-socket joint in which a hemispherical femoral head fits into an ellipsoid acetabular socket within the pelvic bone.

The femoral neck joins the shaft of the femur at an angle of 146.2° (SD 4.8°). This angle has been called the *cervicofemoral angle* or the *angle of inclination* and may be defined as the angle formed at the intersection between the femoral neck axis and the femoral shaft axis on a ventrodorsal radiograph. This measurement depends on the technique of measurement, positioning, and the angle of femoral torsion. As the angle of femoral torsion increases, the apparent angle of inclination increases. An increased apparent angle of inclination may be due to increased femoral torsion, an actual increase in inclination, or a combination of both. When the angle of inclination is corrected for femoral torsion, the range has been reported as 137° to 155°, with a mean of 144.7°. The angle between the plane of the femoral condyles and the axis of the femoral neck is the torsion or declination angle. In dogs, the axis of the femoral neck normally projects cranial to the transcondylar plane. The angle of torsion is positive and is called *anteversion*. Similarly, if the axis projects caudally, the angle of torsion is negative and is called *retroversion*. The normal angle ranges from $+12°$ to $+40°$, with a mean of $+27°$ when measured by direct radiographic technique. A method of indirect measurement using trigonometry and biplanar radiography has demonstrated a normal femoral torsion angle of 18° to 47°, with a mean of 31°. The angle of inclination is not a factor in the development of hip dysplasia in dogs, although some dogs with hip dysplasia have an increased angle of inclination.

The fit of the femoral head within the acetabulum can be estimated from a ventrodorsal radiograph of the pelvis by measuring the Norberg angle. This angle is defined by a line connecting the centers of the femoral heads and a second line from the centers of the femoral heads to the cranial acetabular rims. An angle less than 105° indicates displacement of the femoral head relative to the acetabulum and implies hip dysplasia.

SURGICAL APPROACHES TO THE HIP (pp. 1789–1793)

MANAGEMENT OF HIP DYSPLASIA (pp. 1793–1801)

Canine hip dysplasia is a complex disease characterized by primary hip joint laxity in immature animals, resulting in malarticulation and secondary development of degenerative joint disease. The available treatments for hip dysplasia vary widely and depend on the age of the animal, desired function, pathological condition of the joint, and financial resources of the owner.

Conservative Therapy

A recommendation of conservative therapy in the management of hip dysplasia may be made in immature animals after the diagnosis of hip joint laxity has been verified by physical examination and subluxation of the femoral head has been confirmed by radiographic examination. Similarly, it may be recommended in mature animals with evidence of compromised hip joint function associated with advanced degenerative changes. The primary goals of therapy are to alleviate discomfort and maintain function. Many dogs may live a reasonably comfortable life despite advanced degenerative joint disease. If an animal is overweight, recommendations include weight loss to decrease the load across the hip joints. The judicious use of analgesics may help ameliorate pain. Although analgesics may alleviate pain, they do not alter the degenerative changes that occur in the coxofemoral joint. Nonsteroidal anti-inflammatory drugs (NSAIDs) are the most widely recommended analgesics in the treatment of dysplasia. Acetylsalicylic acid is given (10 to 20 mg/kg PO TID) as necessary. Other orally administered NSAIDs, including phenylbutazone and meclofenamic acid, have been recommended. All NSAIDs have a potential side effect of gastrointestinal irritation and generally are administered with a small quantity of food.

Nonconcussive exercise such as swimming may help maintain muscle mass and joint function without overstressing the hip joints. Highly traumatic exercises including running and jumping may exacerbate discomfort and are not recommended.

Surgical Therapy

Palliative

Transection of the pectineal muscle or tendon has been recommended for the treatment of hip dysplasia in dogs and cats. Generally, this procedure has found merit in immature animals with pain due to subluxation and little or no evidence of degenerative joint changes. The procedure does not improve joint stability, and the effect is temporary. An unstable joint eventually progresses to an osteoarthritic joint, and pain usually recurs. Performance of myotomy versus myectomy or tenectomy seems to have little bearing on the ability of this operation to reduce discomfort. The clinical benefits of this procedure are difficult to predict but generally are related to the degree of degenerative changes in the hip joint at surgery. In animals with an unstable joint and mild degenerative changes, the results are favorable. As the degenerative changes become more severe, the results of this procedure are inconsistent.

The purpose of a pectineal myectomy is to release one of the adductor muscles and allow increased abduction of the femur. Theoretically, spasm of the pectineal muscle could create an upward force on the femoral head, driving it against the dorsal acetabular rim. Although pectineal muscle fiber hypotrophy has been verified in dogs with hip dysplasia, a cause-and-effect relationship has not been established. This procedure is not recommended as a substitute for a corrective osteotomy; however, it may provide temporary relief from pain.

Preventive Procedures

Reconstructive osteotomies of the femur or pelvis have been advocated to increase the stability of the hip joint in immature animals by bringing the femur and acetabulum into closer apposition. Secondarily, these procedures prevent the development or slow the progression of degenerative changes in the hip joint by providing a more congruent articulation. A femoral osteotomy can be performed to place the proximal femur in a varus position (angle of inclination < 145°) and to correct excess anteversion. A pelvic osteotomy allows rotation of the acetabulum over the femoral head to increase dorsal coverage.

Intertrochanteric Osteotomy. *Femoral osteotomy* is usually performed in the intertrochanteric region to correct the angle of inclination or the angle of femoral torsion. A decrease in the angle of inclination to a varus position decreases the hip joint force and abductor force, allowing better centering of the femoral head within the acetabulum and decreasing the abnormal loading of the dorsal acetabular rim that is evident with subluxation. The procedure is recommended in young growing dogs that have radiographic evidence of subluxation and have either an increased angle of inclination or an increased angle of femoral torsion or both. It is not recommended as the treatment of choice in animals that have subluxation and severe acetabular dysplasia. Femoral osteotomy is most effective if performed before the development of degenerative changes in the hip joint. The procedure is recommended at the level of the lesser trochanter so that the femoral malformation can be corrected proximally, without changing the shape of the femoral diaphysis.

Pelvic Osteotomy. An *osteotomy* is performed on the *ilium, ischium,* and *pubis* so that the acetabular segment of the pelvis can be rotated over the top of the femoral head to increase its dorsal coverage. The optimum rotation has not been determined; however, it is readily accepted that excessive rotation compromises extension and abduction of the hindlimb by impinging the femoral neck on the acetabular rim. The amount of rotation necessary to cover the femoral head adequately has been calculated from radiographs, estimated by measuring the angles of reduction and subluxation on physical examination, and determined by direct observation at surgery. Acetabular rotation of 20° to 30° is adequate for most cases, except for those with extreme subluxation. Pelvic osteotomy alone is not recommended if there is an increase in the angle of inclination or femoral torsion. A femoral osteotomy is first necessary to correct these abnormalities. As in a femoral osteotomy, a pelvic osteotomy appears to be most effective in young growing animals with subluxation and minimal evidence of degenerative changes in the hip joint. The procedure has been recommended in mature animals with minimal degenerative changes and has been used in animals with severe osteoarthritis. The results have been less encouraging in these latter two situations.

Salvage

Femoral Head and Neck Excision. Femoral head and neck excision or excision arthroplasty is a salvage procedure in the coxofemoral joint for hip dysplasia; degenerative joint disease; Legg-Calvé-Perthes disease; irreparable fractures of the femoral head, neck, or acetabulum; recurrent luxations; and failed total hip replacements. Although long-term follow-ups on clinical cases have been evaluated subjectively through client questionnaires and physical examinations, the degree of pain associated with the procedure is unclear. Most reports describe evidence of some long-term functional impairment, which may vary from a mild lameness after excessive exercise to intermittent nonweightbearing. Muscle atrophy, limb shortening, and reduction of hip extension are commonly observed, even after extended follow-up periods. The average time to leg use after the surgery is approximately 5 weeks. Return to normal function may take considerably longer. When femoral head and neck excision was performed on dogs with normal hip conformation, objective gait analysis revealed that the dogs had not returned to normal function 16 weeks after the procedure.

Femoral head and neck excision is a viable salvage procedure, with limitations. One should not expect an affected joint to function normally afterward. Providing the physical demands placed on the animal are not extreme, adequate functional results for the majority of patients can be expected. Interpositional materials have been recommended to decrease bone-to-bone contact and to improve the recovery rate. These materials include joint capsule, fat, fascia, and deep gluteal and biceps femoris muscle slings. Although subjective evaluations of muscle slings have been encouraging, objective assessment of function has not demonstrated conclusive benefits from their use.

After surgery, passive physiotherapy consisting of gentle flexion and extension is begun as soon as the animal allows it. Analgesics may be necessary in the immediate postoperative period to control pain. Swimming and slow leash walking are encouraged within the first week.

Total Hip Replacement. Total hip replacement has become a viable alternative to femoral head and neck excision for the treatment of degenerative joint disease, hip dysplasia, chronic hip luxation, and irreparable fractures of the coxofemoral joint in medium-sized to large dogs.

HIP DISLOCATION (pp. 1801–1804)

The hip is the most commonly luxated joint in small animals. The most common cause of acquired hip luxation is trauma, with motor vehicle accidents accounting for approximately 60 per cent. The majority of hip luxations are craniodorsal, presumably because of the type of injury and contraction of the gluteal muscles, which are strong extensors and abductors of the hip joint. The hip occasionally luxates caudoventrally, with displacement of the femoral head into the obturator foramen, or rarely caudodorsally. Caudoventral luxations are more commonly associated with falls. Invariably, the ligament of the head of the femur and the joint capsule are torn, permitting luxation. The deep gluteal muscle is closely applied to the dorsal joint capsule and is often damaged in dorsal luxations. Avulsion of the ligament from the femoral head may include a fragment of bone. Erosion of the articular cartilage of the femoral head is commonly associated with chronic luxation and rubbing of the femoral head against the ilium.

Hip luxation is suspected when an animal has a nonweightbearing lameness of the hindlimb and a history of trauma. The limb is usually held adducted, with some external rotation if the luxation is craniodorsal. If the luxation is caudoventral, the limb is usually held abducted, with internal rotation. Physical examination may reveal pain and crepitus on flexion and extension of the hip joint. In a craniodorsal luxation, dorsal displacement of the greater trochanter may be palpated in reference to the ischial tuberosity and the cranial dorsal iliac spine. Placing the thumb between the greater trochanter and ischial tuberosity and externally rotating the femur causes impingement of the thumb in a normal hip. Caudal extension of the hindlimbs may suggest a relative shortening of the affected limb if the luxation is craniodorsal. Radiographic examination is necessary to confirm the diagnosis. Ventrodorsal and lateral projections are made to evaluate luxation; the presence or absence of avulsion fractures of the femoral head; concomitant femoral neck, femoral head, or acetabular fractures; and degenerative joint disease.

Closed reduction is the treatment of choice for most cases of acquired hip luxation. Indications for open reduction include avulsion fractures of the femoral head; fractures of the femoral neck, greater trochanter, or acetabulum; and unsuccessful closed reductions. Advanced hip dysplasia or degenerative joint disease may preclude successful closed reduction. The majority of successful closed reductions are performed within 10 days of luxation. If the luxation is not treated, a false joint forms, resulting in various degrees of dysfunction.

In recurrent luxation, after open and closed methods of treatment or when irreparable femoral head or acetabular fractures are present, a salvage procedure (femoral head and neck excision or total hip replacement) is recommended.

CHAPTER 136

Fractures of the Femur
(pages 1805–1817)

Because of the proximity of the femur to the trunk, the heavy surrounding musculature, and the complexity of many fractures, adequate alignment and stabilization are difficult if not impossible to achieve by external fixation. The high incidence of internal fixation as the preferred treatment is reflected in studies that report the femur as the most common site of nonunion and osteomyelitis. This high rate of complications demonstrates inadequacies in commonly used methods of repair and frequency of errors in surgical judgement, especially in respect to surgical treatment of complicated femoral fractures.

Because of the heavy surrounding muscle mass and the difficulty in immobilizing the proximal segment and the hip, temporary support or stabilization with a padded bandage (Robert Jones), coaptation splint, or a Schroeder-Thomas splint is not indicated in most cases. Restriction of activity by cage confinement is the most prudent method for protecting the fracture and surrounding soft tissue from further injury.

Growth

The physes of the femoral head and greater trochanter contribute approximately 30 to 40 per cent of the longitudinal growth of the femur. The exact time of physeal closure varies, with most studies reporting beginning closure at approximately 6 months and complete closure between 9 and 12 months. From a clinical viewpoint, the time of closure is not nearly as important as the percentage of remaining growth at any given age. At 5 months, 80 per cent of the proximal femoral physeal growth is completed, and by 7 months, 95 per cent of skeletal growth is completed.

Capital Epiphyseal Fractures (Avulsion Fractures of the Femoral Head)

Avulsion fractures of the femoral head occur most often with coxofemoral luxations in immature animals. In most cases, the small, predominately cartilaginous segment is simply excised with the attached ligament of the head of the femur before reduction of the femoral head. Rarely the avulsed segment is large, with substantial subchondral bone. In these cases, excision of the fragment leaves a major defect in the ventral third to half of the femoral head and predisposes the joint to arthritic changes. Alternative treatment considerations include internal fixation, excision arthroplasty, and hip prosthesis. Internal fixation is preferred, but the procedure is technically demanding.

Capital Physeal Fractures

The physis is the weak point of the immature skeleton, and trauma frequently results in fractures at this site rather than dislocation. Capital physeal fractures are the most common fracture of the proximal femur and are observed in animals between 4 and 11 months of age, with the highest incidence between 6 and 8 months. Most are Salter-Harris type I.

Avascular necrosis of the femoral head is uncommon when the fracture is treated properly by internal fixation. Excision arthroplasty is most justified with chronic injuries and in complex fractures with comminution of the head or neck or both. Internal fixation is not delayed, because remodeling of the neck produces an incongruent, unstable reduction. Multiple small pins or Kirschner wires are most frequently used to stabilize the small epiphyseal segment (femoral head) and offer a simple, comparatively atraumatic technique. Compression screw fixation has been advocated to increase stabilization and promote revascularization. Compression of the physis in an actively growing animal younger than 5 months may promote physeal closure and deformity of the proximal femur.

Femoral Neck Fractures

Fractures of the femoral neck occur predominately in mature animals. Femoral neck fractures are subdivided according to specific location into subcapital, transcervical, and basilar and according to their relationship to the joint capsule into intracapsular (medial) and extracapsular (lateral). These subdivisions are of little clinical value because all neck fractures are treated by similar surgical techniques. Most fractures are basilar and frequently accompany trochanteric and subtrochanteric fractures.

Techniques using lag screws or Kirschner wires are used for internal fixation. Compression screw fixation offers the most rigid stabilization and is preferred in large dogs. Multiple small pins provide satisfactory fixation in small and medium-sized animals. Femoral head and neck excision is always an option and is most indicated in irreparable comminuted fractures.

Greater Trochanter Fractures

Fractures of the greater trochanter are uncommon and occur most frequently at the physis in conjunction with capital physeal fractures. This fracture in mature animals may occur with fractures of the femoral neck or dislocations of the hip. The greater trochanter is subjected to tractional forces from the gluteal muscles and compression forces from the vastus lateralis muscle. Although fixation with a compression screw or multiple small pins and tension band wire is recommended, interfragmentary compression is not always required to provide adequate stabilization of this broad-based angular fracture of trabecular bone.

Fractures in immature animals are treated satisfactorily with multiple Kirschner wires directed diagonally into the medial cortex of the proximal metaphysis and diaphysis. Tension band wire is optional but should be used to increase stabilization when needed without fear of producing substantial functional disturbances due to premature closure of the physis. In mature animals, interfragmentary compression with multiple pins and tension band wire or a compression screw is recommended.

The prognosis for a return to normal function is favorable, but guarded for normal development of the greater trochanter in immature animals. Deformities reported from premature closure of the trochanteric physis include shortened trochanter, coxa valga, and elongated or narrowed femoral neck. These changes generally do not affect limb function.

Subtrochanteric Fractures

Subtrochanteric fractures are uncommon and are most often observed with multiple fractures of the proximal femur. Repair of such fractures can be difficult because of the frequency of comminution, involvement of the femoral neck, comparatively short proximal segment, large medullary canal, and tapered contour of the subtrochanteric region.

Bone plating techniques (compression, neutralization, buttress) provide rigid stabilization of the fracture and are especially indicated in large dogs and comminuted fractures.

Intramedullary fixation has more application in simple transverse, oblique, and spiral fractures, especially in small and medium-sized animals. With simple fractures, a stable anatomical reduction, and proper aftercare, the prognosis for a return to normal function is favorable. Comminuted fractures offer the greatest challenge and have a more guarded prognosis.

FEMORAL DIAPHYSIS (pp. 1810–1813)

Three general groups of fractures occur: transverse, oblique/spiral, and comminuted. Open fractures are rare because of the heavy surrounding musculature. The type of fracture is important in considering the forces that must be neutralized by internal fixation.

Treatment of Diaphyseal Fractures

Diaphyseal fractures of the femur are noted for substantial displacement and over-riding of the fracture segments. The distal segment is usually displaced and pulled caudomedially into the adductor and hamstring muscle groups by the gastrocnemius muscle, and the proximal segment is pulled cranially and rotated externally by the iliopsoas and external hip rotators.

Alignment and stabilization necessary for rapid bone healing and return to function are difficult if not impossible to achieve using external splintage. Conservative treatment (Schroeder-Thomas splint, coaptation splints, cage rest) usually results in side-to-side healing, deformity, and substantial shortening of the limb. Although not the ideal method of treatment, conservative treatment may produce acceptable functional results when recommended internal fixation techniques are not accepted by the owner. Caution must be observed with immobilization of the limb in immature animals because irreversible muscle and stifle joint changes may develop (hyperextended stifle, quadriceps contracture).

Transverse Fractures

Intramedullary pinning is a practical and economical method of treating transverse diaphyseal fractures of the femur, but the detrimental force of rotation is not neutralized with single-pin fixation. Type I external fixators are the most effective technique for controlling rotation. An alternative technique is to use multiple intramedullary pins.

Compression plating is most indicated in large mature dogs but is considered in any mature animal in which a rapid return to normal function is desirable.

Oblique/Spiral Fracture

With oblique and spiral fractures, satisfactory alignment and stabilization can be achieved by combining various internal fixation techniques.

Intramedullary pinning combined with transcortical pins and full-cerclage or hemicerclage wire is the simplest method of treatment and provides adequate stabilization in many cases.

Interfragmentary compression screws, used in conjunction with a bone plate (neutralization plating), provide rigid fixation and accurate alignment with minimal fracture gap.

Comminuted Fractures

These complex fractures require sophisticated repair techniques capable of resisting compression, shear, rotation, and bending. Rebuilding the fracture so that all fragments are accurately aligned and gaps are eliminated is often impossible. Malalignment and substantial osseous defects decrease stabilization and shift stresses from the bone to the appliance, predisposing to failure. Inadequate fixation, extensive soft-tissue damage, and a loss of periosteal and medullary blood supply predispose this type of fracture to nonunion or osteomyelitis or both.

Intramedullary fixation supplemented with full-cerclage wires, as well as transcortical pins, may be used to treat comminuted femoral diaphyseal fractures. Best results with pin and wire fixation are expected when the fragments are large enough to permit anatomical reconstruction.

Bone plating provides the most rigid fixation and is most indicated in mature dogs of large and giant breeds. Fixation of the plate with at least three screws (cortices) in each main segment is desirable and often requires a plate that extends most of the bone length. Cancellous bone grafts promote healing of comminuted diaphyseal fractures and are considered mandatory when substantial gaps are present.

A number of variables affect the prognosis, including signalment, severity of comminution, surgical technique (time, sterility, trauma, alignment, fixation), and patient care. A guarded prognosis is rendered in most cases.

Postoperative Care

Postoperative care is very important and is most critical with comminuted fractures. Restriction to house and leash activity is recommended for at least 4 to 6 weeks. Uncontrolled activity is not allowed until radiographic examination demonstrates adequate bone healing.

DISTAL FEMORAL FRACTURES (pp. 1813–1817)

Fracture Classification

Fractures of the distal femur are classified as metaphyseal, physeal, and epiphyseal. A rigid classification is difficult to establish because of the anatomical and structural differences between mature and immature animals. The term *supracondylar* has referred to both metaphyseal and physeal fractures.

Metaphyseal Fractures

Metaphyseal fractures occur most frequently in mature animals but are not a common fracture. Transverse and mildly comminuted fractures are most common at this junctional area between the (cortical) diaphysis and (cancellous) epiphysis. The short distal segment and the large medullary canal present problems in stabilization for both intramedullary pinning and bone plating.

A single pin, multiple pins, and Rush pins are used for intramedullary fixation. Multiple pins or pins used according to the Rush pin principles provide greater stabilization and are preferred over a single pin.

Bone plating provides the most rigid fixation and is the preferred method of repair for large dogs and for transverse and comminuted fractures. Plate fixation to the short distal segment with three screws may be impossible, and cancellous bone screws are generally used because of the thin cortex and abundant trabecular bone.

The metaphysis has a rich blood supply and source of osteogenic cells. With adequate stabilization of the fracture, bone healing occurs very rapidly. Improper seating of a single intramedullary pin with inadequate stabilization is a common cause of complications.

Physeal Fractures

Most physeal fractures in dogs are Salter-Harris type II. Cats have a high occurrence of Salter-Harris type I. Types III and IV are rare in both species. Type V, compression fractures, may occur in conjunction with any of the other physeal fractures and contribute to growth retardation. The degree of retardation is related to the age of the animal, the method of repair, and the amount of trauma to the physis (type of fracture) and surrounding soft tissue.

Salter-Harris Types I and II and Supracondylar Fractures

The method of treatment should provide sufficient stabilization to allow early use of the leg and should have minimal effect on physeal growth. Anatomical reduction of the fracture is preferred. The protuberances from the metaphyseal segment interdigitate with the corresponding fossae in the epiphyseal segment and contribute to stabilization.

Internal fixation is usually required. Popular methods include single intramedullary pin, double intramedullary pins, Rush pins, and cross pins. External immobilization with a flexion (Ehmer) sling and Schroeder-Thomas splint has been used successfully, but irreversible joint and muscle changes (quadriceps contracture, hyperextended stifle) are major concerns.

Interference with growth is a consideration in immature animals with substantial remaining potential, but its importance overall has probably been overemphasized. Premature closure of the physis commonly occurs as a result of initial trauma regardless of the method of treatment; most physeal fractures occur in animals over 5 months of age that have achieved 80 per cent of their skeletal growth; dogs can lose at least 20 per cent of their total femoral length without substantial functional impairment. In dogs younger than 4 to 5 months, interference with growth is a factor in selecting the method of repair.

Single intramedullary pins are most indicated in small to medium-sized animals and in animals 3 to 4 months of age with substantial remaining growth. Double pins, Rush pins, and cross pins provide more than one point of fixation, increasing stabilization. These techniques are especially indicated for fractures in large dogs.

The age of the animal and the rich blood supply and osteogenic tissue contribute to rapid bone healing. Premature closure of the physis is common and may be promoted by surgical repair. Uniform shortening of the femur rarely causes substantial impairment of function. Complications (quadriceps contracture, hyperextended stifle) due to voluntary or forced immobilization of the stifle are of most concern.

Salter-Harris Types III and IV and Intercondylar Fractures

Salter-Harris types III and IV and intercondylar fractures of mature animals are treated in the same manner. The collateral and cruciate ligaments remain attached to the fractured condyle and maintain some degree of alignment.

Simple intercondylar fractures most often involve the medial condyle. Multiple Kirschner wires, compression screws, and various combinations of the two are used for fixation. Multiple pins provide sufficient fixation in immature animals and small dogs and cats. Compression screw fixation provides the most rigid fixation and is necessary for fractures in medium and large dogs.

Fractures of both condyles (T-Y) are treated by intercondylar fixation with compression screws or Kirschner wires and fixation of the repaired epiphyseal segment to the metaphysis with Rush pins, double pins, or cross pins.

Epiphyseal Fractures

Transcondylar fractures of the epiphysis are rare and occur most frequently in mature chondrodysplastic dogs. These fractures traverse the epiphysis (condyles) close to the intercondylar notch and involve the trochlear groove. An intercondylar component (T fracture) and fragmentation of the trochlear ridges are often present but may not be visible with radiography. Close proximity to the intercondylar notch prevents intercondylar stabilization with a compression screw. Fixation is achieved with multiple Kirschner wires placed through the articular surface of the condyle and into the metaphysis. The pins are set below the articular cartilage.

CHAPTER 137

Stifle Joint (pages 1817–1865)

ANATOMY AND BIOMECHANICS (pp.1817–1824)

The stifle is a complex hinge joint with two functionally distinct articulations. Weightbearing occurs primarily through the articulation between the femoral and tibial condyles. The femoropatellar articulation greatly increases the mechanical efficiency of the quadriceps muscle group and facilitates extensor function.

Stifle Joint Motion

Flexion and extension occur in the sagittal plane, with the normal range of motion being about 140°. Simple uniplanar rotation about a stationary axis does not occur. With flexion, the lateral collateral ligament relaxes and allows the lateral femoral condyle to displace caudally, resulting in internal rotation of the tibia. A small amount of craniocaudal motion also occurs in the sagittal plane as a result of the cam shape of the femoral condyles.

Slight varus (medial) and valgus (lateral) movement of the tibia occurs in the transverse plane. The collateral ligaments are responsible for limiting this motion in the extended joint; with flexion, the cruciate ligaments also contribute to the control of varus and valgus motion.

Excessive joint motion is prevented not only by the ligamentous constraints of the stifle joint but also by a complex system of reflex arcs that involves the major muscle groups around the stifle.

CRANIAL CRUCIATE LIGAMENT RUPTURE (pp. 1824–1846)

Cranial cruciate ligament rupture may be purely traumatic, occurring in a young large dog and associated with an acute history and distinct traumatic event. A small percentage of these dogs avulse a bony insertion of the ligament rather than tear the ligament within its substance; the tibial attachment site fails more often than the femoral. The majority of dogs with cranial cruciate ligament rupture have a more chronic course without a history of distinct trauma. Physical and radiographic examination generally confirms chronic degenerative changes in the affected stifle joint.

Epidemiology and Pathogenesis

Rupture of the cranial cruciate ligament occurs in large breeds of dogs more often than in small breeds, with the rottweiler, bull mastiff, and chow chow particularly at risk. Acute traumatic ligament rupture most often occurs in dogs less than 4 years of age; dogs with the syndrome of chronic lameness and degenerative joint disease usually are between 5 and 7 years of age. There is a trend for small dogs (<15 kg) to rupture the ligament later in life (>7 years of age) than large dogs. Numerous clinical studies have reported a higher incidence of rupture in females than males.

The strength of a dog's cranial cruciate ligament deteriorates with aging, correlating with loss of fiber bundle organization and metaplastic changes of cellular elements. These changes are more pronounced and occur at an earlier age in large dogs, perhaps helping to explain the occurrence of rupture earlier in life than in small breeds.

Abnormal conformation of the limb is implicated as a cause of degenerative joint disease (postural arthrosis) and excessive stresses within the ligament, thereby causing chronic deterioration and eventual rupture.

Partial tears of the cranial cruciate ligament are diagnosed with increasing frequency. Partial tears in dogs consistently progress to complete rupture of the ligament, usually within 1 year of the onset of lameness. Joint instability may not be palpable early in the course but usually becomes apparent as the ligament undergoes progressive failure. Sectioning of either the craniomedial or caudolateral portions of the ligament does not result in clinically detectable instability, and if abnormal cranial drawer motion is present clinically, either the entire ligament is torn or the intact portion has undergone significant disruption.

Clinical Signs and Diagnosis

The diagnosis of cranial cruciate ligament rupture is based on a history of lameness and physical examination findings. Dogs with acute traumatic ligament rupture are severely lame and occasionally do not bear weight on the affected limb. The key to diagnosis of traumatic ruptures is to verify a truly acute onset of lameness, usually with a definite history of injury, and if the joint is examined within a few weeks of injury, the presence of minimal or no degenerative joint disease in the affected stifle.

Dogs with chronic cruciate disease have a more insidious history of lameness, often intermittent and exacerbated by physical activity. The affected joint is thickened, especially medially, and has radiographic evidence of degenerative joint disease. The frequency of bilateral disease is as high as 31 per cent. Cranial instability may be difficult to elicit because of periarticular fibrosis, especially if the ligament is partially torn. Some degree of abnormal movement usually can be detected, especially if the dog is sedated or anesthetized. Joint effusion is invariably present.

Cranial drawer motion may be detected by the cranial drawer test or the tibial compression test. The cranial drawer test can be performed with a dog standing or in lateral recumbency, as preferred by the examiner; a tranquilizer or occasionally general anesthesia is required in nervous dogs or dogs in pain. The cranial drawer test is performed with the stifle in extension and in about 30° of flexion to aid detection of partial tears.

With complete tears of the cranial cruciate ligament, abnormal cranial drawer motion is noted in both the extended position and in flexion. Often the craniomedial band of the ligament is torn, leaving the caudolateral portion intact. The caudolateral portion is taut in extension, therefore preventing cranial tibial displacement. Abnormal cranial drawer motion is evident in flexion because the caudolateral portion is relaxed. Isolated rupture of the caudolateral portion occurs and can confuse diagnosis because the intact craniomedial portion prevents detection of drawer motion, regardless of joint position. The latter cases are typical of partial tears in that degenerative joint changes, although present, are often mild, and the medial meniscus usually is normal.

Radiographic Examination

In dogs with partial tears of the cranial cruciate ligament, cranial drawer motion may be difficult to detect, and high-quality radiographs are important in demonstrating joint effusion and often early signs of degenerative joint disease. Both stifle joints are radiographed for comparison.

Evaluation of the Intercondyloid Fossa (pp. 1827–1828)
Clinical Pathology

The majority of dogs with cranial cruciate ligament rupture have synovial fluid white blood cell counts less than 5,000/mm³, consistent with chronic degenerative joint disease. The cells are generally mononuclear; large numbers of polymorphonuclear cells suggest immune-mediated joint disease. Dogs with partial tears may have elevated total white blood cell counts (mononuclear) in synovial fluid; therefore, arthrocentesis and joint fluid analysis may be valuable in diagnosis of minimal instability but with other signs associated with partial tearing of the cranial cruciate ligament (lameness, joint effusion, pain).

Meniscal Injury

Injury to the medial meniscus is frequently associated with cranial cruciate ligament rupture. Dogs with partial tears have a low frequency of meniscal damage (5 of 25 dogs). With chronicity, the frequency of meniscal damage increases and is as great as 80 per cent in dogs with complete tears.

Guidelines for Meniscectomy

Clinical management of meniscal injuries is controversial. Major meniscal injuries, such as large bucket-handle tears, cause lameness, and the damaged segment should be excised. Routine removal of the entire medial meniscus has been advocated, based on the rationale that progressive meniscal deterioration occurs in all dogs with cranial cruciate ligament rupture, and degenerative changes in the meniscus may not be evident. Conversely, investigators have reported good to excellent results when the menisci were left in place in most or all of the dogs operated on. Preservation of the meniscus is clearly beneficial given the degenerative sequelae associated with its removal. Meniscectomy adversely affected the prognosis after surgery for rupture of the cranial cruciate ligament. Leaving in place menisci that are grossly normal is not without risk; the most common cause of lameness in dogs that have had prior surgery for cranial cruciate ligament rupture is a damaged meniscus. The frequency of lameness developing in dogs that had a grossly normal medial meniscus left intact has not been documented; in my experience, it is uncommon (<10 per cent).

Based on these considerations, the following guidelines for meniscectomy can be given:

1. The meniscus is protective of joint cartilage and is preserved if it is grossly normal.
2. Damaged portions of the meniscus are excised because they can cause lameness.

Treatment

Decisions about the nature of therapy in dogs with rupture of the cranial cruciate ligament are influenced by the animal's age, body size and weight, intended use (e.g., active hunting dog versus sedentary house pet), concurrent orthopedic or medical problems, economic considerations, and anticipated owner compliance.

Conservative (i.e., nonsurgical) therapy is recommended for cats.

Eighteen of 18 cats examined after a mean follow-up period of 20.5 months became clinically normal without surgical intervention. The mean duration before regaining normal limb function was 4.8 weeks, with a range of 1 to 16 weeks.

Small dogs (i.e., < 15 kg) often do well without surgical intervention. Twenty-four of 28 dogs (86 per cent) that weighed 15 kg or less were clinically normal or improved after a mean follow-up period of 36.6 months. Based on the latter studies, it is prudent to wait for at least 6 to 8 weeks before recommending surgery for small dogs. These dogs are older at diagnosis and are often obese, with concurrent medical problems. Small dogs that are lame for 6 weeks after diagnosis and show no improvement often have meniscal tears and are operated on for meniscectomy and joint stabilization.

Large dogs (> 15 to 20 kg) clearly benefit from surgical therapy. In 46 of 57 (81 per cent) large dogs (> 15 kg) with cranial cruciate rupture treated conservatively, lameness persisted or worsened during a follow-up period of 10.2 months.

Surgical Methods of Joint Stabilization

Numerous surgical procedures have been designed to restore stability and minimize secondary degenerative joint disease. Although limb function can be improved in the majority of dogs by using various techniques, none of the procedures has proved clearly superior to any other; a study of the factors affecting the prognosis after surgery for cranial cruciate ligament rupture found that the type of surgical procedure had little influence on the eventual outcome. The common denominator to all of these procedures may be enhancement of periarticular fibrosis, with stabilization coming at the expense of range of motion. The true test of a reconstructive procedure is whether or not it prevents the development of secondary degenerative joint disease. Unfortunately, published studies indicate that degenerative joint disease progresses despite a satisfactory clinical result.

Three basic surgical methods are used for restoring stability in a joint with cranial cruciate ligament rupture: (1) The ligament can be repaired primarily, including suture techniques for midsubstance tears or tension band fixation of bony avulsion injuries. (2) The ligament can be replaced or reconstructed using various materials, and these techniques are classified as intra-articular or intra-capsular methods. (3) The joint can be stabilized by transposition of periarticular structures or placement of suture materials outside of the joint. The latter methods are classified as extra-articular or extra-capsular.

Primary Repair. Primary repair of midsubstance cranial cruciate ligament tears is not feasible in dogs. The ability of the ligament to heal directly with scar tissue is limited; the ligament stumps invariably atrophy, accompanied by collagen degradation.

Avulsion Injuries. Dogs with acute avulsion injuries of a cranial cruciate ligament attachment site can be treated effectively by tension band repair or screw fixation of the avulsed segment, provided that the piece of bone is large enough to support the implant. Suture fixation of these injuries can be attempted if the bone fragment is small or friable, but I found the latter method unsuccessful in two large dogs. Tenuous repairs are supported by extracapsular stabilization and coaptation of the limb for 2 to 3 weeks.

Intra-articular Reconstruction:
General Principles (pp. 1833–1835)

Extra-Articular Reconstruction (pp. 1841–1846)

CAUDAL CRUCIATE LIGAMENT RUPTURE (pp.1846–1852)

Isolated injuries of the caudal cruciate ligament are unusual but are generally diagnosed in young large dogs that have sustained severe trauma.

Surgical Techniques

COLLATERAL LIGAMENT INJURIES (pp. 1852–1854)

Isolated collateral ligament injuries are unusual. More often, collateral ligament injury is a component of a "deranged" or luxated stifle joint in which multiple ligaments and often menisci are damaged.

Injuries that damage ligament fibers are termed *sprains*. First-degree sprains are mild and cause minimal instability. Second-degree sprains involve stretching and tearing of ligament fibers and some degree of instability, although the ligament is grossly intact. Third-degree sprains are complete ruptures of the ligament. Grading the degree of instability helps establish the severity of ligament injury and organize treatment.

Clinical Signs and Diagnosis

Patients usually have a history of acute trauma and lameness, which may be severe, depending on the degree of injury. The stifle joint is usually tender, and various degrees of swelling are present over the involved ligament.

Medial Collateral Ligament

The valgus stress test is used to evaluate the medial collateral ligament. With the stifle joint extended, one hand is used to stabilize the femur and palpate the medial joint line while the other hand is used to abduct the tibia, thereby applying a valgus stress. The medial joint space opening, as well as the stiffness of the motion limit (soft or hard endpoint), is estimated and compared with the contralateral joint. When the medial collateral ligament is completely torn, increased external tibial rotation is possible with the stifle flexed.

Lateral Collateral Ligament

The varus stress test is used to evaluate the integrity of the lateral collateral ligament. With the stifle joint held in extension, one hand stabilizes the femur and simultaneously palpates the lateral joint line. The other hand is used to adduct the tibia, thereby applying a varus stress to the joint. The lateral joint space opening, as well as stiffness of the motion limit, is estimated and compared with the contralateral joint.

Radiographs are useful to detect avulsion injuries and determine the presence of degenerative joint disease. Stress radiographs can be taken to document the instability.

Treatment

Because no clinical studies have investigated isolated collateral ligament injuries in dogs, recommendations for treatment are based on clinical experience and research literature. The concept of primary repair of torn collateral ligaments has been supported by experimental studies, and immediate surgical repair of second- and third-degree injuries in active large dogs has been recommended. In man, conservative treatment of isolated medial collateral ligament tears has been successful, and numerous animal studies involving complete severance of this ligament have demonstrated that conservative treatment of isolated ligament injury produced better results than surgical repair and immobilization.

Based on the latter studies, it is recommended that isolated tears of either collateral ligament be managed conservatively. One week in a lateral splint is advised to limit excessive movement, followed by 6 weeks of limited activity (leash walks only). If lameness and instability persist, ligament reconstruction is advised. Acute avulsion injuries with substantial bone fragments are repaired immediately.

Operative Techniques

STIFLE LUXATION (p. 1854)

Stifle luxation, or derangement of the stifle, refers to severe injuries in which numerous ligaments, the joint capsule, and often the menisci have been damaged. The most common combination of injuries is both cruciate ligaments and the medial collateral ligament.

Diagnosis is based on thorough palpation of the joint under general anesthesia. Because multiple ligaments are involved, the results of palpation can be confusing. It is helpful to hold the joint in extension and gently apply varus and valgus stresses to test the collateral ligaments. Drawer motion is tested with the joint held in slight flexion and neutral rotation. Confirmation of which structures are damaged requires joint exploration. Radiographs are helpful to identify avulsion fractures, and stress views can be used to document instability.

Cats and small dogs have been successfully treated using transarticular pinning to provide temporary stabilization. Extra-articular suture techniques and joint immobilization via external fixation were successful in 12 dogs and 1 cat. Meticulous reconstruction of damaged ligaments followed by external splintage also has been successful in restoring limb function, even in large dogs.

Operative Technique

Chronic severe derangement of the stifle joint with advanced osteoarthrosis is best managed by arthrodesis or amputation.

PATELLAR LUXATION (pp. 1854–1861)

Femoropatellar instability is a common cause of lameness in dogs. The condition varies from complete, irreducible luxation of the patella and severe lameness to mild instability without associated clinical signs. The luxation may be intermittent, lateral or medial, traumatic or developmental.

The most common diagnosis is congenital or developmental medial patellar luxation in small dogs. Medial patellar luxation in large dogs is now a relatively frequent diagnosis. Cats also develop patellar luxation, usually medial, but much less commonly than dogs. The luxation in cats is generally intermittent and associated with a mechanical, nonpainful lameness. Surgical correction is recommended if lameness is frequent.

Lateral luxation in small dogs is rare and is usually congenital. Lateral patellar luxation in large dogs or giant breeds is often a distinct syndrome associated with severe limb deformities and carries a much more guarded prognosis.

Clinical Signs and Diagnosis

Acute traumatic patellar luxation may be medial or lateral and is associated with nonweightbearing lameness and pain on manipulation of the joint. These signs gradually subside and may be mild in an animal with chronic luxation.

The clinical signs associated with congenital or developmental medial patellar luxation vary with the degree or grade of luxation. Acute lameness in a dog with chronic luxation is usually caused by rupture of the cranial cruciate ligament.

Lateral patellar luxation occurs rarely in small dogs and may cause an acute, painful lameness. More often, it is a component of a severe limb deformity in large dogs and giant breeds, characterized by coxa valga, excessive anteversion of the femoral neck, hypoplasia of the vastus medialis, medial bowing of the femur and tibia (genu valgum), and external rotation of the foot. These animals have a crouched posture, awkward gait, and generally unthrifty appearance.

Physical Examination

Careful physical examination is necessary to characterize the patello-femoral instability and rule out cranial cruciate ligament rupture. One hand is placed over the patella, and the other hand used to pick up the tibia and place the joint through a range of motion. Patellar tracking is evaluated, and the presence of crepitation or pain is noted. Spontaneous luxation is easily detected as a snapping or popping sensation. With the joint in extension, the patella is isolated between the thumb and index fingers and pushed medially and laterally. In a normal joint, the patella may subluxate slightly but does not luxate.

Radiography

Radiographs can document the luxation and are useful to determine the extent of bony deformity and degenerative joint changes. Dogs with intermittent luxation may be reduced during positioning, and the radiographs appear normal. Skyline views of the distal femur are useful both before and after surgery to evaluate the depth and contour of the femoral trochlea.

Treatment

Because patellar luxations vary greatly in the degree of pathology present and the potential for degenerative sequelae, it is imperative to individualize the treatment for each patient. Several situations are clear-cut. Grade 1 medial patellar luxation without clinical signs is managed conservatively; if lameness develops, the dog is re-evaluated. Grade 4 medial patellar luxation is corrected surgically early in life to prevent severe bony deformity and disability. Traumatic luxations are repaired by suturing the respective fascial defect (medial or lateral).

The gray zones involve small dogs with grade 2 or grade 3 medial patellar luxation and only occasional lameness. These dogs generally have mild degenerative joint disease, and it does not markedly progress; routine surgical correction is not recommended. Medial patellar luxation is associated with internal tibial rotation and may cause excessive stress within the cranial cruciate ligament and predispose to rupture. The primary criterion for operating on these dogs is the frequency of lameness and disability. If lameness is frequent and a major concern for the owner, the luxation is corrected. If the lameness is mild and infrequent, surgery is discussed and offered as an option if the problem worsens. The combination of medial patellar luxation and cranial cruciate ligament rupture causes significant disability and is surgically corrected if the dog is otherwise sound.

Lateral patellar luxation, when associated with severe limb deformities, is a complex disorder with a guarded prognosis. It is imperative to educate owners about the nature of the limb deformities and not embark on an expensive sequence of operations unless an owner is fully committed and knowledgeable about potential complications.

Surgical Methods

PATELLAR FRACTURES AND PATELLAR TENDON INJURIES (pp. 1861–1862)

Patellar fractures are uncommon and are usually the result of a direct blow. Patellar tendon tears are also unusual, and the cause is often unknown. A direct wound can cause tendon laceration, or the tendon may rupture when quadriceps contraction occurs simultaneously with forced knee flexion. The lameness is often severe, and physical examination reveals marked pain over the site of injury. Patellar tendon rupture is suggested by dorsal displacement of the patella. It is imperative in all such cases to carefully examine the stifle joint for concurrent injuries to the ligaments and menisci.

Patellar fractures require tension band fixation to overcome the distracting forces of the quadriceps muscles. Conservative treatment results in nonunion of the bone and secondary fracture disease in the limb, with a correspondingly worse prognosis. Patellectomy is strictly a salvage procedure for highly comminuted fractures and should be avoided if at all possible because of the critical importance of the patella in providing extensor power to the stifle.

Repair of Patellar Fractures (pp. 1861–1862)

Repair of Patellar Tendon Injuries (p. 1862)

CHAPTER 138

Fractures of the Tibia and Fibula (pages 1866–1876)

Most fractures of the tibia include the fibula, although the fibula is frequently ignored in treatment unless the stability of the stifle or hock is jeopardized. Fractures of the tibia account for 20 per cent of fractures. Motor vehicle accidents are responsible for a large percentage. Other causes of fractured tibias include gunshots, fights, falls, and unknown trauma. Skeletal tumors may predispose the bone to fractures.

SURGICAL TREATMENT (pp. 1866–1867)

Diagnosis of tibial fractures is by physical and radiographic examination. Affected animals usually do not bear weight on the injured limb and have palpable swelling and crepitation at the fracture site. Because of the frequency of multiple organ injury sustained during trauma of sufficient force to cause fractures, the animal is evaluated carefully.

Preoperative treatment includes careful cleaning of open wounds and application of a Robert Jones bandage to protect the fracture and surrounding soft tissues and prevent or reduce limb swelling before surgery.

Applicable reduction and fixation techniques include closed reduction with external coaptation or an external fixation splint and open reduction with fixation using pins and orthopedic wire, an external fixation splint, or plate and screws. Selection of method depends on the type and location of the fracture, signalment of the animal, additional skeletal injuries, and the surgeon's familiarity with the various types of fixation equipment and fixation techniques.

If antibiotics are indicated because of an open fracture or anticipation of a lengthy, complicated procedure, a broad-spectrum antibiotic is administered intravenously at anesthetic induction and continued parenterally for at least 48 hours after surgery until the results of culture and sensitivity testing are known.

FRACTURE FIXATION TECHNIQUES IN IMMATURE ANIMALS (pp. 1867–1870)

FRACTURE FIXATION TECHNIQUES IN MATURE ANIMALS (pp. 1870–1872)

HEALING OF TIBIAL FRACTURES (pp. 1872–1876)

Physeal fractures heal quickly, with either continued production of cartilage or cessation of growth and bridging of the physis with bone. In either situation, the fracture is stable within 3 to 4 weeks and implants can be removed. If the physis is still functional, the implants are removed to eliminate further interference with growth.

Tibial diaphyseal fractures in immature animals varied in time to healing from 3.95 ± 0.98 weeks for cast fractures, to 7.12 ± 2.04 weeks for pinned and wired fractures, to 10.5 ± 3.65 weeks for plated fractures. Healing times for the tibial diaphysis in mature animals were similar for fractures treated with a cast at 3.65 ± 1.38 weeks but were significantly increased to 13.29 ± 8.54 weeks for pinned fractures and 19.38 ± 10.25 weeks for plated fractures.

Rate and type of healing depend on the location of the fracture, type of fixation used, and stability achieved at the fracture site. Primary union occurs when there is absolute stability and contact between fracture segments. As fixation becomes less rigid, bone union occurs through callus production and remodeling. Bridging periosteal callus allows implant removal earlier than with primary bone union. This effect is partially responsible for the shorter healing times reported for fractures stabilized with pins and wires compared with compressive fixation.

In the tibia, most implants are removed after healing of the fracture. Pins may interfere with function of the stifle. Plates have little soft-tissue covering and may cause irritation of the soft tissues or may conduct cold or heat to the bone. Cerclage wire and screws are only removed if associated with loosening of the implant or infection.

COMPLICATIONS (p. 1876)

Complications include infection, implant failure, delayed union, non-union and malunion, and impaired function of the limb. Causes of these problems are instability, improper reduction, wound contamination, or interference with adjacent joints by implants.

Nonunion occurs in approximately 4 per cent of tibial fractures. The cause usually is instability, in some cases complicated by osteomyelitis. Extremely rigid fixation coupled with a large fracture gap may result in nonunion if adequate cancellous bone grafting is not used. Malunions result in angular or rotational deformities and are usually associated with severely comminuted fractures in which the cortex cannot be anatomically reconstructed.

CHAPTER 139
Tarsus and Metatarsus
(pages 1876–1888)

ANATOMY (pp. 1876–1879)

Ligamentous Support of the Tarsus and Metatarsus

The tarsus is supported by medial and lateral collateral ligaments. They originate from the medial and lateral malleoli and are composed of a short and a long part. The short portion of the medial collateral ligament attaches distally to the talus and then extends distally with the long portion to attach to the first tarsal and metatarsal bones.

The short portion of the lateral collateral ligament attaches to the talus and calcaneus. These bands are at right angles to the long part of the lateral collateral ligament and are located under the long part. The long part of this ligament is attached to the fifth metatarsal bone.

The plantar ligaments are better developed than those on the dorsal side, allowing them to withstand the tensile stresses placed on the joint. These plantar ligaments are distinct. One ligament extends from the base of the calcaneus to the fourth tarsal bone and then to the bases of the fourth and fifth metatarsal bones (middle plantar ligament). A second ligament leaves the plantar surface of the sustentaculum tali and attaches to the central tarsal bone on its way to the tarsometatarsal joint capsule (medial plantar ligament). A third plantar ligament leaves the caudolateral surface of the calcaneus and unites with the long lateral collateral ligament before attaching to the base of the fifth metatarsal bone (lateral plantar ligament).

EVALUATION OF THE TARSUS AND METATARSUS
(pp. 1879)

The region is scrutinized for swelling or abnormal joint angles. Each tarsal and metatarsal bone is carefully palpated, and range of motion is noted. The joints are stressed in mediolateral, dorsoplantar, and rotary planes. In some injuries, sedation or general anesthesia is necessary for complete evaluation.

The findings on physical examination dictate the radiographic views necessary to confirm the presence of bony or ligamentous injury. Standard lateral and dorsoplantar views often are inadequate and are complemented with stress views and oblique views when necessary. Using stress radiography, a controlled force is applied on a joint to demonstrate an abnormal spatial relationship between two or more of its components. Stress radiography is especially helpful to demonstrate ligamentous injury in the hock and can help identify osteochondritic lesions of the talus dome.

LUXATIONS OF THE TARSUS AND METATARSUS
(pp. 1880–1881)

The most common luxations involve the tarsocrural joint. These are debilitating injuries that respond poorly when handled conservatively. Reconstructive surgery and in some cases arthrodesis are required to provide tarsocrural stability.

Because both collateral ligaments originate from their respective malleoli, fracture of either malleolus results in a tarsocrural subluxation or luxation. Medial malleolar fractures occur more commonly; the short components of the collateral ligaments may occasionally avulse independently of the long components. Small fragments must be excised, and the remaining soft tissues sutured. Larger fragments are reattached with pins and figure-eight tension band fixation. Lateral malleolar fractures are repaired in a similar way, and when possible a small pin is passed antegrade into the fibula.

Tarsocrural luxations are frequently the result of traumatic rupture of either the medial or lateral collateral ligaments. The tarsus is flexed to examine the lateral collateral ligament. In this position, the long portion of the ligament is relaxed and the short segment is taut. The foot is twisted inward to assess the integrity of the short portion of the lateral collateral ligament. With the tarsus extended, the long portion is taut and the short portion is relaxed. A varus stress is applied to assess the integrity of the long portion of the lateral collateral ligament. When the tarsus is flexed, the short portion of the medial collateral ligament is taut. Applying a valgus stress demonstrates integrity of this ligament. The long portion of the medial collateral ligament is taut when the tarsus is extended, and a valgus stress is used to examine this portion.

In many cases, primary repair of the torn and frayed ligament is either impossible or fails to provide adequate support. Prosthetic material attached to bone screws placed in the tibia and the talus or calcaneus is indicated when ligament reconstruction is impossible.

Aron has demonstrated the advantage of a double prosthetic replacement in tarsocrural luxations. Placing two bone screws distally to anchor the prosthetic ligament more closely mimics the support of the short and long portion of the collateral ligament.

SHEAR INJURIES OF THE TARSUS (p. 1881)

Shear injuries of the tarsus invariably contain dirt, rocks, asphalt, hair, and often feces. Shear injuries require aggressive débridement, joint and soft-tissue lavage, and bacterial culture before attempted primary closure. Most shear wounds are left open to drain and allowed to heal by second intention and contraction. Wet to dry bandages are changed daily, and the injured part must be immobilized. An external fixator can be used to immobilize the joints. When possible, bacterial cultures are obtained at initial débridement; a broad-spectrum antimicrobial regimen is indicated. As the wounds heal and drainage decreases, definitive repair of the ligamentous instability can be undertaken.

PROXIMAL PLANTAR INTERTARSAL LUXATION (p. 1881)

Proximal plantar intertarsal luxations are a result of damage to the plantar ligaments. Disruption of the calcaneoquartal and talocalcaneocentral joints occurs. These injuries respond poorly to conservative management because the damaged ligaments are on the tension band side of the tarsus. Motion results in continuous destructive forces. This injury, although reported in many breeds, most commonly occurs in greyhounds.

Injuries of the plantar ligaments may avulse bone chips from the plantar process of the central tarsal bone or from the base of the calcaneus. Repair of this injury consists of primary arthrodesis of the calcaneoquartal joint by pin and figure-eight tension band wire. With severe instabilities, arthrodesis of the talocalcaneocentral joint may also be accomplished. The tarsus is coapted in a position of function for 6 to 8 weeks. In greyhounds, this injury is debilitating, and despite successful arthrodesis, few dogs return to racing.

DORSAL PROXIMAL INTERTARSAL SUBLUXATION
(pp. 1881–1883)

This is a subtle hyperextension injury, and patients are able to bear weight. Little soft-tissue swelling occurs. Diagnosis is confirmed with stress radiographs demonstrating dorsal opening of the joint space. Most have a medial or lateral component. In performance animals, this subluxation is best treated by primary arthrodesis of the talocalcaneo-central or the calcaneoquartal joints. Bone screws are lagged from the head of the talus through a small portion of the central tarsal bone and into the fourth tarsal bone or from the base of the calcaneus into the fourth tarsal bone, respectively.

In nonperformance animals, some dorsal proximal intertarsal luxations can be treated successfully by coaptation for 6 to 8 weeks.

TARSOMETATARSAL JOINT SUBLUXATION (p. 1883)

Tarsometatarsal joint subluxations can be either dorsal or plantar. Physical examination and stress radiography are required for diagnosis. Plantar subluxations are more common despite thicker and stronger ligaments. Primary arthrodesis is recommended in most cases.

TARSOCRURAL ARTHRODESIS (p. 1883)

Tarsocrural arthrodesis is indicated for failed reconstructions, irreparable soft-tissue injuries, severely comminuted articular fractures, and crippling degenerative joint disease. The angle of arthrodesis is 135° for dogs and 120° for cats. The arthrodesis is splinted for 6 to 8 weeks and monitored radiographically until arthrodesis is successful.

FRACTURES OF THE CALCANEUS (p. 1883)

Calcaneal fractures are common in racing greyhounds and rare in other breeds. In greyhounds, calcaneal fractures are associated with either central tarsal fractures or disruption of the plantar ligaments, resulting in proximal plantar intertarsal luxation.

The type of calcaneal fracture dictates the treatment method. Steinmann pins, tension band wiring, and lag screws are most commonly used. Neutralization plates and cerclage wires have also been used to repair calcaneal fractures.

TALUS FRACTURES (p. 1885)

Isolated talus fractures are rare. Talar head fractures may be encountered with central tarsal fractures. This type of fracture is repaired by lag screw fixation.

Talar fractures in pets often result from trauma. Intra-articular body fractures are surgically repaired and usually can be approached by osteotomy of the appropriate malleolus. The prognosis for head and neck fractures associated with central tarsal fractures is fair to good.

The prognosis for intra-articular fractures of the body is guarded owing to the potential for degenerative joint disease.

CENTRAL TARSAL FRACTURES (p. 1885)

Central tarsal fractures are most commonly reported in racing greyhounds but do occur in other breeds. In dogs racing counterclockwise, compressive forces are concentrated in the right tarsus. Central tarsal fractures frequently show radiographic evidence of compression, subluxation, and comminution but are rarely open. Once the buttress action of the central tarsal bone is lost, the talocalcaneocentral joint collapses. With many severe central tarsal fractures, simultaneous fracture of the fourth tarsal bone and the calcaneus may occur. Second tarsal bone fractures may also be combined with severe central tarsal fractures.

Central tarsal fractures have been graded according to the fracture type and amount of displacement. Undisplaced fractures may be attended by little apparent lameness. Repair of type I and type II fractures requires one 2.0- or 2.7-mm cortical screw placed in lag fashion. These fractures are coapted for 4 weeks, and the prognosis is excellent.

Type III fractures are rare and require the use of one 4.0-mm partially threaded cancellous bone screw for fixation.

Type IV fractures usually have many small posterior comminutions in addition to the two major fragments. Surgical repair consists of a 4.0-mm partially threaded cancellous bone screw lagged into the body of the fourth tarsal bone. A second 2.0- or 2.7-mm cortical screw placed in lag fashion is used to secure the anterior fragment. The prognosis for type IV fractures is favorable.

Type V fractures are usually externally coapted or internally stabilized to salvage the animal for breeding purposes.

METATARSAL FRACTURES (p. 886)

Metatarsal fractures usually cause an acute nonweightbearing lameness with various amounts of swelling, crepitus, and pain. Undisplaced fractures may be treated with coaptation for 4 to 6 weeks. When severe displacement occurs or when multiple bones are fractured, internal fixation is indicated.

FRACTURES OF THE SESAMOID BONES (pp. 1886–1888)

Fracture of the plantar sesamoids occurs primarily in greyhounds. When presented acutely, mild soft-tissue swelling and point pain are noted over the plantar aspect of the affected metatarsophalangeal joint. Chronic fractures are evidenced by soft-tissue proliferation and decreased range of motion of the affected joint. Detailed radiographs are necessary to identify these fractures. Removal of the comminuted bone fragments is indicated because the fragments are too small for repair. The prognosis for return to racing is favorable.

CHAPTER 140

Arthrodesis (pages 1888–1901)

Arthrodesis is the removal of motion from a joint by fusion of the opposing surfaces into a solid bony unit.

GENERAL INDICATIONS (pp. 1888–1889)

Fusion of a joint is usually performed to relieve a painful condition due to instability or inflammatory disease.

The most common indications for arthrodesis in veterinary medicine can be divided into three categories: traumatic, developmental, and congenital. Traumatic injuries to joints consist of both fractures and ligamentous disruptions with or without dislocation. Examples include (1) shearing injuries and fracture-dislocations of the hock or carpus with major bone and ligament loss and (2) severely comminuted condylar fractures of the distal humerus and femur, especially in miniature breeds.

The major developmental diseases can be included under the heading *arthritis* and are further subdivided into idiopathic or secondary degenerative joint disease, septic arthritis, and immune-mediated arthritis (rheumatoid or polyarthritis). Congenital elbow luxations and stifle deformities that are not amenable to primary reconstruction are examples of indications for arthrodesis. A fourth category is the use of arthrodesis to improve the mechanics of a limb rather than to relieve pain and instability—for example, arthrodesis of the carpus for radial nerve paralysis or the talocrural joint in conjunction with a muscle transfer for ischial paralysis.

GENERAL PROCEDURE (p. 1889)

Stability is of prime importance, even more so in arthrodesis than fracture fixation because the mechanical structures of a limb are designed to provide and maintain motion at this location. Therefore, the body is working against maintaining immobility at the fixation point. The type of fixation and the surgical technique are critical, and the use of compression, which provides more rigid fixation, is desirable. Plates, screws, cross pins, tension band wire, and external pin splints used alone or in combination, plus external coaptation, are the common devices used to accomplish rigid fixation.

The articular cartilage is removed down to bleeding subchondral bone to enhance bone contact and facilitate early union. If an angular or rotational deformity exists, it can be corrected at this time by removing a suitable amount of bone.

For added insurance, autogenous cancellous bone grafts are used to shorten healing time and to fill in small defects in the opposing surfaces. Normal angles for different joints have been reported, but the simplest method of determining the correct angle is to measure the opposite normal limb during weightbearing. This angle may have to be adjusted if there will be shortening caused by the procedure.

GENERAL COMPLICATIONS (p. 1889)

When a point of motion is obliterated via arthrodesis, increased stress is transferred to adjacent bones and joints. This is especially true in the carpus and vertebrae. Fusion of the antebrachiocarpal joint without fusion of the adjacent intercarpal joints results in degenerative joint disease of the latter. When performing arthrodesis on a midlimb joint, these stresses are transferred to the long bones themselves, increasing the risk of fracture, especially in large active dogs. The ends of plates and screw holes act as stress risers, further increasing the risk of fracture.

Other possible causes of failure are infection, insufficient fixation, or insufficient removal of cartilage. Any technical error such as poor plate placement or too small or too short a plate can cause implant failure.

SHOULDER (pp. 1889–1890)

Shoulder problems requiring arthrodesis are not common. However, any condition causing severe arthritis and intractable pain can be considered an indication for arthrodesis. Included are intra-articular fractures, osteochondritis dissecans, and chronic luxations in miniature breeds.

ELBOW (pp. 1890–1893)

The most common indication for arthrodesis of the elbow is degenerative joint disease, which in this joint usually is secondary to trauma (fractures and luxations) or developmental diseases such as ununited anconeal process, fragmented coronoid process, osteochondritis dissecans, or premature closure of the distal radius or ulnar growth plates.

Congenital and traumatic fracture luxations that cannot be stabilized while preserving motion are indications for arthrodesis.

CARPUS (pp. 1893–1895)

The most frequent indications for arthrodesis of the carpus are hyperextension injuries and fracture luxations, especially old injuries. Casting alone is often insufficient—especially in large dogs with hyperextension injuries that may have been incurred from falls or leaping from heights or moving vehicles. The antebrachiocarpal joint may be spared or included in the arthrodesis, depending on the extent of the trauma. However, if the antebrachiocarpal joint is fused, the other joints of the carpus must be included, or secondary degenerative joint disease will develop in the latter, causing pain.

Immune-mediated arthritis is especially prevalent in the carpal joint, and in advanced cases these joints become very unstable as a result of ligament damage. Affected dogs have clinical signs similar to hyperextension injuries but without any history of trauma. This condition more frequently affects small dogs.

Another indication for carpal fusion is peripheral nerve damage. If the patient can support weight on the leg but lands on the dorsal surface of the paw, arthrodesis can improve this condition. However, most of these animals suffer from brachial plexus injuries, and too many muscles are affected for arthrodesis to be helpful.

Another situation in which carpal fusion may be necessary is nonunion of fractures of the radius and ulna in miniature breeds. Severe bone atrophy precludes simple handling of these cases. Fusion of the carpus provides adequate bone distal to the fracture to anchor plates or external pin splints in conjunction with cancellous autografts.

STIFLE (pp. 1895–1898)

Indications

Degenerative disease of the stifle is usually secondary to ligament injuries, the two most common of which are old, chronic anterior cruciate ruptures and severe traumatic derangements. In the latter, numerous structures are torn and primary reconstructive procedures may be unsuccessful, or excessive cartilage damage may require arthrodesis. With chronic cruciate tears, the degree of secondary degenerative joint disease determines whether primary repair or arthrodesis is attempted. Open fractures involving the stifle and accompanied by cartilage damage or bone and cartilage loss are another indication. Another indication is ''fracture disease.'' Although this disease can affect any joint, it most commonly occurs in the stifle and usually in young dogs treated for femoral fractures. The quadriceps is tied down to the callus, restricting motion of the stifle and leading to atrophy of the muscles and bones and fibroplasia of the capsule. All motion is eventually lost, and if the joint becomes painful, arthrodesis in a functional position is recommended.

HOCK (pp. 1898–1901)

The tarsal joints are subject to traumatic injury as well as degenerative disease. One of the most common traumatic injuries encountered in this joint is the shearing fracture that may occur when the leg has been dragged along the road by a car, causing significant loss of soft tissue and bone. The collateral ligaments and most of the malleolus are lost in these injuries, leaving the joint open and devoid of soft-tissue coverage and stability. The medial aspect is more frequently affected than the lateral. These wounds usually heal without active signs of infection, and sufficient fibroplasia often occurs to stabilize the joint without further surgery. However, if instability remains and simple replacement of the appropriate collateral ligament is insufficient, pantarsal arthrodesis is indicated. Severe fracture luxations of the tarsocrural, middle tarsal, or tarsometatarsal joints also occur and can be treated with fusions of the involved joints alone. Rupture of the plantar ligament also requires fusion of one or more of these latter joints.

Rupture of the calcaneal ligament not amenable to suture because of either severe trauma to the ligament or fragmentation of the calcaneus can be treated by fusion of the talocrural joint.

Rheumatoid arthritis or polyarthritis also commonly affects the hock, and as with the carpus, arthrodesis can be used as a palliative treatment. Osteoarthritis or septic arthritis, if severe enough, can require arthrodesis. Degenerative joint disease from an osteochondritis dissecans lesion of the talus is one such situation.

CHAPTER 141
Amputations (pages 1901–1910)

Indications for amputation include severe trauma, ischemic necrosis, intractable orthopedic infection, severe disability due to unmanageable arthritis, paralysis, congenital deformity, and neoplasia. However, veterinary surgeons should also consider the adaptability and suitability of the individual animal to amputation and the owner's view of the animal's disabled condition. Preoperative assessment of metastasis by chest radiography in neoplasia is a factor in determining an animal's suitability for surgery. Placing a sling on the affected leg and observing the animal's ability to function on three legs help determine the animal's adaptability. Decisions to amputate based on financial factors or a decision to euthanize instead of amputate must be respected by the veterinarian and handled with great sensitivity and concern.

GENERAL CONSIDERATIONS (pp. 1901–1902)

Level of Amputation

In forelimb amputation, scapular removal is faster and easier than shoulder disarticulation. If the scapula is left in shorthaired dogs, muscle atrophy allows bony prominences of the scapula to be seen, creating a cosmetically unacceptable appearance to some owners.

In the rear limb, amputation at midthigh leaves a stump that can protect the male genitalia and is also easier to perform than disarticulation at the hip. In any case, it is advisable to perform the amputation through normal tissue well above the diseased area and proximal enough in the limb to avoid leaving a dangling, useless stump.

Division of Muscles

Muscles may be severed at origins or insertions or divided through the belly. Electroincision is helpful in controlling hemorrhage.

Major arteries are double ligated with nonabsorbable inert suture material. The artery and vein are not ligated together to avoid the formation of an arteriovenous fistula. Veins may be singularly ligated with nonabsorbable suture. Attention is given to the level of arterial division to guard against necrosis of parts of the stump.

The artery is generally ligated first to allow blood to drain from the limb through intact veins. This technique helps preserve vascular volume, electrolytes, and protein. With diseased limbs that pose a possibility of disseminating the disease by surgical manipulation, it is advisable to ligate the vein first and the artery immediately afterward.

Neuromas after amputation are not generally a problem. As a consequence, there are no special concerns about severance of nerves. Nerve trunks are severed by sharp dissection while held in mild tension.

Correct closures start with a properly planned amputation. Extensive dissection of the subcutaneous space results in dead space that is difficult to close. The bone end must be adequately covered with viable muscle. When muscle is sutured, the fascial covering and not the muscle itself is used to hold the suture. Seromas, common sequelae to amputation surgery, can be prevented by gentle technique, effective hemostasis, secure closure of fascial planes, elimination of dead space, and avoidance of extensive subcutaneous dissection.

PHYSIOLOGICAL CONSIDERATIONS (p. 1902)

Preoperative evaluation of a patient's physiological status is important when a major amputation is planned. Complete hematological evaluation with a biochemistry and electrolyte panel is advisable. When a limb is removed, a large amount of tissue with fluid, electrolytes, and red blood cells is lost. Intravenous fluid administration during the operation is necessary to maintain hydration and blood pressure. Postoperative monitoring is essential to the recognition and treatment of shock.

TECHNIQUES (pp. 1902–1910)

CHAPTER 142

Skull and Mandibular Fractures (pages 1910–1921)

An animal with a mandibular or skull fracture usually has been subjected to significant trauma. Although a client may express great concern over a bloody mouth, a dropped jaw, or facial swelling, the clinician must perform a thorough physical examination of other systems to evaluate life-threatening injuries. Particularly with maxillary fractures, partial airway obstruction can occur and may necessitate immediate oxygen therapy or emergency tracheostomy. A gauze or leather muzzle may temporarily be used to reduce open bilateral mandibular or maxillary fractures and minimize exposure of bone. Many dogs with such injuries must breathe through their mouth because of nasal hematoma and swelling. Muzzling may produce excitement and hyperthermia and exacerbate airway obstruction—such devices must be used with care. Because the majority of mandibular and many skull fractures are open, these animals are routinely placed on systemic broad-spectrum antibiotics, and wounds are débrided and fractures stabilized as soon as the animal can be safely anesthetized.

Pharyngostomy Intubation

Anesthesia is induced, and oral intubation is performed as usual. The hair is clipped, and the skin caudolateral to the angle of either mandible is aseptically prepared. By oral palpation, the piriform fossa of the lateral pharynx caudal to the mandible is tented up. An incision approximately one and one-half times the diameter of the tube is made through the skin into the pharynx either just cranial or just caudal to the hyoid bone. Forceps are passed through the incision from the outside to grasp the cuff inflation tube and pull it to the outside. The endotracheal tube adapter is detached from the tube, and the cranial end of the tube is pulled through the incision using forceps passed from the exterior. The tube is reattached to the adapter and the anesthetic circuit. After surgery and recovery from anesthesia, the cuff is deflated and the tube is pulled out through the pharyngostomy incision. The skin incision is usually left unsutured to heal by second intention.

GENERAL SURGICAL CONSIDERATIONS (pp. 1911–1912)

Fracture reduction and fixation can often be accomplished through the oral wound. Any foreign material is removed, and nonviable tissues débrided. Bone with significant soft-tissue attachment may contribute to callus formation and is retained even if it cannot be rigidly fixed. Likewise, teeth, even if partially involved in the fracture, are left in place because they provide stability and aid alignment.

Although mandibular fractures heal well, if significant bone loss has occurred or defects remain after fracture reduction, autogenous cancellous bone grafts are used to fill the gaps and induce bone formation. If the fracture is grossly infected or avascular, the grafting procedure may be delayed for 10 to 14 days to allow granulation tissue to biologically débride and revascularize the region. If the approach communicates with an open oral lesion, delayed skin closure or closure over a drain is considered to decrease infection.

POSTOPERATIVE TREATMENT (p. 1912)

If rigid stabilization is achieved, relatively few restrictions are made other than feeding soft foods until the fractures heal. If less than optimal fixation is obtained, the repair may be supplemented with a muzzle and pharyngostomy tube used to supply nutrition for 3 to 4 weeks while early fracture healing occurs. Because the majority of these fractures are open, antibiotic therapy is appropriate and reduces the incidence of infection.

MANDIBULAR FRACTURES (pp. 1912–1918)

Two related reports found that canine mandibular fractures were relatively uncommon, accounting for about 3 per cent of the total number of canine fractures. Although approximately 15 per cent of fractures in cats involve the mandible, the majority were symphyseal separations. Most mandibular fractures were traumatically induced (89 to 100 per cent) and open (65 to 70 per cent). However, a significant number of mandibular fractures in dogs (11 per cent) occurred during dental extractions. Malocclusion was the most common significant complication of mandibular fractures in dogs (35 per cent), followed by infection (27 per cent) and delayed union (7 per cent).

Mandibular Symphyseal Fracture/Separation

The majority of these injuries are actually separations of the mandibular syndesmosis and heal by fibrous rather than bony callus. Fixation does not need to be extremely rigid or prolonged; 3 to 4 weeks is usually sufficient. A single stainless steel wire (18 to 22 gauge) encircling the rostral mandibular rami just behind the canine teeth works well.

Mandibular Body Fractures

Mandibular body fractures often involve alveoli, exposing tooth roots. Although bone cannot heal directly to tooth roots, leaving teeth in place assists reduction and fixation of the fracture. If a tooth becomes nonviable, it can easily be removed later.

Treatment

Partial Mandibulectomy

Partial mandibulectomy and hemimandibulectomy for the treatment of neoplastic conditions have resulted in good return to function. Consequently, this technique can be used as a salvage procedure for nonunion associated with intractable infection and bone loss. Enough bone is resected to remove all abnormal tissue and to allow tension-free closure of soft tissue over the resection stumps.

Caudal Mandibular Fractures

Fractures of the vertical ramus and condylar regions are difficult to expose because of the surrounding musculature. Cortical bone of the mandible in these areas is thin, limiting purchase of bone screws or external fixation pins. Consequently, most of these fractures are treated conservatively with tape muzzles or interarcade wiring to maintain proper dental occlusion.

Intra-articular fractures of the temporomandibular joint can be ex-

posed through a lateral approach. These fractures are difficult to stabilize, so conservative treatment is commonly used.

If significant arthritic changes develop and limit mastication, con-
dylectomy can be performed later. A pseudoarthrosis develops and
generally allows good return to function. Analgesics and chewy foods
may be used to encourage motion of the joint.

TEMPOROMANDIBULAR JOINT LUXATIONS (p. 1918)

Temporomandibular joint luxations may occur as isolated injuries or
in association with mandibular fractures. The mandibular condyle can
displace either rostrally or caudally relative to the mandibular fossa of
the temporal bone. If the luxation is unilateral and the condyle displaces rostrally, the mandibular canine teeth shift rostrally and away
from the side of the luxation relative to the maxillary canine teeth. If
the condyle luxates caudally, the mandibular canines shift caudally
and toward the side of the luxation. Most temporomandibular luxations
can be reduced with closed manipulation. In the standard technique, a
wooden dowel (pencil for cats) is placed transversely in the back of
the mouth between the last molars to act as a fulcrum. The rostral
mandible and maxilla are squeezed together to distract the condyle
ventrally. The mandible is pulled rostrally or pushed caudally to move
the condyle into place. Some joints are stable after closed reduction,
but many reluxate if not supported. Consequently, I palpate the joint
and provide additional support if instability is apparent. A muzzle is
adequate in many dogs, but interarcade wiring works better, particularly in cats. The periarticular tissues fibrose well, and the joint becomes stable. Consequently, support is needed for only 7 to 14 days.
Open reduction and stabilization by suture imbrication of the joint
capsule can be accomplished in many patients when closed reduction
is unsuccessful. Delay in treatment can result in significant condylar
cartilage damage, requiring condylar resection.

SKULL FRACTURES INVOLVING THE ORAL CAVITY
(pp. 1919–1920)

CHAPTER 143
Degenerative Joint Disease
(pages 1921–1927)

Degenerative joint disease (DJD, osteoarthritis) is a disease of the
cartilage of joints. Primary clinical signs are joint pain, altered gait,
limited range of motion of the affected joint, and various amounts of
effusion and local inflammation.

PATHOGENESIS (p. 1921)

DJD in man is a heterogeneous group of disorders with many etiological factors that result in a common final pathway leading to changes
in cartilage integrity. DJD has primary and secondary etiologies. This
classification has also been used for DJD of animals. The term *idiopathic DJD* is now preferred to *primary DJD* because it is likely that

specific forms of the disease are due to specific causes that have not been identified. In secondary DJD, alterations of articular tissues are the consequence of known factors and conditions affecting joints. Although idiopathic and secondary DJD are classified separately, the ultimate changes in joint tissue integrity are the same.

PATHOLOGY (pp. 1921–1923)

CLINICAL PRESENTATION (p. 1923)

Animals affected with DJD are usually presented because of lameness or change in gait. Signalment is combined with the information gleaned from the physical and neurological examinations to establish a list of tentative differential diagnoses.

RADIOGRAPHIC EXAMINATION (pp. 1923–1924)

Once the affected joints have been identified, radiographs are taken to determine the relative degree of degenerative change. It is important to obtain high-quality radiographs of the joints in at least two standard views.

The characteristic radiographic features of DJD include subchondral bony sclerosis, subchondral cyst formation, joint space narrowing, and intra-articular or periarticular osteophyte formation. Subchondral cysts are not commonly found in DJD in dogs and cats, although they often occur in large animals.

CLINICAL LABORATORY FINDINGS (p. 1924)

Results of a complete blood count, urinalysis, and serum chemistry studies are usually within normal limits in cases of DJD unless other conditions exist. Results of rheumatoid factor tests and lupus erythematosus clot tests are negative, as is the search for antinuclear antibodies. A decrease in synovial fluid viscosity due to a reduction in hyaluronic acid concentration, an increase in synovial fluid volume, and increased numbers of mononuclear phagocytic cells in the synovial fluid often confirm the presence of a low-grade intra-articular inflammatory process. Total white blood cells in the synovial fluid rarely exceed 5,000/mm^3.

TREATMENT (pp. 1924–1926)

Surgical therapy in dogs is directed at correcting the inciting cause of DJD. It includes stifle joint stabilization after rupture of the cranial cruciate ligament, pelvic osteotomy or intertrochanteric osteotomy in cases of DJD secondary to hip dysplasia, or procedures to correct patellar luxations. In severe cases of DJD, arthrodesis may be considered. Rest and physical therapy decrease inflammation in an affected joint and strengthen the supporting structures of the joint.

Medical Therapy

No drug or combination of drugs now available can consistently prevent or reverse the pathological changes in DJD. Nonsteroidal anti-inflammatory drugs (NSAIDs) are administered primarily for the symptomatic relief of clinical signs by their analgesic and anti-inflammatory activities. These drugs exert their actions by inhibiting the synthesis or release of prostaglandins. In general, these drugs seem to be effective while blood levels are maintained; withdrawal is usually followed by a recurrence of joint discomfort. Although effective in moderating the inflammation of DJD, NSAIDs are symptomatic treatments only.

Aspirin (acetylsalicylic acid) is the basic drug for the treatment of DJD. When used with care, it can be effective and relatively free of side effects. Mild to moderate peripheral pain is relieved by the ability of aspirin to block the effect of inflammatory mediators such as bradykinin. The action of aspirin as an anti-inflammatory agent is due to its ability to inhibit prostaglandin synthesis.

An oral aspirin dosage of 25 mg/kg every 8 hours produces and maintains therapeutic serum salicylate concentrations in normal dogs. Once the desired effects have been obtained, the amount of drug and its frequency of administration may be reduced. Doses reaching 50 mg/kg may produce emesis. Vomiting can occur at lower doses as well and may be prevented by administering the drug with food. Products containing aspirin and magnesium-aluminum hydroxide do not produce gastric lesions when given at therapeutic doses.

At therapeutic doses, aspirin is virtually free of serious side effects. Gross overdoses may produce hyperthermia, severe acid-base and electrolyte disturbances, renal hemorrhage, convulsions, and coma. Treatment for these acute and severe problems includes gastric lavage to remove unabsorbed drug, urine alkalization with sodium bicarbonate to enhance renal excretion of salicylate, and peritoneal dialysis to remove salicylates from the plasma.

In dogs, the most common side effects are vomiting and melena. Other toxic manifestations include skin eruptions, edema, gastrointestinal bleeding and ulceration, hypoprothrombinemia, and deafness. Seizures caused by aspirin overdosing have been reported in dogs.

Phenylbutazone has been used successfully in some animals for symptomatic treatment of DJD. Its mechanism of action is similar to aspirin. It is given orally in dosages ranging from 0.5 mg to 1.0 mg/kg every 8 hours. Bone marrow depression is the most serious of its side effects. Animals on long-term treatment are periodically evaluated with hemograms.

Corticosteroids and Other Agents

Corticosteroids are potent anti-inflammatory agents that may be beneficial in some animals with DJD. They should be reserved for those cases unresponsive to NSAIDs. Steroids for the treatment of DJD are given in low doses and for short periods. Prednisolone may be given parenterally at a dose of 1 to 2 mg/kg, followed by an oral maintenance dosage of 0.5 to 1.0 mg/kg once daily. The lowest possible maintenance dosage is established, such as alternate-day or every-third-day administration of 0.5 to 1.0 mg/kg.

CHAPTER 144
Immune-Mediated Joint Diseases (pages 1928–1937)

The causes of inflammatory arthropathies are diverse and are categorized into two basic groups: infectious (septic) and noninfectious (nonseptic). Noninfectious inflammatory arthropathies include the immune-mediated arthritides, which are subdivided into nonerosive (non-deforming) and erosive (deforming) arthritis.

Immune-mediated arthritides have been identified in dogs and cats, although the incidence is relatively low in cats. The cause of immune-mediated arthritides is unknown. Independent of their diverse origins, a type III (immune complex) hypersensitivity reaction is involved in the pathogenesis of the synovitis. Clinical manifestations are due to persistent inflammatory reactions that are the result of the deposition and phagocytosis of immune complexes and release of damaging lysosomal enzymes within the synovial membrane.

CANINE NONEROSIVE ARTHRITIS (pp. 1928–1934)

Idiopathic polyarthritis is the most common form of immune-mediated joint disease. The disease can occur at any age in either sex, although most occurs in young adults between 1 and 3.5 years of age. Any breed, as well as mongrels, can be affected, particularly large breeds (German shepherd, Doberman pinscher) and various sporting breeds (Labrador, golden retriever, Irish setter).

Systemic lupus erythematosus (SLE) is characterized as a multisystemic disease with various clinical manifestations, with immunological abnormalities that include autoimmunity (type II reaction) and immune complex (possibly nuclear antigen and antinuclear antibody [ANA]) hypersensitivity. SLE in dogs has no age predilection (8 months to 14 years), but females and certain breeds (German shepherds, collies, Shetland sheepdogs, beagles, and poodles) may be predisposed.

The gastrointestinal tract can be associated with an inflammatory joint disease, also referred to as *enteropathic arthritis*. In man, this type of polyarthritis is recognized as a complication of ulcerative colitis and regional enteritis. A similar relationship has been recognized in dogs with fulminating enterocolitis and ulcerative colitis.

Clinical Presentation

Independent of the type of immune-mediated joint disease, the clinical features are similar and include fever (persistent or episodic), inappetence/anorexia, and malaise accompanied by lameness of varying severity. The primary complaint occasionally is chronic lameness without any systemic signs. Joint disease and clinical manifestations tend to be cyclical: the onset is acute, and improvement can be spontaneous. The arthritic manifestations range from overt lameness to subtle signs of generalized weakness. A single (monoarticular, pauci- articular) or shifting (pauciarticular, polyarticular) leg lameness may be observed. Dogs with polyarticular involvement show generalized stiffness (arched back, stilted gait) after rest or exercise and may exhibit difficulty rising and lying down, predominantly involving the hindquarters. Generalized pain and behavioral changes, such as aggression and increased irritability, are often observed when affected dogs are handled. Some severely affected dogs, particularly small or toy breeds, refuse to stand, walk, or exercise. In these instances, appreciation of the joint disease is difficult and often overlooked.

In addition to pyrexia (103° to 106°F [39.4° to 40.8°C]), tachypnea and peripheral lymphadenopathy are common. Regardless of the type of immune-mediated arthritis, distal extremities and stifle joints are most commonly affected. Synovial distension, pain, soft-tissue swelling, or heat in one or more of the joints is a physical finding more frequently associated with acute febrile states. In more chronic forms, swelling and heat are often absent and only subtle signs of discomfort or joint capsule thickening are detectable. Spinal hyperesthesia, involving the neck and back, is a consistent clinical feature. In severely affected dogs, the disease can be debilitating, resulting in generalized muscle atrophy and weight loss. Disproportionate atrophy of the temporal and masseter muscles is often observed.

Specific immune-mediated arthritides cannot be distinguished based on clinical presentation alone. Joint disease tends to be the sole manifestation in idiopathic polyarthritis. The clinical manifestations in dogs with SLE are diverse and depend on organ involvement, but polyarthritis is the most common finding (60 to 90 per cent) and frequently the primary presenting complaint.

Clinical Pathology

Anemia is infrequent in most nonerosive arthritides, the exception being canine SLE (20 to 35 per cent). Nonregenerative anemia is the predominant type of anemia in canine SLE, instead of an autoimmune hemolytic anemia. In nonerosive arthritides, elevated concentrations of fibrinogen (acute phase protein) and increases in the erythrocyte sedimentation rate are consistent. Mild to marked leukocytosis and absolute neutrophilia are common in acute febrile attacks, although the leukogram can be normal.

Serum chemistry profiles are either normal or show variable decreases in albumin and absolute or relative increases in serum globulin. In patients with these abnormalities, serum electrophoresis is valuable to confirm hypoalbuminemia and demonstrate elevations in alpha$_2$- and gamma-globulins.

Findings on urinalysis are unremarkable. Detection of proteinuria is compatible with SLE and present in approximately 50 per cent of the cases. Proteinuria is also present in most cases of polyarthritis associated with bacterial endocarditis and frequently is accompanied by hematuria and renal casts.

Synovial fluid analysis is essential to establish and differentiate between inflammatory and noninflammatory arthropathies. Arthrocentesis of multiple joints, both clinically affected and asymptomatic, is recommended because multiple joints are often pathologically but not clinically affected, and analysis from a single joint occasionally is inconclusive. Therefore, analysis of synovial fluid is the single most helpful test to establish the presence, severity, and distribution of joint involvement in inflammatory joint diseases.

The volume of synovial fluid is often increased in patients with joint capsule distension. Affected joints show variable discoloration and increased turbidity as a consequence of increased cellularity. Normal fluid forms a long (>2.5 cm) ''string'' between the needle and a glass slide before the drop separates. A thin, runny consistency or the inability to form a long string suggests a deficiency in polymerized hyaluronic acid or dilution from excess serum. Nonerosive arthritides generally have low viscosity.

Nucleated cell counts in nonerosive immune-mediated arthropathies are moderately or markedly increased, ranging from 3,000/μl to 100,000/μl or more (reference range, <3,000/μl). Neutrophils (nontoxic) are the predominant cell type, ranging from approximately 30 per cent to 100 per cent (average 80 per cent) of nucleated cells (reference, <12 per cent and frequently ≤5 per cent). An increased number of neutrophils suggests inflammation of the synovial membrane and has no differentiating diagnostic value for specific inflammatory arthritides. Lymphocytes and large mononuclear cells with phagocytic potential account for the remainder of nucleated cells. Lupus erythematosus cells are found on rare occasions and are diagnostic of SLE.

Immune-mediated nonerosive arthritides, excluding SLE, are negative for both rheumatoid factor (RF) and fluorescent ANA (FANA) or have positive titers at insignificant levels. Indirect FANA is the most specific and sensitive serological test for SLE. FANA is not specific for SLE, and low titers can be found in a number of chronic infectious, inflammatory, and neoplastic disorders. A positive FANA test result therefore should be interpreted with caution and correlated with clinicopathological, pathological, and immunopathological findings. Geographic location or other clinical signs, in addition to polyarthritis, may require serological testing for chronic infectious diseases and include occult dirofilariasis, coccidioidomycosis, Lyme disease, ehrlichiosis, and Rocky Mountain spotted fever.

Radiographic Findings

Radiographic findings in immune-mediated nonerosive arthritides are usually normal or limited to nonspecific signs of soft-tissue swelling and joint distension. Even in chronic cases, radiographic signs are minimal: increased periarticular soft-tissue density due to fibrosis, periosteal bone proliferation at ligament or joint capsule attachments, and secondary degenerative joint disease. However, radiographic joint surveys should not be excluded from the initial examination, because the inflammatory process can be superimposed on a joint already affected with osteoarthritis.

Diagnosis

Diagnosis of immune-mediated nonerosive arthritis is based on the history, clinical signs, radiological and pathological features, and clinicopathological findings. Fever and joint pain are usually unresponsive to acetylsalicylic acid (aspirin) or antibiotics, although apparent clinical improvement may be observed owing to the cyclical nature of the disease. A diagnosis of idiopathic polyarthritis can be made when serological abnormalities are absent or detected at insignificant levels, bacterial cultures are negative, and evidence of an underlying disease process is absent.

The diagnosis of SLE in dogs can be exceedingly difficult because of the marked variability in clinical manifestations and laboratory findings. SLE is a multisystemic disease, and simultaneous or sequential involvement of more than one body system should be evident. The presence of two or more main clinical features stated earlier constitutes multisystemic involvement. Pyrexia, lethargy, and inappetence are minor nonspecific features that are not regarded as multisystemic involvement. Central to the diagnosis of canine SLE is the demonstration of a significantly high ANA titer in the blood. When one major sign is present with a positive ANA result, the diagnosis of *probable* canine SLE is justified because involvement of more than one body system may take time. There is disagreement about the justification of probable SLE without the presence of ANA. Approximately 10 per cent of human patients with SLE are ANA negative; however, other autoantibodies, besides ANA, directed against soluble tissue antigens can be demonstrated.

A diagnosis of polyarthritis associated with a chronic infective disease process elsewhere in the body depends on finding a sterile arthritis and identifying an infectious agent remote from the joints. Urinary and respiratory tract infections and bacterial endocarditis are most frequently identified. Chronic and subacute bacterial endocarditis present the most difficulty in differentiating infectious from noninfectious immune-mediated arthritis. Bacterial endocarditis is considered in all dogs with unexplained fevers, lameness, cardiac murmur, and multisystemic involvement compatible with circulating immune complexes or embolic phenomena.

The overlying enteric, hepatic, or neoplastic disease process associated with arthritis is usually apparent and generally precedes or coincides with the onset of lameness. Enteropathic arthritis is diagnosed by detecting an inflammatory bowel disease, such as chronic ulcerative colitis or fulminating enterocolitis, concurrently with sterile arthritis. Hepatopathic arthritis is substantiated when chronic active hepatitis or cirrhosis is identified histologically and no other cause of polyarthritis is found.

Drug-induced arthritis is suspected if the use of any drug is accompanied by a sterile arthritis with or without various dermatological lesions. The most common drugs incriminated are antibiotics, especially sulfonamides and penicillins. In Doberman pinschers with sulfadiazine-induced allergies, clinical signs were delayed 10 to 21 days after initial treatment.

The many similarities shared by inflammatory joint diseases, particularly the immune-mediated forms, should emphasize the importance of a systematic approach and careful interpretation of all test results.

Treatment

The treatment of immune-mediated nonerosive arthritis depends on the primary disease identified. The arthritis generally resolves spontaneously if treatment of the infectious, gastrointestinal, hepatic, or neoplastic disease is successful. Persistent arthritis may necessitate administration of glucocorticoids. In some geographic areas canine ehrlichiosis and borreliosis infections are associated with a nonerosive polyarthritis indistinguishable from immune-mediated nonerosive polyarthritides. For this reason, doxycycline (10 mg/kg once daily) is recommended while awaiting (5 to 7 days) serological test results for suspected infectious disorders. In addition to rest and confinement, idiopathic polyarthritis, SLE, plasmacytic-lymphocytic synovitis, and polyarthritis/polymyositis syndrome are treated with glucocorticoids or combination immunosuppressive drugs.

Prednisone or prednisolone is administered orally at a dosage of 2 to 4 mg/kg (100 mg/m^2 body surface area) in divided doses for 2 weeks. After 2 weeks, the dog is re-evaluated. Clinical signs and physical examination, although helpful, should not be the basis for adjusting glucocorticoid dosage or adding immunosuppressive drugs to the treatment protocol. As in the diagnosis of inflammatory joint disease, arthrocentesis and cytological examination of synovial fluid are essential in evaluating the response to treatment. Those joints containing the most dramatic synovial fluid abnormalities can be monitored and used as reference points on subsequent rechecks.

Treatment is modified depending on whether or not the disease is in remission. Remission is the resolution of clinical abnormalities and the absence of inflammatory changes in the synovial fluid. Remission is observed within 2 to 4 weeks if prednisolone alone is to be successful. If remission has occurred, prednisolone is reduced by 50 per cent at 2-week intervals until maintenance dosage (1 mg/kg every other morning) is attainable. Prednisolone can usually be safely reduced if a dog is clinically stable but synovial fluid cannot be obtained. In such cases, the measurement of fibrinogen, if previously elevated, may be of value in determining a patient's clinical status. If remission has been maintained, alternate-day therapy (1 mg/kg) is continued for an additional 1 to 2 months and rechecks extended to once a month. If complete remission has been maintained after this time, medication is discontinued.

If, after the second week, improvement in either the joint fluid abnormalities or the clinical signs is not substantial, combination therapy (glucocorticoid and cytotoxic drug) is started. Combination therapy can also be used as the initial treatment, avoiding undesirable effects from high-dose glucocorticoid therapy. I prefer a glucocorticoid combined with cyclophosphamide. The dosage of cyclophosphamide is 50 mg/m^2 body surface area given orally once daily on 4 consecutive days or on alternate days for a week. This constitutes one cycle of therapy. Azathioprine (Imuran) can be used for induction therapy, but remission may take longer than when cyclophosphamide is used. Azathioprine is less toxic and preferred for the few cases in which long-term therapy is necessary. The dosage of azathioprine is 50 mg/m^2 body surface area given orally once daily. Chlorambucil (Leukeran, 2 mg/m^2 body surface area daily) and 6-mercaptopurine (Purinethol, 50 mg/m^2 body surface area daily) are alternative cytotoxic drugs that have met with some success. A glucocorticoid is administered simultaneously with cytotoxic drugs at the same dosage or at half the dosage outlined previously.

Bone marrow toxicity is the most common adverse effect of the cytotoxic drugs. Therefore, complete blood cell counts are recommended every week or two until complete remission is achieved.

The prognosis for idiopathic polyarthritis is usually favorable. Glucocorticoid therapy alone can successfully induce remission in many cases. Patients not responding to glucocorticoid therapy usually respond favorably to combined immunosuppressive drug therapy. In all patients, recurrence is common (30 per cent to 50 per cent) for a variable period of time after drug therapy has been discontinued. The prognosis for SLE is guarded, depending on the extent of the systemic involvement, and poor if renal involvement develops. Dogs with SLE can often achieve long-term remission on alternate-day therapy of a glucocorticoid, and some may achieve long-term remission without drugs.

CANINE EROSIVE ARTHRITIS (pp. 1934–1937)

CHAPTER 145

Other Orthopedic Diseases
(pages 1938–1996)

Hip Dysplasia in Dogs (pages 1938–1944)

Malformation of the hip in dogs, or canine hip dysplasia, is a developmental not a congenital disorder of the coxofemoral joints. The disease is a serious medical problem because hip osteoarthritis, restricted joint mobility, pain, and lameness are associated with it. It is particularly common in large breeds such as Saint Bernards, Alaskan malamutes, bulldogs, boxers, collies, rottweilers, German shepherds, golden retrievers, huskies, Labrador retrievers, Old English sheepdogs, and standard poodles, but the smaller breeds are not spared. Males and bitches are affected with similar frequency, although one study identified more females with the disease.

Research during the past 20 years has not elucidated the essential nature of the disease. A genetic basis has been identified, but the pattern of inheritance is multifactorial, not simple mendelian genetics. Because diagnosis based on pelvic radiography can accurately identify the presence or absence of the abnormality only in adults, control of canine hip dysplasia has been limited.

CLINICAL SIGNS AND DIAGNOSIS (pp. 1938–1941)

Clinical Signs

Decreased activity and various degrees of joint pain are early manifestations. These signs are often first observed between the ages of 4 months and 1 year. Affected dogs often run with both hindlegs moving together, the so-called gait of bunny hopping. A dog may have difficulty in rising from a sitting or lying position, and stairs are difficult to climb. Affected dogs may exhibit pain when an affected hip joint is manipulated.

Radiography

Observation and physical examination can arouse suspicion of hip dysplasia; however, the diagnosis of hip dysplasia is established by radiographic examination with the dog under general anesthesia or deep sedation to ensure proper positioning. A ventrodorsal pelvic radiograph is made with the dog's hindlimbs extended to their maximum position, with the femurs parallel to each other and to the spine. The patellae are superimposed over the sagittal plane of the femoral condyles of the stifle by rotating the stifles inward. The pelvis must be positioned symmetrically so that the obturator foramina appear of equal size. Disease-free hip joints have well-formed femoral heads that fit congruently into the acetabula. In large dogs, the center of each femoral head should be located medial to the cranial edge of the acetabulum, and more than 50 per cent of the projected area of the femoral head should be shadowed by the dorsal rim of the acetabulum.

Coxofemoral joints of pups that later become dysplastic appear structurally disease free at birth. The initial radiographic diagnosis can sometimes be made as early as 10 to 12 weeks but frequently is made between 5 and 9 months of age. By 1 year of age, 70 to 80 per cent of susceptible dogs have radiographic signs of dysplasia.

The joint is considered dysplastic when the femoral head conforms poorly to the acetabulum. Increased joint space is commonly observed, and structural abnormalities can be detected in the acetabula and femoral heads. Subluxation, or partial displacement, of the femoral heads from the acetabula is the hallmark of canine hip dysplasia. Radiographic changes characteristic of hip dysplasia sometimes cannot be detected until a dog is 2 years old. The changes often are subtle and can be detected only by an experienced radiologist. In studies of German shepherds and Labrador retrievers, about 40 per cent of dogs disposed to hip dysplasia had radiographic evidence of dysplasia at 6 months of age, 70 to 80 per cent at 1 year of age, and about 90 per cent at 2 years.

The conventional hip-extended position for radiographic examination is unnatural and exerts constraints on the joint capsule, the round ligament, and muscles, perhaps "tightening" some abnormal joints. It is because of this concern that another position was used; anesthetized dogs were placed with their hindlimbs nearly perpendicular to the tabletop, and a distraction force applied to the femurs.

Joint Laxity

A characteristic feature of hip dysplasia is joint instability. The cause of increased laxity in the pathogenesis is unknown, but data suggested that the laxity is associated with mild synovitis and increases in the volume of the round ligament and synovial fluid. Some anesthetized dogs have increased coxofemoral joint laxity on palpation but appear normal on radiographic examination. An anatomical basis for this inconsistency has not been identified, but possible explanations include how precisely the animal is positioned, the force used during palpation, and depth of anesthesia.

Palpation for joint laxity in young dogs is not reliable to predict hip dysplasia. Manipulation of a joint, or palpation, is a subjective procedure. To estimate the extent of laxity, Smith and colleagues measured the distance in millimeters between the center of the femoral head and the acetabulum. Bellkoff and associates measured the percentage of the femoral head medial to the cranial acetabular rim. Both of these quantitative measurements and the Norberg angle are useful in a number of situations when it is necessary to assess the extent of subluxation of femoral heads on pelvic radiographs. Preliminary data of Smith and colleagues and of my own studies suggested that the hip joints of some pups appeared normal on the standard radiographs but had abnormal femoral head displacements by the new method and may later become dysplastic. The exact relationship between increased laxity observed by the force methods and the other signs of disease, or the lack thereof, observed with the legs-extended position is unclear and needs to be explained. For this reason, the forced laxity procedures should be regarded as experimental and unproven. To establish their usefulness in hip dysplasia diagnosis, they require standardization and follow-up studies for correlation with the conventional pelvic radiographic method.

Genetics

Hip dysplasia in dogs has a hereditary basis. It is considered to be a polygenic or quantitative trait with the expression being determined by an interaction of genetic and environmental factors. The practical implication is that breeding dogs for desirable traits such as good temperament or large size may result in the unwitting selection of animals susceptible to hip dysplasia. The incidence of hip dysplasia can be reduced by selecting for breeding only dogs that have disease-free hips as assessed by standard radiographic examination. Selective breeding has led to some decrease in occurrence, but the disease has not been eliminated.

Many investigators involved with the genetics of this disease accept that hip dysplasia is a quantitative trait with a heritability of between 0.25 and 0.40. On a population basis, breeding normal males to normal females resulted in 64 to 81 per cent normal dogs and 19 to 36 per cent dysplastic offspring. For dysplastic-dysplastic matings, 7 to 37 per cent of offspring were normal and 63 to 93 per cent were dysplastic. From these considerations, it cannot be concluded that such matings produce only disease-free offspring, even when both parents are free of hip dysplasia. Despite this uncertainty, it is advisable to breed only disease-free dogs to reduce the incidence and severity of hip dysplasia in the canine population.

Progression of Abnormalities in Hip Joints

Coxofemoral joints of pups that later become dysplastic are structurally and functionally disease free at birth. Hip dysplasia in dogs is a developmental discontinuity of the femoral head and the acetabulum. This relationship between the articulating surfaces allows excessive movement of the femoral head. The effect is to damage, mildly inflame, and eventually weaken the hip joint. In more advanced stages of disease, synovitis and cartilage loss are increased, capsule thickening continues, bone changes occur and osteophytes form on the acetabulum and femoral head, and muscles in the region of the hip atrophy.

It is likely that the pain associated with canine hip dysplasia in its early stages results from stretching or tearing of fibers in the joint capsule and the round ligament. The pain associated with advanced disease is that of osteoarthritis.

Growth Patterns

Several reports in the literature suggested that the development of hip dysplasia can be influenced by food consumption. Nutritional supplements have no proven benefit. Investigators have proposed that the time of appearance and the rate of progression of hip dysplasia can be affected by the rate of weight gain of a dog. Weight gain as a result of increased food consumption accelerated; conversely, slowing weight gain by reducing food during the first several months of life delayed the appearance or diminished the severity of dysplasia.

It has been proposed that susceptible dogs made ''normal'' by dietary restriction would in effect have ''masked'' the disease and can yield dysplastic progeny. It was reasoned that radiographically normal dogs possibly carrying the undesired genes for hip dysplasia can be identified by using high food consumption.

Role of the Acetabulum (pp. 1942–1943)

Osteochondrosis (pp. 1944–1966)

Osteochondrosis is a well-described yet incompletely understood systemic disease of endochondral ossification affecting man, dogs, swine, horses, cattle, chickens, and turkeys. The term *osteochondrosis* describes a disease that affects the normal endochondral ossification of the growth plates, be they epiphyseal, metaphyseal, or apophyseal. Osteochondritis dissecans (OCD), the clinical manifestation of osteochondrosis with which veterinarians are most familiar, denotes a dissecting lesion between bone and articular cartilage. *Osteochondritis* is a misnomer because it implies inflammation of bone and cartilage, a rare condition.

Normal Anatomy (pp. 1944–1945)

Normal Growth (p. 1945)

Pathology

Osteochondrosis is marked by a disturbance in the normal differentiation of cartilage during endochondral ossification, resulting in thickening of the articular epiphyseal complex. The primary lesion in OCD is a dissecting intracartilaginous separation between the calcified and noncalcified tissues.

The possibility of cartilage separation from subchondral bone without communication with the articular surface is consistent with radiographically identifiable lesions not associated with clinical signs. Radiographically, osteochondrosis is identified as a radiolucent zone along the articular margin of the bone. The radiolucent zone is due to bone growth around a local site of retardation of ossification and cartilage. Radiographic evidence of osteochondrosis is often bilateral in animals with unilateral signs.

Articular cartilage normally exhibits poor ability to replace and repair itself. When cartilage suffers a partial-thickness injury, no bleeding and relatively little necrosis result, owing to low oxygen demand of this tissue. Because blood supply to cartilage is poor, little inflammation ensues. Chondrocytes have limited ability to produce matrix and cannot support repair. Repair occurs if the underlying bone, with its blood supply, is involved. The larger the defect, the more likely the animal is to have persistent lameness, and the larger the lesion, the more likely the opposite joint surface is to develop a "kissing" lesion.

During the repair process, subchondral bone formation occurs at the base of the granulation tissue bed but stops at the tidemark. The reparative fibrous granulation tissue undergoes chondrification and even develops some hyaline cartilage. Continuous passive motion during healing may encourage hyalinization of the reparative fibrocartilage.

Pathogenesis

The pathogenesis of osteochondrosis is a disturbance of articular/epiphyseal cartilage growth and endochondral osteogenesis. It is due to slow ossification of cartilage in the deep zone. In addition to increased articular cartilage thickness, chondrocytes of cartilage in this region had an irregular arrangement and were abnormal along the line of cleavage. The normal process of endochondral ossification of the deep cartilage ceases. Articular cartilage thickening leads to poor diffusion of nutrients from the synovial fluid to the deep zones of the articular cartilage. This leads to abnormal metabolism and function of the deep chondrocytes and, with some trauma, separation of the calcified and abnormal noncalcified tissues. Once the articular cartilage dissects free from the underlying calcified tissue, the lesion of OCD has formed.

Vertical fracture of articular cartilage is a later manifestation in the pathogenesis of OCD. If trauma sufficient to cause vertical fracture of the articular cartilage does not occur, the cartilage flap may reattach to the underlying subchondral bone because blood is present in the separation space as a result of bleeding from subchondral bone. This blood allows deposition of fibrin and permits undifferentiated mesenchymal cells to invade the area, leading to reattachment of the cartilage to the underlying bone.

Etiology

The etiology of osteochondrosis in animals is most likely multifactorial. The disease process involves traumatic, environmental, and constitutional aspects.

The process of ossification of the epiphysis may be under hormonal influences. Histological increases in cartilage thickness occur in animals given excessive somatotropin or thyrotropin. Excessive administration of these hormones resulted in a condition similar to OCD. Testosterone also stimulates epiphyseal growth and acts synergistically with growth hormone. Estrogen has the opposite effect, encouraging calcification of cartilage. These observations may account for greater predilection for males to develop osteochondrosis than females.

Overnutrition is directly related to the frequency of osteochondrosis in pigs. Rapid growth secondary to overnutrition results in increased cartilage thickness. Free feeding in young Great Danes leads to multiple skeletal abnormalities and cartilage disturbances, including osteochondrosis. These anomalies were due to excessive dietary calcium, which resulted in hypercalcitoninism, inhibiting cartilage maturation. In swine and poultry, osteochondrosis can be reduced by restricted feeding. Dogs presumably would similarly benefit from normal diet and a slower rate of growth. A familial tendency for development of

OCD exists, but definitive studies showing inheritability have not been completed. Trauma may have a major role in the etiology of the disease.

Species, Breed, and Age Distribution

Osteochondrosis is most frequently encountered in immature dogs whose mature weight is greater than 25 kg. The breeds most commonly affected are the Labrador and golden retriever, rottweiler, Great Dane, Saint Bernard, German shepherd, and Bernese mountain dog, although all large dogs and giant breeds may develop the disease.

OSTEOCHONDRITIS DISSECANS OF THE SHOULDER
(pp. 1947–1957)

Lesions of the shoulder joint usually involve the caudal central aspect of the humeral head articular cartilage, although lesions of the glenoid occur. Although this disease most frequently occurs in large dogs, it also affects small and medium-sized breeds. The age at which animals are presented for treatment varies. Ages ranging from 3 months to 5 years have been reported, although 75 per cent of cases in one study were presented between 5 and 10 months of age. Males are more commonly affected than females (2 to 5:1). The incidence of bilateral disease is reported to range between 20 and 85 per cent.

Clinical Signs

The most common clinical sign is a mild to moderate unilateral front leg lameness. It is unusual for dogs to show bilateral front leg lameness, even when both shoulders are affected. Some atrophy of the supraspinatus and infraspinatus muscles may be present, but it is seldom marked unless the lameness has been severe and protracted.

Extreme flexion and extension of the shoulder joint usually elicit a pain response. Because breeds of dogs presented for shoulder OCD are the same breeds that are typically presented for elbow disorders, one should not overly flex and extend the elbow while examining the shoulder to minimize the chance of confusing elbow pain with shoulder pain.

Diagnosis

The history and physical examination lead to a presumptive diagnosis of OCD, but shoulder radiographs are necessary to confirm the diagnosis. Mediolateral projections of both shoulders are obtained. Most can be diagnosed with this lateral view because the lesion is usually located in the central portion of the caudal aspect of the humeral head. The lesion occasionally is located more lateral or medial to the center of the humeral head. In these cases, obtain two additional lateral views, one while internally rotating the leg and the other while externally rotating the leg.

The typical OCD lesion of the caudal humeral head appears radiographically as a flattened radiolucent defect in the subchondral bone immediately beneath the articular cartilage. A mineralized cartilage flap or joint mice may be seen. Contrast arthrography can be helpful in confirming the presence of joint mice within the biceps tendon sheath and in diagnosing articular cartilage defects.

Treatment

Conservative therapy consisting of strict rest with or without analgesics has been recommended for some patients. Analgesics are used sparingly because they do not help the lesion heal and may cause a dog to become more active by minimizing pain.

We use conservative therapy (i.e., 4 to 6 weeks of strict rest) if the owner is reluctant to have surgery performed on the dog. The owner is asked to return the dog for surgery if there is no improvement during that time or if the lameness worsens. Conservative therapy can also be used if the dog is less than 7 months old, has mild lameness of short duration, and has a small radiographic lesion. I do not recommend conservative therapy if the dog is older than 7 months, if the lameness is severe or protracted, or if a radiographically demonstrable joint mouse or mineralized cartilage flap is present.

Surgical Treatment

Surgical treatment produces the most rapid return to function and minimizes degenerative joint disease. The objectives of surgery are to remove all loose cartilage fragments, including joint mice, and to stimulate the articular surface defect to heal by fibrocartilage formation.

Removal of the Cartilage Flap. Regardless of the approach, the cartilage flap is removed. All or a portion of the flap usually is still attached at the craniomedial extent of the lesion. It is important to remove all of the loose articular cartilage around the periphery of the lesion with a small bone curette. The margins of the remaining articular defect are left perpendicular to the joint surface because beveling the margins results in a larger defect that takes longer to heal and is more likely to cause a concurrent lesion in the glenoid cavity.

Forage (i.e., drilling multiple holes into subchondral bone) offers an alternative to curettage. If the subchondral bone is pale and sclerotic, curettage is necessary but removal of subchondral bone is minimized. Forage also may be useful. The joint is lavaged with sterile saline before closure.

Aftercare, Complications, and Prognosis. Most patients can be discharged the day after surgery. Bandaging is not necessary. Owners are instructed to restrict the dog's exercise to leash walks for the next 4 weeks.

The most common complication after surgical exposure of the shoulder joint is seroma formation. The incidence of seroma formation has been reported to be 0, 6, and 18 per cent. The exact cause of seroma formation is unknown, but several factors contribute, including failure to restrict the dog's activity, inadequate hemostasis, excessive undermining of the skin, and failure to eliminate dead space. Inadequate closure of the joint capsule is not a factor in seroma formation.

The prognosis after surgical treatment is good to excellent. Most dogs return to normal within 4 weeks of surgery. Older dogs with chronic lameness and degenerative joint disease have a more guarded prognosis.

OSTEOCHONDRITIS DISSECANS OF THE ELBOW
(pp. 1957–1961)

The signalment is the same as in dogs with OCD of the shoulder and occurs most frequently in large dogs. The disease is most prevalent in Bernese mountain dogs and in golden and Labrador retrievers.

The age at which dogs are presented for examination varies. Ages ranging from 4 months to 12 years are reported, and most dogs are less than 1 year old. Some dogs are asymptomatic (or lameness is not noticed) until they are older; therefore, one should not rule out elbow OCD simply because a dog is mature. Males are more commonly affected than females (2:1). Bilateral disease ranges between 20 and 50 per cent.

Clinical Signs/Physical Examination

An owner may report that the dog appears stiff in the morning or after periods of rest. Lameness is usually present but may be mild or intermittent. The lameness is worse after vigorous exercise.

A slight lateral swelling of the elbow may be present and is due to increased synovial fluid volume and joint capsule thickening. Crepitus may be felt on joint manipulation. Flexion and extension of the elbow may elicit pain. Because the signalment and clinical signs of dogs with elbow OCD and shoulder OCD are similar, it may be necessary to radiograph both the elbow and shoulder.

Diagnosis

The history, clinical signs, and physical examination lead to a tentative diagnosis of an elbow disorder, but radiographs are necessary to confirm the diagnosis. *Both* elbows are radiographed because the disease is often bilateral. Early radiographic changes are subtle, so high-quality radiographs are essential.

Several radiographic views are necessary for complete evaluation of the elbow. A mediolateral view is obtained by placing the dog in lateral recumbency with the elbow downward. The joint is maximally flexed during film exposure so that most of the anconeal process can be seen. A craniocaudal view is obtained with the dog in sternal recumbency. A slightly medial oblique craniocaudal projection may enhance observation of the medial humeral condyle.

Radiographic changes are varied, depending on the extent of secondary osteoarthritis. One of the first visible radiographic changes is osteophyte formation on the nonarticular cranial surface of the proximal anconeal process. Osteophytes are also frequently seen on the proximal radial head, medial humeral condyle, and medial coronoid process. These radiographic changes are nonspecific and represent secondary degenerative joint disease. Many dogs with elbow degenerative joint disease suffer from a general incongruity of the joint termed *elbow dysplasia.*

Specific radiographic changes are not seen in every patient. A radiolucent defect may be noted in the medial humeral condyle. This lucency is best observed in a craniocaudal, slightly medial oblique projection with the elbow in about 30° of flexion. If the defect is large, it may also be visible on a lateral projection as a flattening of the articular surface of the medial condyle. In most cases, the radiographic changes of OCD of the elbow are not diagnostic; definitive diagnosis often requires exploratory arthrotomy.

Treatment

Treatment consists of a medial arthrotomy and removal of the cartilage flap. A simple medial approach without tenotomy or osteotomy provides excellent exposure of the elbow joint.

Surgical Approach (p. 1959)

Aftercare, Complications, and Prognosis

The wound is covered with a sterile dressing, and a padded bandage is applied to the leg. The bandage remains in place until the sutures are removed in 10 to 14 days. Clients are instructed to restrict the dog's activity to leash walks for 4 weeks.

The only complication is seroma formation. If the bandage remains in place and the dog's activity is restricted, seroma formation is uncommon.

The prognosis after surgery depends on the size of the lesion and the severity of the secondary osteoarthritis present at treatment. Generally, young dogs with small lesions and minimal secondary osteoarthritis have a favorable prognosis. Dogs with more severe lesions, more severe osteoarthritis, and concurrent fragmented medial coronoid have a more guarded prognosis. Most dogs improve clinically after surgery, but the osteoarthritis may progress.

OSTEOCHONDRITIS DISSECANS OF THE STIFLE
(pp. 1961–1962)

Although OCD occurs much less commonly in the stifle than in the shoulder or elbow, it also afflicts young large dogs. Males are more commonly affected than females.

Clinical Signs

The main clinical sign is lameness. The onset of lameness is insidious, and the lameness worsens with exercise. The owners are frequently only aware of a unilateral lameness even though both stifles are affected. Dogs with bilateral disease may assume a crouched stance.

Mild muscle atrophy may be present, particularly in the more chronic cases. A slight joint effusion is often present. Pain and occasional crepitus or an audible click may be elicited on manipulation.

Diagnosis

A diagnosis of OCD of the stifle cannot be confirmed by physical examination. Joint effusion, muscle atrophy, pain, and crepitus could be associated with various causes of osteoarthritis of the stifle. Mediolateral and caudocranial radiographic views of the stifle are necessary to confirm the diagnosis.

A flattened area on the weightbearing surface of the femoral condyle and joint mice may be seen on the mediolateral view. It is difficult but not impossible to determine from the mediolateral view which femoral condyle is involved. The fossa of the long digital extensor tendon can be used to determine which is the lateral condyle. The caudocranial view can help reveal which condyle is involved if the lesion can be seen. The lesion may not always be visible in this view and should not be confused with the superimposed extensor fossa.

Bilateral lesions occur in 72 per cent of cases. The medial femoral condyle alone was involved in 4 per cent. The lesion was located in the medial femoral condyle in 80 per cent in one human study. Most of the lesions in dogs occur in the lateral femoral condyle.

Treatment

The treatment of stifle OCD is similar to treatment in other joints. If the lesion is located in the lateral femoral condyle, a lateral arthrotomy is performed. A medial arthrotomy is performed for medial condylar lesions. All joint mice and loose cartilage flaps are removed. As with all OCD defects, the articular margins are left perpendicular to the articular surfaces.

Aftercare, Complications, and Prognosis

Activity is restricted to leash walks for 4 weeks.

The prognosis depends on the extent of the degenerative joint disease and size of the lesion. As with OCD of the elbow, the degenerative joint disease of the stifle progresses. Dogs with small lesions and late onset of clinical signs have the best prognosis. Dogs with large lesions, advanced degenerative joint disease, and early onset of clinical signs have a worse prognosis.

OSTEOCHONDRITIS DISSECANS OF THE TARSUS
(pp. 1962–1965)

OCD of the tarsus also occurs in large dogs and is most commonly reported in rottweilers and Labrador retrievers. Although most dogs are less than 1 year old when initially presented, one study reports an age range of 5 to 48 months.

Clinical Signs

Hindlimb lameness is the most common clinical sign. Hyperextension of the tarsocrural joint is common. Joint effusion and tarsal thickening are often present, especially on the medial side of the joint.

Diagnosis

Confirmation of OCD of the talus depends on high-quality radiographs. The craniocaudal projection is most helpful in diagnosing OCD of the medial trochlear ridge of the talus. The mediolateral or oblique views are most helpful in diagnosing OCD of the lateral trochlear ridge, because the calcaneus is superimposed over the lateral trochlear ridge, in the craniocaudal view. Both hocks are radiographed because the disease often occurs bilaterally.

Radiographic abnormalities include a radiolucent or flattened area involving either trochlear ridge (occasionally both) and a widened joint space. A widened joint space is more common with lesions involving the medial trochlear ridge. Soft-tissue swelling is invariably present, and degenerative joint disease develops in chronic cases.

Treatment

The most common treatment used for OCD of the tarsus has been removal of the cartilage flap or joint mice with or without curettage of the subchondral bone.

Aftercare, Complications, and Prognosis

If an osteotomy has been performed, a rigid splint is used to support the internal repair for 4 to 6 weeks. Activity is restricted for 4 to 6 weeks after surgery (8 to 10 weeks if an osteotomy has been performed).

The goal of surgical treatment is to limit or halt the progression of osteoarthritis and lameness associated with OCD of the tarsus. Surgical removal of the lesion did not modify progression of osteoarthritic changes. Removal of the cartilage flap may accentuate joint instability and contribute to osteoarthritis. A more rational approach is to reattach the cartilage fragments, which might be feasible in patients with large cartilage flaps or with osteochondral fragments. The long-term prognosis for OCD of the talus is guarded. Most reports suggest that osteoarthritis tends to progress. The prognosis is generally favorable if the lesions are small and treated early.

Elbow Dysplasia (pp. 1966–1977)

The term *elbow dysplasia* was introduced to describe generalized osteoarthrosis of the elbow joint in which the anconeal process was ununited in some but not all affected joints. Later, fragmentation of the medial coronoid process of the ulna and osteochondritis dissecans of the humeral condyle were associated with this arthrosis.

The breeds primarily afflicted are of intermediate size and heavy set, with a high incidence in the Bernese mountain dog, rottweiler, German shepherd, golden retriever, and Labrador retriever.

Dysplastic Elbow Joint: Anatomy

In an elbow joint with fragmentation of the medial coronoid process or osteochondritis dissecans, the medial coronoid process and the distal edge of the ulnar trochlear notch frequently lie slightly above the level of the adjoining radius, creating a step between the radius and the ulna and causing incongruity within the joint. This may mean that either the radius is too short or the ulnar trochlear notch has a smaller than normal diameter. Whatever the reason, it seems likely that weightbearing forces on the ulna are increased, causing excessive loading of the medial coronoid process (especially its lateral edge) and the distal edge of the trochlear notch, leading to fragmentation. The fragment is often the size of a rice grain or larger and may be attached cranially to the annular ligament. A superficial to deeply grooved "kissing" lesion may be present on the humeral articular surface opposite the coronoid fragment.

Secondary osteoarthrosis becomes evident after the age of 6 to 7 months. Osteophytes and articular lipping develop in the following order: dorsal edge of the anconeal process, lateral epicondylar ridge, rim of the medial flange of the ulnar trochlear notch and medial coronoid process, cranial medial edge of the head of the radius, and medial aspect of the humeral condyle.

The early appearance of osteophytes on the anconeal process and the lateral epicondylar ridge (i.e., lateral edge of olecranon fossa), as well as the frequent finding of loss of central or lateral articular cartilage of the ulnar trochlear notch, suggests that the anconeal process skews medially within the olecranon fossa during flexion, resulting in traction on the lateral joint capsule and causing loss of contact between the lateral aspect of the ulnar trochlear notch and the humeral trochlea. This medial skewing may be evident clinically as "paddling" (i.e., supination of the forelegs on flexion), which is frequently observed in affected dogs.

Dysplastic Elbow Joint: Radiographic Appearance

The radiographic appearance of dysplastic elbows is characterized by incongruity and sequential osteoarthrosis. On a lateral radiograph taken at the age of 6 months, the following may be noticed:

1. Increased humeroulnar joint space in the central area of the ulnar trochlear notch
2. Increased humeroradial joint space
3. A break in the normal continuous arc between the ulnar trochlear notch and the radial articulation, with the distal edge of the ulnar trochlear notch lying a step above the level of the radius

4. Cranial displacement of the humerus on the radius
5. Incomplete or irregular outline of the medial coronoid process
6. Mild increase in bone density at the distal end of the ulnar trochlear notch
7. Early osteophytosis at the dorsal aspect of the anconeal process

On the craniocaudal view, an increased humeroradial and decreased humeroulnar joint space or a joint space that is irregular in width may be seen.

Osteochondritis dissecans can usually be seen on an accurately taken craniocaudal radiograph as a flat triangular radiolucent area on the medial articular edge of the humeral trochlea. On a lateral view, it may create a flattening of the medial caudoventral edge of the humeral trochlea.

CAUSES OF INCONGRUITY (pp. 1969–1973)

CLINICAL FINDINGS (pp. 1973–1974)

Affected dogs are frequently lame or have an abnormal gait, the latter especially when both elbows are involved. This gait may be characterized by excessive supination of the front paws. This is not pathognomonic, however, because many apparently normal dogs of affected breeds supinate also. The animal may hold the elbows out or tucked in and often stands with its feet rotated out. Effusion may be palpable beneath anconeal and extensor muscles and may be more pronounced after activity. In chronic cases, thickening of the joint capsule, increased prominence of the medial humeral epicondyle, and muscle atrophy are present. In severe cases, the dog sits or lies down much of the time and plays for shorter periods than other dogs its age. Some dogs can barely walk around the block.

DIAGNOSIS (p. 1974)

In young dogs (5 to 7 months), the diagnosis is primarily based on clinical signs and radiographic evaluation. Radiographs are made of both elbows to allow comparison, especially of subtle findings, and to check for the presence of bilateral elbow dysplasia, which is common.

In *mature* dogs, the diagnosis of elbow dysplasia (with fragmented coronoid or osteochondritis dissecans) is easier than in young dogs because of the presence of osteoarthrosis, especially osteophytosis of the anconeal process. A flexed lateral radiograph is most useful, especially if the examination is requested for the purpose of registration.

TREATMENT (p. 1974)

Therapy may be surgical or conservative, depending primarily on the degree of osteoarthrosis. Moderation of exercise and strict weight control are important for all dogs with elbow dysplasia. Intermittent use of analgesics may be required, depending on the severity of the condition. Aspirin is recommended (10 to 20 mg/kg BID). Phenylbutazone is prescribed if aspirin is not effective; its initial use is supervised because of the possibility of bone marrow suppression. Because severe ulceration of the gastrointestinal tract can occur in dogs given nonsteroidal anti-inflammatory drugs, careful monitoring is indicated.

Joint incongruity causes cartilage damage and osteoarthrosis. With greater incongruity, osteochondritis dissecans, fragmentation of the medial coronoid process, and ununited anconeal process are common, and both the incongruity and the lesions contribute to the severity of the osteoarthrosis.

The onset of pain is usually between 4 and 6 months of age and is in part due to joint fluid entering subchondral bone either via osteochondritis dissecans, chondral fissures or fragmentation of the medial coronoid process, or chondral and physeal fissures within a separate center of ossification of the anconeal process. *In situ* movement of the bony or cartilaginous fragments prevents healing of the exposed subchondral or subphyseal bone, and the pain persists but diminishes with time. Surgical removal of the fragments is recommended before development of severe arthrosis. *Clients should be made aware of the progressive nature of the disease and that improvement but not normality is to be expected.*

SURGICAL CANDIDATES (pp. 1974–1975)

All immature dogs with fragmentation of the medial coronoid process, osteochondritis dissecans, or an ununited anconeal process are surgical candidates, dogs with slight to moderate incongruity and minimal osteoarthrosis having the most favorable prognosis. Even those with marked incongruity and large lesions benefit from surgery because of the decrease in pain.

Dogs that have a combined ununited anconeal process and fragmentation of the medial coronoid process have the worst prognosis. Even with surgery, crippling lameness is usually present by the age of 4 to 5 years; the lameness is often unresponsive to exercise limitation, weight control, or drug therapy.

Mature dogs with mild to moderate osteoarthrosis may also be considered for surgery. Dogs with severe osteoarthrosis (i.e., with stable but painful elbow joints) are not operated on because interference with this stability may aggravate rather than diminish the problem. Analgesic medication or arthrodesis is considered for these patients.

Removal of Fragmentation of the Medial Coronoid Process or Osteochondritis Dissecans of the Humeral Condyle or Both

Adequate exposure with minimal morbidity is achieved by a medial approach to the medial compartment of the elbow joint. Exposure for the arthrotomy can be gained by separation of the flexor muscles and capsulotomy or via an osteotomy of the medial humeral epicondyle. The choice of technique is a matter of personal preference, although better exposure is gained with an osteotomy.

Bilateral Involvement of the Elbow Joints

When surgery is indicated for both joints, they can be operated on at the same time because use of the legs after surgery is not impaired to the extent that a dog is unable to walk.

PROGNOSIS

In moderately affected dogs, with or without surgery, weight control and the animal's natural inclination to limit its exercise allow the animal to cope with this problem. Working dogs are frequently limited in their performance. In severely affected dogs, it is often a crippling disease.

HEREDITY OF ELBOW DYSPLASIA (p. 1976)

Studies of German shepherds and rottweilers have demonstrated that elbow dysplasia is an inherited disease.

IMPLICATIONS AND RECOMMENDATIONS (p. 1976)

Elbow dysplasia is a polygenetic heritable disease, as is hip dysplasia. Mating of normal phenotypes may still produce dysplastic pups, because the parents carry genes for dysplasia (genotypically affected). Better control of this type of genetic disease requires knowledge of the disease incidence in offspring. This implies (1) registration of normal as well as affected individuals and (2) access to this information for analysis.

Ununited Anconeal Process (pp. 1977–1984)

DEFINITION (p. 1977)

Ununited anconeal process (UAP) in dogs is encountered most frequently in juvenile large dogs, in which the anconeal process fails to undergo bony fusion to the ulnar diaphysis. The anconeal process may remain attached by fibrous tissue or it may become physically separated, producing instability and secondary degenerative joint disease.

ETIOLOGY AND PATHOGENESIS (p. 1978)

In initial reports describing UAP, the affected animals all were German shepherds, and many were closely related. Heredity was assumed to be a major etiological factor.

UAP, along with fragmented coronoid process and osteochondritis dissecans, may be a manifestation of osteochondrosis. Osteochondrosis could weaken the attachment of the anconeal process to the ulna and, with the stress of weightbearing, could lead to failure of the process to unite with the ulna. Underdevelopment of the trochlear notch may cause excessive stress on the developing anconeal process and cause nonunion.

The UAP may be attached to the ulna by fibrous tissue or it may be completely separated from the parent bone, producing lateral instability. Instability and the presence of a free fragment of bone within the joint lead to irritation, abnormal wear, and secondary degenerative joint disease. Early changes include joint effusion, disruption of the cartilage in the semilunar notch, joint capsule thickening, and periarticular osteophyte production. Loss of cartilage and eburnation of subchondral bone, remodeling of the process, and joint capsule thickening with reduced range of motion are noted in chronic cases.

The German shepherd was the first breed in which UAP was described. By 1968, however, UAP had been identified in Saint Bernards, Irish wolfhounds, basset hounds, Newfoundlands, bloodhounds, Labrador retrievers, Great Danes, French bulldogs, pointers, Great Pyrenees, weimaraners, and dachshunds. Classic UAP is a disease of large to giant breeds of dogs, and a separate center of ossification for the anconeal process has been documented in a number of these breeds. In chondrodystrophic breeds, premature closure of the distal ulnar physis causes caudal subluxation of the proximal ulna and shearing stress on the anconeal process. Anconeal separation in these breeds should be considered as a type of fracture rather than classic UAP.

CLINICAL SIGNS AND DIAGNOSIS (p. 1978–1980)

Because the anconeal process may not fuse to the diaphysis of the ulna until 4 to 5 months of age, the diagnosis of UAP is premature if made before a dog is 4½ to 5 months old. The usual age of presentation is 6 to 12 months, but affected dogs may not exhibit clinical signs until they are much older.

Intermittent lameness exacerbated by exercise is the most frequent presenting complaint. The lameness usually becomes evident between 6 and 12 months of age. When the disease is present in both elbows, the lameness may be shifting or may even be difficult to detect when both elbows are equally affected. The lameness is more insidious and progressive in older dogs because of the progressive nature of the osteoarthritic changes. Effusion is present early in the course of the disease, and joint capsule thickening becomes predominant with time. Extension and flexion of the elbow elicit pain and crepitation.

Definitive diagnosis is made by radiographic examination. A radiolucent line separating the anconeal process from the diaphysis of the ulna in a dog older than 5 months is diagnostic of UAP. The anconeal process is obscured by the medial epicondyle of the humerus in the standard lateral view of the elbow, so a flexed lateral view is important to observe the process adequately.

The differential diagnosis includes fragmented coronoid process, osteochondritis dissecans of the medial portion of the condyle, osteochondritis dissecans, panosteitis, trauma (including fractures and ligamentous injuries), and osteoarthritis due to other causes.

TREATMENT (p. 1980)

Treatment options include conservative management, removal of the anconeal process, or surgical stabilization of the anconeal process to the ulna. In a young dog with a process that has not formed a bony union with the ulna in the appropriate time but that appears to be stable via a fibrous union, strict rest and immobilization of the limb with a splint or cast for 4 weeks may allow bony union to occur. If the UAP is discovered as an incidental finding in an asymptomatic older dog, it is appropriate not to intervene surgically unless clinical signs develop.

Chondrodystrophic breeds, especially the bassett hound, may exhibit elbow pain and very slight displacement of the anconeal process as a result of early closure of the distal ulnar physis. In such cases, surgical sectioning of the radioulnar ligament may relieve the stress on the anconeal process and allow fusion to occur. If the process is displaced and unstable, excision is recommended. Surgical removal of the process through a modified lateral approach to the elbow is the most common therapy because it is simple to perform and yields generally satisfactory results.

The prognosis after surgical removal is favorable if surgery is performed before extensive degenerative changes have occurred. The osteoarthritic changes present at the time of surgery are not reversible and continue to progress slowly. Some investigators believe that the benefit produced by surgical removal is temporary and that lameness returns.

Perthes' Disease (pp. 1981–1984)

Necrosis of the proximal femoral epiphysis occurs in children and in immature small dogs. More descriptive terms for the disease include *aseptic necrosis of the femoral head, coxa plana,* and *coxa magna.* Perthes' disease in dogs is usually unilateral, and a higher than expected incidence is noted in the Manchester terrier, miniature pinscher, poodle, Lakeland terrier, West Highland white terrier, and Cairn terrier.

CLINICAL SIGNS AND DIAGNOSIS (p. 1981)

Dogs with Perthes' disease become lame, usually between 4 months and 11 months of age. The onset may appear acute; however, muscle atrophy is invariably present in the affected leg, suggesting a more chronic history. Manipulation of the hip evokes pain and guarding, although crepitation is usually absent. Muscle atrophy is most apparent in the hamstring and gastrocnemius muscles. The primary differential diagnosis in young dogs is medial patella luxation, which may occur as an incidental finding. The presence of thigh muscle atrophy and pain in the hip will distinguish Perthes' disease from medial patella luxation.

A tentative diagnosis of Perthes' disease is based on the history and physical findings and confirmed by radiographic examination. Early radiographic signs include irregular densities within the metaphysis and discrete radiolucent areas within the epiphysis. These findings generally precede lameness, thus clinical patients invariably have more advanced changes, including deformity of the epiphysis, thickening of the femoral neck, and increased width of the joint space. More chronic and severe cases demonstrate collapse and fragmentation of the femoral head with periarticular new bone formation. The diagnosis of Perthes' disease is confirmed by radiographic findings that include deformity of the epiphysis, thickening of the femoral neck, and increased width of the joint space.

PATHOPHYSIOLOGY (pp. 1981–1982)

The cause of Perthes' disease is unknown. Histological findings suggest that the disease is the result of infarction of epiphyseal and metaphyseal bone, including the physis. The epiphysis is deformed, growth plate architecture is lost, and subchondral spaces contain necrotic debris surrounded by fibrovascular tissue and osteoclasts.

Vascular alteration may be related to trauma or predisposing anatomical factors. Toy poodles have a subsynovial blood supply to the femoral epiphysis, compared with an intraosseous system in larger mongrel dogs. The subsynovial location of vessels in toy poodles may increase their susceptibility to ischemia with increased intra-articular pressure. Perthes' disease in Manchester terriers has a multifactorial inheritance pattern with a high degree of heritability, as in man.

TREATMENT (pp. 1982–1984)

Most dogs with clinical signs associated with Perthes' disease are relatively severely affected, and surgical treatment is required. Femoral head and neck ostectomy is recommended for dogs with lameness and radiographic signs of femoral head collapse and joint incongruity. The surgery is a salvage procedure; with dedicated owner compliance and physical therapy, the prognosis for pain-free ambulation is favorable.

Miscellaneous Orthopedic Diseases
(pp. 1984–1996)

PANOSTEITIS (pp. 1984–1987)

Panosteitis is a spontaneously occurring self-limiting disease of unknown cause affecting young large or giant breeds of dogs. The disease involves the diaphyseal and metaphyseal areas of long bones and is characterized by medullary enostosis and occasionally subperiosteal new bone formation. It is most common in German shepherds but has also been reported in the bassett hound, Scottish terrier, Great Dane, Saint Bernard, Doberman pinscher, German shorthaired pointer, Irish setter, Airedale, golden retriever, Labrador retriever, Samoyed, and miniature schnauzer. Panosteitis is not a primary bone disease but a disease of the fatty bone marrow, with secondary effects involving bone.

Clinical signs usually occur in large dogs between 5 and 12 months of age but have been documented as early as 2 months of age and as late as 5 years. Males are more commonly affected; if encountered in females, panosteitis is usually associated with the first estrus. Affected animals have acute lameness ranging from slight to severe without a history of trauma. The lameness may be persistent or intermittent and involve one or more limbs. The disease commonly resolves in one location only to shift to another. This cycle typically occurs at 2- to 3-week intervals, with short lapses between episodes. Physical examination reveals discomfort associated with deep palpation of the affected area.

The earliest recognizable radiographic abnormality is an increase in intramedullary density. In the early stages, this increased density is unifocal and has indistinct margins. As the disease progresses, multiple foci of increased radiodensities coalesce within the medullary cavity. In later stages of the disease, areas of increased radiodensity within the medullary canal regress, although the sclerosis may remain apparent for several months. There is no correlation between radiographic signs, degree of lameness, and amount of pain elicted on palpation.

Treatment consists of supportive care and analgesics to alleviate discomfort. We recommend buffered aspirin (10 to 20 mg/kg PO TID). If gastrointestinal upset occurs or aspirin is ineffective, other nonsteroidal anti-inflammatory drugs may be considered; however, dogs are very sensitive to many of these drugs, and caution must be implemented in their use. The prognosis for return to full function is excellent; however, it is important to counsel owners about the cyclical nature of the disease so that they do not become frustrated with its prolonged course.

HYPERTROPHIC OSTEODYSTROPHY (pp. 1987–1988)

Hypertrophic osteodystrophy is a developmental disease of immature large and giant breeds of dogs in which the metaphyseal area of long bones becomes swollen and painful. The distal radius and ulna are the bones most commonly affected, although all long bones are susceptible.

Although the pathogenesis is obscure, this disease exerts its major effect in the region of the growth plate and adjacent metaphysis of long bones. A disturbance of the metaphyseal blood supply leads to a failure or delay in ossification of the hypertrophic zone of the metaphyseal growth plate. The hypertrophic zone may become elongated and extend into the metaphyseal trabeculae. Inflammation, hemorrhage, necrosis, fracture, and extensive remodeling are prominent in the trabeculae adjacent to the metaphyseal growth plate. Fracture of the trabeculae may cause a secondary lifting of the periosteum with subsequent production of new bone that may encircle the metaphyseal area.

Most affected animals are presented between 2 and 8 months of age. Clinically, the presentation may vary from a slight limp to a nonweightbearing lameness. Depending on this presentation, the metaphyseal regions of the long bones may be swollen, warm, and painful when touched. Severely affected animals may be systemically ill and have a history of depression and anorexia with clinical findings of pyrexia and weight loss. The disease is usually bilaterally symmetrical and episodic.

The diagnosis is confirmed by radiographic examination. In the early stages of the disease, an irregular radiolucent line may be apparent in the metaphyses adjacent to the growth plate. This represents necrosis and resorption of metaphyseal trabeculae. The metaphyseal growth plate may be normal throughout the course of the disease or may show irregular widening associated with delayed ossification of the hypertrophic zone.

Treatment of hypertrophic osteodystrophy is largely supportive. Buffered aspirin is recommended for relief of discomfort. In severely debilitated animals, parenteral fluid and electrolyte therapy may be necessary. Attentive nursing care is paramount in successful management of these patients.

The prognosis is good to excellent for animals with only mild lesions but is guarded for severely affected animals. In mild cases, disturbance of normal metaphyseal growth is not a problem. Premature growth arrests are likely in the most severely affected animals.

HYPERTROPHIC OSTEOPATHY (pp. 1988–1989)

Hypertrophic osteopathy is a secondary pathological disease process characterized by bilateral symmetrical swellings primarily affecting the distal portions of all four limbs. Initially, soft-tissue swelling predominates; however, as the disease progresses, a diffuse periosteal reaction may involve the majority of bones in the limbs.

Pulmonary osteoarthropathy, hypertrophic pulmonary osteoarthropathy, and *hypertrophic pulmonary osteopathy* are names given to this condition because of its association with some form of pulmonary disease. Metastatic pulmonary lesions are most commonly linked with this condition; however, primary pulmonary neoplasia, chronic bronchopneumonia, pulmonary abscesses, and pulmonary tuberculosis have been reported. Dogs suffering from bladder tumors (especially rhabdomyosarcoma) and adenocarcinoma of the liver have also been reported to develop the condition; therefore, the pulmonary portion of the name has been eliminated.

The pathogenesis of hypertrophic osteopathy is not understood. Because the majority of cases are associated with underlying pulmonary disease, the pathogenesis is believed to be related to these pulmonary disturbances. The most popular theory suggests that increased peripheral blood flow results from the pulmonary disease. The increase in blood flow results in congestion of many connective tissue structures, including periosteal tissue. The periosteum responds by laying down new bone on the cortical surfaces.

The majority of affected animals are presented for sudden or gradual onset of swelling and lameness involving all four limbs. Physical examination reveals firm swellings of the distal portion of all four limbs that are warm and sometimes painful when palpated.

Radiographic examination of the appendicular skeleton reveals bilateral symmetrical periosteal reactions affecting all bones of the limbs. Early in the condition, the metacarpal and metatarsal bones may be primarily affected. Radiography should include plain films of the thoracic cavity to check for pulmonary involvement and contrast abdominal studies and ultrasonography to rule out abdominal disease.

Treatment involves removal or elimination of the primary lesions. Clinical signs should resolve within 1 to 2 weeks of treatment. Resolution of the bony lesions may take months.

HYPERPARATHYROIDISM (pp. 1989–1990)

Primary hyperparathyroidism and secondary hyperparathyroidism result in increased parathyroid hormone (PTH) production and release, with increased resorption of cortical bone. Primary hyperparathyroidism is an unusual condition occurring most often with hyperplasia or neoplasia of the parathyroid glands. Secondary hyperparathyroidism is a more common disease in dogs and may be associated with renal disease or a nutritional deficiency.

Diagnosis is made on clinical signs, serum chemistry studies, urinalysis, and radiography. Blood test results may show elevated blood urea nitrogen and creatinine levels. Serum calcium levels may be within the normal range owing to bone resorption. Radiography of the skeletal system may delineate diffuse demineralization of the rami of the mandible/maxilla, with loss of lamina dura dentes and localized radiolucent areas, diffuse demineralization of other bones involved, and pathological fractures.

Treatment is directed toward slowing the progression of kidney disease and restoring kidney function, and includes supportive therapy, dietary protein restriction (high quality, low quantity), phosphate binding gels, and various treatments for anemia and acidosis. The prognosis is guarded, depending on the stage of kidney disease.

Nutritional secondary hyperparathyroidism is a metabolic disorder in which PTH is increased as a result of a nutritionally induced hypocalcemia, hyperphosphatemia with normal or low calcium levels, or inadequate amounts of vitamin D. The disease develops in young puppies and kittens fed a predominantly meat diet, which is high in phosphorus and low in calcium and has an imbalanced calcium/phosphorus ratio.

Treatment involves correcting the dietary mineral imbalance and confining the animal to reduce the chances of further pathological fractures. The prognosis is favorable if the condition is treated before the development of significant skeletal deformities.

VITAMIN D DEFICIENCY (RICKETS AND OSTEOMALACIA) (pp. 1990–1991)

CRANIOMANDIBULAR OSTEOPATHY (pp. 1991–1992)

OSTEOCHONDRODYSPLASIA (p. 1992)

RADIAL AGENESIS (pp. 1992–1993)

BONE CYSTS (p. 1993)

MULTIPLE CARTILAGINOUS EXOSTOSES (pp. 1993–1994)

CHAPTER 146

Muscles and Tendons
(pages 1996–2020)

Muscle Injuries

Minor injuries to muscles can be divided into contusions, strains, and lacerations. Unless the contusion is massive, treatment is usually unnecessary. Owing to hematoma formation, a massive contusion results in excessive inflammation and edema that can result in marked muscle dysfunction requiring treatment. Initial first aid consists of immobilization and cold compresses. After 24 hours, therapy consists of warm water compresses or baths, regional compressive wraps, protective bandaging, and immobilization.

A strained muscle is the result of overstretching or overuse of any part of the muscle-tendon unit, causing structural alterations, pain, and lameness. The treatment of muscle strains is similar to that of muscle contusions, consisting primarily of enforced rest.

The treatment of muscle lacerations depends on whether the injury is acute or chronic or if there is potential for loss of function because of fibrous healing. Wounds are irrigated with copious amounts of isotonic fluid and adequately débrided. Sutures are placed in the muscle sheaths rather than the muscle fibers themselves. If the muscle sheath has been severely damaged or if it is necessary to reappose a deeply lacerated muscle belly, muscle fibers can be apposed with interrupted horizontal mattress sutures placed deep into the muscle bellies and reinforced with rubber or Silastic tubing or buttons to prevent sutures from pulling out.

SPECIFIC MUSCLE INJURIES (pp. 1999–2005)

Rupture of the Gracilis Muscle

Rupture of the gracilis muscle (''dropped muscle'') is commonly seen in racing greyhounds. It also occurs in foxhounds and German shepherds.

Rupture of the muscle is characterized by a hematoma on the medial surface of the thigh. Injuries to the gracilis muscle result in various degrees of lameness depending on the severity of the injury. If this condition is diagnosed immediately after injury, surgical intervention is indicated. A small incision is made over the medial thigh and reattachment of the muscle ends, or for a musculotendinous tear, attachment of the tendon of origin or insertion is performed with interrupted horizontal mattress sutures of monofilament nonabsorbable suture material.

If this condition remains undiagnosed or untreated, a fibrous scar or cording develops on the caudomedial midthigh. Muscle fibrosis may result in a contracture of the rear leg and a distinct rear leg lameness because of inability to extend the stifle. Surgical release of the contracture is the treatment of choice. Partial resection of the fibrous tissue bands may cause recurrence of the contracture. It is best to remove the entire muscle and fibrotic tissue, followed by physical therapy to ensure complete range of motion of the stifle joint.

Rupture of the Long Head of the Triceps (p. 2000)

Rupture of the Achilles Mechanism

The Achilles mechanism is composed of five muscles that have three tendinous components forming the common calcaneal or Achilles tendon. The tendon of the gastrocnemius is the major component of the common calcaneal tendon. The other two tendinous components are formed by the tendon of the superficial digital flexor muscle and a common tendon of the biceps femoris, gracilis, and semitendinosus muscles.

Muscular or musculotendinous rupture of the Achilles mechanism primarily afflicts mature dogs of working and racing breeds. The condition may be bilateral and is manifested as tarsal hyperflexion and stifle hyperextension due to inability to extend the tarsus, the degree of which depends on the severity and completeness of the disruption. A diagnosis of Achilles mechanism injury is based on postural changes and flaccidity of the calcaneal tendon. Careful palpation of the gastrocnemius muscle and calcaneal tendon reveals inflammatory changes near the musculotendinous junction.

The origin of the lateral or medial head of the gastrocnemius muscle may avulse or tear as a result of hyperextension of the stifle. The result may be nonweightbearing lameness accompanied by palpable pain and swelling caudal to the distal femur. Extension of the stifle causes discomfort. Radiographic evaluation of the stifle reveals distal displacement of the fabella.

This is a surgically treatable condition requiring reattachment of the head of the gastrocnemius muscle, especially if clinical signs are severe. If possible, the torn muscle is reattached with nylon or polypropylene suture in a mattress, figure-eight, or alternative pattern.

Acute cases of musculotendinous rupture of the Achilles mechanism are treated surgically by apposition of the muscle-tendon junction. It is important to prevent stress on the anastomotic site by rigid immobilization of the tarsus and the stifle.

If an injury to the musculotendinous junction of the Achilles mechanism is not recognized or treated during the acute phase, the animal may be presented with a chronic injury or one that has failed to heal with conservative treatment. Chronic injuries can be treated by shortening the calcaneal tendon to re-establish function of the gastrocnemius and superficial digital flexor muscles.

Infraspinatus Muscle Contracture

Contracture of the infraspinatus muscle has been described primarily in hunting dogs. The history may include trauma with acute onset of lameness that gradually subsides. Although the lameness may decrease, it is accompanied by a characteristic gait that demonstrates persistent outward rotation, adduction of the elbow, and abduction of the distal limb with a carpal "flip." This gait abnormality develops 2 to 4 weeks after the initial injury, as a result of contracture of the infraspinatus muscle. It is usually unilateral but may occur bilaterally.

The exact cause is unknown, but it appears to be a primary muscle disorder rather than neurological in origin. Histologically, affected tissues show degeneration and atrophy of skeletal muscle with fibrous tissue replacement.

Surgical treatment consists of a caudolateral approach to the affected shoulder joint. The affected infraspinatus muscle appears fibrotic, with atrophy of the belly of the muscle. Blunt and sharp dissection is used to free the musculotendinous area of the scarred, fibrotic muscle from where it crosses the scapulohumeral joint. Once the fibrous tissue is freed from the joint capsule, it is incised either in the tendon or musculotendinous portion of the infraspinatus. All evidence of fibrous contracture is incised, and the range of motion of the shoulder joint is improved. The prognosis for full recovery is excellent.

Quadriceps Muscle Contracture

Contracture of the quadriceps muscle can occur with distal femoral fractures in young dogs. It is most often associated with inadequate fracture repair, osteomyelitis, or overzealous handling of tissues surrounding the femur in conjunction with prolonged immobilization in extension. Joint stiffness develops initially as a result of adhesions between the quadriceps muscle and the distal femur. With time, the affected leg is held in marked extension to such an extent that the knee may be bent backward in genu recurvatum, with the hock extended.

The affected leg essentially becomes a "walking stick" for the animal, with little use in locomotion. As the condition becomes chronic, the pathological changes become more complex; degenerative changes and fibrosis occur periarticularly and intra-articularly.

Restoration of motion in the stifle joint is achieved by (1) breaking down adhesions between the quadriceps muscle group and distal femur, (2) loosening adhesions in and around the femorotibial joint, (3) lengthening the quadriceps mechanism, and (4) releasing adjacent extensors of the stifle (e.g., sartorius and tensor fasciae latae). Whatever surgical procedure is chosen, the prognosis remains very guarded for complete return of function of the stifle. Because of the tendency for adhesions to re-form postoperatively, it is critical that the owner recognize the need for postoperative physical therapy.

Fibrotic Myopathy

Fibrotic myopathy of various muscles occurs in horses, cats, dogs, and man. It involves the supraspinatus, gracilis, quadriceps, and semitendinosus muscles of dogs and the semitendinosus muscle of cats. Fibrotic myopathy may be the result of primary neuropathy or myopathy, frequent intramuscular injections, exercise-induced or acute trauma, or congenital causes.

Fibrotic myopathy of the semitendinosus muscle is the condition most frequently reported. The semitendinosus muscle extends the hip, stifle, and tarsal joints and flexes the stifle when the limb does not bear weight. Affected dogs have lameness characterized by external rotation of the hock and internal rotation of the stifle as the rear limb is carried forward. The foot undergoes a characteristic flipping motion at the end of each forward stride.

Surgical release of fibrotic muscle is the recommended treatment for fibrotic myopathy; it has met with limited success. Immediately postoperatively, the lameness is usually absent. Within a few months of surgery, the fibrous band usually gradually returns along with an accompanying degree of lameness. The prognosis for treatment of fibrotic myopathy must remain guarded. If the lameness is not disabling, surgery is not advised.

HEREDITARY MYOPATHY OF LABRADOR RETRIEVERS
(p. 2006)

Surgical Repair of Severed Tendons

The majority of tendon injuries in small animals are related to lacerations rather than rupture. Unless the injury is chronic and tendon segments have severely contracted or the injury has devitalized large segments of tendon, primary end-to-end tenorrhaphy is the best method for restoration.

Severed Digital Flexor Tendons

Severance of the digital extensor and flexor tendons of small animals commonly accompanies laceration of the skin. Trauma to the digital extensor tendons is of less concern because of the many anastomoses after they branch from the main tendon. Because of the duplication of the digital flexor tendons, severance of the superficial digital flexor alone may have little effect on posture, whereas severance of the deep digital flexor results in flattening of one or more digits.

The most common locations of severance of the digital flexor tendons are above and below the metatarsal and metacarpal pads. An injured animal is often presented with profuse hemorrhage and accompanying soft-tissue damage. By having the dog stand on the affected leg or by pushing its foot hard against the palm of the hand, changes in posture of the digits can be detected.

Postural defects, such as flattening of one or more digits or elevation of the toes, are an indication for surgical exploration. Because the deep digital flexor tendon is of primary importance in posture of the toe, injuries to the superficial and deep digital flexor tendons in the metacarpal and metatarsal area and deep digital flexor near the digit require surgical treatment.

Chronic injuries are more difficult to treat in that the soft tissues on the plantar surface of the foot may be heavily scarred. The tendon ends can be reattached as described earlier, but large defects often remain. These defects in the digital flexor tendons can be filled with tendon grafts, fascial grafts, or suture material, but the prognosis for return to normal posture is guarded.

Severed Achilles Mechanism (Common Calcaneal Tendon)

The major cause of rupture of the common calcaneal tendon is direct trauma, usually by a sharp object.

Clinical signs of injury include tarsal hyperflexion and stifle hyperextension. If the superficial digital flexor is severed, the paw becomes more plantigrade than normal. These postural changes along with flaccidity of the tendon on flexion of the hock confirm the diagnosis. If the superficial digital flexor tendon remains intact, the animal assumes a dropped-hock posture with flexion of the digits.

Surgical repair of the severed calcaneal tendon should occur as soon after injury as possible. Restoration of gliding function is not of extreme importance. Surgical correction can be undertaken in open contaminated wounds if proper débridement is practiced. After thorough débridement of the wound, a primary tenorrhaphy is performed on each of the three tendon components. A locking loop (Kessler) or three-loop pulley suture pattern may be used.

Avulsion of a piece of the calcaneus (epiphysis in immature animals) may occur along with the tendon. In this instance, the piece of bone along with its tendon of insertion is reattached with a bone screw or pin and tension band wire.

Avulsion of the Tendon of Origin of the Long Digital Extensor (pp. 2014–2015)

Avulsion of the Origin of the Popliteal Muscle (pp. 2015–2016)

Avulsion of the Lateral or Medial Head of the Gastrocnemius Muscle (p. 2016)

Avulsion of the Origin of the Biceps Tendon

Bicipital Tenosynovitis

Inflammation of the tendon of origin and bursa of the biceps brachii is called *bicipital tenosynovitis*. Inflammation of the tendon may be caused by excessive stress, acute or chronic, or may be associated with the synovitis resulting from osteochondritis of the humeral head. The shoulder joint communicates with the bicipital bursa, and "joint mice" can become lodged adjacent to the tendon in the intertubercular groove.

Clinical signs include forelimb lameness that may be acute or chronic. Acute pain may be caused by local pressure applied directly to the bicipital tendon and bursa.

Initial treatment of bicipital tenosynovitis includes limited activity and nonsteroidal anti-inflammatory medications. Injection of intrasynovial long-acting corticosteroids yields temporary relief in severe cases. The use of corticosteroid injections remains controversial.

In refractory cases, the treatment of choice is surgical obliteration of the bursa and transposition of the biceps tendon. The biceps tendon is transected at its origin. The bicipital bursa is excised. The tendon is passed through a drill hole in the greater tubercle of the humerus and sutured on itself.

Displacement of the Tendon of Origin of the Biceps Brachii (p. 2019)

CHAPTER 147

Limb-Sparing Surgery for Dogs with Bone Neoplasia
(pages 2020–2026)

Limb-sparing surgery aims to provide a functional pain-free limb for the patient after removal of the local disease without adversely affecting survival. The bone or joint removed is usually replaced with a metal endoprosthesis, an allograft, or a combination of the two. Function in most patients has been good, and chemotherapy has improved survival. Limb sparing is preferred to amputation for extremely large dogs, dogs with concurrent orthopedic or neurological disorders, or dogs with owners who refuse amputation.

CASE SELECTION (pp. 2020–2021)

Dogs with osteosarcoma or other primary neoplasms of the appendicular skeleton may be candidates for limb-sparing procedures. Suitable dogs have their primary tumors clinically confined to one appendicular site with no more than 50 per cent of the length of the bone affected as determined radiographically.

Histological diagnosis is made from biopsy material, preferably obtained by a closed technique using a Jamshidi bone marrow biopsy needle.

In addition to biopsy of the primary site, tumor staging includes radiography of the affected limb, regional lymph node palpation with fine-needle aspiration cytological evaluation performed if lymphadenopathy is detected, and thoracic radiography using dorsoventral and both lateral projections. Bone survey radiography is also useful. The incidence of second bone lesions detected by bone survey radiography in dogs with osteosarcoma at presentation is 6.4 per cent, which is a higher yield than the incidence of pulmonary metastasis detected by thoracic radiography in the same dogs (4 per cent).

Suitable candidates for limb-sparing surgery must otherwise be in good health and have good cardiac, renal, and bone marrow function to tolerate surgery and adjuvant chemotherapy.

Location of the primary tumor is an important consideration in case selection because dogs with primary tumors in the hindlimbs generally do not function as well after limb-sparing surgery as dogs with tumors in the front limbs. Primary tumors around the elbow are rare; we have treated only one case with elbow fusion with good functional results. Proximal femoral lesions have been treated with a proximal femoral allograft and concomitant total hip replacement. Knee fusions have had poor functional results, but custom metallic total knees can be fashioned for dogs to fit into an allograft. Distal tibial tumors can be resected with fusion of the tarsal joint, but infection rates are prohibitively high. Considering the generally excellent function of dogs with rear leg amputation and the high complication rate with limb-sparing surgery in the rear leg, we rarely use salvage procedures for tumors of the femur or tibia. The most suitable dogs for limb sparing are those with tumors in the distal radius. These dogs generally function well, and the period of postoperative rehabilitation is generally shorter than for dogs undergoing limb-sparing surgery for proximal humeral tumors.

ADJUVANT TREATMENT (pp. 2021–2022)

SURGICAL TECHNIQUE (pp. 2022–2024)

RESULTS (p. 2024)

In carefully selected cases, limb function can be maintained without adversely affecting survival. Overall function has been satisfactory, with approximately 80 per cent of dogs experiencing good to excellent limb function. Dogs receiving the same dose of cisplatin with either amputation or limb-sparing operations have the same probability of survival. With two intra-arterial doses of cisplatin with or without radiation therapy before limb-sparing procedures, the median survival for dogs is 52 weeks. This is significantly longer than 19.8 weeks when amputation is the only treatment.

COMPLICATIONS (pp. 2024–2025)

The local recurrence rate after limb sparing is approximately 20 per cent, but 70 per cent of these dogs can be salvaged with further surgery (amputation or local resection). Local recurrence of osteosarcoma is rarely the cause of death or euthanasia. The infection rate is approximately 30 per cent, but the limb is preserved in 70 per cent of these dogs when treated with long-term antibiotics. For distal radius sites, if the ulna is still present, prognosis for recovery from infection is good. For humeral sites and distal radial sites where the ulna has been removed at the time of limb sparing, however, the prognosis for saving the leg is poor.

Another complication of limb-sparing surgery has been screw loosening in the allograft and host bone. For the radial location, this is radiographically evident from 3 to 9 months after surgery. The cause is presumed to be related to "normal" revascularization and resorption (creeping substitution) of the allograft.

Shoulder fusions for proximal humeral lesions place tremendous stress on the distal humeral host bone. Spiral fractures of this bone may develop. Some limbs can be resalvaged with a second plate or cerclage wires, but some require amputation.

Oncology (pages 2027–2244)

CHAPTER 148

Biology of Neoplastic Disease (pages 2027–2036)

ETIOLOGY OF NEOPLASIA IN DOGS AND CATS
(pp. 2027–2028)

Various extrinsic and intrinsic causes of neoplasia have been identified. Extrinsic causes include ultraviolet and ionizing radiation, tumor viruses, and chemical carcinogens. Intrinsic causes include diet, hormone effects, genetic predisposition, and age.

Irradiation

Exposure to ultraviolet radiation is a common, well-recognized cause of cutaneous squamous cell carcinoma in white cats, white-faced cattle, and possibly collies and Shetland sheepdogs. White cats and white-haired areas (especially ear tips and nose) of multicolored cats are susceptible to chronic inflammatory dermatitis that is exacerbated by exposure to direct sunlight. These inflammatory lesions may evolve to squamous cell carcinoma. The prevalence of solar-induced skin tumors is higher in cats than in dogs.

Oncogenic Viruses

The most clinically important oncogenic virus is feline leukemia virus (FeLV), which is the cause of lymphoma, leukemia, and myeloproliferative disease in cats. Oncogenic DNA viruses also cause tumors. In dogs, a DNA papovavirus causes multiple wartlike lesions on oral mucous membranes and the tongue (oral papillomatosis). A papovavirus is also suspected of causing cutaneous papillomas in dogs.

Diet, Hormones, and Prostaglandins

The influence of diet on the development of many neoplasms is well accepted. One of the most suspicious components of diet in mammary tumor development is fat.

Diets high in fats may influence gut flora to increase deconjugation and reabsorption of steroid hormones that may initiate or promote neoplasia. The small amount of estrogens normally synthesized by gut flora may be enhanced by diets high in fat. Excess dietary fat and obesity may increase the synthesis of prolactin. Circumstantial evidence suggests a role for prolactin in canine mammary neoplasia but no definitive role for prolactin in mammary tumor development has been established in dogs.

Prostaglandin synthesis may be an important factor in promoting the effects of dietary fat on the risk of mammary tumors by regulating cell proliferation, differentiation, and components of the immune system.

Data from epidemiological studies suggest a longer median survival time after mastectomy for dogs fed low-fat diets (less than 39 per cent, total calories from fat sources).

Chemical Carcinogens

Pet dogs exposed to topical insecticides, particularly flea and tick dips, have been found to have an increased risk of transitional cell carcinoma of the bladder. The risks of developing bladder tumors were highest among dogs receiving more than two applications per year.

Various active ingredients are found in flea and tick dips, including organophosphates, carbamates, pyrethrins, and pyrethroid compounds. Label substances identified as inert ingredients (which may represent up to 96 per cent of many products) are actually petroleum distillates, aromatic petroleum solvents, polyethers, and xylene, which are potential carcinogens.

THE CELL CYCLE AND ITS RELATIONSHIP TO THE TREATMENT OF NEOPLASIA (pp. 2028–2029)

The cell replication cycle is divided into discrete phases. At the beginning of the completion of mitosis, cells enter a phase of RNA and intracellular protein synthesis (G_1). After this, cells enter a phase of DNA synthesis (S) and then enter another phase of RNA and intracellular protein synthesis (G_2). This occurs immediately before mitosis (M). In mammalian cells, M phase is consistently brief (30 to 90 minutes), S phase is usually long (8 to 30 hours), and G_2 is brief (approximately 60 minutes). The duration of the G_1 phase varies. Cells in G_0 are sometimes referred to as *resting* or *nondividing*.

The distribution of cells cycling within a tumor may have important implications for therapy, because active cell division is necessary for sensitivity to cytotoxic drugs and ionizing radiation. Rapidly growing tumors tend to be most sensitive to cytotoxic drug therapy.

Most antineoplastic drugs and ionizing radiation have cytotoxic effects at different phases of the cycle. Antimetabolite and anthracycline drugs have maximum cytotoxic effects in S phase. Vinca alkaloids also have action in S phase but are most active in M phase. Alkylating drugs and ionizing radiation have two periods of maximum activity: near transition between G_1 and S phases and for G_2 phase or M phase.

Regulation and Growth of Normal Cells

Proto-oncogenes are normal genes that control the production of the growth regulatory substances, mainly peptide growth factors that stimulate cell proliferation by binding to specific cell surface receptors.

A cascade of biochemical events, initiated by a growth factor, signals the nucleus for proliferation to begin. At the cell nucleus, expression of specific proto-oncogenes and genes is induced, resulting in cell division. Growth factors are secreted by cells and interact with specific membrane-bound glycoprotein receptors that function as transducers of signals generated by them. Under differing circumstances, the same growth factor may stimulate or inhibit cell proliferation.

Growth factors may act as self-stimulants (autocrine), stimulants of nearby cells (paracrine), or stimulants of distant cells (endocrine). Autocrine secretion of growth factors by neoplastic cells is important in uncontrolled growth of tumor cells.

Signal Transduction

Signal transduction is the process of cellular expression of a proto-oncogene following the interaction of a growth factor with a cell membrane receptor. Common mechanisms of signal transduction involve beta-adrenergic receptors and the signal transducers adenylate cyclase and transducin and cellular kinases and phosphatases. The activation of a kinase known as *maturation promoting factor* is the immediate trigger for cell division.

NEOPLASTIC TRANSFORMATION AND GROWTH OF CELLS (pp. 2029–2031)

Oncogenes are derived from normal proto-oncogenes and are either altered or overexpressed versions of their normal cellular proto-oncogene counterparts. Oncogenes are genes that are capable of inducing or maintaining cell transformation to a malignant phenotype. Oncogenes can be activated from proto-oncogenes.

Oncogenes encode for the synthesis of oncoproteins, which are similar to the normal products of the proto-oncogenes except they have lost important regulatory constraints on their activity and do not need external activation. When oncoproteins replace normal proteins in signal transduction, oncogenesis may occur.

Loss of antioncogenes from a cell's karyotype can promote cell growth. Antioncogenes, also known as *tumor-suppressing* genes, regulate cell growth. Many descriptions of tumor development involve a time-dependent multistep (initiation and progression) process. Initiation may be associated with various stimuli, such as viral, environment, or dietary influences that activate a dominant oncogene or inactivate a pair of recessive antioncogenes.

The events involved in progression of neoplasia are less clear. Amplification of proto-oncogenes (an increased number of copies of the proto-oncogene in the cancer cell genome) has been implicated in progression of the neoplastic phenotype.

Metastasis

Neoplasms are composed of subpopulations of cells that differ in growth rate, karyotype, surface receptors, susceptibility to cytotoxic drugs, and other biological characteristics. They can also have subpopulations that form early in the development of the primary tumor and that have the ability for metastasis.

The transition from an *in situ* to a locally invasive neoplasia is accompanied by angiogenesis. An enzyme known as *collagenase type IV* and other enzymes such as heparinase and cathepsins make it easier for tumor cells to penetrate the often defective basement membrane of newly formed blood vessels within the primary tumor. Tumor cell pseudopodia penetrate the basement membrane and the cell becomes "extravasated" into the surrounding tissue.

Tumor cells extravasated to an extravascular location can proliferate into colonies, but angiogenesis must occur before they can grow to larger than 0.5 mm. Neoplastic cells that do enter lymphatic channels are carried to lymph nodes and quickly (within 10 to 60 minutes) leave by efferent lymphatics. Regional lymph nodes thus do not function as true mechanical barriers to neoplastic cell dissemination. Although patterns of metastasis vary widely, the most frequent localization of metastasis is likely to be in the first capillary bed encountered by the circulating cells.

Metastasis from Cancer of Unknown Primary Origin

Tumors of unknown primary origin are metastases from a primary tumor that cannot be detected.

Although derived from different tissues of origin, these tumors have important common biological characteristics. They display a marked degree of malignancy and metastasis early in primary development when the tumor is still small. The primary tumor may subsequently involute or retain its initial small size because of a slow growth rate while the metastatic sites proliferate aggressively. These tumors are malignant from the outset (type II progression) rather than evolving from benign to malignant (type I progression).

Carcinoma is the most frequent of such tumors in dogs. Affected dogs are usually 7 years or older, large (> 18 kg), physically impaired at the time of diagnosis, and affected with various nonspecific clinical signs such as weakness, cough, pain, and anorexia. Survival is poor.

NEOPLASTIC CELL ADAPTATIONS TO SURVIVE CHEMOTHERAPY (pp. 2031–2032)

Resistance of neoplastic cells to chemotherapy may be acquired after exposure to cytotoxic drugs or may be a property of the cells from the onset of malignant transformation (de novo resistance).

Cellular resistance to individual drugs usually depends on circumvention of a specific intracellular process that is targeted by the drug. In single-drug resistance, the mechanism is usually not effective for different classes of cytotoxic drugs.

Multidrug Resistance

Multidrug resistance occurs when acquired resistance to a single drug simultaneously confers resistance to classes of drugs that are structurally and functionally different. Multidrug resistance is a difficult clinical problem. Although structurally and functionally dissimilar, drugs associated with multidrug resistance all are hydrophobic compounds derived predominantly from plants and fungi.

PARANEOPLASTIC SYNDROMES (pp. 2032–2035)

Paraneoplastic syndromes are diverse systemic disorders associated with neoplasia but due to noninvasive actions of a tumor. The recognition of a paraneoplastic syndrome is important because (1) the observed abnormality may represent a hallmark of a specific tumor and facilitate early diagnosis and treatment; (2) it may help quantify and monitor the response to therapy; and (3) it may aid in the evaluation of tumor recurrence or disease progression.

Neoplasia-Associated Hypercalcemia

Neoplasia-associated hypercalcemia is characterized by persistent elevations of serum calcium (> 12 mg/100 ml). Hypercalcemia can result in mental depression, mental weakness, anorexia, vomiting, and various arrhythmias. Calcium nephropathy and renal failure may follow hypercalcemia if the calcium and phosphorus product (total serum calcium multiplied by serum phosphorus) exceeds 70. Polyuria with a compensatory polydipsia may be an early sign of hypercalcemia.

Because approximately half of the total serum calcium is nonionized and bound to albumin, hypoalbuminemia lowers the normal upper limit of serum calcium by relatively increasing the unbound form.

The most common tumors associated with hypercalcemia are malignant lymphoma, apocrine gland adenocarcinoma of the anal sac, multiple myeloma, and parathyroid adenoma. The general mechanism involved in the pathogenesis is inappropriate production of circulating humoral factors by neoplastic cells, causing osteoclastic bone reabsorption.

The mechanism of hypercalcemia in dogs with malignant lymphoma is unclear. In some cases it is hormonally mediated, whereas in others it may result from production of a locally acting bone-reabsorbing factor.

Hypercalcemia associated with apocrine cell adenocarcinoma of the anal sac is purely humoral because resection of the tumor results in normocalcemia and local or metastatic recurrence results in recurrent hypercalcemia. Hypercalcemia associated with multiple myeloma results from osteolysis caused by bone-reabsorbing factors. Hypercalcemia associated with parathyroid adenoma results from an overproduction of an appropriate hormone (parathyroid hormone).

Hypoglycemia

Hypoglycemia caused by neoplasia is most commonly associated with insulinoma; however, any large mesenchymal tumor may cause hypoglycemia.

The amended glucose-to-insulin (AGIR) ratio is helpful in demonstrating the presence of an insulin-secreting tumor:

$$\text{AGIR} = \frac{\text{Serum insulin (IU/ml)} \times 100}{\text{Serum glucose (mg/dl)} - 30}$$

If the serum glucose level is 30 or less, a value of 1 is used in the denominator. Insulin-secreting tumors are characterized by an AGIR of more than 30.

Hypertrophic Osteopathy

Hypertrophic osteopathy occurs secondary to malignant and nonmalignant diseases in the thorax or abdomen. In dogs, hypertrophic osteopathy is more commonly associated with primary lung tumors than with metastatic tumors.

Clinical signs usually include a history of gradual or occasionally sudden onset of lameness and reluctance to move. All four limbs are usually affected simultaneously. Hypertrophic osteopathy is characterized by periosteal proliferation. Treatment has included lobectomy, tumor removal, vagal resection, intercostal nerve resection, and chemotherapy. Treatment failure is usually related to recurrence of the tumor or metastases.

Hyperviscosity Syndrome

Hyperviscosity syndrome is usually associated with monoclonal gammopathies in patients with multiple myeloma. As the amount of an abnormal protein in the serum increases, the serum viscosity increases. Abnormal serum proteins may be macroglobulins or myeloma-type proteins. Treatment is directed at control of the inciting tumor. Emergency phlebotomy may be performed with concurrent replacement of blood with an equal volume of isotonic fluids.

Fever

When fever is a paraneoplastic syndrome, it is usually low grade and unresponsive to antibiotics. Fever associated with malignancy is due to production of interleukin-1 (endogenous pyrogen) by macrophages or tumor cells, acting on the hypothalamus to increase local synthesis of prostaglandins.

Altered Coagulability

Alterations in normal hemostasis usually accompany tumors that cause platelet dysfunction, disseminated intravascular coagulation, or heparin excess. Platelet dysfunction is most frequently observed with gammopathies from multiple myeloma.

Mast cell tumors, especially multiple or invasive tumors, are associated with hyperheparinemia. Disseminated intravascular coagulation results in hemorrhage from the combined effects of platelet consumption (thrombocytopenia), clotting factor consumption, and increased amounts of fibrin degradation products (anticoagulant effect). Hemangiosarcoma is frequently associated with disseminated intravascular coagulation in dogs.

Hemorrhagic Gastroduodenitis

Histamine from mast cell tumors in dogs and cats stimulates specific receptors (H_2) on gastric parietal cells, resulting in stimulation of hydrochloric acid production.

Pancreatic nonbeta-cell tumors in dogs and cats that inappropriately secrete gastrin (Zollinger-Ellison syndrome in man) may cause gastric and duodenal ulceration. Symptomatic treatment with an H_2-receptor antagonist like cimetidine or ranitidine, combined with a surface protectant such as sucralfate, may palliate symptoms. Sucralfate should be given first because it needs an acid environment to become active. Misoprostol is a synthetic prostaglandin E_1 that has antisecretory and cytoprotective properties that may be of use in treating gastric and duodenal ulceration.

Cachexia

Profound weight loss in patients with neoplasia is known as *cancer cachexia*. Protein catabolism may be a prominent part of cancer cachexia. Amino acids derived from host proteins are used for tumor protein synthesis and, in addition to lactate, gluconeogenesis. Depletion of body fat can be dramatic. Increases in host lipolysis and oxidation of lipids for energy lead to a severe loss of body fat. High serum concentration of growth hormone results in severe lipolysis and weight loss despite the intake of adequate calories. Acromegaly is not a clinical feature.

CHAPTER 149

Diagnosis of Neoplasia
(pages 2036–2048)

SAMPLE COLLECTION (pp. 2036–2042)

A biopsy is required to confirm a diagnosis of malignancy and provide information for planning therapy.

Fine-Needle Aspiration and Cytological Study

Cytological examination of cells from effusion or masses is useful diagnostic procedure. Cytological interpretation of fine-needle aspirates may not yield a definitive diagnosis but may discriminate between a benign and malignant process. Cytological interpretations often require histopathological confirmation.

Potential risks following fine-needle aspiration biopsy include fistula formation, bleeding, spreading of infection, and tumor seeding. A contraindication for fine-needle aspiration biopsy is severe coagulopathy; however, fine-needle aspiration poses the least risk of any biopsy technique to patients with bleeding potential if a small-diameter needle is selected and the tissues are disturbed as little as possible.

Cells are removed from a lesion with a 22- or 25-gauge needle using negative pressure created with a syringe. Alcohol swabbing of the skin and parting of hair facilitate collection from superficial masses without complications. If intrathoracic or intra-abdominal masses are aspirated, a small area of skin is clipped and prepared as for surgery. Negative pressure is created by drawing back on the syringe plunger. Using a jabbing motion, the needle is passed through several secants of the lesion. The tip of the needle should not leave the lesion during the negative pressure phase. Negative pressure is released before removing the needle from the lesion. The needle is detached, the syringe is filled with air, the needle reattached, and the air used to force the needle contents onto several glass slides.

The most common method of evaluating cytological specimens is by light microscopy.

Criteria for malignancy are summarized in Table 149–1. To diagnose malignancy, a minimum of three or four criteria must be prominently displayed within a high proportion of cells examined.

Most cytological specimens are stained with Wright and Diff-Quik stains. Users of Diff-Quik stain must remember that cytoplasmic gran-

TABLE 149–1. CYTOLOGICAL CRITERIA OF MALIGNANCY

General criteria
    Highly cellular specimen of a single cell type
    Pleomorphism but many large cells
    Ectopic cell population
Nuclear criteria
    High nuclear/cytoplasmic ratio
    Variation in nuclear size, shape, and number
    Prominent nucleoli
    Variation in nucleoli size, shape, and number
    Abnormal mitotic figures
    Irregular and/or coarse chromatin

ules within mast cells occasionally fail to stain and that staining time may need to be extended to two to three times longer than for peripheral blood smears.

Transtracheal Aspiration and Tracheal Washing

A long indwelling intravenous catheter capable of sliding through a needle is used. After preparation of the skin and local anesthesia infiltration, the needle is introduced through the cricothyroid ligament and angled down into the trachea. The catheter is gently threaded into the trachea, and the needle withdrawn. Sterile saline (3 to 10 ml) is injected from a 12- to 30-ml syringe into the trachea, and negative pressure is applied. Air, mucus, and some fluid are drawn into the syringe. Aspiration is repeated several times.

Bone Marrow Biopsy

Any unexplained abnormality in peripheral blood and the possibility of neoplastic infiltration of bone marrow are potential indications for a bone marrow biopsy. The most common sites for bone marrow sampling in small animals include (1) the wing of the ilium, dorsally or laterally, (2) the greater tubercle of the proximal humerus, and (3) the trochanteric fossa of the proximal femur. A bone marrow core biopsy can be taken from any of the sites used for bone marrow aspiration. These cores are usually taken with a Jamshidi biopsy needle. The sample is placed between two glass slides and gently rolled back and forth to prepare slides for cytological examination. The core can be placed into a container of suitable fixative.

Lymph Node Biopsy

Local or generalized lymph node enlargement is an indication for lymph node biopsy. Fine-needle aspiration is the quickest and easiest procedure for biopsy of lymph nodes.

Lymph nodes can be removed by surgical excision, which provides the largest and perhaps the best possible specimen for examination. The need for general anesthesia must be considered. Needle biopsy instruments can be used on lymph nodes accessible to aspiration. The instrument most commonly used for this method is the Tru-Cut disposable biopsy needle.

It is generally wise to obtain multiple samples if cytological and histopathological specimens are to be prepared. Hemorrhage can be minimized by applying digital pressure and possibly a pressure dressing to the area.

Percutaneous Lung Biopsy

The Lee needle and the Tru-Cut needle are effective for obtaining small portions of lung tissue. The Lee needle is similar to the Tru-Cut needle but is smaller and has suction capabilities through the inner cutting needle. Tru-Cut needles are used for large solid masses in the thorax. The Lee biopsy needle, which combines aspirating action with cutting action, may be used to sample aerated lung tissue. Complications of lung biopsy include pneumothorax and hemoptysis.

Bone Biopsy

A large core of bone may be removed using a Michele trephine, or a small core may be obtained with a Jamshidi biopsy needle. Large core techniques require general anesthesia and normal clotting parameters.

The sample is placed between two glass slides and gently rolled back and forth to prepare it for cytological examination. The core can then be placed into a container of suitable fixative for histopathological examination. Postbiopsy hemorrhage often results from large core biopsies.

Incisional and Excisional Biopsies

Histopathological examination is usually necessary to establish a definitive diagnosis. Incisional biopsies may be used in any tumor. A wedge of tissue is taken from an area that will be removed during a later excision or that lies within the treatment field if nonsurgical therapy such as radiation is to be applied. If possible, a junction of tumor and normal tissue is sampled. Excisional biopsy is nearly always the procedure of choice if a surgical biopsy is indicated. The surgical margins of an excised tumor should extend at least 1 cm around and deep to the mass. If mast cell tumor or hemangiopericytoma is suspected, a 3-cm margin is recommended.

HISTOPATHOLOGY (p. 2042)

In addition to assessing malignancy, histopathology allows for examination of the neoplasm's architecture and growth pattern (invasiveness). Malignant cells often invade the surrounding tissues, lymphatics, and blood vessels.

Histopathological examination can also be used to provide important prognostic information. Low-grade malignancies frequently are slowly progressive. High-grade malignancies are frequently invasive, rapidly growing, and metastatic in their behavior. Histopathological grading is determined by criteria of tumor differentiation, mitotic index, necrosis, and blood vessel invasion.

Microscopic examination of cut margins of tissue is a common way to determine if a tumor has been completely excised. The presence of neoplastic cells at a surgical margin can influence the decision about the need for further surgery or adjunctive therapy such as radiation or chemotherapy.

IMMUNOHISTOCHEMISTRY (pp. 2042–2043)

MOLECULAR CYTOGENETICS (pp. 2044–2045)

Bronchoalveolar Lavage

Bronchoalveolar lavage is a technique in which the alveoli and smaller airways of a portion of lung are bathed in saline, allowing exfoliated cells to be collected through a bronchoscope. Cytological examination of lavage fluid can be performed after centrifugation. Bronchoalveolar lavage is not the same as tracheal washings. Cells recovered in tracheal wash fluid represent those in large airways. Cells recovered by bronchoalveolar lavage are from deep in the lung parenchyma.

IMAGING (pp. 2045–2047)

Creating diagnostic images with x-rays, ultrasound, computed tomography, magnetic resonance, and scintigraphy has become increasingly important in detecting, diagnosing, and monitoring treatment responses in patients with tumors. Survey radiographs provide excellent spatial resolution compared with other modalities of imaging; however, contrast discrimination between normal and neoplastic soft tissue is poor. Invasiveness and tissue architecture cannot be assessed.

Medical gray scale ultrasonography can be used to create images of a tumor and provide more information about soft-tissue architecture and size than is available from survey radiographs alone. Ultrasonography cannot image through bone or air, so it is not possible to image the brain, spinal cord, lung, or an air-filled gastrointestinal tract directly. Abdominal fluid does not interfere with the creation of an ultrasonographic image as it does with standard radiographs. Cystic structures can usually be identified with ultrasonography, and machines with Doppler capabilities can determine and assess blood flow.

Computed tomography allows excellent contrast discrimination among different tissue types. As with ultrasonography, spatial resolution is poor with computed tomography because only one slice of tissue at a time is available for examination. The unique cross-sectional imaging ability of computed tomography makes it possible to detect soft tissues independent of overlying bony structures.

Magnetic resonance imaging is characterized by poor spatial resolution, but it has contrast capabilities superior to computed tomography, especially valuable in diagnostic evaluation of the central nervous system. Scintigraphic images are made by using a gamma camera to detect the amount of a radiopharmaceutical agent that distributes to the tissue under study. The use of scintigraphy in evaluating dogs and cats with thyroid disease is well documented. Bone scintigraphy is more sensitive than survey radiography for detecting primary and secondary bone tumors. Scintigraphy does not differentiate benign from malignant bone disease and biopsy is required to establish a definitive diagnosis.

CHAPTER 150

Surgical Therapy (pages 2048–2052)

ROLE OF SURGERY IN ONCOLOGICAL THERAPY
(pp. 2048–2049)

Surgery in the overall management of tumor patients includes definitive, palliative, and exploratory procedures, combination therapies, and surgery as immunotherapy. Undetectable metastasis is the major cause of failure of surgical treatment of neoplasia. In most instances, the neoplasm has metastasized by the time it is diagnosed.

Definitive Procedures

Surgery alone may be curative in the treatment of many neoplasms if the neoplasm is confined to a nonvital organ or region and amenable to complete removal. Common examples in dogs include tumors of the skin, mammary glands, and genitalia.

Palliative Procedures

The goal of some surgical procedures is to locally reduce a tumor mass, despite local invasion or metastasis, to provide relief for a patient.

Exploratory Procedures

Surgical procedures are used to establish a diagnosis and prognosis for neoplastic conditions. Biopsy specimens are often taken during exploratory procedures for microscopic examination.

Combination Therapy

Many neoplasms are now managed with a multidisciplinary approach. A surgeon may now be a member of a team that includes immunologists, radiologists, pathologists, oncologists, pharmacologists, and biochemists. The most effective treatments include maximum reduction of tumor cell mass by surgery or radiation.

Surgery as Immunotherapy

Immunotherapy in the treatment of neoplasia involves the stimulation or moderation of a patient's immune system to damage or destroy neoplastic cells. In addition to blocking tumor-specific antigens, a growing neoplasm often causes nonspecific immunosuppression. This immunosuppression is reversed by removing the growing neoplasms. In this respect, surgery is immunotherapy because it effectively decreases neoplastic cell mass and increases patients' immunocompetence.

COMPONENTS OF IMMUNOTHERAPY (p. 2049)

Active Specific Immunotherapy

The basic assumption that tumor cells contain antigens that the host may recognize as foreign is the basis of active specific immunotherapy. Although occasional encouraging results with tumor vaccines have been reported, much research still needs to be done to prove the clinical effectiveness of such an approach.

Passive Immunotherapy

Passive immunotherapy involves administration of immune mediators to the patient.

Successful results have been reported with the administration of immune lymphocytes and immune sera, but the technical problems render them clinically unusable.

Nonspecific Immunotherapy

Nonspecific immunotherapy uses various agents that nonspecifically stimulate the immune system to destroy tumors. These agents are broadly classified as biological modulators or chemical immunostimulators. The biological modulators are bacteria, including a mixed bacterial vaccine of *Streptococcus pyogenes* and *Serratia marcescens*; bacillus Calmette-Guérin, an attenuated strain of *Mycobacterium bovis*; and *Corynebacterium parvum*. Studies using these agents have produced inconsistent results. Include drugs of the imidothiazole class (levamisole and thiabendazole). Clinical results have been discouraging. Interferon may have some antitumor effects that are partly mediated by the immune system.

PREOPERATIVE CONSIDERATIONS (p. 2050)

Individual patients must be completely and objectively evaluated before any treatment is considered or initiated. A thorough history and physical examination are essential, as well as a complete blood count, electrocardiogram, and laboratory assessment of renal and hepatic function. Tumor boundaries are defined before therapy to determine whether the neoplasm is localized, invasive, or metastatic. Thoracic radiographs are evaluated if the neoplasm has a tendency for pulmonary metastasis. A ''negative'' chest radiograph does not ensure the absence of metastasis.

SURGICAL MANAGEMENT (pp. 2050–2051)
Anesthesia

Newer anesthetic agents with minimal cardiopulmonary suppressive effects are ideal. Indwelling intravenous catheters and maintenance fluid therapy are required; these are often lengthy procedures with considerable potential for hemorrhage.

Local anesthetic agents should probably be avoided in tumor resections.

Surgical Technique

Strict aseptic techniques must be maintained to minimize the chances of surgically induced infection. Preoperative prophylactic antibiotics may also be considered. A wide area round the lesion is prepared for surgery, should a larger incision be needed.

Tissue Handling

Minimal, gentle handling of neoplastic tissues is imperative. Excessive surgical trauma may cause exfoliation of tumor cells into the wound and systemic circulation.

Margins

The best opportunity for surgical cure of neoplasia is at the first operation. A wide margin of normal tissue must be excised to ensure total removal of the neoplasm. Normal tissue margins of at least 1 cm should suffice in all but the most highly malignant neoplasms. Histological examination of specimen margins is recommended.

En Bloc Resections

An *en bloc* resection is removal of the primary tumor, intervening lymphatics, and regional lymph node in continuity. It is indicated only when a regional lymph node is in close proximity to a primary neoplasm. Although controversial, it is generally recommended that only those lymph nodes that are clinically affected be removed.

POSTOPERATIVE MANAGEMENT (p. 2051)

Each surgically treated neoplasm is unique and may pose specific postoperative management problems that are as important as the surgical procedure itself. Although adjuvant therapy may be started before surgery, other phases of combination therapies are often implemented in the immediate postoperative period.

STAGING (p. 2051)

To standardize classification and aggressiveness of various neoplasms, staging systems have been designed. The most widely accepted staging system is the TNM designation (T, tumor; N, regional lymph node; M, distant metastasis).

POSTOPERATIVE FOLLOW-UP (p. 2051)

The intensity of postoperative follow-up is dictated by the type of neoplasm being treated. Patients with highly aggressive malignancies are re-evaluated frequently. Careful repeat examinations are important not only for care of individual patients but also for comparison and evaluation of various treatment regimens.

CHAPTER 151

Radiation Therapy (pages 2052–2067)

PRINCIPLES OF RADIATION THERAPY (pp. 2052–2054)
Radiobiology

Radiobiology is the study of the interaction between ionizing radiation and living matter. Therapeutic forms of ionizing radiation include x-ray, gamma-ray, electrons, neutrons, and other charged particles that randomly deposit their energy within matter in discrete clusters of ionization.

Conversion of kinetic energy to biological damage by ionization within the cell can result from direct interaction between the ionizing photon or particle and the critical molecule or from indirect interaction of chemically reactive free radicals of water ionization and their subsequent interaction with regional molecules. Indirect mechanisms of biological damage predominate. Two mechanisms of radiation-induced cell death are recognized: mitotic cell death and interphase death. Mitotic cell death occurs with moderate but lethal doses of radiation and results in the ultimate failure of cells to pass through mitosis. Alternatively, in cells receiving large doses of radiation, a cell may degenerate in interphase and fail to reach its first mitosis.

Radiosensitivity, Radioresponsiveness, and Radiocurability

The radiosensitivity of cells is related to their mitotic rate, further reproductive capabilities, and degree of differentiation and specialization.

Radiosensitivity is also influenced by other factors unrelated to a cell's mitotic activity and degree of differentiation. Radiosensitivity is the ability of radiation to biologically damage cells in normal or neoplastic tissue.

Radioresponsiveness is the time required for visible structural or functional changes to occur and is measured by the rate at which the clinical manifestations of radiation injury take place.

Radiocurability is the ability of ionizing radiation to reduce the number of malignant cells below a critical level so that no further clinical manifestations occur during a patient's remaining lifetime (Table 151–1).

Four factors, called the "four R's" of radiotherapy—repair, repopulation, redistribution, reoxygenation—are involved in designing radiotherapy protocols.

TABLE 151–1. RADIOTHERAPY FOR COMPANION ANIMAL NEOPLASMS*

Tumor Type	Radiosensitivity	Responsiveness	Curability
Canine transmissible venereal tumors	High	Rapid	Excellent
Perianal adenomas	High	Rapid	Excellent
Squamous cell carcinoma	Variable†	Moderate to rapid	Fair to good
Fibrosarcoma	Low to moderate†	Slow	Poor to fair
Mast cell tumors	Moderate	Moderate to slow	Good to fair
Melanocarcinomas	Low	Slow	Poor to none
Osteosarcoma	Low	Slow	Poor to none

*Based on the authors' clinical experience in radiotherapy of companion animal neoplasms.

†Biological behavior after radiotherapy varies with location on the patient and species.

Repair of sublethal injury is possible to a greater degree in normal cells than in neoplastic cells. This advantage is increased by dividing the total dose into a number of smaller doses (fractionation).

Repopulation by regeneration of stem cells may differ between normal and neoplastic cells.

Redistribution of cells within the cell cycle is another possible advantage of fractionated radiotherapy. Cells surviving a dose of radiation tend to synchronize in resistant phases of the cell cycle.

Reoxygenation of hypoxic cells is a result of several complex processes. Oxygenated cells are more sensitive to radiation than hypoxic cells and are selectively killed during fractionated treatment.

METHODS OF RADIOTHERAPY (pp. 2054–2055)

External Beam Radiotherapy (Teletherapy)

External beam radiotherapy uses a source of ionizing radiation separated at a distance from the patient. External beam radiotherapy currently available in veterinary institutions includes orthovoltage x-ray, cobalt 60 (^{60}Co), cesium 137 (^{137}Cs), and linear accelerators.

Orthovoltage Radiotherapy

Orthovoltage radiotherapy uses x-rays with a low to medium energy range of 150 to 400 kVp. Orthovoltage x-ray therapy has many limitations compared with higher-energy x-rays and gamma-rays in the megavoltage range (in excess of 1 MeV). The ability to penetrate tissue and achieve adequate depth of dose is a major limitation. With megavoltage radiotherapy, the maximum dose is below the skin surface, thus achieving a degree of "skin sparing." Another disadvantage of orthovoltage radiotherapy is the disparity of dose distribution between soft tissue and bone in the same field. With megavoltage radiotherapy, minimal differential absorption occurs between bone and soft tissue. The major advantages of orthovoltage are its simplicity, low cost, and reduced requirements for environmental shielding compared with those for megavoltage equipment.

Supervoltage Radiotherapy

Supervoltage teletherapy uses x-rays, gamma-rays, or electrons in an energy range in excess of 500 KeV. Gamma-rays and x-rays are forms of electromagnetic radiation; gamma-rays originate from spontaneous nuclear decay of a radioactive isotope, and x-rays originate from an event outside the nucleus. ^{137}Cs gamma emissions are intermediate in energy between orthovoltage (400 KeV[0.400 MeV]) and megavoltage ^{60}Co emissions (1.25 MeV). Although ^{137}Cs has advantages over orthovoltage radiotherapy, the added advantages of depth dose penetration, skin sparing, and uniform dose distribution for soft tissue and bone, as well as ease of equipment maintenance (compared with linear accelerators), make ^{60}Co the most practical method for veterinary radiotherapy.

Interstitial Brachytherapy

With interstitial brachytherapy, a radioisotope sealed in a metallic container, usually a seed, needle, or applicator, is placed in or on the patient. The primary advantage of brachytherapy is that the sources are placed in the tumor, providing maximum tumor dose while minimizing the dose to surrounding normal tissues. The disadvantages of brachytherapy include (1) exposure to the personnel involved in placing the sources, (2) the necessary isolation facilities required for hospitalization of a patient to prevent environmental contamination with lost sources, and (3) exposure to the animal's owner or trainer.

The radioactive isotopes currently available to veterinary radiotherapists include ^{60}Co, ^{137}Cs, gold 198 (^{198}Au), iridium 192 (^{192}Ir), and iodine 125 (^{125}I).

Systemic Radiotherapy

The internal use of radionuclides resembles interstitial brachytherapy except that the radioactive source is submicroscopic. The radionuclides can be administered orally, intravenously, or into the peritoneal or pleural space. ^{131}I has been used to treat feline hyperthyroidism, as well as metastatic thyroid carcinoma in people and animals. The disadvantages of systemic radiotherapy are similar to those with brachytherapy.

SEQUENCE OF RADIOTHERAPY IN COMBINATION WITH SURGERY (pp. 2055–2056)

Surgery and radiotherapy are the major potentially curative methods available for veterinary tumor treatment. Surgery and irradiation may be used in several combinations. It is logical to assume that surgery and radiotherapy can be complementary, surgery removing the gross mass and irradiation eliminating microscopic foci. Irradiation may be preoperative, intraoperative, or postoperative.

Preoperative Radiotherapy

The arguments in favor of preoperative radiotherapy include the following: rendering a locally diffuse tumor removable, decreasing the required extent of surgical resection of normal tissues, and rendering nonviable any malignant cells that may be inadvertently implanted surgically in the wound or circulatory system. The argument against preoperative radiotherapy concerns impaired wound healing, which is directly proportional to the radiation dose. Preoperative radiotherapy may be of benefit in neoplasms with a high incidence of postoperative recurrence.

Intraoperative Radiotherapy

The major disadvantage is the expense of combined radiotherapy and a surgical facility. Single doses of 1,000 to 3,000 cGy* of orthovoltage x-rays or electrons (from linear accelerators) are currently used. It has been used in selective intra-abdominal tumors with some success.

Postoperative Radiotherapy

The primary indication for postoperative radiotherapy is a local neoplasm that cannot be completely removed. A higher total dose of irradiation can be given compared with preoperative or intraoperative radiotherapy. Postoperative radiotherapy has several disadvantages: (1) Distant metastases may be produced by the surgical procedure, (2) surgery may decrease vascularity and predispose to tissue hypoxia, and (3) tumor proliferation may occur before irradiation is initiated if surgical healing is prolonged.

RADIATION COMBINED WITH NONSURGICAL TREATMENT (pp. 2056–2058)
Hyperthermia

Temperatures of 104°F (40°C) or greater are used to treat tumors. Hyperthermia may be used as a primary treatment method or combined with radiotherapy or chemotherapy. Cell death by heat alone begins at 107.6° to 109.4°F (42° to 43°C) (tissue temperature). For each degree rise in temperature above 107.6°F, the time required to produce the same biological effects was halved. Local or systemic hyperthermia may be used. Radiofrequency, microwave, ultrasound, and water immersion or whole-body chambers are currently used. No definite evidence shows that tumor cells are more sensitive to heat than normal tissues. The primitive vascularity of tumors reduces their ability to dissipate heat. The net result is that the tumor tissue has a higher temperature than the normal surrounding tissues. Hypoxic cells found in a tumor are more resistant to radiation than oxygenated cells but are more sensitive to heat than oxygenated cells. The rationale for combining hyperthermia and radiotherapy is based on their synergistic effects.

Hypoxic Cell Sensitizers (p. 2057)
Chemotherapy

The combination of chemotherapy and radiation has received little attention by veterinarians.

Chemotherapeutic agents such as antibiotics, alkylating agents, and antimetabolites may be used with radiation therapy to prevent metastasis during irradiation of the primary tumor. They do not increase the lethal effects of radiation but probably add to the effect of radiation. The severity of complications encountered when radiation and chemotherapy are simultaneously combined may produce unacceptable complications that are more severe than if either had been used alone. The toxicity of commonly used chemotherapy agents combined with radiation is listed in Table 151–2.

APPLICATIONS (pp. 2058–2060)
Evaluation Before Radiotherapy

Evaluation before radiotherapy is critical and directly influences the decision to accept a patient for radiotherapy. A minimum data base for

---

*Centigray (cGy) = 0.01 gray = 1 rad; 1 gray (Gy) = 100 rad.

TABLE 151–2. MAJOR TOXIC EFFECTS OF DRUGS COMMONLY USED IN CONJUNCTION WITH RADIOTHERAPY

Complication	Vin-cristine	Actino-mycin D	Cyclophos-phamide	Adria-mycin	High-Dose Metho-trexate	Cis-platin
Leukopenia	–	+	+ +	+ + +	+ + +	+ + +
Thrombocytopenia	–	+ + +	+	+	+ +	+ + +
Neurotoxicity	+ +	–	–	–	–	+
Cardiotoxicity	–	–	+	+ + +	–	+
Cystitis	–	–	+ + +	–	–	–
Mucositis	–	+ +	–	+ +	+ + +	–
Gastrointestinal toxicity	+ +	+ +	+ +	+ +	–	+ + +
Cellulitis	+ +	+ +	–	+ +	–	–
Erythema	–	+ +	–	–	+	–
Pulmonary	—	—	—	—	—	+ + +
Renal toxicity	–	—	—	—	—	+ + +
Hepatotoxicity	–	–	–	–	+ + +	—

Increased number of + signs denotes increasing severity and frequency of complications.

Complications represented by + are for combined protocols of chemotherapeutic agents and radiation.

From Suton WW, Chan RC: Irradiation and chemotherapy in pediatric tumors. *In* Fletcher GH (ed): *Textbook of Radiotherapy.* Lea & Febiger, Philadelphia, 1980, p. 639.

each patient is necessary. If lymphadenopathy is identified, a biopsy should be performed to determine if inflammatory or metastatic disease is present. Thoracic radiographs may show if metastases are present. Abdominal radiographs are recommended with tumors of the perineum, anus, and hind legs to evaluate caudal retroperitoneal lymph nodes. A biopsy is a prerequisite to radiotherapy by providing a cell-type diagnosis, thereby determining the overall prognosis.

Selection of Patients

Radiation therapy is not a panacea for all neoplasms, nor should it be considered a last-ditch effort when all other therapies have failed to control a tumor. In general, the physical characteristic of a tumor determines treatment. Surgical resection followed by radiation frequently is appropriate for tumor therapy. Surgical resection is recommended even in invasive tumors to reduce the size of the tumor mass.

Selection of Radiotherapy

The selection of radiotherapy for an individual case depends on the location and physical characteristics of the tumor and the availability of radiotherapy facilities. Superficial lesions up to 5 mm in depth can be effectively treated using low-energy x-rays. However, these low-energy x-rays should not be used to treat superficial lesions directly over bone. Low-energy x-rays are disproportionately absorbed by bone.

For treating deep tumors, high-energy orthovoltage x-ray may be used. High-energy orthovoltage x-rays can be used for the treatment of tumors 3 to 4 cm in depth. The main limitation at these depths is the excessive surface dose. High-energy orthovoltage x-ray also delivers a slightly higher dose to bone than to soft tissue.

High-energy gamma rays from ^{60}Co have an average energy of 1.25 MeV. Photon and electrons from linear accelerators may be in excess of 2 MeV. These megavoltage radiotherapy units have the advantage of delivering tumoricidal doses to deep-seated tumors yet sparing skin because the maximum dose is several millimeters below the skin surface. Bone and soft tissue attenuate radiation similarly with megavoltage radiation.

Specific Application to Selected Tumors

The tumors most frequently treated by radiotherapy are listed in the Appendix (pp. 2062–2067).

FAILURE OF RADIOTHERAPY AND COMPLICATIONS
(p. 2060)

Failure of radiotherapy results from an inadequate field size to cover the primary tumor site and failure to detect regional or distant metastases. Failure of radiotherapy may also result from the inherent resistance of the tumor because of hypoxic cells or because adequate lethal doses could not be delivered without exceeding regional normal tissue tolerance.

Complications of radiation therapy are primarily limited to the site of irradiation. Necrosis is the most common long-term sequel if tissue or organ tolerance is exceeded. Tissue or organ atrophy and fibrosis may be the end result of radiotherapy. Because the surface dose is usually greater than the maximum tumor dose with orthovoltage radiotherapy, the most common sites for injury are the skin and mucous membranes. Epilation, depigmentation, and moist desquamation are the most frequently encountered complications.

CHAPTER 152

Chemotherapy (pages 2067–2075)

The goal of chemotherapy is to cure the disease, but how frequently a true chemotherapeutic cure is obtained in veterinary medicine is debatable.

Clearly, the more effective the chemotherapy in controlling the distant spread of the disease, the longer a patient's survival.

TOXICOSES (p. 2068)

Chemotherapeutic protocols are most often limited by host toxicosis. The most commonly encountered problems relate to gastrointestinal toxicity, bone marrow suppression, and immunosuppression. Vomiting and anorexia may be noted as the gastrointestinal epithelium is affected.

Bone marrow damage may affect all cellular components of blood. Anemia and thrombocytopenia may be life threatening, but leukopenia and the associated risk of infection are more common problems. Recommended leukocyte counts at which to postpone therapy vary. One such guideline is 4,000 total white blood cells per microliter with at least 2,500 granulocytes per microliter. Generally, chemotherapy can be reinstituted in 1 to 2 weeks based on a return to normal white blood cell parameters. When resuming chemotherapy, it may be advisable to decrease the dosage of the offending drug by 25 per cent.

Immunosuppression relates closely to bone marrow toxicosis and myelosuppression. Cyclophosphamide is the most immunosuppressive of the commonly used anticancer agents. Less common problems involve other body systems. Hemorrhagic cystitis associated with cyclophosphamide is a well-known complication that limits prolonged use. The kidneys are subject to damage from methotrexate, streptozotocin, L-asparaginase, and other chemotherapeutic agents. Skin reactions and alopecia are less frequent in animals than in man. Clipped hair may not regrow or may regrow a different color. Wire-haired and curly-coated breeds seem more likely than others to develop alopecia.

SAFE HANDLING OF CHEMOTHERAPEUTIC AGENTS
(pp. 2068–2069)

1. Unpack anticancer drugs carefully. Store them in a locked cabinet.
2. Never eat, drink, smoke, or apply cosmetics where anticancer drugs are prepared or administered.
3. Reconstitute these materials in a well-ventilated area.
4. Prepare and administer anticancer drugs with unpowdered surgical latex gloves.
5. Use syringes and intravenous sets with Luer-Lok fittings.
6. Consult package inserts for directions regarding spills.
7. Ensure that patients are well restrained during administration.

GUIDELINES FOR CHEMOTHERAPY (p. 2069)

Although patients may benefit from a single chemotherapeutic drug, the use of drugs in combination has advantages. Chemotherapeutic drugs kill a constant fraction of tumor cells, and the fraction killed by one drug is independent of that killed by another. Drugs can be used in combination to attack different specific portions of the cell cycle. Drugs that have different major toxicities are chosen. Intermittent treatment schedules allow intensive attack on a neoplasm and a rest period for recovery of normal cells before the next treatment. A few principles of combination chemotherapy follow:

1. Use drugs effective as single agents.
2. Use drugs with different mechanisms of action.
3. Use drugs with different toxicities.
4. Use an intermittent treatment schedule.

DRUGS USED IN CHEMOTHERAPY (pp. 2069–2073)

Comments on selected drugs (p. 2070) aid in effective, rational chemotherapy. Doses are expressed as milligrams per square meter (body surface area) rather than milligrams per kilogram. Weight in grams is converted to body surface area (m²) by a fractional exponential function:

$$m^2 = \frac{Km \times W^{2/3}}{10^4}$$

where m^2 is the body surface area in square meters, W is the body weight in grams, and Km is a species-specific constant (10.1 for dogs, 10.0 for cats). Table 152–1 is a conversion table for dogs. The table is also applicable to domestic cats.

TABLE 152–1. CONVERSION TABLE OF WEIGHT IN KILOGRAMS TO BODY SURFACE AREA IN SQUARE METERS FOR DOGS

kg	m²	kg	m²
0.5	0.06	26.0	0.88
1.0	0.10	27.0	0.90
2.0	0.15	28.0	0.92
3.0	0.20	29.0	0.96
4.0	0.25	30.0	0.96
5.0	0.29	31.0	0.99
6.0	0.33	32.0	1.01
7.0	0.36	33.0	1.03
8.0	0.40	34.0	1.05
9.0	0.43	35.0	1.07
10.0	0.46	36.0	1.09
11.0	0.49	37.0	1.11
12.0	0.52	38.0	1.13
13.0	0.55	39.0	1.15
14.0	0.58	40.0	1.17
15.0	0.60	41.0	1.19
16.0	0.63	42.0	1.21
17.0	0.66	43.0	1.23
18.0	0.69	44.0	1.25
19.0	0.71	45.0	1.26
20.0	0.74	46.0	1.28
21.0	0.76	47.0	1.30
22.0	0.78	48.0	1.32
23.0	0.81	49.0	1.34
24.0	0.83	50.0	1.36
25.0	0.85		

Alkylating Agents

Alkylating agents have an alkyl radical ($R\text{-}CH_2\text{-}CH_2+$) substituted for a hydrogen atom. Alkylation causes breaks in the DNA molecule and cross-linking of the twin strands of DNA. Cross-linking interferes with DNA replication and RNA transcription. The alkylating agents are not specific for the cell cycle phase.

Cyclophosphamide is the most widely used alkylating agent in veterinary medicine. It has been administered for lymphoreticular neoplasia, various sarcomas and carcinomas, mast cell tumors, and transmissible venereal tumors, as a single agent, and with other drugs. Cyclophosphamide must be given orally or intravenously. Hematological and gastrointestinal toxicoses are dose limiting. Leukopenia is most severe within a week or two of administration.

A unique and important problem associated with cyclophosphamide is sterile hemorrhagic cystitis. Patients may show signs of hematuria, pollakiuria, and stranguria. Early recognition of signs, diuresis, and cessation of cyclophosphamide administration help limit the problem. Some cases may persist and require more aggressive therapy, such as instillation of a 1 per cent formalin solution into the bladder.

Chlorambucil is often used in chemotherapy of canine lymphosarcoma as a replacement for cyclophosphamide. Melphalan is most useful in multiple myeloma but also in lymphoreticular neoplasia, mammary and lung carcinomas, and osteogenic sarcoma. Dacarbazine may be useful in lymphoma in dogs but is not widely used.

Antimetabolites

Antimetabolites are structural analogues of normal metabolites required for cell function and replication.

The antimetabolites are S-phase–specific drugs.

Methotrexate acts in S phase and is a folic acid antagonist used in the treatment of lymphoreticular neoplasms and myeloproliferative disorders as well as metastatic transitional cell tumor, transmissible venereal tumor, Sertoli cell tumor, and osteogenic sarcoma.

The purine analogue 6-mercaptopurine interferes with purine synthesis and interconversion and is used for lymphocytic and granulocytic leukemias. Other useful pyrimidine analogues include 5-fluorouracil and cytosine arabinoside. 5-Fluorouracil is used in the treatment of various carcinomas. Hematological and gastrointestinal toxicoses are important. It is not used in cats because of severe neurotoxicosis. Cytosine arabinoside blocks S-phase action and progression of cells from G_1 to S. Myelosuppression is the major dose-limiting toxicosis, although gastrointestinal signs ranging from anorexia to vomiting may be observed.

Antibiotics

The antitumor antibiotics are natural products, derived from strains of the soil fungus *Streptomyces*. They are cytotoxic and nonspecific for cell cycle phase. Doxorubicin is the most frequently used in veterinary medicine. Hematological, gastrointestinal, and cardiac toxicoses are important. Renal disease may be significant in cats. Myelosuppression may be a dose-limiting problem. Cumulative cardiac toxicosis results in a dose-related cardiomyopathy.

Doxorubicin is administered slowly through a free-flowing intravenous line. Extravasation causes serious sloughing and is treated promptly with saline dilution. Slough may be noted in 7 to 10 days. Restlessness, facial swelling, or head shaking may signal excessively rapid administration. Doxorubicin has had wide application in the treatment of canine lymphosarcoma as both a first- and second-line drug and for various carcinomas and sarcomas with limited success.

Bleomycin has had limited use in squamous cell carcinoma in animals. Pulmonary fibrosis may be a lethal complication.

Plant Alkaloids

Vincristine and vinblastine are alkaloids extracted from *Vinca rosea*. They act specifically in M phase. Although vincristine and vinblastine have a common mechanism of action, resistance to one does not imply resistance to the other. They also have different major toxicities. Vincristine affects the nervous system.

Vinblastine toxicity is primarily hematological. These drugs cause sloughing if injected perivascularly.

Vincristine is the treatment of choice for transmissible venereal tumor and is used for sarcomas and carcinomas. Vinblastine is used to treat carcinomas and mast cell tumors.

Hormones

Unlike other chemotherapeutic agents, hormones are not primarily cytotoxic and are more selective in their actions.

Adrenal corticosteroids have important uses in therapy of lymphosarcoma and mast cell tumors and may be of benefit in central nervous system neoplasms because of their ability to cross the blood-brain barrier. Their beneficial actions probably relate more to anti-inflammatory effects than to direct antitumor effects.

Sex hormones have been used in the treatment of hormone-dependent tumors of mammary, prostatic, or perianal gland origin.

Miscellaneous Agents

L-Asparaginase is an enzyme derived from bacteria. Asparaginase acts against cells in G_1. It is effective in canine lymphoreticular neoplasms. Anaphylaxis has been the most dangerous side effect.

The cell cycle–nonspecific drug *o,p'*-DDD directly suppresses both normal and neoplastic adrenocortical cells. With proper management, *o,p'*-DDD may be beneficial in patients with inoperable adrenocortical carcinoma as well as with adrenocortical hyperplasia secondary to a pituitary neoplasm.

Platinum complexes have tumoricidal activity; *cis*-dichlorodiammineplatinum (CDDP) is a cell cycle phase–nonspecific drug that has been used in veterinary medicine for various tumors. The most clearly defined indication for CDDP is adjunctive treatment of osteosarcoma in dogs.

CHAPTER 153

Skin and Subcutis (pages 2075–2088)

The skin is the origin of about one-third of canine neoplasms. Likewise, the skin accounts for one-fourth of feline tumors. Skin tumors in cats are more likely to be malignant than in dogs.

Benign tumors are commonly denoted by the suffix *-oma.* Malignant neoplasms of ectodermal or neuroectodermal origin (epidermis and mucosa) are commonly denoted by the suffix *carcinoma.* Malignancies arising from the tissues of mesoderm or endoderm are most commonly denoted by the suffix *sarcoma.*

DERIVATION OF SKIN TUMORS (pp. 2075–2076)

The deep or basal layer of the epidermis, called the *stratum germinativum,* is composed of melanocytes and basal cells; the latter differentiate into prickle cells. Both benign and malignant *epidermal (skin) tumors* arise from these cells.

The basal lamina and epidermis deeply invaginate into the dermis and subcutis, forming the origin of each gland or hair follicle. Hair follicles and glands are called, corporately, the *adnexa.* The follicles, glands, and ducts are lined by epidermis. Benign and malignant tumors arise here and are referred to as *adnexal tumors.*

Cutaneous sebaceous, apocrine sweat, and merocrine glands, singly or in combination, form specialized glands, some of which have unique locations, such as the caudal tail gland (sebaceous and apocrine sweat), circumanal gland (sebaceous), and anal sac gland (sebaceous and apocrine sweat). Sebaceous glands are most numerous in the lips, anus, and dorsum of the body. The smaller coiled merocrine sweat glands are found in the footpads. Malignant neoplasms of the adnexa are referred to as *adnexal carcinomas.*

The *dermis* is directly beneath the basal lamina and subcutis (hypodermis) is deep to the dermis. Because of the deep invaginations of the hair follicles and glands, these glands appear in the dermis and subcutis in histological sections, and thus epidermal tumors may form "beneath" the epidermis.

REACHING A THERAPEUTIC DECISION (pp. 2076–2078)

Staging

Tumor staging establishes whether local therapy is likely to be sufficient or whether advanced extent of disease requires systemic therapy. *TNM staging* is based on physical characteristics of the tumor (T), palpation and clinical examination of the local and regional lymph nodes (N), and metastasis (M). Mast cell tumor and cutaneous lymphoma are exceptions to this TNM format because of their systemic involvement.

Cytology and Biopsy

Because prognosis and therapy are influenced by cell type and histological grade, early identification of the tumor by cytology and follow-up by histopathological evaluation are optimal.

General Therapeutic Options

Whenever localization of a skin tumor allows, complete *surgical excision* is the treatment of choice because immediate cure is provided. Localized skin tumors that are not resectable or that are incompletely resected may respond to *radiation* therapy with or without the combination of *hyperthermia*. *Chemotherapy* with or without hyperthermia and *immunotherapy* are best suited for use with disseminated neoplasms or to enhance the efficacy of surgery or radiation.

EPIDERMAL AND ADNEXAL TUMORS (pp. 2078–2081)

Epidemiology and Etiology

Epidermal tumors account for up to 28 per cent of canine tumors and include the basal cell tumors, melanocytic tumors (discussed with round-cell tumors), and prickle cell tumors. The incidence in cats is roughly half that in dogs. Although primarily a disease of older animals, these lesions also afflict young animals.

Pathology

Typical epidermal neoplasms are derived from ectoderm and neuroectoderm. The majority of epithelial tumors are composed of pleomorphic cells that are roundish to polyhedral rather than spindle shaped. Some carcinomas can appear scirrhous, so the differential diagnosis of poorly differentiated carcinomas must also include poorly differentiated sarcomas.

Carcinomas are locally invasive. Small carcinomas that have not invaded deeper than the basal lamina are referred to as carcinomas *in situ.* Once they have invaded through the basal lamina, carcinomas metastasize, more likely via local and regional lymphatics than blood vessels. Distant metastases commonly affect the lungs, bones, kidneys, and central nervous system tissue.

Basal Cell Tumors

Basal cell tumors, also known as *basal cell carcinoma, basal cell epithelioma,* and *basiloma,* increase in frequency near the mean ages of 6 years in dogs and 10 years in cats. Poodles, mixed breeds, and cocker spaniels are more commonly affected. The head and trunk of dogs are the most common sites. Microscopically, they are aggressive, but their clinical course is usually benign. Complete surgical excision or biopsy and cryodestruction are the treatments of choice.

Squamous Cell Carcinoma

Squamous cell carcinoma arises from keratinocytes in the *stratum germanitivum/spinosum*. Skin with little or no pigment is more commonly affected. Common locations on dogs include the toes, scrotum, nose, anus, and abdomen. The eyelids, ears, and nose are commonly affected in cats.

The most characteristic lesion is that of a chronic nonhealing wound. The histopathological criterion necessary to diagnose squamous cell carcinoma is the presence of desmosomes. Squamous cell carcinoma may aggressively invade into adjacent tissue including bone. Squamous cell carcinomas of the inguinal area and nail bed metastasize earlier and exhibit a more aggressive behavior.

The treatment of choice is complete excision or biopsy followed by cryodestruction or electrodesiccation. Radiation therapy (45 to 50 Gy; x- or gamma rays) is unpredictable. Intravenous cisplatin (40 to 60 mg/m^2) has yielded partial to complete responses of primary and metastatic lesions for 2 to 15 weeks. The prognosis for tumors detected and adequately treated while localized is favorable; however, for large and invasive lesions, the prognosis is guarded. Application of sunscreens is mandatory for animals after treatment and advised as prophylactic for lightly pigmented animals exposed to intense sunlight.

Sebaceous Gland Tumors

The sebaceous glands are located over the entire body, and other modified sebaceous glands include the perianal glands, tarsal glands of the eyelid, and ceruminous glands of the ears. Sebaceous lesions account for 7.9 per cent of canine skin tumors and are more common in older dogs. Adenomas are firm, well circumscribed, freely movable, frequently hairless, warty, and occasionally ulcerated. These lesions are benign. Larger adenomas may be excised, but biopsy and electrodesiccation or freezing under local anesthesia is the safest and most convenient therapy for smaller lesions. Sebaceous gland carcinoma is a rare tumor of older dogs, especially cockers and poodles. Carcinomas are frequently larger than adenomas, possess more ill-defined borders, and are often ulcerated.

Perianal Tumors

Perianal gland adenomas/carcinomas are the most common neoplasms of male dogs. Malignant perianal tumors are less common (1:10). Tumors of the perianal region of a bitch are more likely to be malignant, possibly of anal sac origin. Perianal glands are modified sebaceous glands. Adenocarcinomas exhibit greater pleomorphism. Rectal palpation, as well as thoracic and especially lateral radiographs of the abdomen, is used for staging. Enlarged sublumbar lymph nodes may cause ventral colonic deviation.

The treatment for adenomas is castration and tumor excision. Although the value of castration for adenocarcinomas has not been completely documented, castration is recommended in conjunction with excision of the tumor and a margin of normal tissue. Adjuvant radiation is recommended for adenocarcinoma that is not resectable or incompletely excised, as well as for sublumbar metastases.

Adenocarcinoma of the Apocrine Glands of the Anal Sac

Adenocarcinoma of the apocrine glands of the anal sac is reported only in bitches. This tumor secretes a parathormone-like substance that raises serum calcium levels above normal in 85 per cent and may cause dystrophic soft-tissue calcification and renal failure. The sacral, hypogastric (intrapelvic), and medial iliac (caudal sublumbar) lymph nodes are the local and regional nodes that are inspected during staging for metastasis (67 per cent). Treatment is by aggressive excision and adjuvant radiation if excision is incomplete. Serum calcium is useful for diagnosing recurrence because metastatic foci secrete the parathormone-like protein.

Sweat Gland Tumors (pp. 2080–2081)

Hair Follicle Tumors

Pilomatricomas, tricoepitheliomas, and tricolemmoma probably originate from hair matrix, primitive hair matrix or basal cells, and the outer root sheath, respectively. Hair follicle tumors are most common in Kerry blue terriers, schnauzers, and poodles. The skin over the tumor is often hairless and thinned or ulcerated. Complete excision of a localized neoplasm is curative.

Intracutaneous Cornifying Epithelioma

Intracutaneous cornifying epithelioma commonly affects Norwegian elkhounds and occurs three times more frequently in males. The lesions are small, firm nodules characterized by a hard keratin plug protruding from a pore.

SOFT-TISSUE SARCOMAS AND MESENCHYMAL NEOPLASMS (pp. 2081–2086)

Soft-tissue sarcomas account for 14 to 17 per cent of canine tumors and encompass more than 20 different tumors and subtypes. The incidence in cats is half that in dogs.

Pathology

Soft-tissue sarcomas are mesodermal tumors usually arising in connective tissue. The tumors take their names from their cells of origin. A number of sarcomas fail to show the characteristics necessary for classification or are so poorly differentiated that they are called *undifferentiated sarcomas*.

The majority of sarcomas are composed of large, elongated malignant cells with a so-called spindle-cell pattern. Sarcomas form their own vascular capillary spaces as they grow. These spaces are usually lined by neoplastic cells, not endothelium, as seen in most carcinomas. Their most typical route of metastasis is by blood.

Diagnosis

Soft-tissue sarcomas are likely to have no clinical sign other than a painless mass. They occasionally cause lameness or other dysfunction because of their location.

Fine-needle aspiration may not be reliable for diagnosis of sarcomas because of their poor exfoliation during aspiration. Very large or rapidly growing tumors may have necrotic centers and be misdiagnosed as abscessation. Negative findings on fine-needle aspirates are verified by biopsy.

Staging

The TNM system, currently advocated for staging soft-tissue sarcomas, is not associated with prognosis. The reason for the inadequacy of clinical staging to provide prognostic support is that it appears that both anatomical site and histopathological grade influence survival. In man, histopathological grade is the single most important prognostic factor. For these reasons, a TNMG system has been recommended to stage soft-tissue sarcomas: G represents the histological grade.

General Therapy and Response

Surgery is the most important form of treatment for soft-tissue sarcomas, primarily in the form of "radical" excisions. The rationale for such surgery is high local recurrence. The primary surgical feature of these tumors is that they frequently appear encapsulated and are often "shelled" or enucleated. The apparent capsule is a pseudocapsule, and the shelling out leaves microscopic neoplastic infiltration within the tissue, a source of recurrence.

Although sarcomas are frequently considered radiation resistant, the most common adjuvant for soft-tissue sarcomas is radiation therapy. Most commonly, the postoperative surgical field is irradiated when resection is incomplete, but preoperative radiation is used to reduce the neoplasia to a resectable volume. Radiation is administered in doses ranging from 3,500 to more than 5,000 cGy in 10 to 18 fractions.

The responsiveness of sarcomas to chemotherapy is variable. In animals, single-agent chemotherapy with doxorubicin and mitoxantrone has shown overall response rates of 22 per cent and 17.7 per cent, respectively. In both man and pet animals, combination doxorubicin and cyclophosphamide or vincristine, doxorubicin, and cyclophosphamide are commonly used. Responses in animals vary from 2 to 6 months in our experience.

Specific Tumor Idiosyncrasies and Prognosis
Fatty Tumors

Lipomas are benign, usually well circumscribed, and easily excised. A subclass of lipomas is infiltrative and possess a benign histological appearance but invade adjacent structures. They may occur in any site but commonly afflict the limbs. Recurrence is likely if excision is inadequate.

Hemangiopericytoma

Hemangiopericytomas are characterized by infiltrative growth, high recurrence rate after incomplete excision, and low metastatic potential. They are most frequently seen on the limbs. The reported recurrence rate with surgery alone is approximately 25 per cent. In our experience, many inoperable hemangiopericytomas regress for 3 to 9 months when treated with gamma irradiation; not all respond.

Lymphangioma/Sarcoma

Lymphangioma/sarcomas are extremely rare tumors. Sarcomas occur frequently on the trunk and metastasize early. Cure is unlikely.

Hemangiosarcoma

Although most commonly a malignancy of parenchymatous organs, hemangiosarcoma is one of the most common soft-tissue sarcomas in dogs, especially German shepherds. Metastasis is common, and death is almost assured; 100 of 104 dogs in one series died.

Mast Cell Tumor

Mast cell tumors account for 7 to 21 per cent of all skin tumors and 11 to 27 per cent of all malignant skin tumors in dogs. In cats, they account for 2 to 15 per cent of all skin tumor types. A breed predisposition is noted in boxers, Boston terriers, bulldogs, and related breeds.

Canine mast cell tumors occur primarily in the dermis and subcutaneous tissues. In cats, mast cell tumors arise from the dermis, subcutaneous tissues, and viscera (spleen or liver).

Mast cell cytoplasmic granules contain several different vasoactive substances, especially histamine and heparin. With toluidine blue staining, heparin stains red and is found in highest concentrations in mature mast cells, whereas histamine stains blue and is found in highest concentrations in immature mast cells.

In addition to histamine and heparin, mast cell granules contain serotonin, leukotrienes, prostaglandins, and proteolytic enzymes. Histamine stimulates H_2 receptors on gastric parietal cells, causing increased acid production, and also increases gastrointestinal motility, leading to gastroduodenal ulceration and vomiting.

The most common sites of involvement of canine mast cell tumors are the trunk and perineum (50 per cent), extremities (40 per cent), and head and neck (10 per cent). Multiple sites are involved approximately 11 per cent of the time. Masses are usually firm and raised. In another form, because of collagen breakdown caused by mast cell granule products, the tumor mass is ill defined, soft, and almost edematous. On palpation, this form is frequently confused with lipoma.

Dogs have a broad range of clinical histories. The appearance ranges from small solitary dermal nodules with well-defined borders, to ill-defined alopecic erythematous, to an ulcerated mass. They may be firm or fluctuant, and palpation can cause degranulation to occur, leading to erythema and swelling in the area. Inguinal and perineal canine mast cell tumors recur and metastasize more frequently than tumors located on other areas of the body. Cats are most likely to have a solitary tumor that is benign. There is no evidence that tumors in one cutaneous site are more aggressive than those at another.

Mast cell tumors are usually easily diagnosed by cytological study, but histological assessment of canine tumors does allow grading of the tumor, which has shown prognostic significance in several studies. In cats, histological evaluation may also afford prognostic information.

Radiographs of the thorax are of limited value because metastasis of cutaneous mast cell tumors to the lungs is rare; however, they may show involvement of intrathoracic lymph nodes. Abdominal radiographs may demonstrate lymph node enlargement. Additionally, they may show splenic involvement in cats. Organomegaly can be further evaluated with ultrasonography and aspiration cytological study.

The primary mode of therapy for mast cell tumors is wide surgical excision with at least 3-cm margins of normal tissue. Radiation therapy is considered as postsurgical treatment for intermediate and poorly differentiated tumors. It is of benefit as the primary therapy for inoperable or recurrent tumors and involved lymph nodes that are not excised.

Once the tumor is no longer localized, treatment becomes palliative and success rates quite variable. Various chemotherapeutic protocols involving vinca alkaloids or cyclophosphamide have been proposed for mast cell tumors, but no studies show that such protocols are more efficacious than corticosteroids alone. Corticosteroid therapy usually involves the use of oral prednisolone or prednisone given at 40 mg/m^2 PO daily for 7 days, then 20 mg/m^2 PO every other day. Triamcinolone is used less frequently but can be used intralesionally at 1 mg/cm^2 of tumor every 2 weeks.

Animals with mast cell tumors are at risk for gastroduodenal ulceration secondary to histamine. This complication is treated with H$_2$ blockers (e.g., cimetidine, 5 mg/kg PO TID to QID; or ranitidine, 0.5 mg/kg PO BID). The most frequently used gastrointestinal protectant for treatment of ulceration is sucralfate (500 mg PO TID for animals <18 kg and 1 g PO TID for animals >18 kg). Sucralfate interferes with the absorption of cimetidine; therefore, cimetidine must be given either 45 minutes before or 2 hours after sucralfate. H$_1$ antagonists such as diphenhydramine (2 mg/kg PO TID) have been suggested to prevent the suppressive effects of histamine on fibroblast activity during wound healing. Several studies of dogs suggest that mast cell tumors are unlikely to recur if they have not done so by 6 months after treatment.

Histiocytoma

Histiocytomas are a common tumor in dogs; a few similar tumors have been reported in cats. These benign tumors arise from the monocyte macrophage population of the skin and account for 10 to 20 per cent of all skin tumors.

Histiocytomas are usually solitary tumors and are rapidly growing, dome-shaped masses with the surface being alopecic and inflamed to ulcerated. They are frequently excised because of their clinical appearance. Recurrence is uncommon, and metastasis does not occur.

Cutaneous Lymphosarcoma

Lymphosarcoma uncommonly involves the skin of dogs and cats. It occurs in older dogs (mean age = 9.5 years) and cats (mean age = 11 years). Cats with the tumor are feline leukemia virus negative. Clinically, the tumors may appear as simple erythema, crusting, ulcers, or nodules.

Therapy of cutaneous lymphosarcoma includes surgery, radiation therapy, and chemotherapy. The response of cutaneous lymphosarcoma to treatment is variable and frequently disappointing. Cats, even with solitary lesions, do poorly.

Plasmacytoma

Plasmacytomas are solitary broad-based, round, circumscribed, alopecic cutaneous or mucocutaneous lesions that occur in older dogs. Cats are also affected. The lips, feet, and ears are most commonly affected. Surgical excision results in cure. Recurrence ranges from 3 to 30 per cent. Recurrent lesions respond to re-excision.

Transmissible Venereal Tumor

Canine transmissible venereal tumor is a transmissible, usually nonmalignant tumor that becomes metastatic in only 5 per cent.

Therapy consists of surgery, radiation therapy, or chemotherapy. Surgery may be effective for localized lesions. Localized or more extensive tumors also respond well to chemotherapy with vincristine

(0.5 mg/m^2 IV weekly) or doxorubicin (30 mg/m^2 IV every 3 weeks). Treatment is continued until remission is complete.

Malignant Melanoma

Melanomas are of neuroectodermal origin and are frequently round or epithelioid, but they are also seen as spindle cells histologically. The degree of pigmentation varies. These features are not associated with prognosis.

Cutaneous melanomas are common in dogs (approximately 6 per cent of all skin tumors) and rare in cats. In dogs, most cutaneous melanomas are benign except for ones of the nail bed and mucocutaneous regions. Eyelid melanomas are usually benign.

The benign forms respond to simple excision. Suspected malignant lesions necessitate complete diagnosis, including thoracic radiographs for metastatic disease. Malignant masses require wide surgical excision, which may include amputation for digital melanomas. Radiation therapy may also be considered. The response of malignant melanomas to treatment is usually poor.

CHAPTER 154
Alimentary Tract, Liver, and Pancreas (pages 2088–2105)

OROPHARYNGEAL NEOPLASIA (pp. 2088–2091)

Neoplasia of the oral and pharyngeal cavities is the fifth most common canine and the seventh most common feline malignancy. Squamous cell carcinoma and malignant melanoma are the most frequent malignant oral tumors in dogs; squamous cell carcinoma and fibrosarcoma are most common in cats. Most oral tumors arise from the gingiva in dogs and from the gingiva or tongue in cats. Canine tongue tumors are uncommon. Older animals have an increased risk. Fibrosarcomas, however, occur more frequently in younger large dogs. The risk of developing oral melanomas and fibrosarcomas is greater in male dogs.

Biological Behavior

Epulides arise from the periodontal stroma, are typically located in the gingiva near the incisor teeth, and are more common in dogs than in cats. Acanthomatous epulides are locally invasive, causing bone destruction, but do not metastasize.

Ameloblastomas, the most common tumors of dental laminar epithelium, are expansile, slow-growing tumors. They are locally invasive and typically do not metastasize. Malignant melanomas grow rapidly and are characterized by early metastases to regional lymph nodes and lungs. Surface ulceration and necrosis are common.

Nontonsillar squamous cell carcinomas are most frequently identified arising from the gingiva rostral to the canine teeth in dogs and under the tongue in cats. Regional lymph node involvement is uncommon. Cell carcinomas appear as plaquelike or cauliflower lesions affecting one tonsil. They are locally invasive and frequently spread to the cervical lymph nodes and to distant sites.

Fibrosarcomas are typically firm, fleshy tumors that arise from the gingiva, hard palate, or buccal mucosa and frequently identified in the maxillary arcade between the canine and carnassial teeth. They are locally invasive but metastasis to regional lymph nodes and distant sites is uncommon.

Clinical Signs and Diagnosis

Clinically, oral tumors produce proliferative or occasionally ulcerative lesions. Associated signs may include decreased appetite, halitosis, tooth loss, and bloody salivation.

Radiographs of underlying bone are obtained in animals with tumors that adhere to bone to aid in determining clinical stage. A negative radiograph does not preclude bone involvement. Chest radiographs are obtained to rule out pulmonary metastasis.

Surgical Therapy

Benign and malignant tumors that do not involve bone are surgically excised. Epulides are cured by aggressive surgical treatment.

In dogs and cats with malignant oral tumors, mandibulectomies and maxillectomies have increased survival times compared with surgical excision alone, but local recurrence and metastatic disease remain significant problems.

Radiation Therapy

Local radiation therapy can produce long-term remissions and cures of radiosensitive tumors (squamous cell carcinoma, acanthomatous epulis, dental tumors). It can be used alone, as an adjuvant to surgical excision, or combined with hyperthermia.

Survival times in cats with oral squamous cell carcinomas are shorter than in dogs. Long-term results of radiation therapy for oral fibrosarcomas and malignant melanomas in dogs are disappointing.

Chemotherapy

Short-term benefits have been documented in dogs with oral squamous cell carcinomas treated with cisplatin[134] and in cats with fibrosarcomas and squamous cell carcinomas treated with doxorubicin and cyclophosphamide.

ESOPHAGEAL NEOPLASIA (pp. 2091–2093)

Esophageal neoplasia is rare in dogs and cats except for osteosarcomas and fibrosarcomas associated with *Spirocerca lupi*. Leiomyoma is the most frequently identified benign esophageal neoplasm. Carcinomas arise from squamous epithelium of the esophagus and may cause annular constriction of the esophagus.

Esophageal sarcomas are frequent in areas of the world where *S. lupi* is endemic. Esophageal sarcomas frequently metastasize to the lungs, and a high incidence of hypertrophic pulmonary osteoarthropathy has been noted.

Clinical Signs

Regurgitation, dysphagia, and weight loss are common. Regurgitation may result in aspiration pneumonia and respiratory signs.

Diagnosis

Esophagoscopy, radiographic evaluation, and thoracotomy can be used to establish a diagnosis of esophageal neoplasia.

Treatment and Prognosis

Neoplasia of the esophagus is associated with a poor prognosis.

GASTRIC NEOPLASIA

Adenocarcinoma is the most common canine gastric tumor but accounts for less than 1 per cent of all canine malignancies. The incidence of gastric tumor in cats is less than in dogs. Lymphosarcoma is the most frequent feline gastric neoplasm.

Benign Gastric Tumors

Leiomyoma is the most common benign gastric tumor in dogs. The average age of dogs with gastric leiomyomas is 16 years. Leiomyomas originate in the muscle layers of the stomach wall. Treatment is by surgical removal. Adenomatous polyps result from benign gastric mucosal proliferation. Both single and multiple polyps have been reported in the canine stomach.

Malignant Gastric Tumors

Malignant gastric tumors of dogs and cats include adenocarcinomas, lymphosarcomas, fibrosarcomas, leiomyosarcomas, and squamous cell carcinomas. Adenocarcinomas account for 42 to 72 per cent of all malignant gastric tumors in dogs. Gastric adenocarcinomas occur in older dogs. Lymphosarcoma is the most frequent feline gastric tumor. Gastric adenocarcinomas are usually located in the pyloric antrum or along the lesser curvature of the stomach. Early metastasis to regional lymph nodes and liver is common. Other metastatic sites include the spleen, omentum, adrenal glands, myocardium, and lungs.

Clinical Signs

Chronic vomiting, weight loss, and anorexia are usually noted. In addition, hematemesis, melena, and abdominal pain may be detected.

Diagnosis

Chronic vomiting and weight loss in an older dog suggest gastric adenocarcinoma. Contrast radiography, either a barium series or double-contrast gastrogram, is usually required to detect gastric lesions. Significant abnormalities persist on multiple films. Gastric lesions can also be detected with a flexible gastroscope. Directed biopsy of lesions can be achieved with biopsy forceps passed through the gastroscope. It is sometimes difficult to obtain diagnostic biopsy samples from submucosal tumors. Surgical exploration is used to confirm a diagnosis of gastric neoplasia. Tissue can be obtained for histopathological evaluation from primary and metastatic lesions.

Treatment

Complete surgical excision is the treatment of choice for gastric adenocarcinomas. Because the pyloric area of the stomach is often involved, a gastroduodenostomy or gastrojejunostomy may be required.

Enlarged regional lymph nodes are removed. Extensive gastric involvement may preclude complete excision of the primary tumor.

In dogs and cats with gastric lymphosarcoma, multiple-drug chemotherapy is indicated if the tumor cannot be removed and is probably indicated after surgical resection of localized lesions.

Prognosis

Most dogs with gastric adenocarcinoma have extensive involvement at diagnosis. Survival time in untreated dogs is generally less than 3 months after the onset of clinical signs. Survival after tumor excision is less than 6 months.

INTESTINAL NEOPLASIA (pp. 2093–2096)

Intestinal neoplasms are uncommon in dogs and cats. Intestinal tumors occur most frequently in the colon and rectum of dogs and small intestine of cats. Intestinal neoplasms usually occur in older animals, and males are more frequently affected than females.

Benign Neoplasms

Leiomyomas occur infrequently in the small and large intestine of dogs and cats. They arise from smooth muscle in the intestinal wall and may obstruct the intestinal lumen.

Adenomatous polyps occur most frequently in the canine rectum. Male and female dogs are equally affected. Rectal polyps are raised, sessile, or pedunculated and may occur in grapelike clusters. Single or multiple polyps may be present. Polyps generally do not recur after surgical removal.

Malignant Neoplasms

Adenocarcinomas occur most frequently in the rectum, colon, and jejunum of dogs and in the ileum of cats. Intestinal adenocarcinomas frequently metastasize to regional lymph nodes, especially mesenteric and iliac nodes. Diffuse metastasis to peritoneal surfaces (carcinomatosis) results in ascites.

Lymphosarcoma is most frequently identified in the jejunum of dogs and ileum of cats. Multiple sites within the intestinal tract are frequently involved. Affected cats are usually feline leukemia virus negative. Leiomyosarcomas have been reported infrequently throughout the intestinal tract of dogs and cats.

Clinical Signs

Intermittent vomiting and diarrhea, weight loss, and inappetence characterize small-intestinal tumors. Tenesmus, bloody mucoid feces, constipation, rectal prolapse, and increased frequency of defecation are frequent signs with large-intestinal tumors. Intestinal bleeding may result in anemia, thrombocytopenia, and hypoproteinemia.

Diagnosis

Intestinal tumors are often identified by abdominal palpation. Diagnosis can sometimes be established by cytological examination of an aspiration biopsy of the abnormal mass. Rectal examination may reveal a polypoid lesion or stricture. Survey abdominal radiographs and contrast studies (upper gastrointestinal series, barium enema) often show abnormalities. Endoscopic biopsy is sometimes possible for proximal duodenal tumors.

Treatment

Polyps in the rectum and distal colon can be surgically removed by pedicle ligation, electrocautery, or cryosurgery after digital exteriorization or rectal prolapse.

Wide surgical excision and intestinal anastomosis compose the treatment of choice for most malignant intestinal tumors. Pelvic osteotomy may be required to gain adequate exposure in animals with midrectal tumors. A rectal pull-through or a dorsal approach to the rectum can be used to expose distal rectal tumors. Radiation therapy may provide an alternative to surgery in some dogs with rectal adenocarcinomas. Chemotherapy has little effect on intestinal adenocarcinomas.

Prognosis

The prognosis after removal of polyps and other benign tumors is usually favorable. Recurrences are infrequent. In general, intestinal adenocarcinomas are associated with a guarded to poor long-term prognosis. In cats with intestinal adenocarcinomas, survival times after surgical resection are short.

HEPATIC NEOPLASIA (pp. 2096–2099)

Primary Hepatic Tumors (pp. 2096–2097)

Primary hepatic tumors are uncommon in dogs and cats.

Hepatocellular Carcinomas (pp. 2097–2098)

Tumors Metastatic to the Liver (Secondary Tumors)

The liver is a major site for metastasis of tumors. Clinical signs associated with metastatic liver tumors are variable. Hepatomegaly, which is common with primary hepatic neoplasms, is uncommon with metastatic tumors. Nineteen to 30 per cent of dogs with metastatic hepatic neoplasia have normal biochemical profiles. Tumors metastasizing to the liver arise from three major sources: hematopoietic cells, epithelium, and mesenchyme. Therapy for these tumors is directed at the primary neoplasm, if possible.

PANCREATIC NEOPLASIA (pp. 2099–2103)

Neoplasms of the pancreas arise primarily from epithelial tissue. The two most important neoplasms are pancreatic adenocarcinoma and pancreatic islet cell adenocarcinoma. Neoplasms of the pancreas are uncommon in both dogs and cats.

Pancreatic Adenocarcinomas

Pancreatic adenocarcinomas arise from both ductular and acinar tissue of the exocrine pancreas. Ductular carcinomas predominate. These tumors metastasize readily, most often in the liver, retroperitoneum, and mesenteric lymph nodes.

Clinical signs are often nonspecific and frequently relate more to the primary metastatic site (liver) than the organ of origin. Pancreatic adenocarcinomas frequently compress the common bile duct, producing jaundice.

A definitive antemortem diagnosis is rarely made except via exploratory celiotomy. Biochemical profiles most often suggest that liver rather than pancreatic disease is present. Abdominocentesis, with or without lavage, may help establish a diagnosis. Pancreatic adenocarcinomas exfoliate readily, and cytological study of peritoneal fluid suggests abdominal malignancy. The prognosis for animals with pancreatic adenocarcinoma is invariably poor owing to the tendency for early and widespread metastases.

Pancreatic Adenoma/Hyperplasia

Pancreatic hyperplasia is a frequent finding in aged dogs and cats. Pancreatic adenoma is rare, although precise microscopic criteria for separation of these two entities are equivocal.

Pancreatic Islet Cell Tumors

Insulinomas

Insulinoma is a functional tumor of the pancreatic beta cell. Insulinomas are less frequently recognized than pancreatic acinar cell carcinomas. Large dogs weighing more than 25 kg are at increased risk.

Clinical signs are variable, but all are related to hypoglycemia induced by excessive production of insulin by the tumor or to catecholamine release secondary to hypoglycemia. Hypoglycemic convulsions or collapse may occur in two-thirds of dogs with insulinomas. Nearly one-third have been treated nonspecifically for an idiopathic seizure disorder before diagnosis. Signs are nearly always intermittent, and long periods may elapse between episodes of clinically apparent hypoglycemia. Signs become more frequent as the disease progresses.

Confirming a diagnosis of insulinoma is uncomplicated. The majority have blood glucose values less than 70 mg/100 ml on initial evaluations. Once hypoglycemia is confirmed, the next step is to validate that it is due to relative or absolute insulin excess and not some other cause. Serum is analyzed for insulin concentration from any hypoglycemic sample in which another obvious cause of the hypoglycemia is not identified. Normal fasting serum immunoreactive insulin concentrations range from 5 to 26 microunits/ml from most veterinary laboratories. Approximately 75 per cent have elevated serum insulin concentrations when initially evaluated, and a diagnosis of insulinoma is highly likely. In the remaining 25 per cent, initial insulin values are in the normal range.

Preoperative treatment of dogs with insulinomas varies. Feeding three to six small daily meals of a diet high in protein and complex carbohydrates often reduces or eliminates clinical signs. Semimoist diets high in simple sugars are avoided. The addition of prednisone or the oral hyperglycemic agent diazoxide may also help preoperatively to stabilize patients that fail to respond to frequent feedings alone.

Patients are given no food for 8 to 12 hours before surgery, and blood glucose concentrations are maintained by intravenous 5 per cent dextrose. Nearly all animals have readily identifiable round 1- to 2.5-cm-diameter solitary (85 per cent) or multiple tumor nodules visible in the pancreas. Approximately 45 per cent of patients also have metastases to regional lymph nodes or the liver at surgery. Tumors are identified with equal frequency within the left (splenic) or right (duodenal) limb of the pancreas.

If no primary tumor is identified and the diagnosis is likely, consider blind resection of 50 per cent of the pancreas in case diffuse islet cell neoplasia is present. Development of diabetes mellitus is a unique paradox of this disease. Prolonged increases in tumor insulin and subsequent hypoglycemia may lead to atrophy of normal islet tissue. Diabetes may develop in 15 to 29 per cent of dogs in the postoperative period. In many cases, the hyperglycemia is transient, lasting from a few days to 2 months. Occasional dogs have persistent moderate to severe ataxia even though hypoglycemia has been corrected.

Medical treatment of dogs with insulinomas is considered in the preoperative period to stabilize their disease before surgery. Methods to control hypoglycemia include frequent feeding, reduced exercise, glucocorticoids, oral hyperglycemic agents, somatostatin analogues, and islet cell cytotoxic drugs. Dogs with recurrent hypoglycemia are fed between four and six times per day, offering a high-protein diet that is low in simple sugars and high in complex carbohydrates. Prednisone or prednisolone is given twice daily to stimulate gluconeogenesis. Initial dosages are 1.0 to 4 mg/kg/day, BID. This dosage may be increased up to 2 mg/kg/day in refractory cases.

The prognosis for dogs with functional islet cell tumors is highly variable but generally poor. Prognostic factors associated with decreased survival are age at the time of diagnosis (younger dogs have shorter survival times), high preoperative serum insulin concentrations, and the presence of distant metastases at surgery. Although dogs in which hypoglycemia persists after surgery generally survive only briefly, combinations of surgical and medical therapy have resulted in animals living as long as 3½ years after surgery.

Gastrinomas

Gastrinomas are functional nonbeta islet cell pancreatic tumors.

Nine cases were reported to document the existence of pancreatic islet cell tumors that secrete gastrin in dogs, and one case in a cat. Presenting complaints usually include depression, anorexia, vomiting, diarrhea, and weight loss. Vomiting of blood or melena and abdominal pain were observed in 11 per cent of cases.

A definitive diagnosis is based on identifying a pancreatic islet cell neoplasm and documentation of elevated fasting serum gastrin concentrations. Normal fasting serum gastrin concentrations in dogs are between 20 and 190 pg/ml and in cats between 28 and 135 pg/ml. Serum gastrin concentrations in dogs with gastrinomas have been from 360 to 2,780 pg/ml and in one cat, 1,000 pg/ml.

Most dogs and cats with gastrinomas are treated by a combination of medical and surgical approaches. Ulcer care usually involves the use of H_2-receptor antagonists such as cimetidine (5 mg/kg four to six times daily) or ranitidine (2 mg/kg TID) and the ulcer protective agent sucralfate. Gastrinomas are generally small, similar to insulinomas, and surgical removal of primary and metastatic tumors is attempted.

The prognosis for animals with gastrinomas is poor. Most have had metastatic disease when the diagnosis was first made and survive briefly.

CHAPTER 155

Cardiovascular System
(pages 2106–2111)

PRIMARY CARDIAC NEOPLASMS (pp. 2106–2107)

Hemangiosarcoma (angiosarcoma, hemangioendothelioma), a highly malignant tumor of endothelial origin, is more commonly found in dogs than cats. A predilection is noted in middle-aged to aged male German shepherds, boxers, and golden retrievers.

Primary cardiac hemangiosarcoma frequently originates in the right atrium at the crista terminalis, a ridge of muscle at the juncture of the right atrium and right auricle, or within the right auricle. Hematogenous metastasis to the lungs, liver, spleen, kidneys, brain, and subcutaneous tissue is common. Right-sided congestive heart failure often develops in dogs. More than 50 per cent of affected dogs are borderline to severely anemic. Patients with hemangiosarcoma may be predisposed to disseminated intravascular coagulation.

Chemodectomas arise from the nonchromaffin paraganglia of the aortic bodies (aortic body tumor, heart base tumor). Although common in older male dogs, they are rare in cats. Clinical signs relate to disease caused by local tissue alteration or metastasis. Aortic body tumors are usually benign, grow slowly, and often become large. Clinical signs are often those of congestive heart failure (e.g., dyspnea, cough, cyanosis, hepatomegaly, venous engorgement, and ascites). A bloody pericardial effusion is often encountered and may cause cardiac tamponade.

Myxomas are rare in dogs. Myxomas are benign neoplasms derived from mesenchymal cells of the subendocardial region. They form polypoid pedunculated masses that arise from the subendocardium of the atria or ventricles. Complete surgical excision is the treatment of choice in dogs.

Fibromas are benign connective tissue tumors that may be of congenital origin and appear less frequently in the heart than elsewhere in the body. Clinical signs of the neoplasm relate to mechanical interference of blood flow. They are found most frequently in the right heart.

Mesotheliomas are rare mesodermal neoplasms that can arise from the pleural, pericardial, or peritoneal cavities. *Rhabdomyoma* is a benign striated muscle tumor that seldom occurs in the heart. *Sarcomas*, other than hemangiosarcoma, are infrequently reported in dogs and cats, although melanosarcoma, fibrosarcoma, chondrosarcoma, and leiomyosarcoma all have been described in dogs.

METASTATIC CARDIAC NEOPLASMS (pp. 2107–2108)

Metastatic cardiac tumors occur less frequently than do primary cardiac tumors in dogs. Hemangiosarcoma, pulmonary adenocarcinoma, mammary gland adenocarcinoma, squamous cell carcinoma, and undifferentiated malignant oral tumors are the most commonly observed metastatic tumors in dogs.

Hemangiosarcoma often arises from the right atrium, but neoplasms may originate from peripheral organs or tissues such as the spleen, liver, or bone and metastasize to the heart and lungs because they have access to vascular channels.

Lymphosarcoma, the most common metastatic heart tumor in cats, rarely invades the hearts of dogs. In the nodular form, the neoplasm is smoothly nodular, with masses sometimes becoming very large. In the diffusely infiltrative form, the myocardium is irregularly thickened and gray-white, resembling myocardial degeneration and fibrosis. The cranial mediastinal form of lymphosarcoma has the greatest tendency to afflict the myocardium. Large cranial mediastinal masses may displace the heart and cause incompressibility of the cranial chest.

PERIPHERAL VASCULAR NEOPLASMS (pp. 2108–2109)

Hemangiomas are more prevalent in older dogs (>9 years) with pigmented skin, Scottish terriers, Airedales, Kerry blue terriers, and Labrador retrievers. These dark-red to reddish-black tumors may develop in any location but are usually found in the subcutis or dermis of the leg, flank, neck, face, eyelid, or scrotum. Tumor recurrence is not a problem after complete resection of the mass.

Hemangiosarcoma may arise from many tissues; however, the most common sites of peripheral origin in dogs are the spleen, liver, bone, and skin. Hemangiosarcomas have a high metastatic potential, and survival rates are discouraging. Frequent metastatic sites include the liver, lungs, heart, and brain. Clinical findings include various signs relating to the degree of organ involvement and metastatic spread. Abdominal palpation is helpful in detecting masses involving the spleen, liver, and kidneys. Hematological evaluation of peripheral blood may help in diagnosis because a majority of dogs with hemangiosarcoma exhibit regenerative anemia.

The treatment of choice for hemangiosarcoma is surgical removal, but because most tumors have metastasized by the time they are recognized, the prognosis is guarded.

Chemodectomas originating from the carotid bodies (carotid body tumor) occur less frequently but are more often malignant than chemodectomas originating from the aortic body. The carotid body tumor is a unilateral mass near the angle of the jaw. Clinical signs of dysphagia or dyspnea due to compression of the esophagus or trachea may be encountered as the mass enlarges and invades surrounding structures.

DIAGNOSIS OF CARDIAC NEOPLASIA (p. 2109)

Clinical signs of heart failure are common to many neoplastic disorders as well as to the usual causes of failure. Radiography may be useful in determining the presence of cardiac neoplasms and in detecting metastasis. An electrocardiogram can provide supportive information relating to the presence of pericardial effusion because the QRS amplitude often becomes dampened or reduced. Echocardiography helps define the presence, location, and size of cardiac masses and documents the presence of pericardial effusion.

Biopsy of cardiac masses is difficult, often requiring exploratory thoracotomy. Tissue from intramural lesions can be obtained by guided transvenous myocardial biopsy catheters. Both angiocardiography and intracardiac pressure measurements can provide valuable complementary information to echocardiography by further defining the location and extent of cardiac luminal involvement and the neoplasm's effect on hemodynamic performance.

TREATMENT OF CARDIAC NEOPLASIA (p. 2110)

Solitary cardiac tumors that have not metastasized may be treated surgically if they are accessible and do not involve large portions of the myocardial wall. Solitary hemangiomas or hemangiosarcomas, which are isolated to the right atrial wall, and fibromas and myxomas located in the right heart are the most surgically approachable.

Aortic body tumors can be resected rarely, but removal of the pericardial sac when pericardial tamponade is a problem can relieve clinical signs and extend an animal's life. Irradiation of these tumors has resulted in remission in a few animals.

CHAPTER 156

Hematopoietic System
(pages 2111–2136)

CANINE HEMATOPOIETIC SYSTEM (pp. 2111–2119)
Lymphoma
Epidemiology

Lymphoma (lymphosarcoma) is defined as a lymphoid neoplasm primarily affecting lymph nodes or other solid visceral organs such as the liver or spleen. Lymphoma accounts for 5 per cent of all canine malignant neoplasia and 83 per cent of all canine hematopoietic malignancies. Middle-aged to older (median age of 5.5 to 9.1 years) dogs are primarily affected.

Etiology

The cause of canine lymphoma is unknown and a viral etiology is unconfirmed.

Diagnostics and Staging

Traditionally, canine lymphoma is classified according to anatomical site; the majority are multicentric. The diagnosis of lymphoma is best established after biopsy. Although fine-needle aspirates of lymph nodes, spleen, or liver can suggest neoplasia, conclusive histological diagnosis from lymph node biopsy is recommended. An entire accessible lymph node should be removed to preserve tissue architecture. Up to 96 per cent of dogs with multicentric lymphoma have one or more hematological, biochemical, or bone marrow abnormalities.

Radiographically, 60 per cent of dogs with lymphoma have sternal lymph node enlargement, 55 per cent splenomegaly, 50 per cent sublumbar lymph node enlargement, and 47 per cent hepatomegaly. These radiographic abnormalities are diagnostic, and they can be useful in staging. Ophthalmic abnormalities are common in dogs with lymphoma. These include uveitis, hemorrhage, and ocular infiltration.

Overall, 15 to 20 per cent of dogs with multicentric lymphoma and approximately half of those with mediastinal forms are hypercalcemic. A thorough investigation for lymphoma is carried out whenever hypercalcemia of unknown origin is encountered.

Prognostic Indicators

Most larger studies fail to reveal a relationship between clinical stage and response to therapy; however, bone marrow involvement (especially with associated CBC abnormalities) is associated with decreased long-term survival. Attempts to correlate survival with histopathological grade have failed.

Therapy of Multicentric Lymphoma

Without treatment, most dogs with lymphoma die in 4 to 6 weeks. With few exceptions, canine lymphoma is a systemic disease, and systemic chemotherapy is the therapy of choice. Single-agent chemotherapy is not as effective as combination chemotherapy. The ideal chemotherapeutic protocol remains in question. Published protocols with reported remission and survival data are presented. These remission and survival times are the longest yet recorded for canine lymphoma treatment, yet dogs with lymphoma are still rarely cured; all protocols apparently reach the same 6- to 8-month remission failure.

Drug therapy for multicentric lymphoma may have to be altered based on the presence of one or more cytopenias. Most important, thrombocytopenia ($<75,000/\mu l$) and neutropenia ($<2,500/\mu l$) are cause for concern.

Lymphoma is a drug-sensitive tumor, so much so that a serious life-threatening sequel of therapy known as *tumor lysis syndrome* can develop. Breakdown of tumor cells releases by-products that must be cleared by renal excretion, hepatic metabolism, or a combination of the two. Therapy for hypercalcemia secondary to lymphoma is best accomplished by attaining disease remission. If necessary, diuresis with high-sodium crystalloids (0.9 per cent sodium chloride) delivered at twice maintenance volumes alone or in combination with furosemide is usually successful.

Rescue therapy, defined as an attempt to re-establish remission once an animal's disease reasserts itself, has not been carefully studied in animals. If the disease returns while an animal is on chemotherapy, those drugs being used should be discontinued in favor of alternatives. However, if a drug used in the past was not currently being used when the disease returned, it may still be an effective choice and can be reinstated if superior alternatives do not exist.

Immunotherapy

MacEwen and colleagues reported on 98 dogs with lymphoma that were randomized into either chemotherapy alone (vincristine, cyclophosphamide, methotrexate, and L-asparaginase) versus chemotherapy plus the nonspecific immunomodulator levamisole. No significant difference in response resulted between therapy groups.

Reports have combined chemotherapy with more specific forms of immunotherapy. Overall remission and survival duration are not significantly altered with autochthonous vaccines. Administration of specific monoclonal antibodies against canine lymphoma cell antigens is now being evaluated.

Alimentary Lymphoma

In a large compilation of alimentary lymphoma cases, the majority arose in the gastrointestinal tract; they were rarely solitary and often metastasized to liver and local lymph nodes and were rarely amenable to surgical extirpation. Clinical signs are nonspecific. The major differential diagnosis for alimentary lymphoma is lymphocytic-plasmacytic enteritis; immunohistochemical stains are the only reliable method to differentiate the two in man. Lymphocytic-plasmacytic enteritis may be preneoplastic. Therapy is usually unrewarding. Clinical responses are noted, but remission usually lasts only a few weeks.

Cutaneous Lymphoma

Cutaneous lymphoma usually begins primarily but occasionally is secondary to multicentric forms of the disease. Lesions can be solitary or multiple, with the majority eventually developing into systemic multicentric disease. Approximately half of the reported cases of cutaneous lymphoma are pruritic.

If a solitary lesion is noted and thorough clinical staging, as previously discussed for multicentric lymphoma, fails to reveal systemic disease, local therapy including surgery or radiotherapy may produce a cure. Fractionated radiotherapy to a total dose of 30 to 45 Gy has been associated with long-term control and is ideally delivered as superficial electron therapy. Topical nitrogen mustard (mechlorethamine) has some efficacy.

Positive treatment responses are few, but the disease can be successfully controlled, with long-term survival. Five of six dogs responded to combination chemotherapy with COAP (cyclophosphamide, vincristine, cytosine arabinoside, and prednisone); median remissions and survivals were 250 and 399 days, respectively.

Mediastinal Lymphoma

Dogs with mediastinal lymphoma are often presented with respiratory signs or precaval syndrome (i.e., facial and forelimb edema) secondary to the mass effect of the tumor. Forty to 50 per cent of thymic lymphomas are associated with hypercalcemia.

Lymphoma of the Nervous System

Lymphoma of the nervous system is an unusual finding in dogs. The majority of central nervous system (CNS) lymphomas reported in dogs are secondary to systemic disease, although primary CNS lymphoma does occur. Diagnosis of nervous system lymphoma includes a complete lymphoma staging procedure as well as a cerebrospinal fluid (CSF) aspirate, computed tomographic (CT) scan, or myelogram if available. Biopsy may be necessary for eventual diagnosis if neoplastic lymphocytes are not present in the CSF.

Surgical intervention for diagnosis or removal of accessible tumors has been successfully performed. More common, surgery must be combined with adjuvant chemotherapy or radiotherapy. Only prednisone and cytosine arabinoside (ara-C) consistently cross the blood-brain barrier in therapeutic concentrations. Ara-C can be delivered intrathecaly (20 mg/m^2) after removing an equal volume of CSF, at a dosage of 100 mg/m^2 SC daily for 4 consecutive days every 3 weeks, or as a continuous 4-day infusion given at 100 mg/m^2/day diluted in saline or a balanced electrolyte solution. If the CNS lymphoma is accompanied by disease elsewhere in the body, the ara-C is incorporated into a more traditional combination therapy protocol. Radiotherapy has also been successfully used for treating CNS lymphoma.

Lymphoid Leukemia

Leukemia is defined as the proliferation of neoplastic hematopoietic cells in the bone marrow; such cells may not be circulating in the peripheral blood. The two general categories of lymphoid leukemia are chronic lymphocytic leukemia and acute lymphoblastic leukemia.

Acute Lymphoblastic Leukemia (p. 2117)

Chronic Lymphocytic Leukemia (pp. 2117–2118)

Myeloproliferative Disorders (pp. 2118–2119)

Plasma Cell Neoplasms

Multiple Myeloma

Multiple myeloma, the neoplastic proliferation of a clone of plasma cells, occurs primarily in aged dogs. Seventy-five per cent of affected dogs have a monoclonal gammopathy, either of the IgG or IgA subtype. Differentials for monoclonal gammopathy include ehrlichiosis and benign hypergammaglobulinemia syndrome. Light-chain (Bence Jones) proteins may be detectable in the urine by phoretic techniques. Clinical signs attributable to multiple myeloma are nonspecific. Most patients have lameness secondary to paresis or pain.

Diagnosis of multiple myeloma usually follows documentation of bone marrow plasmacytosis (> 20 to 30 per cent plasma cells), osteo-lytic bone lesions, and serum or urine myeloma proteins.

The short-term prognosis for multiple myeloma is normally favorable, and long-term remissions are the rule. The long-term prognosis is grave because cures are rare. Combination chemotherapy using melphalan (0.1 mg/kg PO daily for 10 days, followed by 0.05 mg/kg/day) with prednisone (0.5 mg/kg/day for 10 days, then every other day) results in remission rates of 90 per cent and median survival times of 540 days. Rescue therapy is not well documented once remission is lost.

Extramedullary Plasmacytoma

Extramedullary plasmacytoma occurs primarily as a solitary mucocutaneous lesion of the mouth but also can affect the feet, trunk, and ears. Cure was by local surgical resection in 40 of 57 dogs treated, with a median disease-free interval of 11.8 months. The prognosis is very favorable for solitary extramedullary plasmacytoma in dogs.

FELINE HEMATOPOIETIC SYSTEM (pp. 2120–2133)

Approximately 25 per cent of feline leukemia virus (FeLV)-induced diseases are neoplastic, and the majority of these are lymphoid and hematopoietic malignancies. Lymphoid and hematopoietic malignancy account for 30 per cent of all feline tumors, and 90 per cent of these are malignant lymphomas.

Natural History of FeLV

Classification

FeLV is a single-stranded RNA virus of the subfamily Oncovirinae, a group belonging to the family Retrovirinae. These viruses are unique because they contain the enzyme *reverse transcriptase*, enabling the viral RNA genome to be copied into a complementary strand of DNA that is ultimately integrated permanently into the genome of infected cells.

Genetic Pathogenesis of FeLV-Induced Disease

FeLV-infected cat cells are destroyed quickly when large amounts of unintegrated FeLV DNA accumulate within the cytoplasm. This is the pathogenesis for FeLV variant A disease. About 20 per cent of FeLV-induced thymic lymphomas and all fibrosarcomas induced by the feline sarcoma virus (FeSV) are the result of virus-host genetic recombinations. Because virus-host genetic recombination recurs *de novo* in FeLV-infected cats, those cats that develop fibrosarcomas do not pose a risk to other cats for development of fibrosarcomas. However, they are still contagious for the FeLV that gave rise to FeSV by genetic recombination.

Transmission and Pathogenesis of FeLV Infection

FeLV is usually transmitted through the saliva of one infected cat to the oral or nasal mucous membranes of another cat via licking and grooming. Virus is replicated intracellularly for 2 to 4 days in lymphocytes or macrophages. Most cats successfully neutralize the virus by this stage through production of virus-neutralizing antibody and are subsequently immune to FeLV infection. In cats that do not eliminate virus, the infected cells leave the nodes and circulate hematogenously for 2 to 14 days. By 4 to 6 weeks, a cat is persistently viremic and has greater than a 95 per cent chance of remaining infected for life. Virus is shed into the environment in saliva and urine. FeLV can also infect unborn fetuses *in utero* and the virus is also secreted into the milk. Most FeLV-infected cats die within 3.5 years of developing chronic infection.

Latent Infection of FeLV

Latently infected cats do not actively shed virus and are not viremic. However, FeLV can be isolated from the bone marrow of these cats after *in vitro* bone marrow culture. These cats have virus-neutralizing antibodies in their serum and are apparently recovered from FeLV infection.

Latent FeLV infections probably represent a phase of recovery after exposure to FeLV in cats that develop immunity. Cats test negative for cell-associated viremia (by IFA methods), although small numbers are intermittently positive by ELISA testing.

From the clinical perspective, it is important to recognize the risk of these cats reverting to an FeLV-producing status. Should this occur, these cats are sources of infective virus to other cats and increase their own chance for an FeLV-associated illness. Latently infected cats are not usually predisposed to development of diseases associated with FeLV, even after prolonged follow-up.

There is no evidence that latently infected cats routinely transmit FeLV to susceptible cats. Most clinicians are not able to confirm latency for every cat presented for surgical (or medical) problems, so a complete history is essential. ELISA-positive, IFA-negative cats are suspect for latency and should be retested.

The key points of FeLV latency relative to clinical (surgical) care are as follows: (1) The cats are not viremic and thus not contagious. (2) Latency is probably a ''normal'' phase of recovery from FeLV exposure. (3) Minimized stress and immunosuppression probably aid a cat in permanently extinguishing FeLV infection.

Clinical Diagnostic Testing for FeLV

It is recommended that a cat showing any of the myriad FeLV-associated clinical or laboratory abnormalities be tested for FeLV infection before surgery. FeLV-induced neoplasms, composed chiefly of lymphoma/leukemia and fibrosarcoma, are often obvious, so it is unlikely that such cats will inadvertently have surgery. It is more likely that cats with non-neoplastic FeLV-associated immunosuppressive and degenerative conditions will have surgery without prior testing of their FeLV status. FeLV testing consists of two basic types: IFA and ELISA.

Therapy of FeLV Infection

Although no effective therapies can reliably eliminate persistent FeLV infection, several experimental approaches have been investigated. Some of these include reverse transcriptase inhibitors, bone marrow transplantation, whole-body hyperthermia, and staphylococcal protein A.

Vaccination Against FeLV

Strict adherence to the manufacturer's recommended vaccination procedure is essential. Despite the proper vaccination schedule, some cats are not protected. All cats should be FeLV negative before vaccination; however, the possibility of prior FeLV exposure can never be ruled out. Cats at highest risk for FeLV infection, such as those in multicat households or cats younger than 1 year, are most likely to benefit from FeLV vaccination. FeLV vaccination should be considered for cats at risk before they undergo elective surgical procedures.

Lymphomas

Lymphomas (malignant lymphomas, lymphosarcomas) are the most common malignancies in cats and account for approximately one-third of all tumors in this species. FeLV is causally associated with 70 per cent of lymphomas.

Lymphomas are malignancies arising in solid lymphoid tissues such as lymph nodes, spleen, liver, thymus, or Peyer patches. In advanced cases, tumor cells can also infiltrate the bone marrow. By contrast, lymphoid malignancy that originates in the bone marrow is usually classified as lymphoid leukemia. Cats with lymphoma have a better treatment prognosis than cats with leukemia. Lymphomas can also affect nonlymphoid tissues. Alternatively, lymphoma can arise exclusively in sites other than the primary lymphoreticular tissues, presenting as so-called extranodal lymphomas. Frequently involved sites of extranodal lymphoma include the kidneys, skin, CNS, and eyes.

Histological Classification of Feline Lymphomas

The morphological criteria of the Working Formulation have been applied to more than 600 cases of feline lymphoproliferative disease: 8.6 per cent were low-grade, 35.1 per cent were intermediate-grade, and 55.2 per cent were high-grade tumors. The remaining 1.1 per cent were plasmacytomas.

Anatomical Classification of Feline Lymphomas
Mediastinal Lymphoma

The majority of cats with lymphoma in the thoracic cavity are FeLV positive. Structures involved can include lymph nodes in the mediastinum and remnants of the thymus, especially in kittens. This form of lymphoma is common in cats and most often affects young animals between 2 and 3 years of age. Affected cats most often show respiratory signs compatible with extrapulmonary, intrathoracic lung compression owing to the large tumor and malignant pleural effusion it induces. Affected cats cough rarely. Horner's syndrome is occasionally present owing to compression of the vagosympathetic trunk by the mediastinal mass.

Mediastinal lymphoma should always be high on the list of differential diagnoses when young cats are presented with restrictive breathing patterns.

Radiographs of the thorax reveal a space-occupying mass in the mediastinum, elevation of the trachea, and usually pleural effusion.

Definitive diagnosis of mediastinal lymphoma is made by microscopic examination of tumor tissue or pleural effusion. Fine-needle aspiration through the lateral chest wall using a small-gauge needle is a reliable method to sample the mass or fluid.

A complete work-up is always recommended to stage lymphoma in the mediastinum. Lymphoma in the chest is usually confined to that location, but some cats have a leukemic hemogram showing bone marrow infiltration by cancer cells. This carries a poorer prognosis. Chemotherapy is used to treat lymphoma in the chest, and several protocols have been advocated.

Alimentary Lymphoma

Affected cats are usually middle-aged (8 years old), and only a minority (30 per cent) are FeLV positive. Alimentary lymphoma involves the stomach, small intestine, or large intestine. It can be solitary or diffuse. A common site of obstruction is the ileocecocolic area. Alimentary lymphoma often progresses to involve mesenteric lymph nodes, the liver, and spleen.

When the disease has been chronic, physical examination often reveals that cats are underweight and sometimes cachectic. Abdominal palpation may reveal mass(es) associated with the bowel or mesenteric lymph nodes. Hepatosplenomegaly can also be palpated when present.

The diagnosis is confirmed by microscopic examination of tumor cells obtained from a fine-needle aspirate of intestinal wall or mass or via laparotomy with incisional/excisional surgical biopsy. Biopsy specimens can also be obtained with the use of an endoscope inserted *per os* or *per rectum*. The major disadvantages of endoscopic biopsy include inability to obtain samples deep into the mucosa or superficial submucosa. Lymphoma has a tendency to ''preferentially'' affect the lamina propria and submucosa in cats. The treatment of choice for alimentary lymphoma is chemotherapy.

Multicentric Lymphoma

Multicentric lymphoma usually includes lymphomas that are widely disseminated to many lymphoid tissues. The peripheral lymph nodes are most often involved, but additional lymphoid structures affected include the spleen, liver, and bone marrow.

Most cats (80 per cent) with multicentric lymphoma are FeLV positive and are younger (mean age 4 years). Enlarged, nonpainful peripheral lymph nodes often are incidental findings by conscientious cat owners. Hepatosplenomegaly is frequently present. Extranodal involvement is frequently found with primary multicentric lymphoid disease, and sites include the kidneys (usually bilaterally), eyes, CNS, and less often the skin.

Miscellaneous Lymphomas

A group of lymphomas arising in various extralymphoid sites are often referred to as *miscellaneous lymphomas*. Most commonly affected sites are the kidneys, eyes, CNS, and skin.

Treatment and Prognosis of Feline Lymphomas

Feline lymphomas are treated with systemic multiagent chemotherapy because the malignancy usually affects more than one body site and lymphoma cells are sensitive to various drugs. Surgery, radiotherapy, and immunotherapy have limited use.

Chemotherapeutic agents most used to treat feline lymphoma include vincristine, cyclophosphamide, L-asparaginase, methotrexate, cytosine arabinoside, and prednisone.

Regardless of location, 62 per cent of all 103 treated cats in one study experienced complete remission and had a median survival of 7 months. One-third of these cats survived at least 1 year. Clinical stage and FeLV status significantly affected prognosis. Those cats with less advanced stages (stages I and II) lived significantly longer than cats with advanced disease. Cats that were FeLV negative with lymphoma also survived longer than FeLV-positive cats. Advanced tumor stages or FeLV infection carried an equally poor prognosis.

Lymphoid Leukemias

Lymphoid leukemias are characterized by the proliferation of malignant lymphoid cells primarily within the bone marrow. Malignant cells usually do not always circulate in the blood and infiltrate organs of the reticuloendothelial system. Therefore, leukemia is a bone marrow disease that spreads peripherally, whereas lymphoma is a disease that originates peripherally and progresses centrally. The prognosis for lymphoma is usually more favorable than for true leukemia.

In cats, most lymphoid leukemias are an immature, blastic cell type, characterized by rapid onset, fulminant course, and relatively poor response to chemotherapy. The hallmark of the diagnosis is identification of large numbers ($\geq$ 30 per cent) of these cells in a bone marrow aspirate. Clinical signs of acute lymphoblastic leukemia are nonspecific. Most animals are FeLV positive.

Although chemotherapy can effectively lower the cell counts, only a small percentage of treated cats attain complete remission. Unless cats attain complete remission, survival time is short. The chemotherapeutic approach for treating acute lymphoblastic leukemia is usually the same as for lymphoma.

Chronic lymphocytic leukemia is rare in cats, suggesting it is not an important consequence of FeLV infection. Chronic lymphocytic leukemia is characterized by excessive numbers of mature (well-differentiated) lymphocytes that are produced in the bone marrow. Physical examination revealed hepatosplenomegaly but not lymphadenopathy.

A less aggressive chemotherapeutic approach is warranted. Chlorambucil (2 mg/m² PO every other day) plus prednisone (20 mg/m² PO every other day) can improve clinical signs.

Plasma Cell Neoplasms

Most reports of feline plasma cell disease are of multiple myeloma. The abnormal plasma cells secrete large quantities of an identical class of immunoglobulin referred to as a *paraprotein* or *M component*. Most reports of feline multiple myeloma have described the paraprotein as IgG. The large amount of circulating immunoglobulin can cause serum hyperviscosity with neurological abnormalities, retinal hemorrhages/degeneration, and cardiac failure.

Other clinical signs associated with multiple myeloma in cats are nonspecific. The diagnosis of multiple myeloma is confirmed by finding bone marrow infiltration by plasma cells, hyperproteinemia with monoclonal gammopathy on serum protein electrophoresis, and Bence Jones proteins in the urine. Osteolytic lesions are uncommon in cats.

Cats, like dogs, have been treated with a combination of the alkylating agent melphalan (0.5 mg PO once a day for 10 days; then 0.5 mg PO every other day) and prednisone.

Myeloproliferative Disorders

Acute

Myeloproliferative disorders constitute as much as 30 per cent of hemolymphatic neoplasia in cats. The majority (70 to 90 per cent) of affected cats test positive for FeLV infection.

Acute onset of signs is the norm, and cats are depressed, anorectic, and lethargic. The diagnosis of myeloproliferative disease is confirmed by examination of the peripheral blood and bone marrow. The bone marrow contains large numbers of atypical immature blasts and decreased numbers of normal precursor cells. Most cats are neutropenic, thrombocytopenic, and profoundly anemic. Because of the aggressive and rapid clinical course of most myeloproliferative diseases in cats, the majority are classed as acute leukemias. Most of these leukemias affect the white cell series. Chemotherapy for cats with myeloproliferative diseases has not been successful and therefore is not routinely recommended.

Chronic (pp. 2131–2132)

Cats have relatively few chronic myeloproliferative disorders.

Feline Immunodeficiency Virus

Feline immunodeficiency virus (FIV) is a retrovirus (family Retrovirinae), but unlike FeLV, it is a lentivirus, endowing it with more similarities to other immunodeficiency viruses, including those of man and simians. Infections by lentiviruses are characteristically asymptomatic for long periods before clinical signs are evidenced. FIV preferentially infects T-lymphocytes.

FIV, like other lentiviruses, elicits an early antibody response in infected cats. Induction of antibodies does not eliminate viremia, and the presence of FIV antibody is therefore a highly reliable sign of FIV infection. Both IFA and ELISA techniques have been used to detect FIV antibodies, and an ELISA test kit is commercially available. Viral transmission is probably most often accomplished through bite wounds.

Once a cat is infected by FIV, three stages characterize the clinical course. Four to 6 weeks after infection, an initial acute stage is seen, typified by neutropenia and generalized lymphadenopathy in most cats with low-grade fever and malaise in some. A period of relative normalcy, which can last from months to years, follows the acute phase.

The third and final stage is considered the terminal stage. Development of mild to moderate anemia and neutropenia signal the onset of the terminal stage. Cats show various clinical syndromes that can wax and wane from months to years before death. The most frequent (50 per cent) finding is chronic progressive oral infection affecting the gingiva, periodontal tissues, cheeks, or tongue. Chronic upper respiratory tract infections affect about 25 per cent of cats. Chronic bacterial skin infections and otitis externa are noted in about 50 per cent, and chronic diarrhea due to enteritis is present in 10 per cent. Cats develop various infections, some of which are unusual or opportunistic. The role of FIV in the pathogenesis of neoplasia is unknown.

Although approximately 10 to 15 per cent of clinically sick cats with FIV infection are coinfected with FeLV, this finding does not appear to represent an increased risk of FeLV infection in cats infected by FIV.

Treatment of FIV-infected cats is symptomatic and directed at control of secondary/opportunistic infections and providing general supportive care. Spread of FIV is probably best controlled by segregating FIV-positive cats.

CHAPTER 157

Central Nervous System
(pages 2137–2166)

CLASSIFICATION (p. 2137)

Central nervous system (CNS) tumors may be classified as either primary or secondary by their cells of origin. Primary tumors include those arising from neuroepithelial, meningeal, vascular, germ cell, nerve sheath, lymphoid, and malformed tissue. The term *glioma* refers to all tumors originating from cells derived from the medullary (neural) plate. These include astrocytomas, oligodendrogliomas, glioblastomas, choroid plexus papillomas, ependymomas, and medulloblastomas.

Spinal tumors are often additionally classified according to their location relative to the dura as extradural, intradural-extramedullary, and intramedullary.

INCIDENCE (pp. 2137–2138)

Brain tumors occur more commonly in dogs than other domestic species. Astrocytoma or meningioma is the most common brain tumor of dogs. Meningioma is the most common primary brain tumor of cats.

Most spinal tumors in dogs occur extradurally. These tumors generally arise from bone and include osteosarcoma, fibrosarcoma, hemangiosarcoma, multiple myeloma, and chondrosarcoma. Various tumors also metastasize to vertebrae. Lymphosarcoma is the most common soft-tissue extradural spinal tumor in dogs. Nerve sheath tumors (schwannoma, neurofibroma) and meningiomas account for most intradural-extramedullary tumors in dogs. Astrocytoma and ependymoma are the most common primary tumor types, whereas hemangiosarcoma is the most common secondary tumor. Lymphosarcoma is the predominant spinal tumor of cats; most occur extradurally.

The age at onset of brain tumors varies, but most dogs are older than 5 years. CNS tumors occurring in young animals include medulloblastoma, epidermoid cyst, and teratoma. Brachycephalic breeds are predisposed to astrocytomas, oligodendrogliomas, glioblastomas, and pituitary tumors, whereas meningiomas may be more common in dolichocephalic breeds.

Meningiomas are recognized more commonly in male cats.

CLINICAL FINDINGS (pp. 2138–2140)

Clinical signs associated with neoplasia depend on the location, rate of growth, and associated secondary effects of the tumor.

Rapidly growing tumors usually cause acute neurological dysfunction, whereas slowly expanding tumors cause insidious disease.

Several typical clinical patterns are characteristic of localized CNS disease. Signs seen with forebrain lesions include circling (usually ipsilateral to the lesion); head pressing; behavioral abnormalities; sensorium changes; seizures; and contralateral vision, motor, and conscious proprioceptive deficits.

Involvement of the floor of the calvarium can lead to a characteristic set of signs termed *cavernous sinus syndrome*. Dogs with tumors of the cavernous sinuses often have parasympathetic, sympathetic, sensory, and motor deficits in the ipsilateral eye.

When the brain stem is affected, cranial nerve and long tract signs occur. Lesions at the cerebellopontine angle often involve cranial nerves V, VII, and VIII, leading to atrophy of the temporal and masseter muscles and loss of facial and ocular sensation (V); inability to blink and sagging of the lip (VII); and head tilt, nystagmus, and ataxia (VIII). Tumors affecting the middle or inner ear can cause signs of cranial nerves VII and VIII dysfunction and Horner's syndrome. Animals with cerebellar tumors may have dysmetria and intention tremor.

Spinal cord tumors are localized by the presence of upper motor neuron or lower motor neuron signs in the pelvic and thoracic limbs. Some tumors affect specific spinal cord areas; neuroepitheliomas involve the area of the thoracolumbar junction, whereas meningiomas and nerve sheath tumors commonly occur in the cervical area.

Pain is often a feature of extradural and intradural-extramedullary lesions but not usually intramedullary tumors.

Peripheral nerve tumors usually cause monoparesis that may initially be mistaken for lameness arising from a musculoskeletal lesion. Definitive signs of neural involvement, such as knuckling and neurogenic muscle atrophy, suggest the actual cause.

DIAGNOSIS (pp. 2140–2146)

Survey Radiography

Survey radiographs of the skull are of limited value in evaluating intracranial neoplasia. Exceptions are tumors involving the skull; nasal tumors invading the cribriform plate, and either bone atrophy or sclerosis adjacent to tumors such as meningiomas.

Contrast Radiography

Cerebrospinal Fluid Analysis

Tumors are classically said to cause albuminocytological dissociation (elevated protein without a concurrent increase in white blood cells). However, changes reflecting inflammation can be encountered.

Electrophoresis of CSF can help establish a diagnosis of CNS disease. Albumin typically increases because of blood-brain barrier disruption. Globulins also may increase, presumably because of increased endothelial cell permeability. An increase in the globulin fraction alone may be more consistent with a primary inflammatory process.

Brain herniation subsequent to CSF collection is a risk in animals with increased intracranial pressure. Lumbar puncture does not decrease the risk of brain herniation.

Computed Tomography

The features of most brain tumors of dogs and cats have been well characterized. Features are defined before and after intravenous injection of an iodinated contrast medium (meglumine iothalamate, 600 to

900 mg I/kg). Contrast medium is normally excluded by the blood-brain barrier but often leaks through the abnormal or damaged barrier in tumors. Secondary effects, such as vasogenic edema, mass effect, and hydrocephalus, can be detected. Spinal lesions may be defined with CT as well

Magnetic Resonance Imaging

Magnetic resonance imaging (MRI) is superior to CT for viewing intracranial tumors in man. Limited data on the features of individual brain tumors in dogs and cats also have been reported.

Biopsy

Although desirable with all CNS lesions, biopsy often is not practical, particularly when there is a high risk of subsequent neurological impairment. Intracranial biopsy in animals has generally been done by means of craniotomy.

TREATMENT (pp. 2146–2149)

Medical Treatment

Glucocorticoids

Treatment of neoplasia involving the nervous system is directed at both the primary lesion and the secondary effects of the tumor. Glucocorticoids are commonly used to decrease peritumoral edema.

Steroid administration alters the CT appearance of brain tumors and decreases the intensity of contrast enhancement in man and presumably in animals. Concomitant steroid therapy may also decrease the concentration of chemotherapeutic agents within brain tumors. Dogs and cats with rapidly progressive clinical signs receive a fast-acting glucocorticoid (prednisolone sodium succinate [15 to 30 mg/kg IV] or dexamethasone [2 mg/kg IV] repeated BID if needed; not to exceed two doses). Smaller doses are used for maintenance.

Hyperosmolar Agents

If cytotoxic edema is suspected, hyperosmolar agents such as mannitol (1 g/kg at 2 ml/min as a bolus) can be administered. If hemorrhage has occurred subsequent to the tumor, mannitol may leak from the vasculature, drawing water with it. This potentially can increase the overall mass effect and lead to acute neurological deterioration.

Chemotherapy

The efficacy of certain chemotherapeutic regimens in management of brain tumors is limited because the blood-brain barrier impedes passage of some agents.

The nitrosoureas, carmustine and lomustine, are highly lipid soluble and cross the blood-brain barrier.

Intrathecal therapy is used in certain CNS neoplasms in man. The goal is to bypass the blood-brain barrier and achieve higher concentrations of drug in the CSF. Dogs with neural lymphosarcoma have been treated with intrathecal cytosine arabinoside.

Anticonvulsants

Anticonvulsants may be necessary to control seizures secondary to intracranial neoplasia.

Surgery

In our hospital, affected dogs that had surgery had an increase in survival time as compared with dogs receiving only symptomatic care; however, the mean survival time of dogs undergoing surgery was only 2 months.

Irradiation

Dogs treated with irradiation alone or in combination with surgery had improved survival times over dogs treated symptomatically. Clinical improvement may occur within 2 weeks of irradiation; actual reduction in tumor size may not be noted on CT for several months. In some dogs, clinical long-term improvement occurs despite persistence of significant tumor volume on CT examination.

As with any form of therapy, the benefits of irradiation must be balanced against potential complications, such as necrosis of normal brain, damage to extracranial structures including the eyes and skin, and tumor necrosis with associated hemorrhage.

Factors associated with increased survival in a retrospective review of 86 dogs with brain tumors were mode of therapy (surgery and/or cobalt-radiation versus symptomatic), tumor type (meningiomas and primary tumors versus other tumor types and secondary tumors, respectively), CSF results (normal or albuminocytological dissociation versus other changes), degree of initial neurological dysfunction (mild versus moderate/severe), tumor volume (small versus medium/large), and multiplicity of brain involvement (solitary versus multiple).

TUMOR TYPES (pp. 2149–2163)

Meningioma

Meningiomas are tumors of mesenchymal origin. Intracranial, optic nerve, spinal, and paranasal meningiomas occur. Solitary meningiomas are common in both dogs and cats; however, cats may have multiple tumors.

Meningiomas occur more commonly intracranially than in the vertebral canal in both dogs and cats. The frontal lobes, falx cerebri, and cerebellopontine angle are frequent intracranial sites for meningiomas in dogs. Most meningiomas in cats occur over the cerebral convexities.

Clinical Features

Clinical signs encountered with these tumors vary depending on the part of the nervous system involved. A high incidence of seizures has been reported in dogs with paranasal tumors, presumably because of edema and various degrees of hemorrhage and necrosis frequently occurring in adjacent brain. Spinal meningiomas frequently cause hyperesthesia and progressive paresis.

Diagnosis

Hyperostosis of the skull may be seen on survey radiographs in patients with meningiomas, particularly cats. On CT evaluation, the precontrast appearance of meningiomas varies from isodense to either hyperdense or hypodense. Uniform contrast enhancement is noted in most tumors.

Changes usually are not noted on survey radiographs in animals with spinal meningiomas, although thinning of the dorsal lamina may be noted. On myelographic evaluation, either an intradural-extramedullary or intramedullary pattern may be seen.

Treatment

Treatment for meningiomas includes surgical cytoreduction/resection and irradiation, alone or combined. Meningiomas over the cerebral convexities are most easily resected. Tumors on the floor of the skull are difficult to remove without associated clinical deterioration.

Surgical cytoreduction may be beneficial when complete resection is impossible. Irradiation seems to improve survival of dogs with meningiomas. Some dogs with large frontal meningiomas treated by surgery and radiation have survived more than 1 year despite persistent tumor. Results of surgery were poor in dogs that had intumescence lesions, ventrally located tumors, iatrogenic spinal cord injury, or spinal cord invasion.

Astrocytoma

Intracranial astrocytomas afflict both dogs and cats. Astrocytoma is the most common glial tumor in dogs. Middle-aged boxers and Boston terriers are most often affected. Cerebral involvement is common. The spinal cord is also affected relatively often. Astrocytoma is the most common glioma affecting cats but occurs infrequently.

Diagnosis

The CT appearance of astrocytomas varies with the biological behavior of the tumor. MRI may allow clearer tumor delineation. The immunocytochemical marker for human astrocytic tumors is glial fibrillary acidic protein (GFAP) staining. In one study, only 12 of 19 canine tumors classified histologically as astrocytomas were unequivocally positive for GFAP.

Treatment

There have been few reports on treatment of astrocytomas in animals. Benign tumors can be resected. Chemotherapy may also reduce tumor mass or at least delay growth in affected dogs.

Glioblastoma Multiforme

Glioblastoma multiforme is an aggressive tumor that shares many features with high-grade astrocytomas. Necrosis and hemorrhage are especially prominent. This tumor occurs relatively infrequently in dogs and is rare in cats. Tumors classified as glioblastomas are undoubtedly called anaplastic astrocytomas or undifferentiated gliomas.

Although these tumors classically are locally invasive, surprisingly well differentiated masses can be seen. Middle-aged and older brachycephalic dogs are predisposed; most tumors affect the cerebrum or thalamus. Multiple lesions may be noted. Aggressive radiation and chemotherapy may be required for treatment of this tumor.

Ependymoma

Ependymomas arise from ependymal cells. They are more common in the spinal cord in dogs but can also arise intracranially. Ependymomas are rare in both dogs and cats. The CT appearance in the few reported canine cases has been variable. Treatment of affected animals has not been described.

Choroid Plexus Tumors

Choroid plexus tumors are derived from epithelial cells of the choroid plexus. Choroid plexus tumors occur relatively frequently in dogs but rarely in cats. Any part of the ventricular system can be involved; however, the fourth ventricle is affected most frequently.

Clinical Features

Middle-aged and older dogs are generally affected, but tumors can occur in young dogs. Brachycephalic dogs are not predisposed. Signs of vestibular disease are frequently noted.

Diagnosis

Tumors are generally well delineated on CT evaluation. All five choroid plexus tumors in one report were hyperdense on precontrast scans. Choroid plexus tumors usually show marked contrast enhancement and well-defined tumor margins with both CT and MRI. Hydrocephalus is commonly noted when the third ventricle is involved. Large tumors in the fourth ventricle also may obstruct CSF outflow, leading to hydrocephalus.

Treatment

We have unsuccessfully attempted to resect two tumors. Given the epithelial origin of this tumor, radiation could be beneficial.

Oligodendroglioma (pp. 2155–2156)

Pituitary Gland Tumors

Pituitary gland tumors occur relatively frequently in dogs but are rare in cats. Micro- and macroadenomas and adenocarcinomas occur. Because most canine pituitary gland tumors involve the pars distalis of the adenohypophysis, dorsal growth is favored and diencephalic encroachment and hypothalamic dysfunction result.

Clinical Features

The mean time from diagnosis of pituitary-dependent hyperadrenocorticism to occurrence of neurological signs in eight dogs in one study was 12.8 months. Affected dogs generally deteriorated rapidly once neurological signs were observed. Systemic signs of hyperadrenocorticism may also occur.

Diagnosis

On noncontrast CT scans, most pituitary gland tumors are isodense but some are hyperdense. Tumors usually enhance uniformly.

Hyperadrenocorticism may result from excess adrenocorticotropic hormone (ACTH) production. In five of eight cases of large pituitary tumors in dogs, high-dose dexamethasone did not decrease serum cortisol concentrations to a degree necessary to diagnose pituitary-dependent hyperadrenocorticism. The pituitary origin of these tumors was confirmed by evaluating ACTH levels.

Treatment

Trans-sphenoidal surgical approaches to the pituitary gland have been described in dogs. Irradiation is the most effective treatment for large pituitary gland tumors. The mean and median survival time after radiation in one study of six affected dogs was 740 and 743 days, respectively. Secretion of ACTH by the tumor may not decrease for 6 to 12 months, so medication to normalize cortisol levels may be necessary initially.

Lymphosarcoma

Lymphosarcoma affects the nervous system in both dogs and cats. Both primary and secondary involvement occur. Lymphosarcoma in cats most commonly affects the epidural space of the vertebral canal. Most tumors are solitary, but multiple sites may be involved. Many cats with renal lymphosarcoma have CNS involvement.

Clinical Features

Lymphosarcoma typically causes progressive neurological dysfunction. Most dogs with neural lymphosarcoma have additional systemic involvement. Only 11 of 24 cats with spinal lymphosarcoma had extraneural organ involvement.

Diagnosis

Leukemia may be evident on evaluation of peripheral blood in both dogs and cats. Cats without leukemia may still have bone marrow involvement, so examination of an aspirate is indicated. Most affected cats are positive for feline leukemia virus. Neoplastic cells can be seen on CSF evaluation. Brain lesions are identified with CT. Biopsy may be necessary for diagnosis.

Treatment

Treatment of lymphosarcoma may include surgery, systemic and intrathecal chemotherapy, radiation, or combinations of these. Rapid reduction of tumor mass occurs within hours of delivering a single large dose of radiation (500 to 1,000 cGy) in extraneural lymphosarcoma in cats. Laminectomy or craniotomy may be necessary to confirm the diagnosis before chemotherapy and radiation.

Various chemotherapeutic protocols have been used to treat animals with lymphosarcoma. Cytosine arabinoside has been incorporated into some lymphosarcoma protocols to decrease the incidence of CNS metastasis.

Nerve Sheath Tumors

The term *nerve sheath tumor* refers collectively to schwannoma, neurofibroma, neurilemmoma, neurinoma, and neurofibrosarcoma. The Schwann cell is the predominant cell of origin for both neurofibroma and schwannoma. These tumors occur relatively commonly in dogs but are rare in cats. Cervical nerve roots are usually affected in dogs.

Clinical Features

Clinical signs vary with the nerve roots affected but often include thoracic limb muscle atrophy, lameness, ipsilateral Horner's syndrome, hyperesthesia, and licking or chewing at the foot or carpus. Tumors usually originate in the dorsal nerve root, causing pain initially and spinal cord compression later. An axillary mass can be palpated in some animals.

Diagnosis

Diagnosis of peripheral tumors may be difficult unless a palpable mass is present. Electromyographic evidence of denervation aids in defining the underlying neural nature of the lesion. Regardless of whether clinical signs of spinal cord involvement are present, myelography should always be performed to identify potential intradural tumor extension. CT allows more precise characterization of lesions.

Treatment

Treatment has centered on surgical resection or debulking of nerve root tumors. Both peripheral and spinal components must be removed. Surgical resection usually cannot be achieved without causing severe denervation; amputation is often necessary. Limited experience with postoperative radiation has not been promising.

CHAPTER 158

Eye and Orbit (pages 2166–2177)

LID TUMORS (pp. 2166–2168)

Tumors of the eyelids may occur at any age but are frequently encountered in middle-aged and older dogs (8 to 9 years).

Canine Cutaneous Histiocytoma

Cutaneous histiocytoma is unique to canine skin. Tumor cells arise from the monocyte-macrophage cells of the skin. The tumor is commonly noted in dogs younger than 2 years. Cutaneous histiocytoma especially involves the skin of the head.

The tumors are pink, fleshy, circular, epilated lesions that may involve the lids. An immune response to the lesions may occur, and some lesions may spontaneously regress or completely disappear.

Cryosurgery can be performed on small lesions. On larger lesions, especially those involving the lid margin, a split-thickness lid resection can be performed, the skin and associated tumor removed, and the lid skin closed from side to side. Alternatively, a vertical or horizontal pedicle graft can be created if the lesion involves more than one-fourth of the lid margin. Histiocytomas do not recur if completely removed.

Papillomas (Verrucas, Warts)

Papillomas are benign epithelial tumors that are common in dogs. Cutaneous papillomas involving the lids are most commonly encountered in dogs older than 8 years. The tumors do not invade the underlying dermis. Papillomas may be multiple on one lid. Because these tumors involve only the epidermis, these growths can be treated by cryosurgery or split-thickness resection of the skin tumor from the lid. Cutting the pedunculated stalk of a papilloma may remove the mass of the tumor, but the small remaining stalk may regrow.

Basal Cell Tumors (Carcinoma, Epithelioma)

Basal cell tumors account for 10 to 12 per cent of canine skin tumors, with dogs in the 7- to 9-year-old group having the highest incidence. The incidence of basal cell tumors may be higher in cats than in dogs.

Size varies from 0.5 to 10 cm, and the skin is elevated, firm, erythematous, and frequently ulcerated. They frequently extend into the dermis.

Basal cell tumors are benign and if entirely removed do not recur. If a tumor involves the lid margin and can be palpated over the dermis as well as epidermis, full-thickness wedge resection is indicated. Cryotherapy may be used.

Squamous Cell Carcinoma

Squamous cell carcinoma is the most malignant of the epithelial tumors. The tumor is more frequently found in animals with lightly pigmented skin. A lesion starts as an epitheliomatous plaque progressing through stages of carcinoma *in situ* and invasive carcinoma. Diagnosis can usually be based on biopsy of the lesion and histological examination.

ADNEXAL TUMORS (pp. 2168–2170)

Tumors of the sebaceous glands of the lids arise from the tarsal (meibomian) glands of the lids and are common in older dogs. Tarsal gland adenomas involve the lid margin. These tumors are most easily removed when they are small. Full-thickness wedge resection of the lid is performed.

Melanomas

Melanomas involve the skin of older dogs, with an average age of 9 to 10 years. The biological behavior of melanomas in dogs varies depending on their location. Tumors arising at mucocutaneous junctions are malignant, whereas those arising in the skin are usually benign. An exception is the interdigital area, in which the tumors are usually very malignant.

Benign dermal melanomas are well-circumscribed, elevated masses covered by thin, hairless skin. They usually measure 0.5 to 2.0 cm. Malignant melanomas are usually larger than benign dermal melanomas. Most melanomas of the lids of dogs are either benign junctional or benign dermal.

Mast Cell Tumors

Mast cell tumors in dogs represent 7 to 21 per cent of all skin tumors and 11 to 27 per cent of all malignant skin tumors. Lid tumors are elevated, nodular, and firm. Hair is lost from the skin, and the tumors frequently ulcerate on the surface. Diagnosis of mast cell tumor can be made on impression smears or fine-needle aspirates of the tumor.

Treatment of lid tumors is by full-thickness wedge resection. Additional therapy may involve chemotherapy, radiation therapy, immunotherapy, or any combination of these. When a mastocytoma is surgically removed, a wide surgical margin of at least 2 cm is made. Thus, it is much easier to remove lid tumors cosmetically when they are small. Cryosurgery can be used for small mast cell tumors.

TUMORS OF THE CONJUNCTIVA, THIRD EYELID, AND CORNEA (pp. 2170–2171)

Tumors of the conjunctiva may involve the third eyelid or the bulbar or palpebral conjunctiva. Conjunctival papillomas usually occur on the lid margins or the third eyelid. They may be pigmented and tend to be pedunculated.

Carcinoma of the conjunctiva often develops at the perilimbal area or on the third eyelid. The earliest lesion is a leukoplakia or slightly raised fleshy mass. Carcinomas of the conjunctiva spread through the epithelial basement membrane and into the stroma or across the limbus and into the cornea. Dermoids are congenital tumors of the cornea and conjunctiva.

INTRAOCULAR TUMORS (pp. 2171–2173)

A number of clinically significant signs may suggest the development of an intraocular tumor:

1. The iris may be altered in color, shape, thickness, or mobility.
2. Keratitis and corneal edema may be associated with neoplastic growth in the iris and invasion of the anterior chamber.
3. Uveitis commonly accompanies lymphosarcomatous infiltration of the anterior uveal tract.
4. Secondary glaucoma may develop.
5. Conjunctival and deep scleral vascularization may be noted over the area of the tumor cell infiltration.

Intraocular bleeding, lens luxation, and retinal detachments may be observed. Intraocular tumors can be classified as primary or secondary. The most common primary intraocular tumor is melanoma, which occurs in two forms, localized and diffuse.

Epibulbar Melanomas

Black masses that appear in the sclera, usually near or at the limbus, may be an epibulbar melanoma arising in the scleral or episcleral tissues and not invading the sclera to involve deeper intraocular tissues. Epibulbar masses may, however, be extensions of intraocular melanomas arising from the ciliary body or iris and growing into the sclera and episcleral tissue.

Based on a limited study of dogs, epibulbar melanomas may be more aggressive in their growth patterns in young dogs. In older dogs (7 to 11 years), the epibulbar melanomas remained in the sclera and episcleral tissue. If epibulbar melanomas do not invade and do not grow into the cornea or through the sclera, surgical removal is not recommended. If the tumors begin to grow, either complete enucleation, scleral wall resection with a scleral transplant, or cryotherapy is performed.

True melanomas of the posterior choroid are rare in domestic animals. Melanomas usually arise from the pigmented epithelial cells of the ciliary processes, ciliary body, or posterior iridal surface. In dogs, melanomas that involve only portions of the iris and small areas of the ciliary body may be treated by surgical sector iridectomy.

More extensive intraocular melanoma in dogs presents a surgical dilemma. Evidence suggests that intraocular melanomas in dogs grow within the globe but rarely metastasize to regional lymph nodes and lungs. Intraocular melanomas in dogs may grow through the scleral wall or cribriform plate and enter the orbit.

Canine choroidal melanomas are distinct entities compared with anterior uveal melanomas. Posterior choroidal melanoma in small animals is much more rarely encountered than anterior uveal melanoma.

Diffuse Feline Melanomas

In cats, the melanoma is more diffuse, involves the iris stroma, and results in infiltration of the anterior drainage angle with development of secondary glaucoma. Neoplastic cells may be seen in the anterior chamber as well as on the anterior lens capsule. Their metastatic potential is controversial. The treatment of choice is enucleation.

TUMORS OF NONPIGMENTED EPITHELIAL CELLS
(pp. 2173–2175)

The second most frequently observed intraocular tumors are growths arising from the nonpigmented epithelium of the ciliary body and ciliary processes. These are neuroepithelial tumors that are derived from mature neuroepithelium or primitive medullary epithelium. Tumors arising from mature neuroepithelium include adenomas and adenocarcinomas. Tumors arising from more primitive neuroepithelial tissue include medulloepitheliomas and teratoid medulloepitheliomas.

Neuroepithelial Tumors

Neuroepithelial tumors usually are not recognized until they become large enough to be seen through the pupil. More of the tumor mass can be seen if the pupil is dilated. Adenocarcinomas of the ciliary body arising from the nonpigmented epithelium grow within the eye and usually do not spread from the eye. Enlarging tumors frequently grow between the iris and the lens, pushing the lens into a posteriorly subluxated position. Increasing tumor size may partially obliterate the anterior chamber, leading to secondary glaucoma and necessitating enucleation. Tumors of the nonpigmented epithelium of the ciliary body are removed by iridocyclectomy or enucleation.

Secondary Intraocular Tumors

The most common secondary intraocular tumor is lymphosarcoma. Immature lymphocytes commonly infiltrate the third eyelid and anterior uveal tract; infiltration may result in a greatly thickened iris and an irregular, usually miotic pupil. Thickening of the iris with infiltration of immature lymphocytes can lead to narrowing of the anterior drainage angle and secondary glaucoma.

Retinal hemorrhages and vitreal bleeding may also be observed. The ocular manifestations of lymphosarcoma in cats are often bilateral, although one eye may show more advanced changes.

Metastatic neoplasms from distant sites most commonly involve the anterior uveal tract. The most frequent tumor type is secondary adenocarcinoma, with metastasis most frequently from the kidney, thyroid, mammary gland, or nasal cavity.

Cats may be afflicted with a unique form of intraocular sarcoma that may develop secondary to chronic uveitis or ocular trauma. These tumors are usually spindle cell sarcomas with pluripotential cells. Tumor tissue may contain osteoid material. These tumors are locally aggressive and frequently do metastasize to adjacent soft tissue and regional lymph nodes. Early enucleation of globes suspected of having ocular sarcoma formation is indicated after careful evaluation for metastatic lesions.

ORBITAL TUMORS (pp. 2175–2176)

Orbital tumors in animals are uncommon.

Tumors arising primarily from the orbit are sarcomas and meningiomas. Sarcomas spread diffusely, metastasize rapidly to regional lymph nodes and lungs, and often destroy surrounding bone, producing lytic lesions visible on radiographs.

Primary meningiomas originate from intraorbital optic nerve sheath, whereas secondary meningiomas arise within the cranium and extend into the orbit directly through bone or by extension through the optic foramen along sheaths of the optic nerve. Meningiomas are locally invasive but usually do not metastasize.

Secondary orbital neoplasms usually include nasal carcinoma, anaplastic sarcoma, fibrosarcoma, squamous cell carcinoma, chondrosarcoma, rhabdomyosarcoma, osteosarcoma, hemangiosarcoma, chondroma, liposarcoma, and malignant melanoma.

Orbital and retro-orbital tumors usually have the following clinical signs:

1. Slowly progressive exophthalmos.
2. Secondary exposure keratitis.
3. Loss of vision; dilated, unresponsive pupil.
4. Optic nerve edema, atrophy, retinal detachment.
5. Impaired mobility of the globe.
6. Protrusion of the third eyelid.

Orbital tumor can be diagnosed via:

1. Contrast orbital venography.
2. Ultrasonography.
3. Radiography.
4. Retro-orbital aspiration.
5. Surgical exploration of the orbit.

Treatment of orbital neoplasms depends on the extent of the lesion, whether metastasis is present, and the tumor type.

CHAPTER 159

Reproductive Systems
(pages 2177–2200)

The World Health Organization (WHO) clinical staging of animal tumors of the reproductive tract is based on character of the primary tumor (T), lymph nodes (N), and presence of distant metastasis (M)

Female (pp. 2178–2192)

OVARIAN NEOPLASIA

Incidence

The incidence of spontaneously occurring ovarian neoplasia is low. In dogs, ovarian tumors occur with equal frequency in the right and left ovaries and occasionally in both. Risk increases with age.

Ovarian tumors may arise from epithelial, gonadal-stromal, or germ cell tissue in the ovary; primary mesodermal tumors or metastatic tumors also occur. Tumors of epithelial cell origin are most common in bitches, and of gonadal-stromal origin in queens. The granulosa cell tumor is the single most common ovarian tumor of both species.

Granulosa cell tumors may produce estrogen, progesterone, or both, leading to paraneoplastic syndromes of persistent estrus, estrogen-induced pancytopenia, cystic endometrial hyperplasia, or pyometra. Persistent estrus occurs in queens with dysgerminomas or granulosa cell tumors.

Diagnosis

Ovarian tumors may be diagnosed at ovariohysterectomy if small and benign or may be associated with signs of a palpable and sometimes painful abdominal mass, persistent estrus, aplastic anemia, or pyometra. If functional neoplasia is suspected, vaginal cytological study to look for cornification (an indicator of estrogen secretion) and serum progesterone measurement for values exceeding 2 ng/ml are indicated. Ovarian tumors are staged clinically. Regional lymph nodes are the sublumbar nodes.

Adenoma/Cystadenoma

Ovarian adenomas are some of the most common primary ovarian tumors in bitches. Ovarian epithelial proliferation, neoplasia, and metastasis can be induced by prolonged estrogen administration in dogs, but the role of endogenous estrogen in spontaneously occurring tumors is unknown. Diagnosis is by histopathological examination after excision.

Adenocarcinoma/Cystadenocarcinoma

Ovarian adenocarcinoma or cystadenocarcinoma usually occurs in bitches older than 9 years. Metastases to omentum, sublumbar lymph nodes, liver, and lungs are described in approximately half the cases.

Granulosa Cell Tumor

The granulosa cell tumor, which arises from ovarian sex cords, is the most common primary ovarian tumor in dogs and cats. Common clinical signs include abdominal distension and the presence of a palpable abdominal mass. Functional tumors may produce estrogens, progesterone, or both. Metastases occurred in about 20 per cent of affected dogs and in 10 of 17 affected cats.

Sertoli Cell Tumor

Ovarian tumors arising from sex cord stroma demonstrate a histological pattern similar to that of Sertoli cell tumors of the testes. Eighteen were described among 155 canine ovarian neoplasms, and one was found in a cat. In nine bitches in which the uterus was examined histologically, cystic endometrial hyperplasia was present.

Dysgerminoma

Dysgerminomas are malignant tumors arising from undifferentiated germ cells of the ovary; they are comparable to seminomas in males. They constitute about 8 per cent of canine and almost 20 per cent of feline ovarian tumors. Twenty to 30 per cent metastasize to adjacent peritoneum, adrenals, kidneys, mesenteric lymph nodes, pancreas, liver, or mediastinal nodes.

Teratoma (Dermoid Cyst)

Teratomas are germ cell tumors that show somatic differentiation beyond the primordial germ cell stage into masses with three germ layers (ectoderm, mesoderm, entoderm). They have been called *dermoid cysts* because the masses typically include cysts lined by hair and keratinized squamous epithelium; they often contain sebaceous fluid, sweat glands, cartilage, fat, muscle fiber, bone, nervous tissue, connective tissue, teeth, and glandular epithelium.

Treatment and Prognosis

Ovariohysterectomy is the treatment of choice because some ovarian tumors are bilateral, tumor extension to the uterus can occur, and cystic endometrial hyperplasia leading to pyometra is common in aging females in which primary ovarian tumors occur. The prognosis is favorable with benign tumors without aplastic anemia but poor with metastasis or bone marrow suppression.

Chemotherapy of dogs with metastatic adenocarcinomas or granulosa cell tumors has been reported. Cyclophosphamide (2.2 mg/kg PO once daily while the white blood cell count exceeds 2,000/cm^3) has been recommended for metastatic ovarian tumors.

UTERINE TUBE (OVIDUCT) NEOPLASIA (pp. 2181–2182)

Tumors of this organ are rare (2 in a survey of 4,187 canine neoplasms). Tumors of the uterine tube have not been reported in cats.

UTERINE NEOPLASIA (p. 2182)
Incidence

Uterine tumors occur in dogs and cats from 5 to 12 years of age but are relatively uncommon. Uterine tumor types in companion animals include those of epithelial (adenoma, adenocarcinoma) and mesenchymal (fibroma, fibrosarcoma, leiomyoma, leiomyosarcoma, lipoma, and lymphosarcoma) origin. The most common of these in bitches is leiomyoma. Endometrial adenocarcinoma is the most common feline uterine tumor. Endometrial adenocarcinoma in cats may metastasize to the peritoneum, mesentery, ovaries, regional lymph nodes, adrenal glands, liver, diaphragm, lungs, brain, and eyes.

Diagnosis

Because uterine tumors are rare and often benign, diagnosis is generally made at ovariohysterectomy or necropsy. Some uterine masses are detected by abdominal palpation or radiographic/ultrasonographic examination of the uterus in patients suspected of having pyometra.

Treatment and Prognosis

Ovariohysterectomy with routine aftercare is the treatment of choice for canine and feline patients with primary uterine neoplasia, following abdominal and thoracic radiography to seek evidence of metastatic disease. Chemotherapy may be considered after surgery for patients with metastasis and should be chosen on the basis of tumor type. The prognosis is excellent for patients with leiomyomas or other benign tumors.

VAGINAL NEOPLASIA (pp. 2183–2185)
Incidence

Vaginal and vestibular tumors are the most common female reproductive neoplasms in bitches, excluding those of the mammary gland. No feline vaginal tumors were reported in three studies comprising 1,115 tumors from all sites, although single cases of vaginal neoplasia have been reported. Most canine vaginal tumors are leiomyomas and transmissible venereal tumors.

Age of animals with vaginal tumors ranges from 2 to 18 years and depends on tumor type. Transmissible venereal tumors occur more in younger bitches than other vaginal tumor types. Vaginal tumors may occur in sexually intact and spayed bitches. There is no evidence that ovariohysterectomy prevents development of malignant vaginal neoplasia or improves prognosis. Metastases from vaginal tumors are rare, because most are benign. Leiomyosarcomas spread to the regional lymph nodes, spleen, lungs, and spinal cord.

Diagnosis

Vaginal tumors range in diameter from 2 to 20 cm in bitches and 2 to 8 cm in queens. Clinical signs of vaginal neoplasia include bulging of the perineum, prolapse of tissue from the vulva, dysuria, pollakiuria, tenesmus, and obstruction to copulation in intact females. If the tumor becomes irritated, infected, or necrotic, it may be associated with a sanguineous or purulent vaginal discharge.

Digital palpation of the vestibule and vagina and vaginal cytological study are performed in patients with any of these signs. Contrast vaginography may help to determine the site of origin and extent of the mass. Rectal palpation may permit localization and characterization of vaginal masses in toy-breed bitches and queens when vaginal palpation is not possible. Primary vaginal tumors are tentatively distinguished from vaginal prolapses based on the age of the bitch, the origin of the mass, and time of occurrence of the mass in relation to the estrous cycle.

Leiomyoma

Vaginal and vestibular leiomyomas are slow growing and are associated with tenesmus and dysuria.

Leiomyosarcoma

Vaginal and vestibular leiomyosarcomas occur in bitches older than 9 years and have not been described in cats. These tumors may recur after excision and metastasize to the regional lymph nodes, lungs, and cervical spinal cord.

Transmissible Venereal Tumor

Transmissible venereal tumors are transplantable tumors of which the tumor transmission, growth, and metastasis depend on the immunological status of the animal to which it is transplanted.

Treatment and Prognosis

Because most vaginal neoplasms are benign, surgical excision is the treatment of choice, with a guarded to favorable prognosis. Most vaginal tumors in bitches are round, well circumscribed, and easy to remove surgically via an episiotomy. Complete vulvovaginectomy and perineal urethrostomy have been described in three dogs with malignant, infiltrative vaginal neoplasia.

Transmissible venereal tumors may regress spontaneously in patients with normal immune systems. They respond well to surgical excision, chemotherapy, and orthovoltage radiotherapy.

Wide surgical excision of the vaginal tumor via episiotomy is usually recommended when the tumor is a single one that is easily accessible. Surgical excision of a large primary tumor may be used with later chemotherapy or radiotherapy with good success.

Chemotherapy with vincristine (0.025 mg/kg IV, not to exceed 1 mg), administered once weekly after a hemogram, is effective. Of 41 dogs of both sexes with primary or recurrent transmissible venereal tumor, 39 experienced complete tumor regression after 2 to 7 weeks of vincristine therapy.

MAMMARY NEOPLASIA (pp. 2185–2190)
Incidence

Dogs. The mammary glands are the most common site of neoplasia in female dogs; tumors of these glands accounted for 42 per cent of 2,917 tumors in all sites and 82 per cent of 1,086 tumors of the female reproductive organs. Mammary neoplasia is rare in bitches younger than 2 years; its frequency increases dramatically after 6 years and peaks at 10 to 11 years, thereafter declining.

Intact bitches have a three- to sevenfold greater risk of developing mammary cancer than neutered females. Ovariectomy has a detectable sparing effect on the incidence of mammary tumors when it is performed before the first estrus (0.5 per cent), after one but before the second estrus (8 per cent), or after two but less than four estrous cycles (26 per cent). After 2.5 years of age or four estrous cycles, ovariectomy has a slight or no sparing effect. Mammary tumors may occur in any of the five pairs of mammary glands and are most common.

Cats. Mammary tumors are the third most common neoplasm in cats, following skin and lymphoid tumors, and may account for up to 76 per cent of reproductive tumors. Age incidence increases most dramatically after 6 years and peaks at 10 to 11 years in intact females, thereafter declining.

Incidence of Tumor Type and Patterns of Metastasis

Dogs. About half of all canine mammary tumors are benign; most benign tumors are fibroadenomas, and most malignant tumors are adenocarcinomas. Regional lymph nodes for the three cranial pairs of mammary glands are the axillary nodes, and for the two caudal pairs the superficial inguinal nodes.

Cats. Nearly 90 per cent of feline mammary tumors are malignant, and most are adenocarcinomas. Metastases are present in more than 90 per cent of cats with malignant mammary tumors and may occur in the lungs (84 per cent), regional lymph nodes (83 per cent), pleura, liver, spleen, omental fat, pancreas, adrenals, kidneys, ovaries, heart, brain, and vertebral column.

Influence of Reproductive Hormones on Occurrence

Receptor assays of mammary tumor tissue in humans, dogs, and cats have demonstrated that some tumor cytosols are rich in estrogen and progesterone receptors.

Of canine mammary adenocarcinomas, 50 to 53 per cent are estrogen receptor rich, and 44 per cent are rich in both estrogen receptors and progesterone receptors. In 87 malignant canine mammary tumors, survival of patients with receptor-rich tumors was significantly greater than for those with receptor-poor tumors.

Diagnosis

Mammary tumors in both dogs and cats are firm, well-demarcated nodules that vary in diameter from several millimeters to 10 to 20 cm.

Large tumors may be traumatized and ulcerated. Differential diagnosis in cats includes nodular mammary hypertrophy.

Cytological examination of fine-needle aspiration biopsy samples are interpreted with caution. In one study, false-positive diagnoses were made in 3 and 0 per cent of the cases by two cytologists, respectively, and false-negative diagnoses were made in 22 and 36 per cent; the positive predictive value of the procedure thus was 90 to 100 per cent, and the negative predictive value was 59 to 75 per cent.

Diagnostic tests for evidence of metastasis include thoracic and abdominal radiographs and ultrasonography of the abdomen. Radionuclide imaging of the skeletal system of dogs with mammary neoplasia has also been advocated. Definitive diagnosis is based on histopathological examination of an excision biopsy specimen. In general, the more highly differentiated tumors have a more favorable prognosis.

Mammary tumors in dogs and cats are staged according to the behavior of the primary tumor (T), regional lymph node involvement (N), and the presence of distant metastasis (M), if any.

Treatment and Prognosis

Surgical Excision

Surgical excision of all canine and feline mammary tumors is recommended for patients undergoing treatment for this tumor, with the possible exception of dogs with inflammatory mammary carcinoma. Six categories of surgical excision of canine mammary tumors have been reported:

1. Removal of the tumor alone (lumpectomy)
2. Removal of the affected gland only (simple mastectomy)
3. Removal of the affected and ipsilateral glands (regional mastectomy)
4. Removal of the affected gland, the regional lymph nodes, and all intervening glands and lymphatics (*en bloc* dissection)
5. Removal of all glands on the affected side (unilateral mastectomy)
6. Bilateral mastectomy (simultaneous or staged)

The type of surgery does not influence survival time or cancer-free survival time. Lumpectomy or simple mastectomy of affected glands, with excision of regional lymph nodes for staging, may be the surgical treatment of choice. Concurrent ovariectomy or ovariohysterectomy of an affected intact bitch should be considered. If performed at the same time, ovariectomy precedes mastectomy to avoid seeding the abdomen with exfoliated tumor cells.

En bloc dissection or unilateral mastectomy has been advocated for surgical management of feline malignant mammary neoplasia, in which frequent lymphatic penetration occurs. Ovariectomy is not indicated for intact affected patients of this species, because most feline tumors are receptor poor.

Chemotherapy

Antiestrogen treatment (tamoxifen citrate [Nolvadex], 10 to 20 mg PO BID) may be indicated for receptor-rich mammary adenocarcinomas after ovariectomy. A chemotherapeutic protocol using doxorubicin (30 mg/m^2 IV on day 1) and cyclophosphamide (100 mg/m^2 on days 3 through 6) repeated at 21-day intervals until remission or death has been advocated for dogs, without documentation of its effectiveness.

Radiation Therapy

Radiation therapy is suggested as the treatment of choice for inflammatory mammary carcinoma in dogs, based on results of this treatment in women.

Prognosis

Prognosis for cats and dogs with mammary cancer is influenced by tumor size, histological type of the tumor, mode of growth, and clinical stage. Inflammatory mammary carcinomas have an extremely poor prognosis, with estimated survival times of less than a few months.

In cats, average survival time after mammary tumor detection was reported as 12.3 months in 56 cats, and 1-year survival rates were significantly higher in cats with well-differentiated tumors.

For both dogs and cats, lymphatic infiltration (with peripheral lymphedema or satellite nodules between the tumor and regional nodes), metastatic lesions, infiltration of the body wall, rapid tumor growth, or recurrence augurs a poor prognosis.

Male (pages 2193–2200)

TESTICULAR NEOPLASIA (pp. 2193–2195)

Incidence

Testicular neoplasia is the second most common tumor of male dogs (following skin) and is more common than in any other domestic mammal or man.

The three major tumors of the canine testicle are the Sertoli cell tumor, seminoma, and interstitial cell tumor, which occur with approximately equal frequency. Testicular tumors cause noticeable testicular enlargement, have a low incidence of metastasis, and are cured by castration. More than one testicular tumor of the same or different type per dog or per testis is fairly common. Cryptorchidism increases the risk of testicular neoplasia in dogs by as much as 13.6 times; risk factors reported by tumor type are 23 times for Sertoli cell tumors, 16 times for seminomas, and 1.6 times for interstitial cell tumors. Tumors occur in dogs from 2 to 17 years old. Risk increases for all intact male dogs until 10 to 14 years of age and then declines. Miniature schnauzers have a syndrome of cryptorchidism, Sertoli cell tumor in the abdominal testis, and persistence of the müllerian duct in individuals that are phenotypically and chromosomally male. Testicular tumors are rare in cats.

Diagnosis

Testicular neoplasia in dogs or cats is diagnosed by palpation of a testicular mass in a scrotal or ectopic testis, followed by excision biopsy and histopathological evaluation. Interstitial cell tumors are the smallest of the canine testicular tumors and may be detected by testicular ultrasonography in a patient with abnormal testicular texture on palpation or abnormal semen quality.

Other abnormalities that are androgen dependent and associated with testicular neoplasia in older male dogs include prostatic disease, perineal hernia, perianal gland adenoma, and perianal gland adenocarcinoma. These concurrent disorders also afflict older intact male dogs without testicular neoplasia. Torsion of a neoplastic scrotal or cryptorchid testis occurs occasionally.

Metastasis is uncommon in canine testicular neoplasia. Clinical staging of canine testicular tumors is by behavior of the primary tumor (T), regional lymph node involvement (N), and the presence of metastasis (M). Regional lymph nodes are the sublumbar and inguinal nodes.

Sertoli Cell Tumors

Sertoli cell tumors are the largest of the three types, are most likely to occur in ectopic testes, and are most likely to secrete estrogens and be associated with paraneoplastic syndromes. Feminizing signs in dogs with Sertoli cell tumors include gynecomastia with or without mammary gland secretion, a pendulous prepuce, attraction of males, and loss of libido. Bilaterally symmetrical alopecia in these dogs has been attributed to estrogen-induced atrophy of hair follicles and sebaceous glands.

Sertoli cell tumors in cats may be unilateral or bilateral and may cause gross gonadal enlargement; they are not associated with paraneoplastic syndromes.

Seminoma

Paraneoplastic syndromes attributable to hormone secretion by seminomas are less common than with Sertoli cell tumors, but a few cases of feminization, alopecia, or blood dyscrasia have been described. Metastases of seminomas were present in 8 of 204 (4 per cent) dogs. Seminoma has not been reported in cats.

Interstitial Cell Tumor

Canine interstitial cell tumors are smaller than other canine testicular tumors. A few dogs with interstitial cell tumors have shown feminization, alopecia, or blood dyscrasia, which are most characteristic of dogs with Sertoli cell tumors. Metastasis is rare in interstitial cell tumors. Interstitial cell tumors have not been reported in cats.

Treatment and Prognosis

Treatment of canine and feline testicular neoplasia is bilateral castration. The tumor regressed in all four dogs, and the dogs survived for 6 to 57 months. The prognosis for patients with testicular neoplasia is favorable in the absence of metastasis and blood dyscrasia. Signs of feminization disappear 2 to 6 weeks after castration unless metastases are present. Pancytopenia at surgery or as late as 2 months afterward is associated with a poor to grave prognosis.

PROSTATIC NEOPLASIA (pp. 2195–2197)

Prostatic neoplasia occurs more often in dogs than in other domestic species. Most canine prostatic tumors are adenocarcinomas. Prostatic adenocarcinoma generally is diagnosed in older dogs. This tumor occurs in both neutered and intact males. There is no evidence that the canine tumor is hormonally dependent.

Prostatic adenocarcinoma has been reported in older cats (10 to 17 years).

Diagnosis

The major clinical signs in dogs with prostatic neoplasia are emaciation, tenesmus, dysuria, and urethral bleeding/hematuria. On physical examination, the prostate usually is palpably enlarged and firm and may be asymmetrical, cystic, or irregularly nodular; enlarged sublumbar lymph nodes may be palpable per rectum.

Survey radiography generally reveals prostate enlargement. Prostatic ultrasonography of ten dogs with prostatic adenocarcinoma revealed increased echogenicity in six, decreased echogenicity in two, and a mixed, mottled appearance in one. Thoracic metastases appear as diffuse structured or nonstructured interstitial lung disease.

Diagnostic methods to evaluate dogs with suspected prostatic adenocarcinoma include cytological examination of ejaculate, prostatic massage, and biopsy by urethral brush, aspiration, punch, incision, or excision of the prostate gland. An iliac lymph node is aspirated at biopsy if possible. Metastatic lesions are common with canine prostatic adenocarcinoma.

Treatment and Prognosis

The only treatments available for prostate neoplasia in dogs are surgical excision and radiotherapy during surgery. Neither procedure is associated with a favorable prognosis, because metastasis usually has occurred before diagnosis. Prostatectomy is associated with a high incidence of urinary incontinence. Results suggest that intraoperative radiotherapy may effectively treat some patients without metastasis.

NEOPLASIA OF THE PENIS AND PREPUCE (pp. 2197–2198)

Tumors of the canine penis and prepuce include epithelial tumors (papilloma, squamous cell carcinoma), fibropapillomas (fibroma), transmissible venereal tumor, and other mesenchymal tumors (fibrosarcoma, lymphosarcoma, hemangiosarcoma, mast cell sarcoma), including a chondrosarcoma of the os penis. The incidence of penile neoplasia is not influenced by neutering, except for decreased risk of acquiring transmissible venereal tumor venereally after castration. Tumors of the penis and prepuce have not been reported in cats.

Diagnosis

Patients with penile or preputial neoplasia may be presented for a preputial mass, preputial hemorrhage, lack of libido, phimosis, or stranguria secondary to urethral obstruction.

Diagnosis of penile or preputial neoplasia is based on observation of a preputial or intrapreputial mass followed by histological examination of a fine-needle aspirate or excision biopsy of the mass. Regional lymph nodes are the superficial inguinal nodes.

Treatment and Prognosis

Tumors of the penis and prepuce are removed by wide surgical excision, using electrocautery to minimize bleeding. With recurrent, invasive, or metastatic transmissible venereal tumors, chemotherapy with vincristine (0.025 mg/kg IV, not to exceed 1 mg) once weekly after a hemogram to look for leukopenia may be administered until there is no longer evidence of disease. Orthovoltage radiotherapy using a single dose of 1,000 rad is effective. Penile amputation and urethrostomy are indicated when tumor involvement is extensive or when urethral patency cannot be maintained. The prognosis for benign tumors of the penis and for transmissible venereal tumors is favorable in the absence of central nervous system metastasis; the prognosis is guarded to poor with carcinomas and sarcomas.

MAMMARY NEOPLASIA IN MALES (p. 2198)

CHAPTER 160

Urinary System (pages 2200–2212)

NEOPLASMS OF THE KIDNEY (pp. 2200–2206)

Benign renal neoplasms are less common than malignant renal tumors in dogs and cats and are primarily observed in older animals. Renal adenoma is one of the more commonly encountered benign neoplasms. Renal interstitial cell tumors have been recognized in dogs. Other benign renal neoplasms include hemangioma, papilloma, lipoma, and fibroma.

Tubular cell carcinomas are the most common primary malignant neoplasms of the kidneys. The incidence is higher in males. The tumor may be hormonally induced, and originate from the renal tubular epithelial cells. Bilateral and multiple renal cystadenocarcinomas have been associated with a syndrome of generalized nodular dermatofibrosis in German shepherds. The disease is hereditary, with an autosomal dominant pattern.

Nephroblastoma is a congenital neoplasm derived from the pluripotential metanephrogenic blastema, which allows production of epithelial and connective tissue elements. The neoplasm occurs more often in young dogs and cats, although many cases have been observed in dogs and cats 4 years of age and older.

Transitional cell and squamous cell carcinomas of the canine renal pelvis are much less common than the same types of tumors in the urinary bladder and are rare in cats.

Renal fibrosarcomas, hemangiosarcomas, and undifferentiated sarcomas are frequently encountered neoplasms of the kidneys of dogs. Metastatic neoplasms are commonly found in the kidneys. Renal lymphomas are generally considered metastatic and are the most common renal neoplasms of cats.

Clinical Signs and Laboratory Findings

Clinical signs vary with location, size, and duration of neoplasia. Neoplasms of the renal pelvis are usually associated with local signs (hematuria, hydronephrosis, and others) that precede polysystemic signs. This pattern is often opposite to that in patients with renal parenchymal neoplasms.

Enlarged kidneys caused by neoplasia must be differentiated from enlarged kidneys caused by hydronephrosis or polycystic disease. Extensive bilateral involvement of the kidneys that destroys 70 to 75 per cent or more of the nephrons is associated with signs of progressive renal insufficiency.

Polycythemia has been observed in dogs and cats with renal adenomas and renal tubular cell carcinomas that elaborated excessive quantities of erythrocyte-stimulating factor. Invasion and growth of renal tubular cell carcinomas into renal veins can occur. One study revealed that 48 per cent of dogs with renal tubular cell carcinomas had pulmonary metastasis on initial radiographic examination. Hypertrophic osteopathy has been observed in dogs with renal tumors.

Nephroblastomas are usually unilateral. The most common site of metastasis is the lung, followed by the liver, mesentery, and lymph nodes. In cats, alimentary lymphoma may be associated with extensive renal involvement. Both kidneys are usually affected and may be palpated as enlarged asymmetrical structures in the abdominal cavity.

Diagnosis

Plain abdominal radiographs often reveal an abdominal mass. Intravenous urography not only allows localization of the neoplasm but may permit estimation of the extent of renal parenchymal involvement. Thoracic radiographs are taken when a renal neoplasm is suspected, to aid in clinical staging for therapy.

A definitive antemortem diagnosis may be established by microscopic identification of neoplastic cells from biopsy specimens of the kidney or detection of neoplastic cells in urine sediment. Exploratory laparotomy is advised because a biopsy sample may be obtained with less risk of metastasis, the abdomen may be explored for metastases, and nephrectomy can be performed for treatment.

Treatment

Therapy is based on clinical staging. If the tumor has not metastasized and if the opposite kidney is not neoplastic and has adequate function, nephrectomy and partial ureterectomy are indicated. In addition to complete removal of the tumor, the associated ureter is removed, because metastasis may occur anywhere along its length. Little information in the veterinary literature describes the use of x-ray or chemotherapeutic agents in the treatment of renal tubular cell carcinomas.

The use of radiotherapy for nephroblastoma is limited in veterinary medicine but has significantly improved survival times in man.

Prognosis

The prognosis depends on the type, location, and extent of neoplastic involvement, the presence or absence of metastasis, and the biological behavior of the neoplasm. Long-term survival has been reported after complete surgical extirpation of a unilateral malignant neoplasm.

NEOPLASMS OF THE URETER (p. 2206)

Primary neoplasms of the canine ureter are rare.

NEOPLASMS OF THE URINARY BLADDER (pp. 2206–2210)

Bladder tumors are more frequent than tumors in other sites of the urinary tract but account for less than 1 per cent of all canine and feline neoplasms. Bladder tumors are more common in dogs than cats, possibly because of a difference in the metabolism of potentially carcinogenic agents, including tryptophan.

In both dogs and cats, malignant tumors are identified more frequently than benign tumors, and malignant epithelial tumors are more common than malignant connective tissue tumors.

Papillomas typically occur in older dogs and may be single or multiple. Clinically, papillomas may be difficult to distinguish from polyps associated with polypoid cystitis. Fibromas are most common in older dogs, may be single or multiple, and are usually associated with bacterial urinary tract infection. Prognosis after surgical removal is favorable.

Transitional cell carcinomas are the most common primary malignant tumors of the urinary bladder in dogs and cats. They typically arise from the trigone region. Invasion of the bladder wall is common, and the mucosa and underlying muscle layers may be completely replaced by neoplastic tissue. Most grow slowly and metastasize relatively late in their course.

Sarcomas are much less common than carcinomas and are characterized by diffuse invasive growth into the bladder wall and metastases. Rhabdomyosarcomas are seen in young large dogs. They are typically located at the neck of the bladder, are locally invasive, often do not metastasize, and frequently result in hypertrophic osteopathy.

Clinical Findings and Diagnosis

Clinical signs commonly associated with bladder tumors include persistent or intermittent hematuria, increased frequency of urination, dysuria, and urinary incontinence. No sign is pathognomonic. Partial or complete obstruction of the urethra or ureters may result in signs referable to renal failure. Signs may be present from a few days to months before a diagnosis is established.

Early and potentially curable neoplasms do not produce abnormalities that can be detected by physical examination alone. Later, thickening of the bladder wall or a firm mass within the bladder can be palpated. Sublumbar lymph nodes are occasionally enlarged. Urinary obstruction has resulted in azotemia. Hematuria and mild proteinuria are consistently noted in urinalyses.

Cytological examination of the urine sediment is useful in establishing a diagnosis, especially in patients with transitional cell carcinomas. Clusters of large anaplastic epithelial cells with prominent nuclear membranes and nucleoli, high nucleus/cytoplasm ratio, and variability in nuclear size are seen.

Survey abdominal radiographs may appear normal or may reveal calcification of the bladder wall, urolithiasis, bladder distension, bladder displacement, or increased size of the sublumbar lymph nodes. Tumors are readily demonstrated by contrast cystography (pneumocystography, positive-contrast cystography, or double-contrast cystography). Carcinomas typically appear as space-occupying masses arising from the bladder trigone and protruding into the bladder lumen.

Thoracic radiographs are obtained to determine the presence or absence of metastatic disease. With transitional cell carcinomas of the bladder or urethra, a diffuse unstructured interstitial pattern is most frequent. Ultrasonography can be used to demonstrate bladder tumors, to determine the extent of disease, and to document ureteral obstruction.

Biopsy is required to establish a definitive diagnosis and to determine histological type. Material for histopathological examination can be obtained by catheter biopsy of the tumor, cystoscopy, or exploratory celiotomy.

Treatment

Animals with benign bladder tumors can often be successfully treated by surgical removal of the tumor if the tumor does not involve the bladder trigone or neck.

The optimum therapy for animals with malignant bladder tumors has not been determined. Clinical staging for bladder tumors aids in defining appropriate therapy. Partial cystectomy can be used to remove tumors without extensive trigonal involvement. More than 80 per cent of the bladder can be removed without significant loss in capacity. Ureteral transplantation to the body of the bladder may be necessary.

Techniques for total cystectomy and urinary diversion have been described, but complications from the diversion procedure or the presence of metastatic disease have resulted in short-term benefit. Complications from the diversion procedure include intermittent vomiting, anorexia, neurological abnormalities, hyperchloremic metabolic acidosis, and pyelonephritis.

Radiation therapy (external beam or during surgery) has been attempted with bladder tumors. Tumor control has been short, and complication rates are high. Postradiotherapy complications, which were severe in some cases, included increased frequency of urination (46 per cent), urinary incontinence (46 per cent), cystitis (38 per cent), and stranguria (15 per cent). Increased frequency of urination probably resulted from bladder wall fibrosis.

Prognosis

The prognosis for benign tumors that can be completely resected surgically is favorable. The long-term prognosis for most malignant bladder tumors is poor because of extensive bladder wall invasion at diagnosis and a high incidence of metastasis.

NEOPLASMS OF THE URETHRA (pp. 2210–2211)
Epidemiology

Primary tumors of the urethra are uncommon. More females are affected than males, and tumors usually occur in older animals.

Pathology and Biological Behavior

Transitional cell carcinoma is the most common urethral tumor. Local invasion into the bladder occurs in one-third of cases. Metastasis to local lymph nodes or the lung occurs in approximately 30 per cent of dogs with urethral tumors.

Clinical Findings and Diagnosis

Chronic dysuria is a frequent clinical sign. Hematuria, urinary incontinence, and urethral discharge may also be noted. Vaginoscopy may reveal a mass protruding from the urethral orifice. Urethral catheterization is often difficult or impossible. Neoplastic cells may be seen in urine sediment.

Urethral tumors are readily demonstrated by contrast radiography. A positive-contrast urethrogram is the technique of choice if the urethra can be catheterized. If catheterization is impossible, a positive-contrast vaginogram or intravenous urogram may enhance observation of the urethra. Extension of contrast medium into periurethral tissues may be noted. Chest radiographs are obtained to rule out pulmonary involvement.

Urethral tumors are definitively diagnosed by biopsy. Material for histopathological examination can be obtained by catheter biopsy of the urethra or surgical exploration of the pelvic urethra.

Treatment

Therapeutic options include surgical excision, radiation therapy, or chemotherapy. Complete urethrectomy, cystectomy, and urinary diversion are associated with the same problems described for bladder neoplasia. Cisplatin chemotherapy produced stabilization of disease in two dogs for 4 and 8 months. Cyclophosphamide and doxorubicin may also be valuable for palliation.

Prognosis

The long-term prognosis for dogs with urethral tumors is poor because of extensive local disease at diagnosis and a high rate of metastasis.

CHAPTER 161

Musculoskeletal System
(pages 2213–2230)

In dogs and cats, primary bone tumors far outnumber secondary bone tumors. The majority of canine and feline primary bone tumors are malignant. Neoplasms of joints are less common than bone neoplasms. Neoplasms of skeletal muscle are rare.

The most frequent clinical signs in dogs and cats with appendicular bone tumors are pain or lameness referable to the primary tumor. Pathological fracture associated with bone neoplasms may cause sudden onset of nonweightbearing lameness.

Radiographic changes such as cortical destruction and periosteal new bone formation may support a diagnosis of bone neoplasia but are seldom pathognomonic for a histological type. Bone biopsy is important in the diagnosis and management of bone tumors in dogs and cats. Two techniques of closed biopsy have received the most attention: Michele trephine and Jamshidi needle biopsy. Both techniques yield a diagnosis of tumor in more than 90 per cent of neoplastic lesions.

A biopsy diagnosis of osteosarcoma may be accepted with great confidence, and biopsy accurately identifies tumor in more than 90 per cent of neoplastic lesions. A biopsy diagnosis of reactive bone or a histological type of bone tumor other than osteosarcoma is interpreted with caution, because more than 50 per cent of these lesions are ultimately identified as osteosarcoma on further histological evaluation.

The majority of primary bone tumors arise from within the medullary cavity or cortical bone, so-called central or medullary bone neoplasms. A subset of primary bone tumors distinct from these classic tumors arises from outside the cortex (presumably from the periosteum), so-called juxtacortical, parosteal, or periosteal bone neoplasms.

Invasion of the joint space by primary sarcomas of bone occurs infrequently. This characteristic has been useful in distinguishing primary sarcomas of bone from conditions such as rheumatoid arthritis, septic arthritis, and synovial sarcoma.

TREATMENT OF BONE NEOPLASMS (p. 2215)

After thorough evaluation of patients, amputation with or without adjunctive therapy is the standard treatment for tumors of the appendicular skeleton. Thoracic radiographs are performed so that pulmonary metastases may be detected, although negative radiographs do not rule out metastatic disease. Survey skeletal radiography or bone scintigraphy may assess involvement of other parts of the skeleton.

PRIMARY BONE TUMORS IN DOGS (pp. 2215–2218)

Osteosarcoma of the Canine Appendicular Skeleton

Osteosarcoma is the most common canine bone neoplasm, accounting for approximately 80 per cent of primary bone tumors. It is more common in the appendicular than axial skeleton. The distal radius is the most common primary site. Large and giant breeds may have up to 150 times greater risk than dogs weighing less than 10 kg.

Although monostotic disease (one bone lesion) is most frequently encountered, multiple bone involvement has been reported. It remains undetermined whether multiple skeletal lesions in dogs represent multiple primary neoplasms or metastatic lesions.

Appendicular osteosarcoma in dogs has a high metastatic rate, with micrometastatic disease or detectable metastases present in most individuals at initial presentation. The lungs are the most frequent site of metastases, although more intensive adjuvant chemotherapy protocols have been associated with an apparent change in metastatic pattern.

Treatment and Prognosis

Data from 62 dogs with appendicular osteosarcoma are frequently cited as the historical standard for survival. Median survival for these dogs after amputation was 18 weeks, with a 6-month survival rate of 26 per cent and 1-year survival rate of 10.7 per cent.

Prolonged survival has been reported in dogs after amputation and postoperative chemotherapy. Dogs treated with amputation and postoperative adjuvant cisplatin had significantly longer median survival time (43 weeks) than dogs treated with amputation alone (14.5 weeks). Cisplatin administration before amputation also prolonged survival but offered no advantage over postoperative cisplatin therapy.

In another study, adjuvant chemotherapy was initiated 2 weeks after amputation as follows: doxorubicin (30 mg/m^2 IV) on day one, cisplatin (60 mg/m^2 IV) on day 21, followed by a second cycle repeated 3 weeks later. Median survival of 19 dogs treated with amputation alone was 25 weeks. Median survival of 19 dogs (17 appendicular, 2 axial) that underwent amputation and adjuvant chemotherapy was 43 weeks.

Limb salvage, consisting of *en bloc* tumor excision, cortical allografting, and bone plate application, combined with preoperative radiation therapy and intravenous or intra-arterial cisplatin, has also prolonged survival in dogs with osteosarcoma. Median survival in 20 dogs was 32 weeks.

Amputation followed by adjuvant immunotherapy using liposome-encapsulated muramyl tripeptide (MTP-PE) prolongs metastasis-free interval and survival in dogs with appendicular osteosarcoma. Median metastasis-free interval in dogs treated with amputation and MTP-PE was 24 weeks, versus only 8 weeks in dogs treated with amputation alone. Median survival in MTP-PE–treated dogs was 32 weeks. Median survival in 13 dogs treated with amputation alone was 11 weeks.

Surgical resection of pulmonary metastases has been reported in man and dogs with osteosarcoma. The rationale for surgical management of pulmonary metastases is that measurable metastatic disease (i.e., nonmicrometastatic disease) in the lungs responds poorly to chemotherapy and immunotherapy.

Pulmonary metastectomy has been reported in 16 dogs with appendicular osteosarcoma. Approximately 50 per cent of dogs developed new pulmonary lesions within 3 months of metastectomy.

Osteosarcoma of the Canine Axial Skeleton

Axial skeletal involvement is present in approximately 25 per cent of dogs with osteosarcoma. Tumor-related death has usually been a consequence of inadequate local tumor control rather than metastatic disease. More radical surgical techniques such as mandibulectomy, rib resection and thoracic wall reconstruction, and hemipelvectomy have shown acceptable morbidity.

Osteosarcoma of the Skull

Osteosarcoma of the skull is most common in boxers; giant breeds are under-represented. Complete surgical excision of these tumors may be difficult or impossible.

Osteosarcoma of the Mandible

Osteosarcoma is one of the five most common tumors of the canine mandible, along with melanoma, squamous cell carcinoma, fibrosarcoma, and acanthomatous epulis. Median survival for six dogs after mandibulectomy was 1.5 months.

Osteosarcoma of the Rib

Osteosarcoma is the most common rib tumor in dogs. Intrathoracic expansion of these tumors may result in a "tip of the iceberg" phenomenon in which only a scarcely discernible mass may be externally palpable. Treatment consists of *en bloc* excision of the tumor followed by thoracic wall reconstruction using polypropylene mesh or alternative materials. Expected survival after surgical excision of these tumors is unknown.

Osteosarcoma of the Vertebrae

Osteosarcoma is the most common canine extradural spinal neoplasm. Surgical excision of these tumors is often impossible.

Extraskeletal Osteosarcoma in Dogs (pp. 2218–2219)

Osteosarcoma arising in nonosseous tissues is termed *extraskeletal osteosarcoma*; it is rare in dogs, accounting for less than 2 per cent of all canine osteosarcomas.

NONOSTEOGENIC PRIMARY MALIGNANT NEOPLASMS OF THE CANINE APPENDICULAR SKELETON
(pp. 2218–2220)

Fibrosarcoma, chondrosarcoma, and hemangiosarcoma are the most prevalent nonosteogenic primary appendicular skeletal neoplasms.

Fibrosarcoma of the Appendicular Skeleton

Fibrosarcoma is the third most common primary bone neoplasm in dogs, accounting for up to 9 per cent of all canine bone tumors. Appendicular skeletal involvement is present in 30 to 40 per cent. Radiographically, fibrosarcoma is predominantly lytic.

Histological evaluation of multiple tissue sections is critical to distinguish fibrosarcoma from osteosarcoma forming scant quantities of osteoid. The absence of osteoid in a single tissue section may erroneously lead to a diagnosis of fibrosarcoma. Appendicular fibrosarcoma is less malignant than oronasal fibrosarcoma and slower to metastasize than appendicular osteosarcoma.

Treatment and Prognosis

The prognosis for cure after surgical treatment of central fibrosarcoma of the appendicular skeleton is poor.

Chondrosarcoma of the Appendicular Skeleton

Chondrosarcoma is a malignant cartilage-producing neoplasm that usually arises *de novo* within bone. It occasionally occurs at the site of a previous bone lesion (e.g., secondary chondrosarcoma associated with an osteochondroma).

Treatment and Prognosis

Appendicular chondrosarcoma may be the canine primary malignant bone neoplasm with the best prognosis for cure after amputation.

Hemangiosarcoma of the Appendicular Skeleton

Hemangiosarcoma is a malignant neoplasm arising from endothelial cells, with highest frequency in male German shepherds. Less than 5 per cent of dogs with hemangiosarcoma have bone involvement. The proximal humerus, femur, ribs, and vertebrae are the most frequently affected skeletal sites. Radiographically, hemangiosarcoma is predominantly lytic and may demonstrate considerable intramedullary extension without dramatic cortical or periosteal changes. A sizable soft-tissue mass may accompany limb lesions in more than 50 per cent. Because of the lytic nature of this neoplasm, pathological fracture may be a sequel.

Treatment and Prognosis

If hemangiosarcoma of bone is suspected, a thorough search for other osseous and extraosseous lesions is indicated; ultrasonographic evaluation of the liver, spleen, and heart is recommended. Because of the aggressive nature of this neoplasm and the frequent presence of extraosseous disease, the prognosis for dogs with appendicular hemangiosarcoma is guarded. Mean survival time in five dogs after amputation was less than 5 months.

NONOSTEOGENIC MALIGNANT NEOPLASMS OF THE CANINE AXIAL SKELETON (pp. 2220–2221)

Multilobular Osteochondrosarcoma

Multilobular osteochondrosarcoma is an osteocartilaginous tumor in dogs. It arises from the mandible, maxilla, or cranium. Radiographically, it displays a lobulated appearance with well-defined borders. Previous descriptions include *chondroma rodens, calcifying aponeurotic fibroma,* and *multilobular osteoma/chondroma.* Although it was once considered benign, evidence now suggests this tumor to be a low-grade malignancy.

Treatment and Prognosis

Despite radical surgical excision, tumor location may make tumor-free margins impossible to achieve. In one study, metastatic disease developed in six of eight dogs with incomplete surgical excision. The lungs were the most frequent site of metastases.

The median interval from surgery to local recurrence was 14 months.Thus, prolonged survival in dogs with multilobular osteochondrosarcoma is possible despite metastatic disease.

Chondrosarcoma of the Rib

Chondrosarcoma has a predilection for the axial skeleton and is the second most common canine primary rib neoplasm. Clinically, this neoplasm is often indistinguishable from rib osteosarcoma. Metastatic rate was 50 per cent in six dogs that had rib chondrosarcoma and underwent necropsy.

Treatment and Prognosis

Treatment consisting of surgical excision and thoracic wall reconstruction may result in long-term survival. Local recurrence 4 to 5.5 years after surgical excision has been reported and may respond to a second surgical excision.

Nonosteogenic Vertebral Neoplasms

Approximately 50 per cent of vertebral neoplasms are metastatic lesions, 25 per cent are osteosarcomas, 15 per cent are chondrosarcomas, and the remaining 10 per cent are other nonosteogenic primary malignant bone neoplasms, including fibrosarcoma, hemangiosarcoma, and myeloma. Complete surgical excision of vertebral neoplasms is often impossible. Responsiveness of chondrosarcoma to radiation therapy is controversial and cytotoxic chemotherapy is ineffective. Chemotherapy and radiotherapy are unproven in treatment of fibrosarcoma of bone.

Sinonasal Chondrosarcoma

In 285 dogs with sinonasal neoplasms, chondrosarcoma was the most common nonepithelial tumor reported, accounting for 34 of 285 (12 per cent) sinonasal tumors. Cytoreductive surgery or radiation therapy has been used in the treatment of dogs with sinonasal chondrosarcoma.

SECONDARY BONE TUMORS IN DOGS AND CATS
(pp. 2221–2222)

Secondary bone tumors may involve bone either via local invasion or distant metastasis.

Bone Metastases

Bone metastases represent tumor cell foci that have become established within bone after hematogenous dissemination from a remote primary neoplasm. The prevalence of bone metastases in dogs is generally low. There is convincing evidence that bone destruction associated with bone metastases is mediated by local factors and that direct bone lysis by tumor cells is generally a late event.

Although many of the radiographic features of bone metastases are nonspecific, certain considerations such as signalment, history, and anatomical site may distinguish these lesions from primary bone tumors or other tumor-like lesions of bone. Metastatic bone tumors may be osteolytic or osteoproductive. Serum calcium concentrations in most dogs with metastatic bone neoplasms are normal.

Definitive diagnosis of bone metastases relies on histopathological evaluation of appropriate tissue specimens. Management of patients focuses on primary tumor control and assessment of the extent of metastatic disease.

FELINE BONE TUMORS (pp. 2222–2224)

Primary bone tumors are uncommon in cats, representing only 20 of 395 (5.1 per cent) feline neoplasms. As in dogs, most feline bone tumors are malignant. Feline bone neoplasms are characterized by a lower metastatic rate.

Feline Osteosarcoma

Osteosarcoma is the most common primary bone tumor of cats, representing 70 per cent of primary bone tumors. Appendicular skeletal neoplasms are more prevalent than axial skeletal neoplasms. Unlike in dogs, lesions of the distal radius are uncommon. Although the radiographic features of feline osteosarcoma are variable, long-bone lesions are predominantly lytic whereas skull lesions are osteoproductive. Osteosarcoma in cats behaves less aggressively than canine osteosarcoma. A metastatic rate of 16 per cent was reported in 32 cats that had osteosarcoma and underwent necropsy.

Treatment and Prognosis

Wide surgical excision or amputation is the treatment of choice for feline osteosarcoma; the prognosis depends on location. In one study, 6 of 12 (50 per cent) cats that had appendicular osteosarcoma and underwent amputation were alive at 13 to 64 months after surgery; median survival of cats that died was 49 months.

Feline Parosteal (Juxtacortical) Osteosarcoma

Parosteal osteosarcoma is distinct from central osteosarcoma because it arises from tissue (presumably periosteum) outside the cortex or medullary cavity. In cats, parosteal osteosarcoma is a painless growth on the surface of the skull or long bones. Radiographs reveal a well-circumscribed osteoproductive lesion. Metastases have been reported but are uncommon. Amputation or wide surgical excision is recommended.

FRACTURE-ASSOCIATED SARCOMA IN DOGS AND CATS (pp. 2224–2225)

Fracture-associated sarcomas are primary bone tumors that develop at the site of previous fractures. Cases have occurred when no fracture fixation was used. Fracture-associated sarcoma should not be confused with pathological fractures, which are fractures occurring in abnormal bone.

Both internal and external fixation devices have been incriminated in the pathogenesis of fracture-associated sarcoma. The increased frequency with which bone plates are implicated most likely reflects the increased use of these implants in comminuted and complicated fractures.

Metastases were reported in 6 of 42 (14 per cent) dogs with fracture-associated sarcoma. It is unclear whether dogs with fracture-associated osteosarcoma have a more favorable prognosis than dogs with classic osteosarcoma. An attempt to prevent fracture-associated sarcoma is *not* the rationale for plate removal after repair of uncomplicated fractures.

NEOPLASMS OF THE DIGITS (p. 2225)

Squamous cell carcinoma, melanoma, and mast cell sarcoma are the most common neoplasms involving the digits. Squamous cell carcinoma is most frequently associated with bone involvement.

Digital squamous cell carcinoma may be solitary or involve multiple digits. Radiographs typically reveal a destructive process with soft-tissue swelling. Clinically and radiographically, this condition may mimic osteomyelitis.

BENIGN BONE TUMORS (p. 2225)

Benign tumors are a small percentage of primary bone tumors. Osteoma, osteoid osteoma, ossifying fibroma, enchondroma, chondroma, and osteochondroma are reported. Complete surgical excision is curative, although tumor location may make this impossible.

NON-NEOPLASTIC BONE TUMORS (pp. 2225–2227)

Radiographic features and biological behavior of non-neoplastic lesions are important because these lesions may mimic bone neoplasms and may be difficult to distinguish. Biopsy and histopathological examination may be necessary.

Osteomyelitis

Radiographic features of osteomyelitis may mimic bone neoplasms.

A syndrome of septic arthritis and osteomyelitis of the coxofemoral joint occurs in mature dogs. In advanced cases, radiographs revealed an osteolytic lesion involving the proximal femur, with periacetabular new bone formation extending along the ilium and ischium. The presence of radiographic changes on both sides of the coxofemoral joint is helpful in distinguishing this syndrome from primary bone tumors or ischemic necrosis of the femoral head. Positive bacterial cultures from synovial fluid or adjacent bone are useful in distinguishing this syndrome from villonodular synovitis or synovial sarcoma. Surgical drainage and débridement of the affected joint, with femoral head and neck excision and systemic antibiotic therapy, were successful in maintaining or restoring acceptable limb function.

Simple or Benign Bone Cyst

The distal radius and ulna of young (<18 months) large dogs are most frequently affected. Multiple bone cysts are found in approximately 40 per cent of affected dogs, particularly Doberman pinschers.

Aneurysmal Bone Cyst

Aneurysmal bone cysts are rare in dogs and cats. This lesion is not a true cyst because it has no epithelial lining.

The ideal therapy for dogs and cats with aneurysmal bone cysts has not been established.

Bone Infarction

Multifocal medullary infarctions are reported in dogs with bone neoplasms. Radiographically, bone infarctions are medullary radiopacities that represent bone proliferation secondary to hypoxia.

NEOPLASMS OF JOINTS (SYNOVIAL SARCOMA) (p. 2227)

Synovial sarcoma is uncommon in dogs and rare in cats. These neoplasms consist of two cell types: synovium-like (epithelioid) cells and a sarcomatous (spindle cell) element. Lameness is the most common presenting sign in dogs with synovial sarcoma. Radiographic lesions may be limited to soft-tissue swelling but frequently include cortical destruction and periosteal reaction. The stifle and elbow are sites of predilection.

Treatment and Prognosis

Although amputation is the recommended treatment, data regarding prognosis after amputation are limited.

NEOPLASMS OF SKELETAL MUSCLE
(pp. 2227–2228)

CHAPTER 162

Respiratory System (pages 2231–2244)

NEOPLASMS OF THE NASAL AND PARANASAL SINUSES
(pp. 2231–2235)

Intranasal tumors generally occur in older animals, with a median reported age of 10 years in dogs and 12 years in cats. Soft-tissue tumors involving the nasal cavity have been reported in dogs as young as 1 year.

Male dogs and cats have a higher incidence of sinonasal neoplasms than females, irrespective of histological diagnosis.

Dolichocephalic breeds may have a higher incidence of nasal tumors than brachycephalic dogs, but dolichocephalic and mesencephalic breeds appear to be equally affected.

Sinonasal tumors may be classified histologically as epithelial, non-epithelial, or miscellaneous. Neoplasms of epithelial origin are the most common, with adenocarcinomas being the single most frequent histological diagnosis in dogs.

The metastatic rate of nasal tumors is low, with metastasis occurring late in the natural course. In one survey, 49 of 120 dogs had metastasis; the most common site of metastasis was the brain (28.3 per cent).

Clinical Presentation

Clinical signs in dogs with tumors involving the nasal cavity include epistaxis, swelling of the facial region (including exophthalmos), nasal discharge, sneezing or snuffling, dyspnea, ocular discharge, bleeding from the oral cavity, and seizures. Epistaxis or nasal discharge is usually unilateral. In bacterial and fungal infections, by comparison, the nasal discharge is usually bilateral and purulent. Foreign bodies and bleeding diatheses may also cause unilateral nasal discharge.

Neurological signs may be the predominant clinical finding in dogs and cats with nasal tumors. Neurological signs are related to erosion of the cribriform plate by the tumor and invasion and compression of the olfactory and frontal regions of the brain.

Diagnostic Evaluation (pp. 2233–2234)

If epistaxis has been severe or chronic, anemia may be noted. Affected animals are carefully evaluated for clotting abnormalities by assessing platelet numbers, bleeding from venipuncture sites, or the presence of ecchymoses, petechiae, melena, hematuria, or retinal hemorrhages. Coagulation is assessed by activated clotting time, prothrombin time, or partial thromboplastin time. Cats are evaluated for feline leukemia virus and feline immunodeficiency virus infections.

Thoracic radiography and aspiration of regional lymph nodes are performed and evaluated for the presence of metastasis. Radiographs of the skull usually require general anesthesia to obtain satisfactory positioning. Of various views, the open-mouth ventrodorsal view consistently provides the most information by allowing examination of the entire turbinate region and reducing superimposition of the mandibles.

Radiographs are evaluated for the presence of increased soft-tissue density of the nasal cavity or frontal sinuses, bone lysis, destruction of the normal turbinate pattern, new bone formation, and the presence of foreign bodies.

Computed tomography (CT) may be helpful in defining the extent of disease in animals with nasal tumors, both for prognosis and for planning of radiation therapy. Both plain and contrast-enhanced CT studies may be useful. Definitive diagnosis is made by cytological or histopathological evaluation of specimens obtained by nasal flushing techniques or by biopsy. When the previously described techniques do not result in a diagnosis, surgical exploration and biopsy may be necessary.

Surgery as the sole treatment of dogs with nasal tumors has not resulted in prolonged survival times. Surgery may palliate clinical signs in some dogs by removing tissues that are obstructing respiration and by decreasing epistaxis.

Radiotherapy appears to be the most effective treatment for nasal tumors. Most studies have investigated orthovoltage (125 to 400 KeV) irradiation, although occasional reports have described the use of megavoltage (>1 KeV) x-irradiation. Adams compared megavoltage irradiation (cobalt or linear accelerator) with softer deep radiation (cesium or orthovoltage) and found that the dogs with the longest median survival (15.2 months) were those that had adenocarcinomas and were treated with cytoreductive surgery and softer deep radiation.

Whether radiation therapy should be combined with surgical debulking is controversial. One study found that survival times of dogs that were treated with softer radiation alone (without surgery) were shorter than those that were treated with the two modalities combined. However, cytoreductive surgery did not improve survival times of dogs that were treated with megavoltage irradiation.

Complications associated with megavoltage irradiation include keratitis, conjunctivitis, cataracts, keratoconjunctivitis sicca, alopecia, changes in skin texture, and bone necrosis.

The prognosis for dogs with nasal tumors is generally poor. In patients not treated and those treated with surgery, chemotherapy, immunotherapy, and cryosurgery, the mean survival time is generally 3 to 5 months. Improvement in this survival period has been accomplished with radiation therapy combined with surgical debulking (discussed earlier), with mean reported survival times of 8 to 25 months.

NEOPLASMS OF THE LARYNX AND TRACHEA
(pp. 2235–2237)

Tumors of the larynx and trachea are extremely rare in dogs and cats. Laryngeal tumors generally occur in older animals. Tracheal tumors often occur in adolescent dogs. In cats, lymphosarcoma is most commonly identified; squamous cell carcinoma and adenocarcinoma have also been reported.

Filaroides osleri (Oslerus osleri) is a nematode that forms nodules in the trachea and mainstem bronchi of dogs. These lesions must be differentiated from neoplastic lesions. The diagnosis is based on identifying eggs, larvae, or adult worms in bronchoscopically obtained biopsy specimens or by identifying the larvae in feces.

Laryngeal and tracheal tumors are often well advanced at diagnosis. The most common signs in dogs are a hoarse bark or loss of voice, with subsequent onset of exertional dyspnea and cough. Patients with tracheal tumor generally have respiratory distress, coughing, and exercise intolerance. With laryngeal tumors, radiography usually reveals a reduction in diameter of the laryngeal air space by an intraluminal mass. Under general anesthesia, these tumors can be sampled by biopsy.

Tracheal tumors usually appear radiographically as a mass that is narrowing or obstructing the tracheal lumen. Biopsy of tracheal tumors is more difficult than that of laryngeal tumors but can usually be performed using either a fiberoptic endoscope or a rigid bronchoscope.

Because of the advanced stage of most laryngeal tumors at diagnosis, therapy is difficult; however, oncocytomas and rhabdomyomas warrant a favorable prognosis after partial laryngectomy.

Although prognosis is related to histological type, the prognosis for many tracheal tumors is excellent, primarily because the trachea can be readily resected and anastomosed. In adult dogs, 12 per cent of the total tracheal length (approximately four rings) may be resected and anastomosed without generating undue tension at the anastomosis. In puppies, as much as 25 per cent of the total trachea length may be removed. Successful treatment of tracheal tumors in cats with tracheal resection and anastomosis has also been reported.

PRIMARY PULMONARY NEOPLASIA (pp. 2237–2240)

The development of spontaneous primary pulmonary neoplasia is uncommon in dogs and cats. The average incidence has been estimated to be 1.24 per cent for dogs and 0.38 per cent for cats.

The average age of dogs with primary lung tumors is 10 to 11 years; these tumors seldom occur in animals younger than 7 years. Cats are often slightly older when primary lung tumors are diagnosed (12 years).

Adenocarcinomas are the most common histological type found in dogs and cats, with squamous cell carcinoma and anaplastic carcinomas being identified more rarely. The diaphragmatic lobes are most frequently involved, with the right lung lobes more often affected than the left. Cavitation may be a feature due to tumor necrosis.

Primary lung tumors metastasize early and aggressively. A necropsy study showed that 100 per cent of squamous cell carcinomas and 90 per cent of anaplastic carcinomas had metastasized by the time of primary lesion detection, whereas approximately 50 per cent of adenocarcinomas had metastasized. One of the most common sites of metastasis is the lungs themselves. Regional lymph nodes are common metastatic sites, and their involvement is an important prognostic factor. Feline tumors metastasize most commonly to long bones, vertebrae, and skeletal muscle.

Clinical Presentation

Pulmonary neoplasia sometimes is an incidental finding when thoracic radiographs are evaluated for an unrelated problem. The most commonly reported clinical sign is a nonproductive cough. Other signs include hemoptysis, fever, lethargy, exercise intolerance, weight loss, dysphagia, and anorexia. Signs referable to the respiratory tract are noted in only one-third of cats, and coughing is only occasionally encountered in cats. Lameness or swollen legs may be associated with metastasis to bone or skeletal muscles or with the development of hypertrophic osteopathy. Paraneoplastic syndromes are rare in animals, with the most commonly associated change being hypertrophic osteopathy.

Diagnostic Evaluation

Thoracic radiography is a valuable noninvasive diagnostic tool. The most common presentation is a solitary nodular density in a dorsal caudal lung lobe; peripheral lesions are more commonly observed than perihilar disease in animals. Neoplasia is more commonly found in the larger, right lung lobes of dogs but is more evenly distributed between the right and left caudal lobes in cats.

Despite their diagnostic value, thoracic radiographs are insensitive in detecting primary or metastatic lung tumors. The nodules must be at least 1 cm in diameter to be reliably recognized with conventional radiography. Intrathoracic calcification of lesions can occur with inflammatory as well as neoplastic masses. Other important factors to note radiographically are intrathoracic lymphadenopathy and pleural effusion, but the absence of enlarged hilar lymph nodes does not rule out metastatic disease.

An additional noninvasive technique that can be performed at many referral centers is a pulmonary perfusion scan. Most scans are performed by venous administration of ^{99m}Tc-labeled macroaggregated albumin.

Collection of specimens for cytological evaluation and culture and sensitivity testing can be accomplished by transtracheal lavage, percutaneous fine-needle aspirates, and bronchoscopy.

Biopsy of a pulmonary mass may be accomplished by bronchoscopy, a percutaneous approach, and exploratory thoracotomy. A thoracotomy is often necessary for definitive diagnosis of a pulmonary mass. Surgical resection is not indicated with intrapulmonary metastasis, distant metastasis of a primary lung tumor, or lung metastasis of a distant primary tumor.

Therapy

Wide surgical resection is the treatment of choice for solitary nodules confined to one lobe or one lung after the anesthetic risk to the patient has been assessed.

Chemotherapy is routinely used for particular histological types of neoplasia in man, but its use in animals with pulmonary neoplasia has been limited. Chemotherapy may be considered when lesions are inoperable, surgery is contraindicated for other reasons, or lesions recur after surgical resection. Cisplatin and vincristine have been used on a limited basis and have resulted in a measurable response.

Course of Disease and Prognosis

The best prognosis is for patients with solitary lesions of small diameter (<5 cm), negative lymph nodes, no malignant pleural effusion, and diagnosis before the development of respiratory symptoms. Under these circumstances, more than 50 per cent of dogs can live at least 1 year after surgery. Dogs with respiratory signs at the time of diagnosis and surgery have shorter survival times than dogs without signs.

The prognosis for most cats with primary lung tumor is poor owing to the advanced nature of disease at the time of diagnosis and aggressive metastatic behavior.

METASTATIC PULMONARY NEOPLASIA (pp. 2241–2242)

Metastasis is a major cause of treatment failure in cancer patients. The lung is second only to regional lymph nodes in incidence of metastatic disease. Metastatic pulmonary neoplasia is encountered far more commonly than primary lung tumors in dogs and cats and represents an important differential diagnosis for nodular lung disease.

Diagnostic Evaluation

Clinical findings supporting metastatic disease rather than primary pulmonary neoplasia are multiple pulmonary masses, the presence of a nonpulmonary mass, and the previous excision of a malignant mass. Compared with primary lesions, metastatic tumors are generally smaller and more circumscribed. Metastatic nodules are usually located in the peripheral or middle portions of the lung and do not cause noticeable displacement or obstruction of bronchi. Cavitation is usually not encountered with pulmonary metastatic disease. Multiple nodules associated with primary lung tumors often consist of one large mass and smaller secondary nodules. When multiple nodules are metastases, several large masses and various smaller lesions are usually present. Because of the varied patterns of metastatic spread to the pulmonary parenchyma, not all metastatic lesions appear as distinct nodular densities.

Therapy

Chemotherapy has been the standard for treating metastatic disease because of its ability to be distributed throughout the body. Surgical management of solitary or slow-growing metastases has been attempted with some success.

MALIGNANT PLEURAL EFFUSION (p. 2242)

Pleural effusion may be associated with either primary thoracic neoplasia, such as pleural mesothelioma, or metastatic pulmonary tumors.

Identification of neoplastic cells in pleural effusion of cats and dogs is uncommon. Additionally, malignant cells are difficult to differentiate from reactive mesothelial cells, which exfoliate in response to the pleural effusion.

Treatment of malignant pleural effusion is directed at controlling the primary tumor. When there is no effective systemic treatment and clinical signs related to the effusion predominate, treatment of the effusion may be indicated to prolong an animal's life. Pleurodesis has been used in dogs to treat pleural effusion; however, its effectiveness is unproven.

Mesotheliomas are rare tumors in dogs. They arise from mesodermal cells of the pleural, pericardial, and peritoneal surfaces. These tumors are highly effusive, and clinical signs are usually related to the presence of large amounts of serosanguineous fluid, which inhibits normal respiration. Diagnosis of mesothelioma is generally made by open biopsy.

Metastasis of mesotheliomas to intrathoracic organs is common in dogs, and therapy is generally restricted to controlling pleural effusion. The prognosis in dogs for long-term survival is similarly poor.

TUMORS OF THE THORACIC WALL AND STERNUM
(pp. 2242–2243)

Primary tumors of the ribs are uncommon in dogs; however, these tumors are usually malignant, have a high metastatic rate, and generally develop in young dogs. Most rib tumors cause a localized swelling of the thoracic wall.

A tentative diagnosis of the cell type can usually be made by fine-needle aspiration of the mass, but definitive diagnosis usually requires histological examination of a biopsy specimen.

Although also rare, both metastatic and primary tumors of the sternum have been reported in dogs. When a diagnosis of sternal neoplasia is made, the diseased bone as well as normal surrounding tissue should be removed. Unlike most bones in the body, the sternebrae can be removed with little decrease in function.

Anesthetic Considerations in Surgery (pages 2245–2309)

CHAPTER 163

Anesthetics and Techniques
(pages 2245–2251)

Chemical restraint refers to a drug-induced state that produces favorable behavior modification, sedation, analgesia, or muscle relaxation. Anesthesia includes two of these qualities, analgesia and muscle relaxation, but also incorporates hypnosis or unconsciousness.

Drugs used for chemical restraint can be placed into one of three broad categories: sedatives, nonopioid analgesics, and opioid analgesics. The combination of a sedative or an alpha$_2$-adrenoceptor agonist (xylazine or another nonopioid analgesic) with an opioid analgesic (e.g., morphine, meperidine) makes up a fourth drug combination group referred to as *neuroleptanalgesics.*

Tranquilizers and Sedatives

Acepromazine is the only phenothiazine sedative (tranquilizer) in common use in small animal practice. All phenothiazine tranquilizers produce calmness and indifference, reduce aggressive behavior, and bring about muscle relaxation by depressing the reticular activating system and brain stem and inhibiting effects of the central neurotransmitters norepinephrine and dopamine. Phenothiazines are also noted for their alpha$_1$-adrenoceptor blocking effect, which is important systemically in producing hypotension. Other pharmacological activities of phenothiazine tranquilizers include antiadrenergic, antiarrhythmic (they abolish halothane sensitization to catecholamines), antifibrillatory, antihistaminic, antiemetic, antipyretic, antishock, and anticonvulsant effects. This anticonvulsant property makes phenothiazines effective in inhibiting ketamine and tiletamine/zolazepam-induced seizures even though they are also known to lower seizure threshold by a separate mechanism. The ability of phenothiazines to lower seizure threshold is important in patients with organic brain disease (neoplasia), inherited or familial epilepsy, or encephalitis. Dogs and cats have accidentally received massive overdoses (10 to 20 times the recommended dose) of acepromazine without ill effect other than pronounced and prolonged depression and hypotension. Fluid therapy, occasional administration of an alpha$_1$-adrenoceptor agonist (phenylephrine), and supportive therapy are generally all that is needed to ensure complete recovery.

The butyrophenone tranquilizers are typified by droperidol, the tranquilizing portion of the neuroleptanalgesic Innovar-Vet, and offer few if any real practical advantages over acepromazine.

Benzodiazepines

Recommended doses of diazepam and midazolam produce no better sedative or calming effects than the butyrophenones. All the benzodiazepines are appetite stimulants. The major advantages of these drugs are their lack of significant cardiopulmonary depressant effects, their muscle relaxant properties, and their ability to inhibit seizures. Rapid intravenous administration of diazepam to dogs and cats may produce bradycardia, hypotension, and transient periods of cardiac arrest. Midazolam is slightly more potent than diazepam but has a shorter duration of action. All benzodiazepines are potentially reversible with a benzodiazepine antagonist, flumazenil.

Nonopioid Analgesics

The nonopioid analgesics xylazine and medetomidine produce analgesic, sedative, and muscle relaxant effects by combining with central nervous system alpha$_2$ adrenoceptors. These drugs also stimulate peripheral alpha$_1$ and alpha$_2$ adrenoceptors, potentially producing marked cardiopulmonary depression. Arterial blood pressure first increases and then decreases. Xylazine-induced bradycardia is partially responsive (atropine or glycopyrrolate) but may require more specific therapy by administering an alpha$_2$-adrenoceptor antagonist. Yohimbine and tolazoline are alpha$_2$-adrenoceptor antagonists that specifically antagonize xylazine's effects by competitively blocking and displacing it from alpha$_2$ adrenoceptors. Doxapram, a central nervous system and specifically a respiratory center stimulant, also speeds recovery in dogs and particularly in cats and returns patients to a higher level of consciousness without eliminating analgesia.

Opioid Analgesics and Neuroleptanalgesia

Opioid analgesics produce their diverse effects, including analgesia, by interacting with one or more opioid receptors. These drugs not only affect multiple receptors but produce both opioid agonistic and antagonistic effects. Butorphanol can be used as an analgesic or to antagonize the opioid agonist morphine. The combination of excellent analgesic properties and poor sedative effects has led veterinarians to become adept at combining opioids with sedatives.

Anticholinergics

The anticholinergic drugs atropine and glycopyrrolate are frequently administered as preanesthetics. They reduce salivary and tracheal secretions, dilate airways, prevent or reverse parasympathetically induced bradycardias, and cause mydriasis. Glycopyrrolate has a longer duration of action than atropine and does not cross the blood-brain or placental barriers. Routine use of anticholinergics in dogs and cats is controversial because the majority of anesthetic techniques in current use do not produce excessive salivation or bradycardia. Anticholinergics are useful in preventing or reversing bradycardia caused by xylazine and opioid analgesics.

DRUGS USED TO PRODUCE GENERAL ANESTHESIA
(pp. 2248–2251)

Barbiturates and Other Hypnotics

Thiamylal and thiopental are ultrashort-acting thiobarbiturates that are popular for producing short-term intravenous anesthesia, inducing general anesthesia before inhalation anesthesia, and reinducing anesthesia in animals that have become light during inhalation anesthesia. They produce hypnosis and muscle relaxation by depressing all areas of the central nervous system and inhibiting polysynaptic reflexes. Thiobarbiturates can produce ventricular arrhythmias and augment cardiac sensitization to catecholamines produced by halothane. If cardiac arrhythmias persist, they are treated with lidocaine (0.5 to 1.0 mg/kg). One of the most disturbing properties of the thiobarbiturates is that they are cumulative. Recovery is prolonged in sight hounds (greyhounds, whippets, borzois, Afghans) after thiobarbiturate administration. The reason for this is unclear but is partially related to the slow liver metabolism of both drugs.

Alternatives to thiobarbiturate induction include methohexital (an ultrashort-acting barbiturate), etomidate, and propofol. These drugs are rapidly metabolized in both the plasma and liver, are not cumulative, and can be used in sight hounds without prolonging recovery.

Cyclohexylamines

The dissociative anesthetics ketamine and tiletamine/zolazepam are used as preanesthetic medication for restraint, as general anesthetics, and intraoperatively as adjuncts to anesthesia. Cardiovascular function is usually maintained or improved. Inadequate muscle relaxation, the potential for seizures during induction and recovery from anesthesia, and the development of emergence delirium during recovery from anesthesia have caused ketamine to be used in combination with acepromazine, xylazine, and diazepam. Ketamine and tiletamine are relatively safe drugs but almost always produce significant increases in arterial blood pressure and tachycardia. Ketamine and tiletamine/zolazepam are contraindicated with severe liver or renal disease because of their extended action due to prolonged drug elimination. Their use in dogs or cats with urethral obstruction is not contraindicated provided renal function is normal.

Inhalation Anesthetics

Inhalation anesthetics provide safe and effective long-term general anesthesia. Methoxyflurane is an excellent muscle relaxant and analgesic but is noted for its prolonged recovery periods *if dosage is not controlled correctly.*

Halothane is a fair analgesic and muscle relaxant but generally provides excellent anesthesia when preanesthetic medications are used. Halothane sensitizes the myocardium to catecholamine-induced arrhythmias.

Isoflurane produces excellent short- or long-term anesthesia in small animals, birds, and reptiles. It does not sensitize the myocardium to catecholamines like halothane but can produce marked hypotension and respiratory depression. Recovery from anesthesia can be so rapid in some dogs and cats that excitement and delirium may occur, requiring resedation. Isoflurane is less potent and more volatile than methoxyflurane or halothane, requiring higher concentrations to maintain anesthesia.

Nitrous oxide can be used to add analgesia and muscle relaxation. It must be administered as at least 40 to 70 per cent of the inspired gas concentration if any real beneficial effect is to be derived, and it should not exceed 70 per cent of the inspired gas concentration if hypoxia is to be avoided.

NEUROMUSCULAR BLOCKING DRUGS (p. 2251)

The peripheral neuromuscular blocking drugs can be used as adjuncts to anesthesia and surgery but are infrequently used in veterinary surgery. Depolarizing (succinylcholine) and nondepolarizing drugs are available, although nondepolarizing (pancuronium, vecuronium, atracurium) drugs are currently preferred because of their predictable duration of action and reversibility with acetylcholinesterase inhibitors.

CHAPTER 164

Equipment and Techniques for Inhalation Anesthesia
(pages 2251–2257)

THE ANESTHETIC MACHINE (pp. 2251–2252)

A generic anesthetic machine consists of (1) a source of oxygen and anesthetic and (2) a breathing circuit through which the mixture of anesthetic and oxygen is delivered to a patient's airway in exchange for exhaled CO_2.

A full high-pressure cylinder of oxygen is pressurized to approximately 2,000 psi, whereas the pressure within a nitrous oxide cylinder is 750 psi. A pressure regulator reduces incoming cylinder pressure to approximately 50 psi. An additional regulator for nitrous oxide may be present. The flowmeter assemblies receive gas from the regulators at a pressure of 50 psi.

Volatile liquid anesthetic is transformed into a vapor within the anesthetic vaporizer. The other type of vaporizer, referred to as a "draw-over" type, is limited to a location within a circle breathing circuit. Examples of this type of vaporizer include the Ohio Number 8 Vaporizer and the Stephans Universal Vaporizer.

ANESTHETIC BREATHING CIRCUITS (pp. 2252–2257)

Mapleson Circuits

Mapleson circuits depend on the fresh gas flow to remove exhaled CO_2. If relatively high fresh gas flow rates are used, these circuits are nonrebreathing circuits.

The Mapleson A system, also called a *Magill system*, allows fresh gas to enter the system near the breathing bag, and excess gas is discharged through a pressure relief valve located near the attachment of the endotracheal tube. The disadvantage of this system is that it cannot be used reliably during controlled ventilation because high fresh gas flow rates are necessary to prevent rebreathing of CO_2.

The Mapleson D and F circuits are functionally similar. An example of the Mapleson D circuit is the coaxial or Bain circuit. Fresh gas flows through the inner hose of the coaxial tube and passes to the patient near the endotracheal tube connection. Exhaled gas flows around the inner tube, through the corrugated tube, toward the reservoir bag. The Jackson-Rees modification of the Ayres T piece is an example of the Mapleson F system. Fresh gas is delivered to the patient near the endotracheal tube connection, and exhaled gas flows through the corrugated tube to exit through the tail of the reservoir bag. The D and F systems can be used with spontaneous or controlled ventilation.

Circle Rebreathing Systems

The advantage of the circle system is that relatively low fresh gas flow rates are used. Fresh gas flow can be low because of the presence of CO_2-absorbent material within the circuit.

Components of the Circle System

Exhaled CO_2 is removed from the circle breathing circuit via a chemical reaction. Exhaled CO_2 reacts with water and a hydroxide of the alkaline earth metals to form carbonate and water.

The paired breathing hoses conduct inhaled gas to and exhaled gas away from the patient. The pressure relief valve vents gas to the atmosphere via the waste gas scavenging system.

The breathing bag provides visual assessment of ventilation. The bag can be compressed to deliver a breath manually. Too large a bag makes visual assessment of ventilation difficult and also adds unnecessary volume to the circuit; too small a bag provides an inadequate reservoir for large tidal volumes.

The fresh gas inlet delivers oxygen and anesthetic gas to the breathing circuit. If fresh gas flow rate is in excess of that removed by the patient, the excess gas fills the breathing system and exits through the pressure relief valve (semiclosed system). If the fresh gas inflow matches uptake by the patient, no gas flows out of the pressure relief valve (closed system). An anesthetic vaporizer can be located outside or within the anesthetic circle.

Fresh Gas Flow Rates

The minimum flow rate of oxygen that can be used with the circle system just equals a patient's minute oxygen consumption: $10 \times$ body weight $(kg)^{3/4}$, or approximately 3 to 6 ml/kg. This low flow rate can be used immediately after anesthetic induction and intubation and continued throughout the anesthetic period when an in-circle vaporizer is used. When an out-of-circle vaporizer is used, relatively high oxygen flow rates (1 to 3 L/min) are initially needed to rapidly deliver the anesthetic vapor leaving the vaporizer into the circle. Oxygen flow rate can be decreased within 20 minutes of induction to closed-system flow rates. Maintenance vaporizer settings for out-of-circle vaporizers during closed-system anesthesia are high because the low fresh gas flow carrying anesthetic into the circle carries only small volumes of volatile anesthetic with it.

CHOICE OF ANESTHETIC BREATHING CIRCUITS (p. 2257)

The choice of anesthetic breathing circuit is primarily determined by a patient's size. Studies confirm that patients as small as 2.5 kg can be safely anesthetized using a circle system.

CHAPTER 165

Anesthesia for Elective Soft-Tissue and Orthopedic Procedures (pages 2258–2262)

A classification system for veterinary patients based on that established by the American Society of Anesthesiologists can be used to classify the risk of anesthesia (Table 165–1).

The laboratory data required to perform anesthesia safely are based on physical status and age (Table 165–2).

ANESTHETIC TECHNIQUES (pp. 2260–2262)

The following examples represent anesthetic plans for routine elective operations. An understanding of the pharmacology of the anesthetic drugs (Chapter 163) is necessary for safe anesthetic administration.

Aggressive Dog

Signalment. A 4-year-old 50-kg intact male rottweiler was presented for prophylactic dental cleaning and polishing.

History, Physical Examination, and Laboratory Data. Current vaccinations; no current problems; unable to handle; PCV = 39, TP = 7.4, heartworm negative.

Premedication. Innovar-Vet, 3 ml IM (60 mg droperidol + 1.2 mg fentanyl).

Induction. Thiamylal sodium, 200 to 400 mg IV.

Maintenance. Halothane; semiclosed circle rebreathing system; 1 L/minute oxygen flow; lactated Ringer solution, 500 ml/hour.

TABLE 165–1. CLASSIFICATION OF PATIENT'S PHYSICAL STATUS

Category	Description	Example
I	Normal, healthy patient	Six-month-old patient presented for elective sterilization with no discernible systemic disease
II	Patient with mild systemic disease	Uncomplicated fracture, compensated heart disease (mitral regurgitation)
III	Patient with severe systemic disease, limiting activity but not incapacitating	Anemia, fever, cachexia, compensated renal disease
IV	Patient with severe, incapacitating systemic disease that is a constant threat to life	Trauma (pneumothorax, uroabdomen), noncompensated heart disease or uremia
V	Moribund patient not expected to live 24 hours with or without surgery	Terminal malignancy, severe trauma

TABLE 165-2. MINIMUM LABORATORY DATA BASED ON PATIENT'S PHYSICAL STATUS

Physical Status Category	Minimum Laboratory Data
I	Packed cell volume, total protein
II	Packed cell volume, total protein, Azostick
III*	Complete blood count, blood urea nitrogen, creatinine
IV*	Complete blood count, chemistry profile, urinalysis
V*	Complete blood count, chemistry profile, urinalysis, blood gas

*Laboratory data obtained are determined by the signalment, physical examination, and history.

Routine Soft-Tissue Surgery—Dog

Signalment. A 6-month-old 12-kg alert female mixed-breed was presented for ovariohysterectomy.

History, Physical Examination, and Laboratory Data. Current vaccinations, normal on examination; no previous estrus; PCV = 44; TP = 7.9; heartworm and fecal negative.

Premedication. Acepromazine, 1.5 mg IM.

Induction. Thiamylal sodium, 50 to 100 mg IV.

Maintenance. Halothane; semiclosed circle rebreathing system; 250 to 500 ml/minute oxygen flow and lactated Ringer's solution.

Routine Orthopedic Surgery—Dog

Signalment. An 8-year-old 4-kg neutered male poodle was presented for repair of ruptured anterior cruciate ligament.

History, Physical Examination, and Laboratory Data. Three-day duration of lameness; positive anterior drawer in right rear limb; otherwise normal on physical examination; PCV = 38; TP = 7.1; blood urea nitrogen = 15; creatinine = 0.7; heartworm and fecal negative.

Premedication. Midazolam, 0.8 mg IM + butorphanol, 0.8 mg IM, or oxymorphone, 0.4 mg IM.

Induction. Thiamylal sodium, 16 to 32 mg IV.

Maintenance. Methoxyflurane; Bain circuit nonrebreathing system; 600 to 800 ml/minute oxygen flow; lactated Ringer solution, 40 ml/hour; fentanyl, 0.009 mg IV when dog shows signs of inadequate analgesia.

Soft-Tissue Surgery—Sight Hound

Signalment. A 6-month-old 32-kg intact male greyhound was presented for castration.

History, Physical Examination, and Laboratory Data. Normal on examination, PCV = 44; TP = 7.5.

Premedication. Acepromazine, 2 mg IM.

Induction. Combination of diazepam, 9 mg, + ketamine, 175 mg IV.

Maintenance. Halothane; semiclosed circle rebreathing system; 650 to 1,000 ml/minute oxygen flow.

Routine Soft-Tissue Surgery—Cat

Signalment. Eight-month-old 4.4-kg Siamese cat was presented for elective ovariohysterectomy and front onychectomy.

History, Physical Examination, and Laboratory Data. Normal on examination, PCV = 41; TP = 7.3.

Premedication. Ketamine, 24 mg, oxymorphone, 0.3 mg, + acepromazine, 0.2 mg IM.

Induction. Thiamylal, 25 mg IV; cat unable to be intubated—additional thiamylal 5 mg IV.

Maintenance. Halothane; Bain nonrebreathing system; 750 to 900 ml/minute oxygen flow.

Aggressive Cat

Signalment. A 4-year-old 7-kg intact male cat was presented for abscess drainage; extremely aggressive.

History, Physical Examination, and Laboratory Data. Current vaccinations including feline leukemia virus; normal on examination; unable to sample blood.

Premedication. Combination of ketamine, 50 mg, + acepromazine, 0.35 mg IM; still unable to restain for catheterization.

Induction. Induction chamber with 4 per cent halothane delivered with 100 per cent oxygen (6 L/minute).

Maintenance. Halothane; Bain nonrebreathing system; 1.0 to 1.5 L/minute oxygen flow.

Routine Orthopedic Surgery—Cat

Signalment. A 10-year-old 6-kg castrated male cat was presented for a fractured femur.

History, Physical Examination, and Laboratory Data. Cat was hit by a car hours earlier and is lame on rear leg; radiographs confirm pneumothorax and a femur fracture; all else normal; PCV = 32; TP = 6.4. Forty-eight hours later, the pneumothorax has resolved; the electrocardiogram is normal.

Premedication. Combination of butorphanol, 1.2 mg, + midazolam, 1.2 mg IM.

Induction. Thiamylal, 40 mg IV.

Maintenance. Isoflurane; Bain nonrebreathing system; 1.0 to 1.5 L/minute oxygen flow; lactated Ringer solution, 60 ml/hour.

Postoperative Analgesia. Butorphanol, 24 mg IM.

CHAPTER 166

Anesthesia for the Trauma or Shock Patient (pages 2262–2266)

PREOPERATIVE EVALUATION (p. 2262)

Airway, breathing, circulation, and neurological status are quickly assessed after the patient's arrival. Traumatized patients are often presented close to cardiopulmonary collapse or cardiac arrest. Because many anesthetic drugs depress cardiopulmonary function, anesthesia enhances the likelihood of cardiovascular collapse or cardiac arrest. As a general rule, anesthesia is not undertaken until the patient's condition has been assessed and stabilized.

ANESTHETIC MANAGEMENT OF TRAUMA PATIENTS
(pp. 2262–2266)

Premedication

Anticholinergics are not recommended for routine use in trauma patients because they often increase heart rate and oxygen consumption while predisposing to cardiac dysrhythmias. A full stomach should be assumed, and measures to prevent aspiration before anesthesia induction need to be considered. Aspiration of acid gastric contents (pH < 2.5) can result in pneumonitis.

Analgesics or sedatives can be given to help allay pain, fear, and apprehension during the preoperative period. Butorphanol (0.1 mg/kg IV) or oxymorphone (0.05 mg/kg IV) may be administered in small incremental doses if analgesia is needed. Diazepam (0.2 mg/kg IV) or midazolam (0.2 mg/kg IV or IM) can be combined with the opioid if greater central nervous system depression is desirable. Ketamine (1 to 3 mg/kg IV or IM) can also be given preoperatively (cats) or in combination with diazepam or midazolam (dogs or cats). A 1:1 combination of tiletamine and zolazepam (Telazol) also produces dose-dependent central nervous system depression and muscle relaxation.

Anesthetic Induction

The most commonly used induction drugs are the ultrashort-acting barbiturates thiopental and thiamylal. Thiobarbiturates are used cautiously in patients with pre-existing cardiac arrhythmias because they are arrhythmogenic when given rapidly or in large doses. Alternatives to thiobarbiturates should be used in severely hypovolemic, hypotensive patients or when severe cardiac disease or pre-existing dysrhythmias are present. Simultaneous administration of diazepam (0.2 mg/kg) or lidocaine (2.0 mg/kg) decreases barbiturate requirement and the incidence of cardiac arrhythmias.

Inhalation anesthetics are as hypotensive as barbiturates and are only safer as induction agents because they are more controllable and homeostatic mechanisms have longer to compensate for the depressant effects of inhalants during induction.

Ketamine is not recommended for anesthetic induction of trauma patients with severe closed head injury because it can increase intracranial pressure. Diazepam (0.2 mg/kg IV) and ketamine (2 to 3 mg/kg IV) can be given in rapid sequence to induce anesthesia in traumatized dogs or cats. Delivery of low concentrations of halothane or isoflurane (0.5 to 1.0 per cent) by face mask completes the induction if the patient is not sufficiently depressed after diazepam-ketamine administration.

Opioid induction usually necessitates concomitant use of an adjunctive tranquilizer-sedative (neuroleptanalgesia) or inhalation anesthetic. Oxymorphone is commonly given intravenously to depressed trauma victims, in small increments (0.05 mg/kg) along with diazepam (0.2 mg/kg) until intubation is possible. Alternatively, midazolam (0.2 mg/kg) and oxymorphone (0.1 to 0.2 mg/kg) can be administered intramuscularly to induce neuroleptanalgesia.

Etomidate is useful for induction in patients in shock or with severe chronic cardiac disease. Etomidate produces minimal hemodynamic alterations and cardiac depression at 0.5 to 2.0 mg/kg IV.

Anesthetic Maintenance

The first priority during maintenance of anesthesia is adequate ventilation. Mechanical ventilation may be necessary for normal gas exchange. Second, preservation of hemodynamic stability is essential. This is achieved by providing adequate intravascular volume, administering positive inotropes if necessary, and using anesthetic drugs judiciously.

Dissociatives

Ketamine given with diazepam or midazolam can be used to maintain anesthesia for short periods in cardiovascularly unstable patients. Ketamine is repeated at an approximate dosage of 1 to 2 mg/kg/IV every 20 to 30 minutes or as necessary to keep the patient anesthetized. Diazepam or midazolam can also be repeated (0.2 mg/kg/IV) every 30 to 60 minutes or as necessary to provide adequate muscle relaxation. Similarly, tiletamine plus zolazepam (Telazol) may be useful when given in low doses for minimal restraint. These injectable regimens are often supplemented with low concentrations of halothane or isoflurane (0.5 to 1.0 per cent) if anesthesia is extended.

Inhalation Agents

The use of high concentrations of nitrous oxide (70 per cent) cannot be routinely recommended because trauma patients frequently have pulmonary contusions with increased venous admixture, and large arterial-alveolar oxygen gradients.

Isoflurane, like halothane and methoxyflurane, is hypotensive but does not sensitize the myocardium to the arrhythmogenic effects of catecholamines as does halothane. Isoflurane depresses the myocardium less and is a more potent vasodilator. Consequently, isoflurane is the preferred inhalation agent in patients with congestive heart failure or those with severe dysrhythmias.

Regional and Local Anesthesia

Epidural or spinal blocks are contraindicated in trauma patients with severe hemorrhage. Sympathetic blockade induced by local anesthetics can cause acute hypotension. Epidural or intrathecal administration of opioids or alpha$_2$ agonists may prove effective alternatives to local anesthetics in providing analgesia without sympathetic blockade. Superficial lacerations and wounds of the extremities can be managed with infiltration of local anesthetic (e.g., lidocaine) in severely depressed, calm, and stoic patients.

Anesthetic Support

Contraction of extracellular volume occurs with hemorrhage as the intravascular compartment is autotransfused with interstitial fluid. Intravenous administration of a crystalloid solution such as lactated Ringer restores this depletion and expands intravascular volume to help maintain cardiac output. Patients generally should be given 20 to 40 ml/kg IV before anesthetic induction. Fluids can be given rapidly into the intraosseous space of the tibia and femur if necessary. Patients in hypovolemic shock can be given one blood volume (80 ml/kg dog; 60 ml/kg cat) of isotonic electrolyte solution in the first hour.

Colloid solutions probably have little advantage in resuscitating hypovolemic patients, although this opinion is controversial. Increasing evidence suggests that hypertonic saline may be beneficial in the early treatment of hypovolemic and hemorrhagic shock. Intravenous administration of small volumes (4 to 6 ml/kg) of 7.5 per cent hypertonic saline results in beneficial cardiovascular effects in dogs and cats.

Red blood cells are administered when extreme blood loss (>40 per cent of blood volume) occurs. Fresh whole blood (<6 hours old) is preferable. Regardless of age, whole blood is preferred to packed red blood cells. Fresh-frozen plasma is reserved for specific coagulation disorders. Surgery and anesthesia are delayed until the packed cell volume can be increased to above 20 per cent.

Traumatized dogs and cats often have metabolic acidosis due to shock, hypothermia, and generalized stress. Ventilation of the lungs to induce a mild respiratory alkalosis helps normalize blood pH. Improved tissue perfusion (fluids) and renal and hepatic function should resolve the problem. Treatment with sodium bicarbonate is reserved for severe metabolic acidosis.

Normal urine output is maintained to prevent acute oliguric renal failure. Maintenance of renal function and diuresis is necessary to reduce intracranial pressure if head injury has occurred. Mannitol can be administered (0.5 g/kg IV bolus) once fluid volume and blood pressure are normal. Furosemide (1 mg/kg) and dopamine (2 to 5 µg/kg/min) can be used to increase renal blood flow and water and solute excretion.

CHAPTER 167

Anesthesia and the Urinary System (pages 2267–2271)

EFFECTS OF ABNORMAL RENAL FUNCTION ON ANESTHESIA (p. 2267)

Few anesthetic drugs rely on the kidneys for primary elimination. There are a few exceptions to this rule (Table 167–1).

The most important effect of renal disease on the pharmacokinetics of anesthetic drugs results from changes in body fluid composition. Azotemia influences the plasma protein binding of thiobarbiturates. Less protein binding results in a higher concentration of unbound (active) thiopental, making more drug available to cross the blood-brain barrier and produce an anesthetic effect. Other drugs that are

TABLE 167–1. AZOTEMIA: DIFFERENTIATION AND ANTICIPATED METABOLIC CHANGES

	Prerenal	Primary Renal	Postrenal
Blood urea nitrogen	Increased	Increased	Increased
Creatinine	Increased	Increased	Increased
Urine specific gravity	>1.040	<1.030	Variable
Urinalysis	Normal	Abnormal	Abnormal
Urine volume	Decreased	Variable	None/decreased
PCV/Total protein	Increased	Anemic (CRF)	Increased
Potassium	Normal	Increased (ARF)	Increased
Phosphorus	Normal	Increased	Increased
Metabolic acidosis	Slight	Compensated	Uncompensated

ARF, acute renal failure; CRF, chronic renal failure; PCV, packed cell volume.

highly protein bound, such as diazepam and midazolam, may also be affected in this way, and reduced doses are usually indicated.

EFFECTS OF ANESTHESIA ON RENAL FUNCTION
(pp. 2267–2269)

The effects of anesthetic drugs on renal function in animals with impaired kidneys are of concern because the potential exists to inadvertently exacerbate the renal disease with anesthesia. This can occur through direct effects of certain anesthetic drugs that are nephrotoxic or it can occur with relatively nontoxic drugs by indirect effects on hemodynamics, neuroendocrine responses, and urine production.

Among anesthetic drugs, only the inhalation agent methoxyflurane directly causes nephrotoxicity. Methoxyflurane can be especially deleterious when used in combination with other nephrotoxic drugs.

Renal blood flow is a product of systemic arterial blood pressure and compliance of the renal vasculature. Therefore, renal blood flow and glomerular function may be depressed as a consequence of systemic hypotension, renal vasoconstriction, or a combination of the two. Irreparable kidney damage can occur in an animal that suffered from only mild renal compromise preoperatively.

Renal blood flow diminishes markedly if the mean arterial blood pressure drops below 80 mm Hg. Even with adequate mean blood pressure, renal perfusion can be inadequate if renal vascular resistance is too high. The blood vessels of the kidneys are richly innervated by sympathetic nerve fibers that mediate vasoconstriction through alpha-adrenergic receptors. Stress, excitement, pain, and light anesthetic planes all can result in sympathetic stimulation. Animals with renal disease respond most favorably if given adequate sedation, analgesia, and stress-free handling.

All general anesthetic drugs in animals with or without renal disease temporarily depress renal function as a result of diminished cardiac output. Epidural anesthesia may produce minimal alterations in renal function. Epidural anesthesia blocks sympathetic fibers in the thoracolumbar spine and prevents renal vasoconstriction.

It is important to remember that the renal effects of anesthetics are dose related and are favorably influenced by adequate repletion of extracellular fluid with intravenous fluid therapy.

FLUID THERAPY FOR PATIENTS WITH RENAL DISEASE
(p. 2269)

One of the keys to successful anesthetic management of animals with renal disease is maintaining proper intravascular volume throughout the anesthetic and operative period. Many patients with acute renal diseases, such as acute renal failure or acute obstructive disease of the urinary tract, present with significant dehydration and oliguria. Preoperative administration of intravenous fluids is a necessity in these animals. A balanced electrolyte solution such as lactated Ringer's is usually appropriate to restore circulating blood volume. Depending on preoperative electrolyte concentrations, 0.9 per cent sodium chloride may be suitable to stimulate urine production. Adequate urine production is 1 to 2 ml/kg/hr. If less than 0.5 ml/kg/hr of urine is produced despite efforts at rehydration, diuretics should be considered before anesthesia. Mannitol (0.25 to 0.5 g/kg) is a good choice for operative diuresis. Its peak effect occurs within 30 minutes. Mannitol should not be used in an animal that is already overhydrated, has renal hypertension, or suffers from congestive cardiac disease.

Fluid therapy is maintained at an initial rate of 10 ml/kg/hr during anesthesia. Useful indices for determining the adequacy of operative fluid therapy include systemic blood pressure (mean blood pressure >80 mm Hg), central venous pressure (<10 cm H_2O), or urine output (>0.5 ml/kg/hr).

Patients with chronic renal damage may be deficient in erythropoietin, a hormone that is produced by the kidneys and stimulates red blood cell production. If the hematocrit falls to 15 per cent or less, blood transfusion is recommended.

Azotemia can also be associated with prolonged bleeding time despite normal platelet numbers. Azotemia interferes with platelet function. Pretreatment with desmopressin acetate (DDAVP, 1 μg/kg SC) may be beneficial in minimizing the risk of prolonged bleeding.

ACID-BASE AND ELECTROLYTE DISORDERS OF RENAL DISEASE (pp. 2269–2270)

Metabolic acidosis is a common finding with most types of renal disease. If an animal has a metabolic acidosis with a pH greater than 7.25, the appropriate preanesthetic treatment is fluid therapy to improve both tissue perfusion and urine production, reducing the base deficit. If an animal's pH is less than 7.20, fluid therapy is warranted, followed by sodium bicarbonate therapy if the response to fluid therapy is inadequate. To minimize the likelihood of these complications, treat with only half of the calculated extracellular fluid bicarbonate deficit:

$$\frac{\text{body weight (kg)} \times 0.3 \times \text{base deficit}}{2}$$

A relatively safe dose of sodium bicarbonate to use if the base deficit is unknown is 0.5 mEq/kg.

Hyperkalemia is sometimes found in patients with renal disease and can be extreme and immediately life threatening in acute obstructive renal disorders. If an animal has a serum potassium level greater than 6 mEq/L, preoperative fluid therapy with a balanced electrolyte solution reduces the potassium to normal levels through improved urine production and dilutional effects. If the serum potassium is greater than 6.5 mEq/L and cardiac effects such as bradycardia or spiked T waves are evident on an electrocardiogram, then treatment might include one or more of the following: intravenous 5 per cent dextrose and regular insulin, sodium bicarbonate administration, administration of calcium gluconate, or the use of ion-exchange resins.

SUGGESTED ANESTHETIC TECHNIQUES FOR RENAL DISEASE (pp. 2270–2271)

Premedication

Premedication is a wise idea, unless the animal is extremely depressed as a result of its disease.

Induction and Anesthesia

All intravenous induction drugs used in veterinary medicine are acceptable for use in patients with urinary tract disease. Thiobarbiturates are safe provided that a reduced dose is used and adequate volume replacement is carried out to prevent significant hypotension. Mask inductions with inhalation anesthetics can also be used and may be the technique of choice in an animal that is depressed or well sedated. Methoxyflurane should not be used because of its potential to cause nephrotoxicity. Both halothane and isoflurane are effective inhalation agents; however, isoflurane offers the advantage of minimal biotransformation and little likelihood for tissue toxicity.

CHAPTER 168

Anesthesia for Central Nervous System and Ophthalmic Surgery (pages 2271–2278)

Central Nervous System (pages 2271–2276)

PHYSIOLOGICAL CONCERNS (pp. 2271–2273)

The brain and spinal cord are protected within the bony skull and vertebral column. Increases in blood flow within the noncompliant cranial vault cause an increase in intracranial volume and pressure. Once increases in cerebral blood flow cause the intracranial volume to exceed the limits of effective compliance, intracranial pressure sharply increases. The results of substantial increases in intracranial pressure include life-threatening systemic manifestations, worsening of cerebral ischemia, and eventually brain herniation.

Anesthetic-induced depression of the central nervous system is usually accompanied by decreased cerebral metabolic rate or cerebral metabolic oxygen requirement. This decrease in oxygen requirement can be protective in possible relative ischemia during anesthesia and neurosurgery. Isoflurane and barbiturates contribute substantially to reduced cerebral metabolic oxygen requirement and afford some cerebral protection.

Cerebral blood flow increases when arterial oxygenation decreases below 50 mm Hg. Cerebral blood flow increases by about 2 ml/min/100 g of brain tissue for every 1 mm Hg increase in Pa_{CO_2}. Hyperventilation electively reduces cerebral blood flow, resulting in cerebral vasoconstriction and reduced tissue bulk. Deliberate hyperventilation to reduce intracranial pressure can be risky as an adjunct to deliberate hypotension when mean arterial blood pressures are less than 50 mm Hg.

Fluid Therapy

Restriction of intravenous fluids to only that volume necessary to maintain adequate circulating volume is recommended in neurosurgical patients with increased intracranial pressure. Diuretic therapy is frequently indicated in medical management of patients with intracranial masses and elevated intracranial pressure or cerebral edema.

Hyperglycemia is contraindicated in animals with cerebral ischemia, and cerebral edema can be exacerbated by administration of isotonic dextrose.

Glucocorticoid Therapy

Glucocorticoids are effective in treating some forms of cerebral edema. Corticosteroids reduce the increased intracranial pressure resulting from brain tumors and hydrocephalus. Steroid therapy is probably of little value once cerebral ischemia has occurred. Glucocorticoid therapy should optimally begin the day before neurosurgery when possible. Dexamethasone is recommended at 0.25 mg/kg every 8 hours, with a dose of 0.25 to 1 mg/kg IV after induction of anesthesia.

Positional Effects

Jugular venous occlusion increased intracranial pressure in patients with pre-existing increases. Slight elevation of the head above the level of the heart with the neck in a neutral position facilitates venous drainage and reduces intracranial pressure.

DELIBERATE HYPOTENSION (p. 2273)

Deliberate hypotension is occasionally indicated during neurosurgery.

However, reduction of arterial blood pressure is rarely necessary in anesthetized animals, particularly if volatile anesthetics are used.

ANESTHETIC CONCERNS (pp. 2273–2274)

Volatile Anesthetics

Volatile anesthetics increase cerebral blood flow and alter cerebral metabolic oxygen requirement to various degrees. Because increased cerebral blood flow and intracranial pressure are also influenced by carbon dioxide retention, respiratory depression associated with volatile anesthesia can be responsible for clinically significant increases in intracranial pressure. Halothane blocks autoregulation. Methoxyflurane, enflurane, and isoflurane all interfere with autoregulation less than halothane.

Modest hyperventilation to reduce arterial carbon dioxide to about 30 mm Hg eliminates the volatile anesthetic-induced increase in cerebral blood flow. Nitrous oxide has substantial cerebrovascular effects, profoundly increasing in cerebral blood flow and intracranial pressure.

Injectable Anesthetics

Most injectable anesthetics cause significant reductions in cerebral metabolic oxygen requirement, cerebral blood flow, and intracranial pressure. The value of barbiturates as therapy for cerebral ischemia/hypoxia is controversial.

The dissociative anesthetics increase cerebral blood flow, intracranial pressure, and cerebral metabolic oxygen requirement. Patients with a history of seizure-related disorders, intracranial masses, craniocerebral trauma, and other conditions potentially increasing intracranial pressure should not receive dissociative anesthetics.

SPECIFIC ANESTHETIC MANAGEMENT (pp. 2274–2276)

Electroencephalography and Seizure Disorders
(Table 168–1).

Myelography and Intervertebral Disc Disease
(Table 168–2).

Intracranial Masses and Elevated Intracranial Pressure (Table 168–3).

TABLE 168–1. ANESTHETIC MANAGEMENT FOR SEIZURE-PRONE PATIENTS AND FOR DIAGNOSTIC ELECTROENCEPHALOGRAPHY

Control of seizures

Treatment or avoidance of hypoglycemia.
Avoid phenothiazine (e.g., acepromazine) and butyrophenone (e.g., droperidol) tranquilizers.
Benzodiazepine (diazepam, 0.4 mg/kg IM or IV) tranquilization or barbiturate (phenobarbital, 2 to 5 mg/kg IM) sedation.
Intravenous induction with thiobarbiturate (thiamylal or thiopental) but not methohexital.
Inhalational induction with isoflurane or halothane but not with enflurane.
Avoidance of increases in cerebral blood flow and intracranial pressure.

Diagnostic electroencephalography

Avoid preanesthetic tranquilizers and sedatives.
Intravenous induction with thiobarbiturate.
Maintain light plane of anesthesia with halothane or incremental thiobarbiturate if necessary to prolong duration.
Infiltration of temporal muscles with lidocaine as an alternative to general anesthesia.

Anesthesia for Ophthalmic Surgery
(pages 2276–2278)

The two goals for anesthetic management of patients undergoing ophthalmic surgery are (1) to avoid increases in intraocular pressure and (2) to support cardiopulmonary function.

INTRAOCULAR PRESSURE (pp. 2276–2277)

Intraocular pressure is influenced by several major physiological factors, including aqueous humor fluid dynamics, choroidal blood volume, central venous pressure, vitreous humor volume, and extraocular muscle tone.

TABLE 168–2. ANESTHETIC MANAGEMENT FOR MYELOGRAPHY AND INTERVERTEBRAL DISC DISEASE

Myelography and surgical decompression

Benzodiazepine tranquilization (e.g., diazepam, 0.4 mg/kg IV).
Low-dose opioid agonist-antagonists (e.g., butorphanol, 0.4 mg/kg IM).
Anticholinergics if indicated.
Intravenous induction with thiobarbiturate or inhalational induction with isoflurane or halothane by mask.
Avoid hyperflexion/extension of neck in patients with cervical trauma, instability, and disc disease.
Maintenance of protected airway and spontaneous ventilation (for recognition of side effects of myelography and to minimize vertebral sinus blood flow during surgery).
Fluid therapy with dextrose for metrizamide myelography.
Positioning to avoid venous occlusion.
Postoperative analgesics as needed.

TABLE 168–3. ANESTHETIC MANAGEMENT FOR PATIENTS WITH ELEVATED CBF/ICP AND FOR INTRACRANIAL SURGERY

Preanesthetic critical care management and stabilization (including glucocorticoid and diuretic therapy as indicated).
Fluid therapy limited to minimize cerebral edema but adequate to support circulation.
Avoid potent respiratory depression, jugular venous occlusion, and coughing at induction of anesthesia and during recovery.
Avoid dissociatives, halothane, enflurane, and nitrous oxide.
Intravenous barbiturate induction of anesthesia.
Minimal concentrations of isoflurane, supplemented with opioids or barbiturates for maintenance of anesthesia.
Modest hyperventilation (30 mm Hg) to reduce CBF/ICP.
Postoperative critical care with support of ventilation and circulation as indicated.

Most anesthetic medications decrease intraocular pressure by reducing cardiac output or systemic blood pressure or both, relaxing extraocular muscles, or increasing aqueous outflow. Barbiturates and narcotics are acceptable induction agents.

Early studies demonstrated that ketamine caused an increase in intraocular pressure. Studies now suggest that intraocular pressure is actually decreased.

PREANESTHETIC ASSESSMENT AND MEDICATION
(p. 2277)

Adequate ventilation is important for patients with eye disease. Patients with ophthalmic disease are frequently medicated with a carbonic anhydrase inhibitor such as acetazolamide (Diamox) or dichlorphenamide (Daranide) for control of intraocular pressure. These drugs can produce a significant metabolic acidemia, and hyperventilation is a normal compensatory mechanism. Anesthetic-induced hypoventilation worsens a patient's acidosis and complicates anesthetic management.

Severe bradyarrhythmias and cardiac arrest due to stimulation of the oculocardiac reflex have been documented and occur infrequently. The oculocardiac reflex is due to direct pressure or traction on extraocular muscles. As a protective measure against the oculocardiac reflex and other vagally mediated cardiac arrhythmias, patients are premedicated with an anticholinergic such as atropine (0.02 mg/kg IM or SC) or glycopyrrolate (0.01 mg/kg IM or SC).

ANESTHETIC MANAGEMENT (pp. 2277–2278)

A quiet, struggle-free recovery is important to avoid trauma to the eyes.

The combined effects of a tranquilizer and narcotic (neuroleptanalgesia) may be used to both calm and provide pain relief, facilitating management of patients with increased intraocular pressures or corneal lacerations. Anesthesia can be induced with any standard anesthetic induction technique.

Intubation is always recommended for animals under general anesthesia. Gentle intubation with the animal at an appropriate level of anesthesia minimizes laryngeal stimulation and reduces the chance for increases in intraocular pressure.

All inhalant anesthetics—methoxyflurane, halothane, isoflurane, and nitrous oxide—reduce intraocular pressure as much as 35 to 50 per cent of awake values. A patient's head is frequently covered with surgical drapes, making it difficult to monitor traditional signs of anesthetic depth such as jaw tone, mucous membrane color, capillary refill time, lingual pulse, and ocular reflexes.

Central or peripheral muscle relaxants may be used to ensure a quiet eye and as an alternative to deep general anesthesia. Routine use of such newer peripheral muscle relaxants such as atracurium and vecuronium offers specific advantages such as an intermedied duration of action (10 to 20 minutes), minimal cardiovascular effects, minimal if any histamine release, and no effect on intraocular pressure. The combination of atropine (0.02 mg/kg IV) followed by neostigmine (0.02 mg/kg IV) is used to reverse the effects of peripheral muscle relaxants.

CHAPTER 169
Anesthesia for Upper Airway and Thoracic Surgery
(pages 2278–2284)

MANAGEMENT OF RESPIRATORY PATIENT DURING ANESTHESIA (pp. 2279–2280)
Airway Management Techniques

Several techniques are available for ensuring a patent airway. The most common is orotracheal intubation using a cuffed endotracheal tube. A high-volume, low-pressure cuff is preferred to seal the airway should ventilatory support be necessary. Alternate techniques of airway management increase tracheostomy or pharyngostomy intubation. The animal is initially intubated after anesthetic induction, and tracheostomy or pharyngostomy is performed aseptically. Oxygen and an anesthetic gas can be adminstered by face mask if intubation is not possible during the initial period.

Ventilatory Support

The goal of ventilatory support is to mimic normal ventilation. Tidal volume is approximately 15 ml/kg. Normal respiratory rate is 6 to 12 breaths per minute. The maximum airway pressure during ventilation is 15 to 18 cm H_2O in the dog and 12 to 15 cm H_2O in the cat. Increased airway pressure of 20 to 30 cm H_2O may be required to maintain adequate volume in open chest procedures. The ratio of inspiration to expiration is 1:2 or 1:3.

Ventilation can be provided by manual compression of the reservoir bag or by mechanical ventilation. A volume-cycled ventilator has a preset tidal volume delivered regardless of airway pressure generated in delivering the breath. A pressure-limited ventilator delivers the gas volume until a preset pressure value is reached.

Ventilatory support is usually administered as intermittent positive-pressure ventilation, which mimics normal breathing. Additional techniques may be used with intermittent positive-pressure ventilation. Positive end-expiratory pressure can be used with intermittent positive-pressure ventilation to help keep small airways open. A similar technique, continuous positive airway pressure, can be used in patients who are ventilating spontaneously. Continuous positive airway pressure allows the animal to take spontaneous breaths while maintaining a basal positive airway pressure. The scavenging hose of the pressure-relief (pop-off) valve can be mechanically restricted to produce the desired degree of positive end-expiratory pressure.

Resistance to ventilation may be encountered during ventilatory support. Inadequate anesthetic depth may be the cause; however, increased anesthetic depth may be undesirable. Supplemental analgesia can be provided. Muscle relaxants may be indicated to overcome patient resistance and allow surgery to proceed. Atracurium besylate or pancuronium bromide are the drugs of choice.

Reversal of muscle relaxation may be necessary after surgery to reestablish spontaneous breathing.

Monitoring

The parameters to monitor in the respiratory patient are similar to those monitored in other patients. Additional emphasis is placed on the assessment of oxygenation and tissue perfusion in patients with special considerations regarding their pre-existing cardiorespiratory disease.

Color and refill of mucous membranes provide information regarding oxygen delivery to tissues. Arterial blood gas evaluation provides information regarding adequacy of ventilation and gas exchange. Pulse oximetry is a technique that works by noninvasive placement of a sensor on the skin or mucous membranes. Normal hemoglobin saturation value, as measured by pulse oximetry, is 98 to 100 per cent, moderate desaturation occurs at less than 90 per cent, and severe hypoxemia occurs at or below 85 per cent. Capnometry measurement of carbon dioxide (in expired gas) can be used to evaluate overall integrity of the respiratory tract.

MANAGEMENT OF RESPIRATORY PATIENT DURING RECOVERY (pp. 2280–2281)

Availability of equipment to provide supplemental airway support and oxygenation following extubation is important to prevent hypoxemia and hypoventilation in the immediate postoperative period. Evaluation of the patient following extubation should continue for 15 minutes. Assessment of mucous membrane color and refill, respiratory rate and effort, and heart rate and pulse quality provides information regarding patient stability.

Patients undergoing thoracotomy require additional consideration. In most cases, a chest drain is inserted through the thoracic wall prior to closure. The tube is used to remove air and fluid from the pleural cavity.

Pain relief following thoracic surgery may be necessary to ensure adequate gas exchange. Intercostal nerve block after lateral thoracotomy is useful for providing analgesia. Bupivacaine hydrochloride (Marcaine 0.5%) is recommended for analgesia because it provides 6 to 8 hours of analgesia per administration. An injection of 0.5 ml per nerve is used. Bupivacaine may also be infused through the chest drain to provide analgesia by intrapleural analgesia. Bupivacaine is combined with saline (1:1 v/v) prior to injection into the thoracic chest tube. The duration of analgesia ranges from 4 to 12 hours with this technique.

Opioids can also be used for pain relief in the post-thoracotomy patient. Butorphanol's analgesic duration is shorter than that of oxymorphone; buprenorphine is longer in duration than butorphanol. Oxymorphone or butorphanol in combination with a tranquilizer works well in the cat for postsurgical pain management. Buprenorphine does not produce central nervous system depression.

Upper-Airway Corrective Procedures. Laryngeal procedures such as partial laryngectomy for laryngeal paralysis and removal of everted laryngeal saccules are usually performed through an oral approach. These procedures may require an unguarded airway or alternate airway management. Oral intubation, airway suctioning, and recovery with oxygen support are performed. The endotracheal tube cuff is inflated to help minimize introduction of blood into the trachea. The cuff is kept partially inflated during extubation to remove blood clots.

Tracheal Procedures. Tracheal lacerations, tracheal collapse, and tracheal neoplasia are the most common diseases encountered that require anesthetic support. Anesthetic induction is rapid and airway control is achieved. Orotracheal intubation is accomplished as quickly as possible. Supplemental oxygen administered by nasal catheter or face mask can prevent hypoxemia in the immediate postanesthetic period.

Chest Wall Injuries. Chest wall injuries are often associated with trauma and require special consideration because of their effects on respiratory mechanics and gas exchange. Traumatic myocarditis is often associated with chest wall injury. Arrhythmogenic anesthetics such as xylazine hydrochloride, thiobarbiturates, and halothane are avoided if traumatic myocarditis is present.

Preoxygenation is provided during the preparation and induction periods to facilitate oxygen transport. Anesthetic techniques that provide rapid induction are selected; orotracheal intubation is immediately initiated. Anesthetic maintenance is usually provided by inhalational agents. Monitoring techniques associated with the high-risk patient include analysis of arterial blood gases and electrocardiography. Supplemental oxygenation maintains systemic oxygenation during postoperative hypoventilation and ventilation/perfusion mismatching. Pain management by local nerve blocks and by parenteral analgesics facilitates normal breathing in the postsurgical period.

Pleural Space Disease. Space-occupying lesions such as hemothorax, pyothorax, pneumothorax, chylothorax, and intrapleural masses create abnormal pulmonary compliance and dynamics.

Drainage of fluid or air from the pleural space by thoracentesis or placement of a thoracostomy tube re-establishes cardiorespiratory stability prior to anesthesia. Supplemental oxygen administration by nasal catheter or face mask is important in the preoperative period. Induction techniques that permit rapid control and management of the airway are preferred in cases with no or minimal cardiovascular dysfunction. Anesthetic maintenance with inhalation anesthesia is acceptable.

Postoperative management includes continued drainage of the pleural cavity until air or fluid cannot be withdrawn. Supplemental oxygenation is critical.

Diaphragmatic Hernia. Supplemental oxygenation by nasal catheter or face mask is beneficial preoperatively. If gastric entrapment and dilation have occurred, percutaneous gastrocentesis can be performed to reduce intragastric volume prior to surgical correction.

Ventilation is supported immediately following induction and orotracheal intubation. Positive-pressure ventilation should not exceed 15 to 20 cm H_2O pressure, at which level too rapid re-expansion of atelectatic lung regions and subsequent pulmonary edma may occur.

Primary Pulmonary Disease. The lung may undergo several disease processes that require surgical correction. Foreign bodies, abscesses, neoplasia, and lung lobe torsion may require partial or total lobectomy as part of the treatment.

These patients are considered at risk for anesthetic complications. Preoxygenation is provided during the preparation and induction period to facilitate oxygen transport. Anesthetic techniques that provide rapid induction are selected. Orotracheal intubation and initiation of ventilatory support by intermittent positive-pressure ventilation are immediately performed. Low levels of positive end-expiratory pressure (5 cm H_2O) may be added during surgery to maintain alveolar inflation.

Patent Ductus Arteriosus. Dogs can be premedicated with an opioid and atropine or with a low dose of acepromazine intramuscularly. Cats can be premedicated with ketamine, a ketamine-tranquilizer combination, or a neuroleptanalgesic. Anesthesia is maintained with inhalation anesthesia. Once the animal is intubated, intermittent positive-pressure ventilation is begun. Trial ligation of the patent ductus arteriosus indicates the potential of reflex bradycardia. Administration of anticholinergic drugs to inhibit vagal reflexes usually reverses reflex bradycardia.

Pericardial Disease. Cardiac tamponade can cause significant hemodynamic changes that can be aggravated during anesthesia. Bradycardia, if present, increases the severity of cardiac dysfunction. Drugs providing inotropic support are commonly used during surgery and postoperatively.

CHAPTER 170
Anesthesia for Gastrointestinal Surgery
(pages 2284–2289)

GASTROINTESTINAL PHYSIOLOGY AND EFFECTS OF ANESTHESIA (pp. 2284–2286)

Hepatic Blood Flow. To function properly, the liver depends on a dual blood supply from the portal vein and the hepatic artery. Isoflurane produces the least reduction in portal blood flow, and increases hepatic artery blood flow. Halothane decreases blood flow from both sources in proportion to the dose-related decrease in cardiac output. Methoxyflurane also causes a marked reduction in hepatic blood flow.

Drug Metabolism. Both halothane and methoxyflurane induce hepatic microsomal enzymes, particularly with prolonged or multiple exposures. Under conditions in which the enzymes are induced, the level of potentially harmful metabolites generated from the biotransformation of the inhalant anesthetics may be increased, leading to organ toxicity. If hypoxia exists, metabolism of halothane can lead to the production of free radicals, rather than to the nontoxic trifluoracetic acid produced under aerobic conditions. The free radicals can in turn lead to lipid peroxidation of the hepatocyte.

Isoflurane is an inhalant anesthetic that undergoes no measurable hepatic metabolism. Nitrous oxide undergoes no hepatic metabolism and is useful in the management of patients with liver disease.

Acepromazine is a phenothiazine tranquilizer that undergoes extensive and prolonged hepatic metabolism. Acepromazine in patients with severe liver disease may have a prolonged duration of action and increases the metabolic demand placed on the already compromised liver. The primary advantage of the opioids in patients with liver disease is the ability to reverse the effects of the drug with a specific antagonist. Hepatic disease prolongs the duration of action of thiobarbiturates and can also prolong the recovery of dogs from large doses of cyclohexylamines.

Carbohydrate Metabolism. Glucose homeostasis depends on normal hepatic function. In cases of severe liver disease, hypoglycemia is possible and dextrose supplementation should be considered. Xylazine is capable of producing marked hyperglycemia. This response is probably blunted in the patient with liver disease because of inadequate glucose reserves, but significant hyperglycemia may result if dextrose is administered supplementally.

Coagulation. Most of the coagulation factors are produced in the liver. Tests for adequate coagulation are performed prior to surgery, and replacement therapy is initiated if coagulation is impaired.

Protein. The liver is also responsible for production of albumin. Replacement therapy is appropriate for severe reductions in albumin (<1.5 g/dl). The dose of anesthetic drugs that are highly protein bound should be reduced (thiobarbiturates, benzodiazepines).

Cerebral Sensitivity. Sensitivity to certain anesthetic agents is increased in many patients with liver disease. Drugs that act via the α-aminobutyric acid receptors (barbiturates and benzodiazepines) may therefore have a greater effect under these conditions.

Alimentary Tract

Salivary Glands. Indications for the use of anticholinergics include oral surgery, mask induction in brachycephalic breeds when airway security could be compromised, animals that salivate excessively prior to anesthesia, and animals that have laryngeal disease and have previously undergone or are considered at high risk for pathologic aspiration. Glycopyrrolate is less likely to produce dysrhythmias, and its antisialogogue effect is two to three times that of atropine.

Gastrointestinal Motility. The anticholinergics decrease gastrointestinal motility and pressure across the lower esophageal sphincter, potentially making regurgitation easier for the patient.

Morphine, oxymorphone, and meperidine have a spasmogenic effect on the gastrointestinal system. Morphine, oxymorphone, and fentanyl can also frequently cause transient vomiting shortly after administration, secondary to stimulation of the central nervous system. Xylazine is also associated with emesis and, when administered as a premedicant, consistently produces vomiting in cats, and to a lesser degree in dogs.

Gastrointestinal Secretions. Both atropine and glycopyrrolate decrease gastric acidity and volume in patients in which vomiting and aspiration, or gastric reflux, is probable. Glycopyrrolate is more effective than atropine in increasing pH.

Gas Distension. Distension of the gastrointestinal tract can be increased by the addition of nitrous oxide. Nitrous oxide is avoided when significant amounts of gas are known or suspected to be present in the gastrointestinal tract (or other closed space).

PREANESTHETIC CONSIDERATIONS (pp. 2286–2287)

The most effective approach to managing many of the potential anesthetic problems associated with the gastrointestinal system consists of withholding food from the patient if possible, for 8 to 12 hours prior to anesthesia. This recommendation is modified in neonates, aged patients, and animals weighing less than 3 kg. Emetics are never indicated except in cases of ingested toxins. These agents do not reliably empty the stomach, are stressful to the patient, and risk aspiration.

Assessment of hepatic function usually involves the evaluation of liver enzymes, direct and indirect bilirubin, and albumin (total protein or solids). Blood urea nitrogen is often decreased in patients with portosystemic shunts. More elaborate tests of hepatic function can be pursued if liver disease is suspected, but not confirmed, from these screening tests. These tests include the analysis of bile acids, urinary bile pigments, and clearance of organic anion dyes removed from the circulation by the liver (sulfobromophthalein sodium and indocyanine green). Evaluation of a patient with a portosystemic shunt often includes a determination of baseline ammonia level and an ammonia tolerance test.

Patients that have chronic vomiting or diarrhea, gastric dilatation–volvulus, or an obstructive lesion can all be expected to have some degree of acid-base and electrolyte disorder. Analysis of blood gases, when possible, is useful in the evaluation of these patients. Electrocardiography is performed prior to anesthesia if significant electrolyte imbalances are present, and in all cases of gastric dilatation–volvulus.

ANESTHETIC MANAGEMENT CONSIDERATIONS
(pp. 2287–2289)

Liver

Potential complications of anesthesia administered to a patient with hepatic dysfunction are related to alterations in the normal liver processes (Table 170–1).

TABLE 170–1. ANESTHETIC COMPLICATIONS ASSOCIATED WITH HEPATIC DISEASE

Anticipated Problems	Anesthetic Considerations
Decreased hepatic blood flow	Administer adequate fluid therapy. Use isoflurane, nitrous oxide, opioids, and diazepam to maintain blood flow.
Decreased drug metabolism	Minimize doses of anesthetic agents. Use drugs not dependent on hepatic metabolism (isoflurane, nitrous oxide). Use reversible drugs (opioids).
Hypoglycemia	Supplement dextrose-containing fluids (5% or 2.5%, 10 ml/kg/hr). Avoid xylazine.
Coagulation defects	Administer vitamin K therapy. Administer fresh plasma or cryoprecipitate.
Hypoproteinemia	Administer fresh or stored plasma. Administer dextran 40 or 70, or hetastarch.
Biliary spasm	Avoid certain opioid agonists (oxymorphone).
Anesthetic-induced hepatitis	Avoid repeated, prolonged exposure to halothane and methoxyflurane.

Oral Cavity

The major anesthetic problems associated with oropharyngeal surgery are related to mechanical difficulties that may be encountered during the procedure.

The endotracheal tube can be introduced into the pharynx through the site used for a pharyngotomy tube. If insufficient, a tracheostomy can be performed, and the airway secured with a tracheostomy or endotracheal tube.

Cuffed endotracheal tubes should be securely in position whenever feasible. The patient is extubated with the cuff partially inflated, and the head positioned lower than the body. Steroids or furosemide are often used if edema or inflammation is expected.

Esophagus

Esophageal masses in some patients may partially obstruct the trachea. Animals with an obstructive esophageal lesion or megaesophagus are at high risk for regurgitation and aspiration. To reduce this possibility, induction and intubation are performed rapidly to secure the airway. The tube is positioned well below the site of esophageal injury (beyond the thoracic inlet). Preoxygenation of patients with aspiration pneumonia is indicated.

Stomach and Intestines

The choice of anesthetics is discussed using the patient with gastric dilatation–volvulus as an example. Gastric decompression of the patient is performed as soon as possible after presentation. Treatment of the dysrhythmias consists of lidocaine (1 to 2 mg/kg IV bolus) followed by infusion at 40 to 80 μg/kg/min procainamide (0.5 mg/kg) in refractory animals. Premedication may not be needed in very depressed patients. Butorphanol (0.2 mg/kg) or oxymorphone (0.1 mg/kg) is effective.

The severely depressed patient can often be induced by mask. Other acceptable techniques for induction include slow intravenous titration of oxymorphone (up to 0.2 mg/kg) or a combination of diazepam (0.2 mg/kg) and ketamine (2 to 4 mg/kg) administered intravenously. Maintenance is accomplished with isoflurane. Nitrous oxide is avoided.

Arterial blood gases are monitored if possible. Operative use of a positive inotropic agent (dopamine or dobutamine, 2 to 5 μg/kg/min) may be needed to support patients with severely depressed myocardial contractility and cardiac output.

Peritonitis and Ascites

Animals with peritonitis may be severely ill, exhibiting varying degrees of shock, abdominal fluid accumulation, and endotoxemia. Positioning the patient in dorsal recumbency inhibits the patient's ventilation. The abdominal fluid may contain a substantial amount of protein. Rapid withdrawal of this fluid during surgery can result in dramatic falls in blood pressure and in hypoproteinemia.

Protein must be replaced by the administration of plasma if hypotension and rapid crystalloid therapy results in dilutional hypoproteinemia. Hypertonic saline has been suggested for the treatment of hypovolemic shock.

Respiratory depressants are avoided in patients with depressed ventilation. The patient is placed in lateral recumbency for as long as possible, and two intravenous catheters are placed. Ventilation is monitored in recovery to ensure that it is adequate.

CHAPTER 171

Anesthesia and the Endocrine System (pages 2290–2294)

THE PANCREAS (pp. 2290–2291)

Diabetes Mellitus

The most important goal in the anesthetic management of the diabetic animal is to prevent hypoglycemia, which can result in brain damage. A practical approach is to produce moderate hyperglycemia (100 to 250 mg/100 ml) for a short time. Prolonged hyperglycemia is avoided.

The diabetic patient is investigated for evidence of hyperadrenocorticism or decreased renal function.

The patient is fed and treated normally on the day before surgery. On the morning of surgery, food is withheld, and only half the usual dose of insulin is administered. Blood glucose is measured before anesthesia, and if the value is less than 80 mg/100 ml, syrup or dextrose solution is administered before proceeding. Infusion of 5 per cent dextrose in water at 5 ml/kg/hr during anesthesia should maintain adequate blood glucose concentration. A non–dextrose-containing solution, such as lactated Ringer's solution, is also given at 5 ml/kg/hr to maintain blood volume. Blood glucose is measured at least every 2 hours during long procedures.

Preoperative anxiety and the surgical procedure may cause hyperglycemia through sympathetic stimulation and release of glucocorticoids. Most anesthetic drugs, with the exception of xylazine, cause only a minor change in blood glucose. Administration of xylazine causes a decrease in serum insulin and an increase in plasma glucose (200 to 500 per cent increase in cats and 69 per cent increase in dogs) for 3 to 4 hours.

A poorly regulated diabetic patient should be hospitalized and stabilized for 2 to 3 days before anesthesia. Blood glucose may need to be measured every 30 minutes during anesthesia.

Insulinoma

Avoidance of hypoglycemia is the main concern in the management of anesthetic patients with a beta-cell tumor of the pancreas. Fasting the patient before anesthesia is necessary but can result in dangerously low blood glucose levels. Hypoglycemia occurs within 4 to 6 hours of beginning a fast in some dogs with insulinoma. Therefore, monitoring of blood glucose levels and infusion of 5 per cent dextrose solution begin during the preanesthetic preparation.

A theoretical argument can be made for choosing anesthetic drugs that decrease cerebral metabolic rate and therefore presumably decrease cerebral metabolism of glucose. Ketamine produces a marked increase in cerebral metabolic rate.

Obese dogs with insulinoma benefit from controlled ventilation during anesthesia. Infusion of 5 per cent dextrose, in addition to balanced electrolyte solution, continues during anesthesia. Blood glucose is measured hourly. Severe hypoglycemia may occur during manipulation of the tumor, whereas a marked increase in blood glucose may occur after its removal. Consequently, blood glucose is measured frequently during and after surgery, and treatment is adjusted accordingly.

Pancreatitis

Patients with pancreatitis are often dehydrated and azotemic, and they may be in hypovolemic or endotoxic shock. Treatment before anesthesia should ensure replacement of blood volume, restoration of urine production, and correction of hypocalcemia.

Anesthetic drugs are chosen for an individual patient, and dose rates are decreased according to the degree of pre-existing central nervous system depression. The combination of tiletamine and zolazepam (Telazol) is contraindicated in patients with pancreatic disease.

Arterial blood pressure is monitored constantly throughout surgery, because manipulation of the inflamed pancreas may cause release of vasoactive substances, resulting in vasodilation and hypotension. Aggressive treatment with fluids, vasoconstrictive drugs, or cardiac stimulants may be indicated.

THE THYROID GLAND (pp. 2291–2292)

Hypothyroidism

Hypothyroidism increases the sensitivity of the central nervous system to anesthetic drugs. Hypothyroidism may be accompanied by hypotension and a decrease in cardiac output as much as 40 per cent because of reductions in heart rate and stroke volume. Hypothyroid patients are usually hypothermic and vasoconstricted and may have a low blood volume. Therefore, anesthetic drugs that cause vasodilation may precipitate hypotension.

Preferably, elective procedures should be postponed until the patient is rendered euthyroid. Severe hypothyroidism increases the risks associated with anesthesia and surgery. A single intravenous injection of L-thyroxine (20 to 40 μg/kg), given several hours before anesthesia, has been suggested for patients that have severe untreated hypothyroidism and require emergency anesthesia and surgery. Anesthesia can be maintained with low concentrations of an inhalation agent. Controlled ventilation may be necessary during anesthesia because hypothyroidism decreases respiratory function and hypoxic ventilatory drive.

Patients with overt hypothyroidism may have a 40 per cent decrease in metabolic rate, which results in a subnormal body temperature and an inability to increase core temperature in response to low-temperature stress. During anesthesia and the early postoperative period, the hypothyroid patient is particularly susceptible to hypothermia.

Hyperthyroidism

Cardiovascular abnormalities are common in hyperthyroid patients. Tachycardia, congestive heart failure, and left ventricular enlargement and atrial ventricular dysrhythmias are seen.

Heart rates exceeding 240 beats/min can be decreased by administration of propranolol, a beta-adrenergic blocking agent. Propranolol is recommended for cats at 2.5 to 5.0 mg every 8 hours as required to decrease the resting heart rate to within the normal range. Propranolol is not given to patients in congestive heart failure. Because of the cardiovascular effects of preoperative administration of propranolol, anesthetic drug delivery is decreased. Intraoperative administration of propranolol may cause significant myocardial depression and hypotension. The required dose of propranolol during anesthesia is extremely small (0.1 mg).

Atropine and glycopyrrolate potentiate tachycardia in hyperthyroid patients and are avoided. Thiobarbiturates have an antithyroid activity and may be the induction agent of choice. Acepromazine (0.1 mg/kg) and ketamine (5 mg/kg), given intramuscularly, provide satisfactory sedation before induction of anesthesia with halothane or isoflurane. Xylazine is used cautiously, as it may increase the incidence of dysrhythmias.

The electrocardiogram is monitored for dysrhythmias, and balanced electrolyte solution (5 ml/kg/hr) is infused during anesthesia. Hypocalcemia can occur 24 to 72 hours after surgery, even when an effort is made to preserve the parathyroid glands; this condition requires treatment with calcium and vitamin D.

THE ADRENAL GLANDS (pp. 2293–2294)

Hyperadrenocorticism

The metabolic and biochemical changes characteristic of hyperadrenocorticism present specific anesthetic problems. Approximately 10 per cent of dogs with hyperadrenocorticism, and a higher proportion of cats with hyperadrenocorticism, also have diabetes mellitus, requiring additional management. Hypokalemia can complicate anesthesia by causing muscle weakness, bradycardia, ventricular dysrhythmias, and hypotension. There is no reason for choosing one anesthetic agent over another on the basis of adrenal disease.

Surgery for adrenalectomy may be associated with acute massive blood loss; therefore, two venous catheters are placed in preparation for rapid fluid infusion. Once the tumor has been identified, dexamethasone is added to the intravenous fluids and administered at 0.02 to 0.04 mg/kg over approximately 6 hours, as adrenalectomy may result in an acute decrease in circulating cortisol level. Mineralocorticoid and glucocorticoid replacement therapy is instituted after surgery.

Hypoadrenocorticism

Adrenocortical insufficiency may be caused by adrenal failure (Addison's disease) or may be secondary to a pituitary or hypothalamic lesion, long-term administration of glucocorticoids, treatment with mitotane, or bilateral adrenalectomy. Hyponatremia and hyperkalemia are frequently present. Severe hyponatremia affects the central nervous system and may cause seizures or coma. Hypovolemia and decreased cardiac output result from sodium and water depletion. Blood volume must be restored before anesthesia, and anesthetic agents must be administered carefully to minimize cardiovascular depression. Hyperkalemia slows heart rate and conduction velocity, and may result in atrioventricular block. Bradycardia may progress to sinus arrest or ventricular fibrillation. Fluid therapy should precede anesthesia to decrease the serum potassium concentration to less than 6.5 mEq/L.

One of four dogs with hypoadrenocorticism may have hypercalcemia. Before anesthesia, serum calcium is restored to near normal by treatment with 0.9 per cent saline infusion and glucocorticoid therapy.

Thus, the preoperative assessment of the patient with hypoadrenocorticism includes measurement of serum electrolytes. Surgery is delayed, if possible, so that treatment to correct abnormal electrolyte values and to expand blood volume can be provided. An additional dose of corticosteroid is usually administered before anesthesia to patients that have been on long-term steroid therapy.

A solution of 5 per cent dextrose in water is given if hypoglycemia is present. Smaller amounts of anesthetic drugs than are usually administered are needed for induction of anesthesia. Stress from surgery is minimized by providing a quiet induction of anesthesia, adequate depth of anesthesia, sufficient fluid therapy during surgery, and prevention of pain postoperatively.

Pheochromocytoma (pp. 2293–2294)

Pheochromocytoma is an adrenal medullary tumor that secretes norepinephrine, both norepinephrine and epinephrine, or, in a few cases, dopamine. Large tumors may constantly secrete catecholamines, resulting in persistent hypertension that leads to venous congestion, cardiomyopathy, and congestive heart failure.

CHAPTER 172

Pediatric and Geriatric Anesthetic Techniques
(pages 2295–2300)

The term *pediatric* is applied to the first 12 weeks of postnatal life in puppies and kittens. Defining the term *geriatric* is more difficult because aging is a gradual process with much species and individual variation. One suggestion is that dogs and cats can be considered aged when they have completed 75 to 80 per cent of their expected life spans. Physiological changes of pediatric animals are summarized in Table 172–1 (see p. 2295).

Puppies and kittens are distressed easily and resist handling. Painful manipulations must be minimized, and handling must be performed gently.

Some pathophysiological changes are expected in older animals because of the aging process and they are summarized in Table 172–2 (see p. 2296). Age-related decline in function of body systems is progressive and often well tolerated. The degree of degeneration and the impact of intercurrent diseases, however, influence the ability of the older animal to tolerate the stress of anesthesia.

Injectable drugs are usually given intramuscularly to young and old dogs and cats. Subcutaneous absorption of drugs may be delayed or incomplete in old animals. Major factors affecting distribution of drugs include differences in body composition, fluid compartments, fat stores, plasma binding, blood-brain barrier permeability, and cardiac output (see Tables 172–1 and 172–2).

PREANESTHETIC ASSESSMENT (pp. 2296–2297)

Elective procedures on puppies and kittens require a minimum preoperative data base that includes history, physical examination including an accurate body weight, and packed cell volume and plasma protein; expected values are listed in Table 172–3 (see p. 2296).

Preoperative assessment of all geriatric animals should be thorough and directed to evaluation of cardiac, renal, and hepatic systems. If cardiac disease, renal disease, or diabetes mellitus is diagnosed, the animal is treated and stabilized before anesthesia, if possible.

The basic principles of anesthetic management are similar for pediatric and geriatric animals. Large or multiple doses of injectable drugs, undue handling, stress and alarm, and overhydration with excess intravenous fluids are avoided. Oxygenation, ventilation, heart rate and rhythm, blood pressure, fluid balance, and body temperature are monitored and maintained.

EARLY NEUTERING (p. 2297)

Early neutering is gaining widespread acceptance. The usual age at which the procedure is performed is 6 to 8 weeks. The combination of acepromazine, xylazine, and ketamine has proved to be the most effective and efficient method. The combination is 10 ml (1000 mg) ketamine, 2 ml (200 mg) xylazine, and 1 ml (10 mg) acepromazine. The intramuscular dose is 0.22 ml/kg of body weight. Atropine is not used as a routine preanesthetic agent. Puppies are awake and active within 30 minutes; kittens recover more slowly, in 1 to 2 hours. When tiletamine-zolazepam (Telazol) is used, recovery is slower.

Tiletamine-zolazepam (6 to 13 mg/kg IM) can be used for ear cropping.* Several adjunctive drugs have been used with tiletamine-zolazepam, including xylazine and butorphanol in dogs, and acepromazine. Another alternative is a combination of acepromazine, diazepam, and ketamine, injected intravenously. Acepromazine (0.9 ml [9 mg]) is combined in the bottle with ketamine (10 ml [1000 mg]). For procedures lasting less than 15 minutes, the combination is given intravenously (0.5 ml/4.5 kg of body weight), along with diazepam (0.25 ml [1.25 mg] per 4.5 kg of body weight). In procedures of longer duration, the puppy is intubated, and anesthesia is continued with either halothane or isoflurane.

HIGH-RISK PEDIATRIC PATIENTS AND COMPLEX PEDIATRIC PROCEDURES (p. 2297)

Simple inhalation anesthesia using either a chamber or mask for induction of anesthesia is often preferred in depressed or sick puppies and kittens. Preoxygenation with a face mask is desirable. Isoflurane is now the inhalant of choice because of rapid induction and recovery from anesthesia, relative stability of the cardiovascular system, and freedom from toxic effects.

Xylazine and high doses of acepromazine are not used in high-risk pediatric animals. Sedative-analgesics are useful in puppies. Oxymorphone (Numorphan) in a dose of 0.1 to 0.2 mg/kg IM, and atropine, in a dose of 0.04 mg/kg IM are suitable. Restraint and immobilization can be produced in kittens or puppies by combinations of ketamine (6 to 11 mg/kg IM) and midazolam (0.1 mg/kg IM) with or without butorphanol (0.4 mg/kg IM) or oxymorphone (0.05 to 0.1 mg/kg IM) for analgesia.

THORACOTOMY FOR CONGENITAL CARDIAC ANOMALY (pp. 2297–2298)

Healthy puppies with patent ductus arteriosus can be treated like healthy animals undergoing elective procedures with certain exceptions, noted later.

Hypotensive drugs such as acepromazine, meperidine, and halothane are best avoided. Anesthetic drugs that are arrhythmogenic should be avoided. These include xylazine, halothane, thiobarbiturates, and ketamine. If ketamine is used in kittens, only small preanesthetic doses (4 to 10 mg/kg IM) are used.

Because the chest is so compliant in pediatric patients, overinflation of the lungs by positive-pressure ventilation should be avoided. Airway pressures of 15 to 18 cm H_2O are sufficient when the chest is closed. The pressure can be increased to 20 to 25 cm H_2O when the chest is opened. Most surgeons prefer to have these young animals ventilated manually.

Fluid therapy at 4 ml/kg/hr may consist of lactated Ringer's solu-

*Editor's Note: For humane and ethical reasons, ear cropping is to be avoided.

tion, Plasmolyte-148, which contains no lactate, or a mixture of dextrose and electrolytes (e.g., one-half strength lactated Ringer's solution plus 2.5 per cent dextrose, or 0.45 per cent saline plus 2.5 per cent dextrose). Dextrose is particularly valuable in preventing hypoglycemia. Oxygen therapy can be continued postoperatively using a mask or oxygen chamber.

Postoperative pain relief is vital. Opioids can be used for analgesia; butorphanol, morphine, or oxymorphone can be used in puppies and kittens.

ELECTIVE GERIATRIC PROCEDURES (pp. 2298–2299)

All older patients should be considered "high-risk," even those undergoing dental work or other short procedures.

If preoperative sedation is needed in dogs for tooth extractions and other painful procedures, one of the opioid analgesic drugs (oxymorphone, 0.1 mg/kg IM, or morphine, 1 mg/kg IM) can be administered. Diazepam (Valium) (0.2 mg/kg IV) or midazolam (Versed) (0.1 mg/kg IV or IM) provides good preoperative sedation with minimal side effects.

Rapid anesthetic induction without premedication can be accomplished using thiobarbiturates in healthy dogs and cats. Ketamine (4 to 6 mg/kg IV) and diazepam (0.2 mg/kg IV), or ketamine and midazolam (0.1 mg/kg IV), can be used. Oxymorphone (0.1 mg/kg IV) and diazepam (0.2 mg/kg IV), or oxymorphone and midazolam (0.1 mg/kg IV), are also effective. Propofol (Diprivan) (6 to 8 mg/kg IV without premedication, 1 to 4 mg/kg IV after premedication) is a relatively new drug that is approved for use in man and produces smooth induction and recovery from anesthesia.

For geriatric patients, isoflurane is the drug of choice for maintenance of anesthesia. A balanced electrolyte solution at a low rate of replacement (1 ml/3 kg/hr) is recommended. If the patient has heart disease, a non–sodium-containing solution such as 5 per cent dextrose can be used.

HIGH-RISK GERIATRIC PATIENTS AND COMPLEX GERIATRIC PROCEDURES (p. 2299)

Simple anesthesia using mask induction with isoflurane and continuing with isoflurane for anesthetic maintenance may be satisfactory for many depressed older patients. Neuroleptanalgesia with the combinations of benzodiazepines (diazepam, midazolam) with opioids (oxymorphone, fentanyl, butorphanol) can produce sedation, analgesia, and sleep, the effects depending on route of administration and dose.

Preoxygenation with a face mask and 100 per cent oxygen before anesthetic induction greatly benefits geriatric animals. Thiobarbiturates are best avoided in these animals. Ketamine may produce tachycardia, which is undesirable in animals with heart failure.

All animals should have an intravenous catheter in place. Continuous monitoring of the electrocardiogram starts before induction of anesthesia. Blood pressure and body temperature are monitored in all patients. Dinamap and Doppler blood pressure monitors can be used for indirect measurements. Heart rate and heart sounds can be monitored continuously via an esophageal stethoscope. Blood component therapy is indicated if packed cell volume is less than 20 per cent, total plasmaproteins is less than 4.0 g/dl, or platelet count is less than 2×10^5 per μl. Urine production is monitored in uremic animals and in those undergoing prolonged or radical procedures. A minimum of 1 ml/kg of body weight of urine should be produced each hour.

Postoperative analgesic drugs may be necessary as described for pediatric animals.

CHAPTER 173

Anesthesia for Cesarean Section (pages 2300–2304)

MATERNAL PHYSIOLOGICAL CHANGES (pp. 2300–2301)

In the normal dam, increased blood volume provides an adequate reserve to compensate for large quantities of blood and fluid lost at delivery. Dogs, and presumably cats, are resistant to supine hypotension at term. Decreases in maternal cardiac output and arterial blood pressure during anesthesia reduce uterine and placental blood flow and threaten fetal viability. Inotropic agents with predominately beta-adrenergic activity are chosen when augmentation of cardiac output and arterial blood pressure is required.

Cranial displacement of the diaphragm by the enlarging uterus is primarily responsible for the mechanical changes in respiratory function. Resting lung volume, particularly functional residual capacity, is decreased. The resulting ventilation/perfusion inequalities and intrapulmonary shunting increase the tendency for maternal hypoxemia. Limiting the time spent in dorsal recumbency and increasing the inspired concentration of oxygen minimize the effects of reduced functional residual capacity.

All dams, particularly those presented for emergency cesarean section, are considered to have a full stomach and be at high risk of regurgitation and aspiration. The risk of regurgitation and aspiration continues into the postoperative period; therefore, extubation should be performed only after return of swallowing reflexes.

SPECIFIC ANESTHETIC DRUGS (pp. 2301–2302)

Anesthetic Premedications. Glycopyrrolate does not cross the placental barrier and therefore does not alter fetal heart rate. Anticholinergics may be administered intravenously as needed.

Phenothiazines (acepromazine, promazine) cross the placenta rapidly and can be found in fetal blood within 2 minutes of intravenous administration. The hypotensive effects of the phenothiazines are aggravated by the large amount of fluid and blood lost by the dam during caesarean section. Acepromazine administered in low doses (0.025 to 0.05 mg/kg IM) in combination with an opioid usually sedates a nervous dam adequately for epidural analgesia. Phenothiazine tranquilizers are used only in low dosages, and when absolutely necessary.

Although xylazine is used in small animals for routine surgical procedures, its use in the dam is contraindicated. Diazepam and midazolam may produce mild calming and muscle relaxation. They produce minimal cardiopulmonary depression. They are most beneficial when administered intravenously prior to induction of anesthesia.

Narcotic agonists are frequently used alone or in combination with sedatives and tranquilizers to produce analgesia and sedation. Opioids readily cross the placenta and concentrate in the fetus, producing central nervous system depression and respiratory depression. Maternal and fetal hypoxemia can be avoided by administering oxygen to the dam if respiratory depression becomes significant. Naloxone, an opioid antagonist, completely reverses all opioid-induced effects, including respiratory and central nervous system depression and analgesia.

Ketamine is frequently administered intramuscularly to cats as an anesthetic premedication. Low doses of ketamine (1 mg/kg IV, 5 mg/kg IM) administered to cats cause minimal neonatal depression. Concurrent administration of diazepam is beneficial in decreasing ketamine-induced muscle rigidity.

Induction Drugs. Ultrashort-acting barbiturates affect the fetus minimally if administered in low doses (less than 8 mg/kg) as a single bolus. Ketamine, administered intravenously in low doses, is a useful induction anesthetic in dogs and cats.

Inhalant Anesthetics. All inhalant anesthetics rapidly cross the blood-brain barrier and placental barrier. Neonatal depression is related to the duration and depth of anesthesia. Halothane and isoflurane are preferred over methoxyflurane, because they are more controllable and because recovery from anesthesia, both maternal and fetal, is more rapid with these agents. Isoflurane has a greater margin of cardiovascular safety than halothane. Both halothane and isoflurane cause profound uterine relaxation, which may increase uterine hemorrhage and prolong surgery.

ANESTHETIC TECHNIQUES (pp. 2302–2303)

The physical status of animals presented for cesarean section varies widely. If the dam is tractable, the surgery site is clipped and scrubbed prior to induction of anesthesia to minimize the interval between induction and delivery. Dams are given a crystalloid solution (e.g., lactated Ringer's solution) intravenously at 10 to 20 ml/kg/hr throughout the anesthesia. Preoxygenation prior to induction of anesthesia is recommended.

Dams presenting for emergency cesarean section usually exhibit varying degrees of dehydration, hypovolemia, hypotension, metabolic acidosis, and shock. Hypovolemia may be treated with an intravenous crystalloid solution administered at 50 to 100 ml/kg/hr. Maternal acidosis is treated with hyperventilation following endotracheal intubation.

CARE OF THE NEWBORN (p. 2303)

Immediately on delivery, each neonate's head and airway is cleared of membranes and fluids. A bulb syringe may be used to aspirate fluids from the oral pharynx. The neonate is gently rubbed with a towel; this action dries the neonate and stimulates its breathing. The neonate is kept in a warm environment, preferably 85° to 90°F (30° to 32°C), and it is placed with the dam as soon as she has recovered from anesthesia.

Respiratory depression may be treated with doxapram or naloxone administered sublingually, intramuscularly, or intravenously. Neonates administered naloxone to reverse opioid-induced respiratory depression must be observed closely over the next few hours for signs of a recurrence of the opioid effects.

CHAPTER 174

Common Complications and Anesthetic Emergencies
(pages 2304–2309)

SLOW INDUCTION (p. 2304)

Absorption of drugs from intramuscular sites is often unpredictable and depends on the blood flow in relation to local tissue. For example, an anesthetic dose of ketamine injected into the epaxial muscles may accidentally be deposited subcutaneously or in fat. The subcutaneous and fat tissues have a poor blood supply, and the drug is poorly absorbed.

There are several reasons for slow induction of anesthesia with inhalation agents. Common causes for a low inspired anesthetic concentration include an empty vaporizer and patient disconnection from the anesthetic system. Excessively high fresh gas flow rates (oxygen, nitrous oxide) delay the rate of anesthetic rise in a breathing system using an in-the-circle vaporizer, and low fresh gas flow rates delay rate of anesthetic rise in a breathing system using an out-of-the-circle vaporizer.

Apnea or hypoventilation can slow anesthetic induction. The high solubility of inhaled anesthetics in rubber or plastic components of the system may contribute to slowing of induction and delayed recovery. Slow induction of inhalation anesthesia may be due in part to the use of a relatively soluble anesthetic (methoxyflurane). Anesthetics of intermediate solubility (halothane, isoflurane) provide faster induction. A high blood solubility means that a large amount of inhaled anesthetic must be dissolved in the blood before equilibrium is reached with the gas phase.

SLOW RECOVERY (pp. 2304–2305)

Metabolism of the inhaled anesthetic can influence the rate of decline of alveolar partial pressure. Metabolism is a principal determinant in the rate of decline of methoxyflurane. Metabolism with halothane is as important as ventilation, whereas the isoflurane alveolar partial pressure decline is due to ventilation.

A slow recovery from thiobarbiturates or ketamine anesthesia may reflect acidosis, low plasma protein concentration, or compromised kidney and liver function. Long recovery from thiobarbiturate anesthesia in greyhounds is probably due to a decrease in tissue distribution and metabolic clearance. Slow recovery from anesthesia could also be due to accidental hypothermia that results in slow metabolism of anesthetic drugs.

INADEQUATE ANESTHETIC DEPTH (p. 2305)

When a patient awakens prematurely from inhalation anesthesia, the anesthetist should first evaluate the anesthetic equipment. The endotracheal tube is inspected for proper insertion or for leaks in the endotracheal tube cuff.

Surgical stimulation is one of the primary reasons for a patient's awakening during surgery. Administration of supplemental anesthetic drugs may be necessary to maintain adequate anesthetic depth.

BREATHING PROBLEMS DURING ANESTHESIA
(pp. 2305–2306)

Hypoventilation

Hypoventilation or apnea may occur in anesthetized animals as a result of an overdose of anesthetics, obstruction of the airway, a space-occupying lesion in the thorax (diaphragmatic hernia or chylothorax), or the peculiar effects of certain drugs. An anesthetic overdose results in a slow respiratory rate and small tidal volumes. Premedicants such as xylazine and the opioids can induce significant hypoventilation during inhalation anesthesia.

Airway obstruction can occur from aspiration of regurgitated stomach contents, kinking of the endotracheal tube, or small larynx, elongated soft palate, and redundant pharyngeal tissue in brachycephalic breeds. Hypoventilation during surgery can also result from physical pressure on the thorax.

Cheyne-Stokes respiration is characterized by periods of apnea of 15 to 20 seconds separated by approximately equal periods of hyperventilation with tidal volumes that wax and wane. Cheyne-Stokes breathing is caused by an abnormally functioning respiratory control mechanism. *Biot's breathing* is an abnormal respiratory pattern in which respirations are faster and deeper than normal with interspersed pauses. *Kussmaul's breathing* is characterized by deep regular breaths that resemble sighs. Apneustic breathing, a deep inhalation followed by breath holding and then an exhalation followed immediately by another inhalation, usually occurs after administration of ketamine or tiletamine-zolazepam.

Hyperventilation

Hyperventilation can occur at the beginning of anesthesia when the patient is lightly anesthetized. Surgical stimulation may also cause a period of hyperventilation. Increasing anesthetic depth prevents hyperventilation.

Tachypnea

Halothane and isoflurane occasionally increase respiratory rate, which is characterized as rapid, shallow, and regular.

HYPOTENSION (p. 2306)

Preanesthetic drugs such as phenothiazine tranquilizers and intravenous opioids can cause hypotension. Induction drugs, including the barbiturates, can cause hypotension, especially if a relative overdose has been administered.

When administered intraoperatively as anesthetic adjuncts, ketamine and butorphanol induce hypotension. Surgical maneuvers leading to hypotension include obstruction of venous return and hemorrhage, either acutely or over long periods. Hypotension can result from cardiac dysrhythmias. Treatment of hypotension involves eliminating its cause, for example, lightening anesthesia, restoring venous return, increasing intravascular volume, inducing vasoconstriction with alpha-adrenergic agonists, stimulating cardiac output with positive inotropic agents (dopamine, dobutamine), reversing drug effects if an antagonist is available, and re-establishing normal cardiac rhythm.

DYSRHYTHMIAS (pp. 2306–2308)

Bradycardia

Xylazine, phenothiazine tranquilizers (acepromazine), opioids, and inhalant anesthetics can cause bradycardia. A declining heart rate of less than 60 beats/min is treated with intravenous atropine or glycopyrrolate.

Tachycardia

Tachycardia occurs during anesthesia as a result of surgical stimulation, administration of atropine or glycopyrrolate, hyperthermia, or anesthetic effects. Ketamine causes tachycardia because it stimulates

TABLE 174–1. SIGNS OF CARDIAC ARREST

No palpable heartbeat. Heartbeat may be present but is not strong enough to be
palpated (i.e., electrical-mechanical dissociation)
No palpable pulse
Apnea
Lack of jaw tone/no muscle tone
Lack of surgical hemorrhage
Cyanosis in the surgical field
Cyanosis or paleness of the mucous membranes
Dilated pupils (after 3 to 4 minutes of arrest)

the sympathetic nervous system. Treatment of tachycardia is not required in the healthy patient.

CARDIOPULMONARY ARREST (pp. 2308–2309)

Cardiopulmonary arrest is the most dreaded of the anesthetic complications. Less than 25 per cent of arrest victims return to normal. The
mechanism of blood flow during cardiopulmonary resuscitation (CPR)
is still the cause of some debate. Lack of success with external thoracic
massage requires an early decision to switch to internal thoracic massage.
  Diagnosis of cardiac arrest involves recognition of the obvious
symptoms (Table 174–1). After confirmation of a diagnosis of cardiac
arrest, the guidelines *A* through *D* for CPR are followed: *Airway,
Breathing, Cardiac* massage, and *Definitive* or *Drug* therapy. A patent
airway is always obtained or confirmed through intubation. The patient
is ventilated at a rate of 4 to 5 breaths per minute. External thoracic
massage is initiated with the patient in right lateral recumbency. An
early decision must be made to switch to internal thoracic massage if
external efforts are ineffective. Internal thoracic massage may be initiated after no more than 2 to 3 minutes of external thoracic massage,
by making an incision through the left fifth intercostal space. The
massage rate for either external or internal massage is approximately
100 compressions per minute. Figure 174–1 shows a simplified protocol for administering CPR (see p. 2309).
  The most important drug to administer during CPR is epinephrine
(adrenalin). Epinephrine is given early and in high doses (1 mg/10 kg).
A central injection of epinephrine is recommended. Alternate routes to
intravenous injection are intratracheal or intracardiac injection.
  Conversion of ventricular fibrillation to normal sinus rhythm is best
accomplished by direct current countershock. For internal defibrillation, 20 to 40 joules are used, and for external defibrillation, 200 to
400 joules are used.
  Sodium bicarbonate is given if the arrest has been present for longer
than 5 minutes. Paradoxical acidosis of the cerebrospinal fluid is not a
problem if sodium bicarbonate is administered during administration
of CPR. Approximately 1.0 mEq/kg of sodium bicarbonate is administered every 10 minutes during resuscitation.
  Aftercare requires good nursing with attention to adequacy of ventilation, fluid load, blood pressure, and arterial pH. Animals with the
best prognosis show fast and steady recovery from the hypoxic insult.

Dentistry (pages 2310–2358)

CHAPTER 175

Introduction to Veterinary Dentistry (pages 2310–2315)

DENTAL CLASSIFICATION (p. 2311)

Teeth are classified into simple or complex types based on the inter-relationships of dental anatomic structures including enamel, cementum, dentin, and pulp. Simple teeth and complex teeth are also known as brachydont (short crown) and hypsodont (high crown). All the teeth of the dog, cat, and man are simple, or brachydont, teeth.

DENTAL STRUCTURES AND FUNCTION (pp. 2311–2312)

The teeth are derived from ectodermal and mesodermal tissues. The basic histologic structures of the simple tooth are enamel, dentin, pulp, and cementum, which are arranged in a definite pattern. Enamel, the outer covering of the tooth is found only on the crown and completely covers and protects the dentin from external exposure.

Dentin, which forms the bulk of the tooth, is just deep to the enamel and separates this structure from the pulp cavity. In an intact normal tooth, dentin is not visible. Dentin is perforated by numerous canals called dentinal tubules, which contain dentinal fibers. These fibers form the cytoplasm of the cells located within the pulp chamber. These special cells of the pulp cavity, which are shared by both the dentin and pulp chamber, are called odontoblasts.

The central structure of the tooth is the pulp cavity or chamber. The pulp contains blood vessels and nerves that enter the tooth through an apical foramen located at the apex of the root. Cementum is a hard bony tissue that covers the dentin of the tooth root and contains crystallized minerals. Cementum attaches the tooth to the alveolus with the periodontal ligaments and to the surrounding alveolar bones. The gingiva may be described as the oral mucosa attached to the alveolar process (the bone surrounding the tooth) and to the neck of the tooth at a crevice or crevicular groove.

The teeth are surrounded by the mandible and maxilla, and the specific bone that surrounds and supports the teeth is called the alveolar process. The alveolar process is composed of the lamellated bone and the supporting bone. The lamellated bone is the bone of the wall of the tooth socket or dental alveolus, whereas the supporting bone is composed of the cortical plate and trabecular bone.

DENTAL ANATOMY (pp. 2312–2313)

The four types of teeth are incisors, canine teeth, premolars, and molars. Incisor teeth are located in the rostral part of the mouth, embedded in the incisive bones of the maxilla or mandible. All incisors have single roots. The four canine teeth have a large root that is nearly twice as long as the crown.

In the permanent dentition, there are four premolar teeth on each side of the jaw, numbered from rostral to caudal. The first premolar may have one or two roots, whereas the remainder of the premolar teeth have two roots. The only exception is the upper fourth premolar or carnassial tooth, which has three roots. Occasionally, premolar teeth are absent, a condition called anodontia.

Molar teeth are located caudal to the premolar teeth and have no deciduous predecessors. There are two molars on each side of the upper jaw and three molars on each side of the lower jaw. Each upper molar tooth has three diverging roots. All the mandibular molars have two roots.

The upper fourth premolar tooth is the carnassial tooth in the maxillary arcade, whereas the lower first molar tooth is the carnassial tooth in the mandibular arcade.

DENTAL FORMULAS AND NOTATION (pp. 2313–2315)

The formula for the permanent dentition of the dog is:

$$\frac{3I \quad 1C \quad 4P \quad 2M}{3I \quad 1C \quad 4P \quad 3M} = 42 \text{ teeth}$$

The formula for the permanent dentition of the cat is:

$$\frac{3I \quad 1C \quad 3P \quad 1M}{3I \quad 1C \quad 2P \quad 1M} = 30 \text{ teeth}$$

The deciduous dental formula for the dog is:

$$\frac{3i \quad 1c \quad 3p}{3i \quad 1c \quad 3p} = 28 \text{ teeth}$$

The deciduous dental formula for the domestic cat is:

$$\frac{3i \quad 1c \quad 3p}{3i \quad 1c \quad 2p} = 26 \text{ teeth}$$

The sequence for eruption of primary deciduous teeth is:

1. Dog is born edentulous (without teeth).
2. Central incisors, intermediate incisors, and canine teeth erupt during first 4 weeks.
3. Lateral incisors erupt at 5 to 6 weeks of age.
4. Premolars erupt at 4 to 8 weeks of age.

The permanent teeth erupt at different times, and the eruption dates are given in Table 175–1.

Different systems have been described for recording dental lesions on medical records.

DENTAL TERMINOLOGY (p. 2315)

Common veterinary dental terms are:

Rostral —toward the nose (cranial)
Caudal —toward the tail
Labial —toward the lips
Lingual —toward the tongue
Buccal —toward the cheek
Facial —toward the face or lips

TABLE 175–1. ERUPTION SCHEDULE FOR PERMANENT TEETH
IN THE DOG

Basic Tooth Group	Eruption Time
Incisors	
Central incisor	2 to 5 months
Intermediate incisor	2 to 5 months
Lateral incisor	4 to 5 months
Canine Teeth	5 to 6 months
Premolars	
First premolar	4 to 5 months
Second premolar	6 months
Third premolar	6 months
Fourth premolar	4 to 5 months
Molars	
First molar	5 to 6 months
Second molar	6 to 7 months
Third molar	6 to 7 months

In general, permanent teeth erupt earlier in large-breed dogs.

Mesial   —toward the center line of the dental arch
Distal   —away from the center line of the dental arch
Contact —where a tooth touches an adjacent tooth
Occlusal—biting surface
Coronal —toward the crown
Apical   —toward the root

CHAPTER 176

Dental Pathology and Microbiology (pages 2316–2326)

DEVELOPMENTAL ANOMALIES OF TEETH (pp. 2316–2318)

Gemination, Fusion, and Concrescence

Gemination, fusion, and concrescence are developmental disturbances
in the shape of teeth. Gemination (or dichotomy) refers to an attempt
at division of a single tooth bud. Fusion and concrescence of teeth
denote a joining of two tooth buds to form a single structure. These
anomalies are rare in animals. Most documented dichotomous teeth in
the dog involve incisor teeth. Extraction may be indicated.

Dilaceration and Supernumerary Roots

Dilaceration is a sharp curve in the root, which is probably caused by
trauma to the dental follicle. Supernumerary roots are anatomical var-

iations that mainly affect the upper premolars, and the third premolar in particular.

Anodontia and Oligodontia

Anodontia is the complete congenital absence of teeth, which may involve both the deciduous and the permanent dentition. This condition is extremely rare in the dog and cat. Oligodontia, or partial anodontia, is the congenital absence of one or more teeth. This condition is common, observed more often in the permanent dentition than in the deciduous dentition. If deciduous teeth are missing, the corresponding permanent teeth are likely to be absent. The first premolar and the third molar are most often affected in the dog.

Polyodontia

Polyodontia, or supernumerary teeth, are less common than missing teeth. In both man and dogs, supernumerary teeth are more common on the upper jaw. A well-recognized entity is the mesiodens, which is a supernumerary upper incisor found between the two first incisors. It is common in the bulldog and boxer.

Retained Deciduous Teeth

Delayed exfoliation of deciduous incisors and canine teeth is common in the dog, especially in toy breeds. In the extreme form, deciduous teeth may persist after the eruption of the permanent teeth.

In most cases, the permanent tooth develops normally, and erupts at a site immediately caudal to the retained deciduous incisors. Retained deciduous canine teeth cause deviation of the erupting canine teeth. Retained deciduous teeth alter the gingival contour, with plaque and debris accumulating between the deciduous and permanent teeth.

Embedded and Impacted Teeth

Embedded teeth are individual teeth that are unerupted, usually because of a lack of eruptive force. An impacted tooth is prevented from erupting by some mechanical barrier in the eruption path.

Enamel Hypoplasia

Enamel hypoplasia is the incomplete or defective formation of organic enamel matrix of teeth. Enamel hypoplasia occurs as a result of damage to the ameloblasts while the teeth are developing. Epitheliotropic virus infections, particularly distemper, are the most important causes.

Mild enamel hypoplasia is characterized by irregular enamel, the areas of which initially appear as opaque but soon become brown-stained. Small irregular pits may be present. In the more severe form, a band-shaped absence or extreme thinning of the enamel is visible.

Tetracycline Staining

Tetracycline administered during tooth development becomes incorporated in the enamel and dentin and causes a permanent brown-yellow-orange discoloration. This drug should not be administered to dogs and cats before the age of 5 months or to pregnant female animals.

INJURIES TO TEETH (pp. 2318–2320)

Attrition is the wearing away of dental substance due to occlusal contact and mastication. Attrition is usually normal but may be abnormal and enhanced because of malocclusion, with one or more teeth wearing abnormally against others. As wear continues, dentin is exposed, and sclerosis of the exposed dentinal tubules takes place. The slightly yellowish dentin contrasts with the surrounding white enamel.

Abrasion refers to the pathological wearing away of dental substance through an abnormal mechanical process. This condition predisposes the animal to fractures of the affected teeth. Dental fractures are common in the dog and cat.

Enamel fractures and uncomplicated crown fractures are of little clinical importance in small animals. The exposed dentin becomes insensitive but is rougher than enamel and facilitates plaque and calculus accumulation.

Crown-root fractures involve the periodontal ligament and may lead to periodontitis because of the altered gingival contour. Complicated crown fractures cause pulp exposure and ensuing endodontic disease. Root fractures of traumatic origin are infrequently seen; iatrogenic fractures are common. Injuries to periodontal tissues are rarely diagnosed, with the exception of lateral luxation, extrusive luxation, and exarticulation.

Response to Trauma

Secondary dentin is formed by the odontoblasts after root formation has been completed. Tertiary dentin (also referred to as irregular secondary dentin or reparative dentin) results from the irritation of odontoblastic processes within the dentinal tubules. Tertiary dentin is produced by the odontoblasts that are directly affected by the irritation.

In attrition, abrasion, and uncomplicated dental fractures, the formation of tertiary dentin usually seals off the pulp cavity effectively. The tertiary dentin may become clinically evident as a brown spot in the center of the occlusal surface. This condition can be differentiated from an exposed root canal through use of a dental explorer. Exposed dentin is painful. Pain eventually disappears as the calcification of the primary dentinal tubules is followed by sclerosis.

Resorption

Internal resorption is poorly understood and may accompany endodontic disease. If resorption occurs in the crown, discoloration and enamel perforation may take place. Internal resorption indicates endodontic treatment. External resorption refers to resorption that begins on the root surface. This type of resorption is characteristic of periodontal disease in cats.

CARIES (pp. 2320–2321)

The reported prevalence of caries in the dog varies from 0.5 to 35 per cent. Caries in the dog may occur as pit or fissure caries (class I cavities) on the occlusal surface, or as smooth-surface caries (class V cavities) around the tooth neck. Fissure caries are the most common and usually affect the upper and lower first molars. An early carious lesion usually appears brown or black and feels slightly soft or sticky when probed with a fine dental explorer. Clinical signs associated with intermediate carious lesions are difficulty in eating and jaw chattering.

ODONTOGENIC TUMORS (pp. 2321–2324)
Epulides

The epulis has been described as the most common benign oral tumor in the dog. The common origin of these tumors is the periodontal

ligament. Generalized gingival hyperplasia has been called an epulis, but the term is a misnomer. Generalized gingival hyperplasia is occasionally seen in the boxer and collie.

Central Ameloblastoma

The most common odontogenic tumor, except for the peripheral odontogenic fibroma (WHO type) and the peripheral ameloblastoma is the central ameloblastoma, which is occasionally referred to incorrectly as adamantinoma. This tumor usually appears as a locally invasive neoplasm with osteolysis around the tooth roots and with cystic changes. Metastasis has not been described.

Odontoma

An odontoma is a tumor in which both the epithelial and the mesenchymal cells are well differentiated, resulting in the formation of all types of dental tissue. An odontoma is probably a hamartoma rather than a neoplasm. Odontomas have been diagnosed in young dogs and in cats.

Ameloblastic Fibroma

This tumor is characterized by ameloblastic epithelial cells arranged around dental pulp–like stroma. The rostral maxilla is the most common site. This tumor may be locally invasive; however, metastasis has not been recorded.

DENTAL MICROBIOLOGY (pp. 2324–2325)

Diverse aerobic, facultative, and anaerobic bacteria are present in the canine oral cavity. In normal dogs, *Streptococcus* spp., *Staphylococcus aureus* and *Staphylococcus epidermidis, Pasteurella multocida, Simonsiella* spp., the Enterobacteriaceae, and many other bacterial organisms have consistently been found.

The high incidence of *P. multocida* is important in the pathophysiology of bite wounds. Anaerobic bacteria are also important and outnumber aerobic bacteria. Those isolated include *Bacteroides* spp., *Fusobacterium* spp., *Veillonella* spp., and *Lactobacillus* spp. Although the bacterial population in periodontitis is the same as is found in the normal mouth, the proportions differ largely. The flora associated with periodontitis is predominantly anaerobic. The subgingival flora mainly includes gram-negative bacteria such as *Fusobacterium nucleatum* and *Bacteroides asaccharolyticus*, whereas the supragingival flora comprises a greater proportion of gram-positive bacteria. Spirochetes are present in great numbers.

Bacteremia may occur during and following periodontal treatment and dental extraction. Dental procedures should not be performed at the same time as other surgical procedures.

The normal oral flora of the cat has not been well documented. *P. multocida* was found in 80 per cent of cats. Anaerobic gram-negative rods such as black-pigmented *Bacteroides* spp. similar to *B. gingivalis* were isolated in increasing numbers with severe periodontitis.

CHAPTER 177

Dental Extractions and Complications (pages 2326–2332)

INDICATIONS FOR DENTAL EXTRACTIONS (pp. 2327–2328)

1. Gross decay or caries
2. Fractured crown or root with the fracture extending into the pulp
3. Advanced periodontal disease
4. Supernumerary teeth
5. Malocclusion
6. Retained deciduous teeth
7. Teeth in the fracture line (mandible or maxilla)
8. Periapical abscess

Carious lesions too advanced to undergo restoration, such that decay invades the pulp chamber, require extraction. A fractured crown or root with exposure of the pulp chamber may require extraction; however, the tooth may be partially restored or endodontically treated if the root is undamaged.

Advanced periodontal disease is one of the most common indications for extraction of teeth. Usually, teeth are loose, and if two-thirds of the supporting structure has been destroyed, restoration is impossible and extraction is necessary.

Supernumerary teeth are extracted to allow appropriate occlusion and interdigitation of cheek teeth. Malocclusion can result from a variety of causes. Whenever possible, the primary cause of the problem is addressed. Selected extractions may resolve the problem. Retained deciduous teeth act similarly to supernumerary teeth. When a deciduous tooth is retained, it is extracted immediately. Teeth located in the fracture line of a traumatized maxilla and mandible are extracted. Removal of teeth from the fracture site prevents interference with the normal healing process. Periapical abscess formation may be another indication for dental extraction when endodontic restoration is inappropriate.

TECHNIQUES FOR DENTAL EXTRACTION— MUCOPERIOSTEAL FLAPS (p. 2328)

An important consideration in dental extraction is whether the entire crown and parts of the root of the tooth are exposed. The first step is to remove the overlying soft tissue away from the bone, using a mucoperiosteal flap. Various mucoperiosteal flaps have been described.

Full mucoperiosteal flaps are used for extractions and periodontal surgery. Limited mucoperiosteal flaps have specific applications such as retrieval of a retained root fragment or exposure of the apical delta for an endodontic procedure.

PRINCIPLES OF DENTAL EXTRACTIONS (p. 2328)

Radiography of the dental arch is performed, especially if the teeth are thought to be primary and if the surgeon is uncertain whether secondary teeth will erupt at the same site.

The surgical site is properly prepared. Ultrasonic scaling or cleaning of the adjacent teeth may be necessary if advanced periodontal disease is present. Chlorhexidine can be sprayed on the extraction site or applied topically. In multirooted teeth, consideration must be given to division of the crown to facilitate extraction.

Crown division can be performed with dental engines and handpieces, power drills and burs, or manual saws. After the crown is divided, a dental elevator can be inserted to apply leverage using the other cusps or crown fragments of the same tooth. This technique prevents damage to the crowns of adjacent teeth.

EQUIPMENT FOR DENTAL EXTRACTIONS (pp. 2328–2330)

The most important instrument for the extraction of teeth is the dental elevator. The goal is to stretch, break, or cut peridontal fibers or ligaments, a small number at a time, until the tooth is loose enough to extract.

Extraction Forceps

Extraction forceps are to grasp the tooth after elevation and withdraw it from the alveolus.

Principles for the application and use of forceps are:

1. Select the correct forceps.
2. Grasp the forceps near the ends of the handle.
3. Apply the long axis of the forceps beak parallel to the long axis of the tooth.
4. Place the forceps on the root structure.
5. Grasp the root firmly to prevent slippage.
6. Place the forcep beak so that impingement on adjacent teeth does not occur.

Dental drills, burs, and discs are used as aids in extractions. After creating a mucoperiosteal flap, a bur on a high-speed or low-speed handpiece can be used to remove the alveolar crest and allow elevation of the tooth.

After the tooth is removed, the dental bur may be used to reduce the alveolar crest and the bone located at the furcation, the space between the roots of a multirooted tooth. This bone, called intraradicular bone, may protrude through the healed gingiva after extraction, and removal of the intraradicular bone facilitates wound closure. A dental drill, bur, or disc can be used to divide the crown of a tooth to be extracted. A dental drill and burs are used to remove root fragments retained in the alveolus after extraction.

An alternative to previously described extraction techniques is the use of a dental drill and burs to obliterate teeth completely. This avoids manipulation and leverage of teeth with elevators and extraction forceps, which may result in fracture of the mandible or maxilla.

COMPLICATIONS OF EXTRACTIONS (pp. 2330–2332)

The following complications are the most common:

1. Hemorrhage
2. Fracture of the mandible
3. Root retention
4. Necrosis of bone around extraction site
5. Oronasal fistula
6. Functional abnormalities

Serosanguineous drainage is expected after extractions, but excessive hemorrhage is abnormal. Small dogs, cats, and animals with chronic periodontal disease are at greatest risk for maxillary or mandibular fracture. Root retention and breakage of teeth during extraction may occur because of improper elevation, underlying dental disease, caries, necrotic pulp, or previous endodontic therapy.

Necrosis of bone occasionally follows extraction. If the remaining alveolar socket does not form a clot, it may become a source of infection and irritation, and in extreme cases, osteomyelitis may occur.

Oronasal fistula may occur after extraction and is usually associated with upper canine teeth or lateral incisors with advanced periodontal disease. If an oronasal fistula occurs, it is best corrected using a buccal flap or a double reposition flap.

Various other complications of extractions have been described and include the following:

1. Gingival abrasions, tears, and lacerations
2. Fractures of the alveolus
3. Temporomandibular joint dislocation
4. Broken instruments
5. Bacteremia and systemic infection
6. Alveolar osteitis (dry socket)

Gingival abrasions, lacerations, and tears occur when dental elevators and extraction forceps are used improperly. Fractures of the alveolus may be desirable if they facilitate removal of intraradicular bone. Conversely, alveolar fractures may weaken the supporting bone and lead to a complete fracture, especially of the mandible.

Temporomandibular joint dislocation occurs in small breeds of dogs and cats when excessive force is used to elevate or extract teeth. To prevent this complication, the mandible is supported carefully with manual pressure during elevation and extraction. Temporomandibular joint dislocations are usually managed by manual reduction and support with a muzzle.

During the extraction, instruments can break within the alveolus. If an instrument is broken, the piece is retrieved by root pulverization or by preparation of a mucoperiosteal flap with an apical approach. Bacteremia and septicemia have been reported as probable complications to dental extraction. Surgical procedures should probably not be performed in conjunction with dental prophylaxis and extraction. If the two procedures must be performed concurrently, appropriate administration of an antibiotic is indicated. Alveolar osteitis is an extension of one of the previous complications, necrosis of bone at the extraction site. This condition is also known as fibrinolytic alveolitis, alveolitis sicca dolorosa, or dry socket.

Various techniques have been recommended to reduce the incidence of infections and alveolar osteitis following extraction. One report recommends soluble tetracycline powder applied topically to the extraction sites during surgery. Other materials including soluble gelatin sponge (Gelfoam) and oxidized regenerated cellulose (Surgicel) have been advocated as biological dressings, and polylactic acid shows promise in preventing alveolar osteitis.

CHAPTER 178

Periodontal Disease (pages 2332–2339)

Periodontal disease is an oral infection that results from the chronic retention of bacteria at the junction of the tooth and the gingiva. The term *gingivitis* refers to swelling, redness, tenderness, and bleeding in the soft tissue around the tooth. It can be resolved by removing accumulated bacteria from the neck of the tooth.

Periodontitis may develop around teeth with gingivitis because of the chronic presence of bacterial products around the teeth. Periodontitis involves deep inflammation, loss of supporting alveolar bone, and destruction of fibrous connective tissue attachment at the neck of the tooth. Treatment of periodontal disease is primarily surgical.

EXAMINATION (pp. 2332–2333)

Changes in color and contour of the gingiva suggest periodontal disease. Red and purple areas signify inflammation. Swelling of the gingival margin is another early indicator of periodontal disease.

With gingivitis, there is a tendency to bleed when the gingival margin is touched lightly with an instrument. Teeth with periodontitis show a similar tendency to bleed when probed underneath the gingival margin and may exhibit a purulent exudate from the gingival space.

Periodontitis that has destroyed support for the teeth can be seen on dental radiographs as resorption of bone around the neck of the tooth. Radiographs showing that bone support has receded more than 2 mm from the cementoenamel junction usually indicate periodontitis.

The periodontal probe measures the depth of the gingival crevice when it is inserted between the gingiva and tooth. The depth of the gingival crevice is measured, and a second line is drawn that is apical to the free gingival margin. The line is the attachment level, the anatomical point at which the periodontium and the tooth are attached. When this distance is greater than 2 mm below the cementoenamel junction, loss of periodontal attachment has occurred.

DIAGNOSIS (pp. 2333–2334)

When the gingiva is inflamed but no loss of tissue attachment to the root has occurred, the diagnosis is gingivitis. To diagnose periodontitis, loss of attachment and inflammation must be demonstrated. Thus, gingivitis may be diagnosed on visual examination based on change in tissue color, but a diagnosis of periodontitis requires measurement.

TREATMENT (pp. 2334–2339)

Periodontal disease is preventable if the teeth can be kept clean. Toothbrushing, antiseptic mouth rinses, and regular professional prophylaxis are recommended to keep the teeth clean to prevent disease.

Systemic problems that predispose patients to periodontal disease must be identified. Diabetes mellitus due to defects in neutrophil function decreases the patient's resistance to periodontal infection.

Initial periodontal treatment involves removing plaque and calculus from the teeth above and below the gingival margin. Ultrasonic scaling along with copious water irrigation is the fastest method of removing gross accretions from the teeth. Because the root surface is softer than the crown, it is important not to use the point of the instrument against the root. The depth of the gingival space is subsequently measured. After ultrasonic scaling, the root is probed with a number 17 explorer to identify residual roughness or calculus that was missed. These areas are smoothed with a number 13 or number 14 Columbia curette until they feel hard and even.

After being thoroughly cleaned and smoothed by scaling and root planing, the teeth are polished. Polishing occurs slightly under the gingival margin if a rubber cup is loaded with polishing paste and pressed gently against the tooth as it rotates in the handpiece.

After the cleaning, the mouth is irrigated, and the patient is discharged with a 2-week supply of 0.1 to 0.2 per cent chlorhexidine solution. Owners are instructed to rinse the mouth twice daily for 30 seconds. Toothbrushing can begin the day after cleaning. A hard diet is offered because it decreases plaque mass on teeth.

About 1 month after cleaning, re-evaluation should occur, and any periodontal surgery necessary can take place. Surgery is indicated when pocket depth is 5 mm or greater and bleeding on probing does not resolve after thorough tooth cleaning. Opening the area by surgery provides better access to the root surface so that hidden calculus can be exposed to view and removed.

Inverse-Bevel Repositioned Flaps for Root Débridement

The goal of inverse-bevel repositioned flaps is to reflect the soft tissue away from the teeth, remove granulation tissue around the roots, and thoroughly clean the roots down to the periodontal attachment.

During the first 2 weeks after surgery, the dentogingival junction is irrigated with 0.1 to 0.2 per cent chlorhexidine twice daily for 30 seconds. Surgical patients should undergo tooth cleaning every 3 to 12 months.

Inverse-Bevel Apically Positioned Flaps for Pocket Reduction

Inverse-bevel apically positioned flaps are indicated to expose the root surface, decrease pocket depth, and increase the amount of attached gingiva. Postoperative care is the same as for other periodontal surgery.

Osseous Flap Surgery

Osseous flap surgery is similar to inverse-bevel flap surgery except that it is intended as an approach for bone surgery. The primary difference between this operation and other flap operations is that it involves bone removal. This operation is seldom used except for treating deep pockets with intractable inflammation below the bony crest that borders them. When supporting bone is removed, the operation is called ostectomy. Postoperative care is the same as for other periodontal surgery.

Crown Lengthening

When teeth are fractured below the gingival margin, normal tooth structure must be exposed to allow an accurate restoration. This operation involves removing bone and soft tissue to reposition the margins of a flap below the fracture line. It is also used on resorptive lesions in cats ("neck lesions") to restore teeth damaged by root resorption. Postoperative care is the same as for other periodontal surgery.

Gingivectomy

Gingivectomy eliminates periodontal pockets through excision of excessive tissue above the alveolar crest. It is indicated when excessive tissue can be removed without creating abnormal gingival tissue contour. The incision is started below the marks and is directed toward the depth of the pocket on the tooth. The resected tissue is removed with tissue nippers and curettes, the area is irrigated, and the roots are cleaned. Postoperative care is the same as for flap surgery.

Gingivoplasty

Gingivoplasty reshapes the gingiva. The intent is to create normal tissue contour rather than to resect soft-tissue pockets. Recurrence of gingival hyperplasia indicates repetition of the operation at a later date.

Mucogingival Surgery

Mucogingival surgery increases the amount of attached gingiva or repositions the attached gingiva and alveolar mucosa. It is indicated when periodontal inflammation persists after cleaning because of an inadequate barrier of attached gingiva between alveolar mucosa and the periodontal attachment to the tooth.

Gingival recession over prominent roots may be treated by rotating a pedicle of adjacent attached gingiva to the denuded area. The margins are sutured, and the postoperative management is the same as for other types of periodontal surgery.

Soft tissue may be harvested from one area of the mouth and transferred to bone or connective tissue in another area to increase tissue at the new site. Postoperative care is the same as for other periodontal surgery except that care is taken to ensure that the graft is not dislodged from the recipient site by vigorous irrigation or by chewing hard objects.

Reconstructive Surgery for Intraosseous and Furcation Defects

Crushed oral cancellous bone or frozen red marrow from the same individual is most effective in stimulating regeneration of new support.

Placing of a bone graft or implant is initiated by inverse-bevel flap exposure. The soft tissue in the bone defect is removed, the roots are cleaned, and the defect is filled with the chosen material. The flaps are carefully adapted to the teeth, and the patient is given tetracycline for 3 weeks. Chlorhexidine solution is used to irrigate the mouth for the first 2 weeks after surgery.

Maintenance Therapy

Each patient has different requirements for how often the dentition must be professionally cleaned.

One way to establish an appropriate recall interval is to re-examine treated patients at 3-month intervals. If the clinician recognizes established gingivitis and bleeding on subgingival probing, the dentition is cleaned, and a new appointment is made for 1 month. Most animals with severe periodontitis require cleaning approximately every 6 months.

Maintenance cleaning only requires supragingival scaling with inspection of the subgingival environment for bleeding. All teeth are polished, and for 2 weeks, 0.1 to 0.2 per cent chlorhexidine rinses are used twice daily for 30 seconds. Radiographs can be used in chronologically evaluating the attachment level on the rostral and caudal surfaces of teeth.

Treatment of Combined Periodontal and Endodontic Lesions

Roots so severely affected by periodontal disease that they are painful or cause periodic abscess should be removed. When little periodontal attachment remains, the offending tooth is extracted. When a multi-rooted tooth has one or more roots that are solid with little bone loss, the decision is more difficult. When the tooth is not valuable, extraction is best.

When a tooth is considered valuable, the surgeon can amputate the involved root and allow the tooth to survive. The tooth is first treated endodontically to prevent pain, contamination of the remaining canals with bacteria, and retarded periodontal healing, which might occur if the root were amputated first. The tooth must be treated by conventional endodontic techniques in all the remaining roots.

Periodontal Prosthesis

When attachment loss has been extensive and mobility of teeth prevents mastication without pain, the surgeon can join teeth together and use their combined support to avoid discomfort. Individual crowns are constructed for the involved teeth, and these are joined together by soldered or cast joints.

Another indication for splinting teeth together with a prosthesis is food impaction between loose-touching teeth. These teeth can be joined together with cast crowns, which prevent food impaction.

CHAPTER 179

Endodontics and Root Canal Therapy (pages 2339–2345)

Endodontic therapy is needed to retain a tooth with a necrotic pulp. Early endodontic therapy on teeth with pulp disease can be used to retain these functional teeth in comfort.

PATHOGENESIS OF THE ENDODONTIC LESION
(pp. 2340–2341)

The term *pulpal hyperemia* refers to reversible inflammation of the pulp due to trauma, and the term *pulpitis* refers to irreversible damage of the pulp due to trauma. Teeth with pulpal hyperemia are engorged with blood and inflammatory cells. Unfortunately, early pulpal hyperemia is rarely diagnosed in veterinary patients because of their stoic nature and inability to communicate. It is much more common to diagnose pulpitis, because clinical signs of the disease become evident.

Pulpitis involves an irreversible lesion that leads to pulpal death. The only part of the tooth that remains vital after pulpal death is the cellular cementum that covers the exterior surface of the root. Death of the pulp does not affect tooth function. When the pulp is secondarily affected as a result of periodontitis, the process is given the term *periodontal-endodontic involvement.* When pulpitis is caused by dental disease, the pulp is affected first. This process is given the term *endodontic-periodontal involvement.*

The two most common drainage patterns for primary endodontic lesions are (1) through the bone and exiting through the mucosa into the mouth and (2) along the periodontal ligament and exiting into the mouth by creation of a periodontal pocket between the gingiva and tooth. Without treatment, the pathological processes associated with endodontic disease rarely resolve.

EXAMINATION (p. 2341)

Teeth with pinpoint exposures of the pulp require tactile confirmation that exposure of the pulp has occurred. A fine, sharp probe is used to explore the suspected area while the patient is under general anesthesia or is sedated and the tooth is locally anesthetized.

Radiography is useful in confirming endodontic disease in chronic lesions. Early lesions simply appear as an interruption of the lamina dura, usually at the apex but occasionally along the side of the root. Later, lesions have some periapical radiolucency, usually in a circular or ovoid pattern.

CONVENTIONAL ENDODONTIC TREATMENT
(pp. 2341–2343)

Conventional endodontics entails removal of contaminated debris from the root canal by a coronal approach and subsequent filling of the canal with biocompatible material so that the area around the tooth heals. The purpose of conventional endodontics is to seal the nutrient foramen in the root so that no further seepage of necrotic debris or bacteria comes from the root. The focus of treatment is usually sealing of the apex of the root.

Endodontic treatment is begun by gaining access to the root canals in a straight line. Surgical-length 1557 carbide burs can be used in a high-speed handpiece to make an opening into the pulp above each root canal.

Once the access preparation has been cut, a number 10 or number 15 file is inserted to ensure that the operator can reach the apex without further modification. When access to the apex is assured, a barbed broach or file is used to remove as much of the pulp as possible. The canal is flushed with a 10 per cent solution of household bleach mixed with water.

As each successively larger file is used, the operator ensures that the working length of the original file is maintained by obtaining an initial radiograph with the thinnest file in place and using a rubber stopper on the shank of the file as a marker.

The operator should cease instrumentation when the canal is clean and the apex has been prepared to a uniform size. At this time, the canal is irrigated a final time with hypochlorite solution and dried with paper points. This process of cleaning and preparing the apex is completed on every root of multirooted teeth.

The most traditionally acceptable, and usually the easiest, technique is the gutta-percha fill technique. The operator selects a preformed gutta-percha point of the exact width and shape of the last file used in instrumentation of the apex. This process continues until the canal does not admit further cones and radiography demonstrates complete filling.

Conventional endodontic treatment is completed by filling the pulp canal with condensed gutta-percha and high compressive-strength cement (e.g., zinc phosphate) and placing a permanent filling (e.g., silver amalgam) in the access preparation. All endodontically treated teeth are covered with a cast metal crown to prevent breakage.

SURGICAL ENDODONTICS (pp. 2343–2345)

The term *surgical endodontics* connotes an approach to the endodontic system through the apex—a "reverse fill." The goal is to approach the apical area laterally or apically, to cut off a section of the apex, and to fill the root canal at the apex with an inert biocompatible material. Because this approach enhances exposure and access, it can improve the outcome of endodontic therapy in difficult cases. Conventional endodontics and surgical endodontics can be performed at the same time, but on different roots of multirooted teeth.

The first re-examination is performed at 7 to 14 days, at which time the area is inspected for proper healing and sutures are removed. Radiographic evaluation is performed at 6 months, and yearly thereafter, for apparently successful cases. Crowning of all endodontically treated teeth is prudent, as structural failure is more likely when endodontically treated teeth are stressed.

COMBINED ENDODONTIC–PERIODONTIC LESIONS (p. 2345)

When both types of lesions are present, the question of which to treat first arises. In practice, both lesions often need to be treated concurrently. Theoretically, the best strategy is to treat the endodontic lesion first, wait for periodontal healing to determine the extent of the persistent periodontal lesion, and complete therapy with periodontal treatment. The presence of chronic periodontal lesions communicating with and responsible for devitalized pulpal tissue indicates a poor prognosis for extensive periodontal repair after endodontic treatment.

CHAPTER 180

Restorative Dentistry (pages 2346–2349)

RESTORATIVE MATERIALS (pp. 2346–2347)

Amalgam

In the past, amalgam had a composition within specified limits: silver 65 per cent (minimum), tin 29 per cent (maximum), copper 6 per cent (maximum), zinc 2 per cent (maximum), and mercury 3 per cent (maximum). Copper is now added as a blended alloy, or as a single silver-copper particle alloy. The amount of copper in amalgam ranges from 12 to 30 per cent, depending on the manufacturer.

The advantage of higher copper content is that mercury has a chemical preference for bonding to copper instead of to tin. The mercury-tin bond was the "weakest, softest, and most corrodible phase in the set metallurgical structure."

A major disadvantage of amalgam in dentistry is the lack of any chemical bond with either enamel or dentin. Amalgam must be held in place by mechanical undercutting of the tooth with an inverted cone-shaped or pear-shaped bur, which weakens the tooth.

When amalgam is used for restorations, cavity varnish liner is applied to all cavity preparations in vital teeth. The layer of varnish seals the open dentinal tubules and fills in the microscopic space between the amalgam and the cavity wall, until the corrosion reaction that seals the restoration to the margin has occurred.

Deeper carious lesions, which extend within 1 mm of the pulp chamber, require a rigid base to protect the pulp tissues. Satisfactory bases include various cements such as zinc phosphate, polycarboxylate, glass ionomer, or reinforced zinc oxide–eugenol.

Composite Resins

Composite resins are of two types. Chemical-cured resins rely on benzoyl peroxide–tertiary amine mechanisms and are self-curing. Two paste systems polymerize when mixed and must be placed quickly into the prepared site. The light-cured composite resins eliminate some of these problems. Visible light is used to initiate the diketone polymerization reaction. Light-cured restorative materials allow the operator more time for accurate placement and result in decreased porosity of the restoration.

Composite resins have many applications in veterinary dentistry, including cosmetic restorations, correction of enamel hypoplasia, and restoration of slab fractures of the upper fourth premolar teeth. Composite resins can also be used to close access openings after endodontic procedures.

Glass Ionomer Cements

Glass ionomer cements are the newest restorative material and are unique in that they form a chemical bond to the dentin and, to a lesser degree, the enamel. The glass ionomer bond occurs in two phases. Calcium polycarboxylate gel is formed initially, followed by aluminum polycarboxylate gel during the next 24 hours.

Major advantages of glass ionomer cements include hard surface translucency, bonding to dentin, release of fluoride, and little accumulation of plaque. These cements are preferred for restoration of cervical line lesions (neck lesions) in feline teeth. Glass ionomer cements are also excellent choices for filling access openings after endodontic procedures.

Glass ionomer cements with silver particles incorporated into the powder have been developed to provide extra strength. These mixtures are called cermets. In veterinary treatment of feline cervical line lesions, this product has little advantage, because an occlusal surface is not involved in the procedure.

ACCESSORY MATERIALS (pp. 2347–2348)

Cements

Cements are used as luting agents to hold restorations in place, and they are used as restorative materials if heavy filling is required. Cements can also be used as interfaces between restorative materials and normal dental tissues. The four basic types of cements are based on the type of bonding to teeth: phosphate-bonded, phenolate-bonded, polycarboxylate-bonded, and polymer-bonded.

Zinc phosphate is a phosphate-bonded cement. It is used as a luting agent, in temporary restorations, and for protection of vital dental tissues against thermal changes. Zinc oxide–eugenol is a phenolate-bonded cement. It is used as a root canal filling material, as a temporary filling material, and as a base for thermal insulation. Duralon is a polycarboxylate cement usually used for luting of restorations. Glass ionomer cements are polymer bonded.

Liners

A cavity liner is a material used to protect vital pulp tissue and over which a restoration is to be placed. Two thin layers of a cavity varnish are often used to seal dentinal tubules. Examples of cavity varnishes used as liners are Copanol and Copanol-F. Glass ionomer restorative materials usually do not require liners because they bond to dentin and are usually not irritating to the pulp when used properly.

RESTORATION OF CARIES AND CERVICAL LINE LESIONS (pp. 2348–2349)

Caries are the organic breakdown of tooth enamel from the by-products of certain microorganisms in the mouth. Carious lesions are usually found in the occlusal surfaces of the molar teeth, where food can become trapped in the enamel pits and fissures, rather than on exposed root surfaces.

In the cat, cervical line lesions (also called cervical line erosions, neck lesions, or caries) are characterized by "progressive, subgingival, osteoclastic resorption." The usual location of these lesions is the gingival margin or neck of the tooth. The buccal surfaces of the teeth are most often affected. Cervical line lesions are either shallow (not into the pulp chamber) or deep (invading the pulp chamber).

Radiographic examination of the affected teeth is necessary, as shallow cervical line lesions should not be restored unless radiographs indicate solid root structure.

Teeth with cervical line lesions that extend into the pulp tissue are usually removed by extraction or pulverization with a high-speed drill and round bur. If a canine tooth is affected and has sufficient root structure, an endodontic procedure may be performed.

Glass ionomer cements are extremely useful for the restoration of certain cervical line lesions. Shallow cervical line lesions may be treated conservatively (not given full restoration) with an application of ScotchBond II, a light-cured material that seals the dentinal tubules. Patients with cervical line lesions are rechecked every 6 months.

CHAPTER 181

Occlusion and Orthodontics
(pages 2349–2358)

Normal occlusion is based on the mesaticephalic skull and is characterized by a scissors bite. The scissors bite is a shear mouth, that is, the mandibular incisors are in minimal contact with the lingual surfaces of the maxillary incisors.

TOOTH ERUPTION AND RETAINED DECIDUOUS TEETH
(pp. 2349–2351)

The retention of these teeth for as short a period as 2 weeks can produce occlusal defects in the permanent teeth. Malocclusions produce early wearing of the teeth (attrition); rotation and crowding of the teeth, resulting in periodontal disease; and in many instances, soft tissue trauma. Occasionally, malocclusions prevent the mouth from closing completely.

The permanent teeth have a characteristic eruption pathway when the deciduous teeth are retained. The incisors, lower canine teeth, and premolars erupt at positions lingual or palatal to the deciduous teeth. The lower canine teeth are "base narrow" and tend to damage the tissues of the hard palate as they erupt. Eruption of the maxillary canine teeth is rostral to the deciduous canine teeth, so that the interdental space between the lateral incisors and the canine teeth is closed. The lower canine teeth are forced in a forward (rostral) and lingual dissection to maintain their position anterior to the maxillary canine teeth. In addition, the attrition produced as a result of striking of the maxillary lateral incisors by the mandibular canine teeth leads to complete destruction of both teeth.

INTERCEPTIVE ORTHODONTICS (p. 2351)

The term *interceptive orthodontics* refers to instances in which a manifest malocclusion is developing because of hereditary patterns or extrinsic or intrinsic factors.

In minor differences of jaw length in the young puppy, extraction of the deciduous incisors or canine teeth is often beneficial. This extraction allows the full genetic potential for growth of the mandible and maxilla to be expressed. Shedding of the deciduous dentition is not left to chance but is kept on schedule through extraction of the tooth or teeth that have not been shed on time via normal processes.

MALOCCLUSION (pp. 2351–2353)

Class I Malocclusion (Neutroclusion)

Class I malocclusion, or neutroclusion, is characterized by irregularities of individual teeth, but with a normal mesiodistal or rostral-caudal relationship of the mandibular and maxillary dental arches. Class I malocclusion is the largest single group of malocclusions.

In class I malocclusions, there is not enough space to accommodate all teeth. This situation may be due to prolonged retention of deciduous teeth, retained root tips of deciduous teeth, micrognathia, and extreme variations in tooth size, as in toy breeds of dogs. Interceptive orthodontics including serial extractions can prevent a substantial number of these malocclusions if performed at the proper time.

Class II Malocclusion (Distoclusion/Brachygnathia)

In class II malocclusion, the upper dental arch is in a rostral or anterior relationship to the lower dental arch, as reflected by the permanent premolars and the permanent canine teeth in the permanent dental arch. The upper premolars drift over the top of their mandibular counterparts. This drift is also referred to as "overshoot" and occurs frequently in dolichocephalic breeds, such as the dachshund, collie, Italian greyhound, and Russian wolfhound.

Brachygnathia, or the lack of growth of the mandible compared with the growth of the maxilla, results in an increase in space between the upper and lower incisors. In some instances, the mandibular canine teeth are completely caudal and palatal to the maxillary canine teeth.

Class III Malocclusion (Mesioclusion/Prognathism)

The upper dental arch is caudal or posterior to the lower dental arch in class III malocclusion, as reflected by the molars, premolars, and canine teeth in their permanent dentition. Prognathism is normal for brachycephalic breeds of dogs such as boxers and bulldogs, but it is an aberration in mesocephalic and dolichocephalic breeds.

The American Kennel Club and most veterinarians consider orthodontic therapy unethical when efforts are made to camouflage genetic malocclusions. At least 50 per cent of all malocclusions are acquired and have no genetic basis.

Malaligned teeth are moved into a more normal configuration to reduce the abnormal wear from one tooth's striking another, to allow the patient to close its mouth and chew more comfortably, and to reduce the high incidence of periodontal disease in animals with malocclusion. Ideally, the 6-month-old to 1-year-old animal is preferred, and most movements can be accomplished in as little as 2 to 16 weeks.

The movement of teeth has three basic prerequisites: sufficient space, adequate pressure, and the necessary anchorage. When constant pressure is applied to a tooth surface, bone is resorbed ahead of the drifting tooth and deposited behind it. Constant pressure must be maintained to reposition the tooth properly. Retention of the tooth in its proper position is sometimes necessary for about 4 weeks.

Oral Appliances

Oral appliances can be used successfully to treat malocclusions. Orthodontic acrylic (polymethyl methacrylate) may be used to form an active appliance or may be used as a retainer. Acrylic appliances are almost always formed on an oral model to prevent thermal damage to the oral tissues during the curing phase, which produces an exothermic reaction. Forming the appliance on a model also allows for a more accurate and easier design of the appliance.

The most common use of the acrylic appliance is for an inclined bite plane indicated for lingually displaced mandibular canine teeth. The acrylic should encompass the lingual aspect of the incisors, extending just beyond the distal margin of the maxillary canine teeth. A buildup of acrylic at the contact points of the lower canine teeth allows the force of mastication to move the teeth along an inclined plane into proper apposition.

Direct Bonding

Improved cements and composite bonding techniques allow orthodontic movement through direct application of brackets or bands. The most common orthodontic problem for which this type of therapy is appropriate is rostral protrusion of the maxillary canine teeth.

Depending on the size and age of the dog, a period of 8 to 12 weeks is required to move a tooth to the new position. Once the tooth is in place, it is retained with ligature wires or an acrylic splint for at least 4 weeks to allow the bone and tissue to reorganize.

Dental Impressions

Indirect applications of orthodontic appliances must be preceded by the development of a working model to enable the veterinarian or the dental laboratory technicians to fabricate the appliance. Impression trays are used to carry the putty-like alginate mixture to the mouth and hold it in position until it sets. The most common impression material is dental alginate, which is supplied in fast and regular setting.

Stone Model Production

The various stone powders that are available differ in strength, setting time, and ability to reproduce detail. Pink stone is most often used in animals. The alginate impression, while still in the tray, is placed on an investment vibrator, and small amounts of the stone mixture are flowed into the impression with the vibrator running. Several hours are necessary for the stone to harden, after which the alginate can be carefully removed or cut away.

Fixed Appliances

Once a study model is produced, designing the appliance to address the orthodontic problem is usually a simple task. The various types of appliances are as follows:

1. Acrylic splints
2. Expansion or jackscrews
3. Bands with hooks or buttons
4. Memory wires
5. Maryland bridge

The expansion screw is more substantial than the microscrew device and can be used to move one tooth or the entire arch segment. Acrylic can also be used to embed elastic ligature thread (power thread), or to retract a tooth and also act as a stop to prevent the tooth from moving too far caudally. Orthodontic bands with hooks or buttons can be constructed on the model to attach the power chain or elastic ligature thread.

Memory wires were developed to return to the original shape no matter how much distortion occurred. This wire can be shaped into a "W" configuration and soldered to bands connected to the mandibular canine teeth on the prepared model. When placed and cemented in the patient's mouth, the "W" wire returns to its original shape. The force produced gives an even, steady pressure to move the lingually displaced canine teeth to their normal position.

Maryland bridge techniques involve a combination of cast-metal and resin-bonded restorative materials. Numerous refinements and improvements have been reported. The Maryland bridge can be used to protrude some or all of the maxillary incisors. It can also be applied to moving rostrally displaced canine teeth caudally. The appliance is made of light, polished metal that offers little area for food, hair, or other debris to accumulate, and is easily cleaned by brushing and flushing.

Full client cooperation is required in keeping the appliance clean, adjusting it if necessary, and keeping appointments needed for evaluation and monitoring of the progress of the procedure.

Surgical Formulary

Agents listed are those most commonly used in small animal surgical patients. Infrequently used medications or those not used in surgical patients are not included. A cross index of common trade names is shown in Appendix II. Dosages shown may be used for both dogs and cats unless separate rates are shown for each species, or unless there is a warning against use in either species. *All dose rates should be checked for accuracy, and specific indications, contraindications, and warnings. The doses of many agents used in surgical patients are extrapolated from use in man, and these should be checked carefully, as use and experience in animals may be limited.*

References: Slatter D (Ed.): Textbook of Small Animal Surgery, Second Edition, Volumes 1 and 2. WB Saunders, Philadelphia, 1993; Ettinger SJ (Ed): Pocket Companion to Textbook of Small Animal Internal Medicine. WB Saunders, Philadelphia, 1993; Kirk RW (Ed): Current Veterinary Therapy IX, X. WB Saunders, Philadelphia, 1986, 1989.

Drug (Trade Name)	Route	Dose	Effects and Medications	Side Effects	Comments
Acepromazine (*Acepromazine*)	PO, SC, IM, IV	0.02–0.4 mg/kg	Sedative, preanesthetic, antiemetic, muscle relaxant. Surgical hypertension. postoperative hyperthermia and pain, aggression.	CNS depression, hypotension.	Phenothiazine derivative. Do not use in patients with seizures.
Acetaminophen	PO	10 mg/kg BID	Antipyretic, analgesic. Causes methemoglobinemia in cats.	Gastric irritation. Toxic to cats.	Antidote is acetylcysteine. In dogs, reduces postoperative pain and swelling but use is *not* recommended.
Acetazolamide (*Diamox*) (*Vetamox*)	IV	20–30 mg/kg	Carbonic anhydrase inhibitor. Reduces aqueous production in glaucoma.	Vomiting, panting, acidosis, anorexia, disorientation.	For emergency use. Avoid oral use to prevent vomiting.
Acetohydroxamic acid	PO	12.5 mg/kg BID (dog)	Urease inhibitor. For struvite urolithiasis.		Rarely used alone.
Acetylcysteine (*Mucomyst*)	Inhalation	10% (drops) or nebulized solution	Protease inhibitor, mucolytic (ocular, bronchial). Acetaminophen toxicosis.	Irritation on instillation.	Rarely used alone. Adjust pH to 7.4 when added to eye drops. Acetaminophen toxicosis, 70 mg/kg PO q6l1h; may be given IV with first dose of 140 mg/kg. Nebulize 3–10 ml of 10% TID-QID or instill 0.25–2 ml into airway hourly.

Drug	Route	Dosage	Indications/Action	Side Effects	Comments
Acetylsalicylic acid (*Aspirin*) (*Ascriptin*)	PO	10–25 mg/kg SID–TID (dog), q48h (cat)	Analgesic, anti-inflammatory, antipyretic. Reduces aqueous protein prior to intraocular surgery. Prevents thrombosis after vascular surgery. Inhibits prostaglandins E_2 and F_2. Degenerative joint disease.	Depresses platelet number. Gastric ulceration, vomiting, melena, skin eruptions, edema, deafness. Side effects rare at therapeutic dosages.	Note dosage in cats. Gastric effects can be reduced by simultaneous administration of oral misoprostol and food. Histamine antagonists do not affect gastric irritation.
Actinomycin D (*Cosmegen*)	IV	0.015 mg/kg	Nephroblastoma (direct) and radiosensitizer.	Leukopenia, thrombocytopenia.	
Allopurinol (*Zyloprim*)	PO	10 mg/kg q8h, then reduce to 10 mg/kg/day	Urate urolithiasis.		TID for 30 days, then SID.
Alloxan	IV	65 mg/kg—single dose	Metastatic insulinoma. Toxic to pancreatic islet cells and renal tubular epithelium.	Nephrotoxicity in 10% of patients.	
Amikacin (*Amikin*) (*Amiglyde-V*)	IM, IV, SC	5–10 mg/kg TID	Bactericidal, broad-spectrum aminoglycoside antibiotic.	Ototoxicity, nephrotoxicity, poor GI absorption, neuromuscular blockade.	Can be combined with ampicillin for sepsis.
Aminocaproic acid (*Amicar*)	PO, IV	50–90 mg/kg loading dose over 1 hr; 15 mg/kg/hr	Inhibitor of fibrinolysis. Hematuria after nephrotomy.	Myopathy and muscle necrosis reported in man.	Given IV followed by PO or IV maintenance. Questionable efficacy. Thrombi formed during treatment are not lysed. Dose rates are for MAN. Maximum human dose 0.4 g/kg/day.
Aminopentamide (*Centrine*)	PO, SC, IM	0.02 mg/kg q8–12hr	Anticholinergic, GI antispasmodic.	Dry mouth.	

Drug (Trade Name)	Route	Dose	Effects and Medications	Side Effects	Comments
Aminophylline	PO, IV	1.5–10 mg/kg SID–TID (dog); 2–4 mg/kg SID–BID	Bronchodilator, diuretic.	Hyperexcitability, gastric irritation, anorexia.	Administer IV slowly.
Aminopropazine (Jenotone)	IM	2.2–4.4 (dog), 6.25–12.5 mg/kg (cat) SID–BID	Urethral obstructions, smooth muscle relaxant.	Not used in cystic atony.	
Ammonium chloride	PO	100 mg/kg divided TID (dog); 20 mg/kg BID (cat)	Urinary acidifier, struvite urolithiasis.	GI irritation, poor palatability.	
Amoxicillin (Amoxi-tabs) (Amoxi-drops)	PO, SC, IM, IV	10–20 mg/kg BID–TID	Broad-spectrum bactericidal antibiotic.	As for penicillins.	Inactivated by beta-lactamases.
Amoxicillin (Clavamox) (Augmentin)	PO	10–20 mg/kg BID	Broad-spectrum bactericidal antibiotic. Clavulanic acid inhibits beta-lactamases.	As for penicillins, vomiting in cats.	Must remain in foil until used.
Amphotericin B (Fungizone)	IV	0.15–1 mg/kg in 5–20 ml of 5% dextrose	Systemic mycoses, fungal corneal ulceration.	Nephrotoxicity, emesis.	Use antiemetics, monitor blood urea nitrogen. Administer rapidly IV 3 times per week for 8–16 wk. Do not exceed 2 mg/kg.
Ampicillin	Subconj. inj.	50–250 mg	Ulcerative keratitis, endophthalmitis.		

Drug	Route	Dose	Action/Indication	Side Effects	Notes
Ampicillin	PO, SC, IM, IV	10–20 mg/kg BID–TID	Broad-spectrum bactericidal antibiotic. Use 4–6 wk for discospondylitis due to beta-hemolytic *Streptococcus*.	As for penicillins.	Inactivated by beta-lactamases. Can be combined with amikacin for sepsis.
Amrinone (*Inocor*)	IV	1–3 mg bolus IV, then 10–100 µg/kg/min	Low-output congestive heart failure.	Tachycardia, anxiety, GI side effects, hepatotoxicity, fever, reversible thrombocytopenia.	Monitor pulse and blood pressure.
Apomorphine	IM, SC	0.08 mg/kg	Emetic.	Contraindicated in cats	Tablet can be administered beneath the third eyelid.
Ascorbic acid	PO	100–500 mg SID–TID (dog), 30 mg/kg QID (cat)	Urinary acidifier. Acetaminophen-induced methemoglobinuria, copper hepatotoxicity.		
Asparaginase (*Elspar*)	IP	10,000 units/m^2 (400 units/kg) IP	Lymphoreticular neoplasia.	Anaphylaxis, leukopenia, pancreatitis.	
Atenolol (*Tenormin*)	PO	0.5–1 mg/kg SID–BID (dog); 1/8–1/4 tab SID (cat)	Beta-1 adrenergic blocker. Supraventricular arrhythmias, systemic hypertension.	Hypotension, depression, beta-blockade–induced congestive heart failure.	
Atracurium (*Tracrium*)	IV	100–250 µg/kg	Nondepolarizing neuromuscular blocker.	Respiratory arrest.	Reversal agents: neostigmine, pyridostigmine, edrophonium.
Atropine	Eye drop	1%	Cycloplegia, mydriasis.	Salivation.	Note: Salivation is due to bitter taste. Contraindicated in glaucoma patients. Use as ointment in cats to limit salivation.

791

Drug (Trade Name)	Route	Dose	Effects and Medications	Side Effects	Comments
Atropine sulfate	IM, SC	0.01–0.04 mg/kg	Preanesthetic to prevent salivation, supraventricular bradyarrhythmia, oculocardiac reflex. Anticholinergic for organophosphate toxicity.	Mydriasis, ileus, tachycardia.	Can be used at systemic doses for preoperative treatment of glaucoma patients. Used with neostigmine to reverse peripheral muscle relaxants.
Auranofin (Ridaura)	PO	0.05–0.2 mg/kg BID	Treatment of idiopathic polyarthritis.	Proteinuria, thrombocytopenia, hemolytic anemia, pruritus, rash, stomatitis, GI side effects.	Used in combination with gold therapy and a glucocorticoid.
Aurothioglucose (Solganol)	IM	1 mg/kg/wk (dog)	Rheumatoid arthritis.		
Aurothioglucose (Solganol)	IM	1 mg/kg/wk	Rheumatoid arthritis—delay of 6–12 wk to improvement.	Blood dyscrasias, liver and kidney toxicity.	Use 0.25 mg/kg to test for anaphylaxis. Decrease dose from weekly to monthly. Monitor renal and hematological parameters every 2 wk.
Azathioprine (Imuran)	PO	1–2 mg/kg every other day	Immunosuppressive agent. Rheumatoid arthritis, renal transplant rejection.	Leukopenia, thrombocytopenia, bone marrow suppression. Hepatotoxicity rare.	Monitor CBC.
Bacitracin	Subconj. inj.	10,000 units	Intraocular infections, ulcerative keratitis, irrigation of bone graft recipient bed (25–50 mg/ml). Bactericidal. Gram-positive cocci and bacilli Neisseria, Pseudomonas, Nocardia, and Candida resistant.	Nephrotoxicity after systemic administration.	

Drug	Route	Dose	Use	Adverse Effects/Contraindications	Comments
Betamethasone (*Betasone*)	IM, PO	0.2–0.4 mg/kg	Long-acting steroid. Potency 7–10× prednisolone.	Polyuria, polydipsia, hunger, adrenocortical suppression.	
Betamethasone (*Betasone*)	Subconj. inj.	3–5 mg	Uveitis, trauma, specific disorders.	Polyuria, polydipsia, hunger, adrenocortical suppression.	Contraindicated if fluorescein positive, infection present, or specific diagnosis lacking. Different salts have different durations.
Betaxolol (*Betoptic*)	Eye drop		Glaucoma. Beta-adrenergic–blocking agent.		Efficacy poor. Not suitable alone.
Bethanecol (*Urecholine*)	PO, SC	Dog, 5–25 mg TID PO; 2.5–10 mg TID SC (dog); 2.5–5 mg PO BID (cat)	Nonobstructive cystic atony, detrusor hypotony in feline urologic syndrome.	Contraindicated in cystic obstruction or areflexia.	
Bleomycin (*Blenoxane*)	IV	10 mg/m² for 3–9 days, then 10 mg/m²/wk	Squamous cell, other carcinomas.	Allergic reactions after administration, pulmonary fibrosis.	Do not exceed 200 mg/m² total dose.
Bretylium tosylate (*Breylol*)	IV	5–10 mg/kg	Reduction of ventricular fibrillation during CPR.		
Bupivicaine (*Marcaine*)	IM	0.5% 0.5 ml/nerve	Local anesthetic for intercostal block after thoracotomy.		Lasts 3–4 hr. Add epinephrine (5 µg/ml) for 6–8 hr of effects. Can be given for epidural anesthesia.
Buprenorphine (*Buprenex*)	IM, IV, SC	5–10 µg/kg	Analgesic, sedative. Antagonizes opioid agonists such as morphine, oxymorphone. Postoperative pain after thoracic surgery.		Opioid agonist/antagonist. Duration 8–10 hr.

793

Drug (Trade Name)	Route	Dose	Effects and Medications	Side Effects	Comments
Butorphanol (Torbugesic) (Torbutrol)	PO, SC, IM, IV	0.2–1 mg/kg QID (dog); 0.2–0.5 mg/kg BID-QID (cat)	Analgesic, sedative. Antagonizes opioid agonists. Cough suppressant. Preanesthetic for gastrointestinal, orthopedics, and trauma patients. Postoperative pain after orthopedic, intervertebral disc surgery.	Vomiting, sedation. Overexcitement in cats.	Opioid agonist/antagonist. Duration 3–4 hr. Combined with ketamine and midazolam at 0.4 mg/kg for restraint in puppies and kittens.
Calcitonin	IM, IV, SC	4–8 μg/kg BID	Reduces serum calcium in hypercalcemia, especially cholecalciferol toxicity.	Irritation at injection site. GI side effects possible.	
Calcium chloride	IV, intracardiac	0.1 ml/kg	Ventricular asystole.	Arrhythmias.	
Calcium EDTA—see EDTA-Ca					
Calcium gluconate 10% (Calcet)	Intralesional	0.5 ml/cm^2	For hydrofluoric acid burns of less than 20% of body surface area, to precipitate fluoride ion and prevent penetration.		Copious lavage; wash with aqueous benzylkonium chloride first.
Calcium gluconate 10% (Calcet)	IV	10–30 ml (dog).	Hypocalcemia, tetany in acute pancreatitis. Uterine atony (0.3 mg/kg) IV. Ventricular asystole (0.5–2 ml/kg over 15–30 min). 15 mg/kg for postoperative hypercalcemia after removal of a parathyroid tumor.	Arrhythmias.	Balanced electrolyte solution safer unless signs of hypocalcemia (prepartum eclampsia) present.

Drug	Route	Dose	Indications	Adverse effects/Notes
Captopril (*Capoten*)	PO	0.5–1.5 mg/kg BID–TID (dog); 3–6.25 mg SID (cat)	Angiotensin-converting enzyme inhibitor, antihypertensive, vasodilator. Congestive heart failure.	Hypotension-depression, anorexia.
Carbenicillin (*Geopen*)	PO, SC, IM, IV	100 mg SC, 15 mg/kg IV, PO	Enophthalmitis. Susceptible to beta-lactamases, useful for *Pseudomonas* and *Proteus* spp.	
Carmustine (*BICNU*)	IV	50–80 mg/m²/6–8 wk	Confirmed glial tumors.	Bone marrow suppression, nausea, vomiting, CNS toxicity, and others reported in man.
Cefadroxil—see cephalosporins				
Cefamandole—see cephalosporins	Subconj. inj.	75 mg	Endophthalmitis. Broad-spectrum bactericidal.	
Cefotetan—see cephalosporins				
Cefoxitin—see cephalosporins	IV	20 mg/kg	Sepsis. Broad spectrum. Useful if renal function compromised. Useful for anaerobic bacteria.	
Cephalexin—see cephalosporins				
Cephaloridine—see cephalosporins	Subconj. inj.	100 mg	Endophthalmitis. Broad-spectrum bactericidal.	Bacteria more likely to develop resistance than to an aminoglycoside. Identify bacteria quickly. Less susceptible beta-lactamases from gram-positive.

795

Drug (Trade Name)	Route	Dose	Effects and Medications	Side Effects	Comments
Cephalosporins	PO, SC, IM, IV	10–30 mg/kg BID	Broad-spectrum bactericidal group.	GI side effects. Possibly nephrotoxic at high doses with aminoglycosides.	
Cephalothin—see cephalosporins					
Cephradine—see cephalosporins (Velosef)	Subconj. inj.	100 mg	Endophthalmitis. Broad-spectrum bactericidal.		Beta-lactamase resistant.
	PO	20 mg/kg TID for 4–6 wk	Discospondylitis due to *Staphylococcus intermedius*.		
Chlorambucil (Leukeran)	PO	2–8 mg/m² 2–4 days wk	Lymphoreticular neoplasms, chronic lymphocytic leukemia, macroglobulinemia, arthritis, ovarian tumors.	Mild leukopenia, thrombocytopenia, anemia, nausea, vomiting (uncommon), bone marrow suppression.	Often used with prednisolone and other antimetabolites. Used SID for 3 wk beyond remission, then 1.5 mg/m² SID for 15 days and then every 3rd day.
Chloramphenicol	Subconj. inj.	50–100 mg	Endophthalmitis. Broad-spectrum bacteriostatic.		Sodium succinate preparation.
Chloramphenicol (Chloromycetin)	PO, SC, IM, IV	25–50 mg/kg TID	Broad-spectrum bacteriostatic, *Mycoplasma, Rickettsia, Chlamydia,* and anaerobes. Discospondylitis, keratitis, wound, and urinary tract infections.	Hepatic microsomal inhibitor. Anorexia in cats. Anorexia, vomiting, reversible bone marrow suppression with aplastic anemia. Inhibition of hepatic microsomal enzymes.	Monitor CBC and chemistries. Do not use with bactericidal antibiotics.
Chlorothiazide (Diuril)	PO	20–40 mg/kg BID	Diuretic.	Hyponatremia, hypokalemia.	Use cautiously with digitalis.

Drug	Route	Dosage	Description	Notes
Chlorpheniramine (Chlor-Trimeton)	PO	2–4 mg BID–TID (dog); 1–2 mg (cat)	Antihistamine, decongestant.	Drowsiness.
Chlorpromazine (Thorazine)	PO, SC, IM, IV	1–3 mg/kg PO QID; 0.5–5 mg/kg parenteral	Tranquilizer, antiemetic.	CNS depression with overdosage. May potentiate seizures.
Chymotrypsin	Lavage	50,000 units/100 ml lavage	Pleuritis, pyothorax.	
Cimetidine (Tagamet)	PO, IV	5–10 mg/kg BID–QID PO; 5 mg/kg BID IV, 2–5 mg/kg BID–TID PO	H₂ receptor antagonist. Used to increase gastric pH in gastritis of various causes; septic shock, prostatic abscess, hypercalcemia before parathyroidectomy, reflux esophagitis, mast cell tumors, Zollinger-Ellison syndrome, esophagitis, gastric reflux, chronic gastritis, GI ulceration, hypergastrinemia, during chemotherapy for mastocytoma.	See also ranitidine. Give 45 min before or 2 hr after sucralfate. Administer slowly IV.
Ciprofloxacin (Cipro)	Eye drop	QID	Broad-spectrum bactericidal antibiotic. Corneal ulceration.	See also enrofloxacin.
Ciprofloxacin (Cipro)	PO, IV, IM	4–10 mg/kg BID	Broad-spectrum bactericidal antibiotic. Discospondylitis, wound and urinary tract infections.	See also enrofloxacin. Approved for human use; dose extrapolated from use in man.

Drug (Trade Name)	Route	Dose	Effects and Medications	Side Effects	Comments
Cisplatin (Platinol)	IV	50–70 mg/m² q28 days (do not use in cats)	Osteosarcoma, squamous cell carcinoma, various sarcomas, carcinomas.	Nephrotoxicity, myelosuppression, GI side effects, anaphylaxis. Constipation.	Administered with saline diuresis. Use antiemetic. Wear gloves.
Clindamycin (Cleocin) (Antirobe)	PO	5–10 mg/kg BID	Gram-positive organisms: Staphylococcus, anaerobes, Bacteroides, toxoplasmosis, osteomyelitis.	Minor GI side effects in cats. Dose-dependent neuromuscular blockage causing skeletal muscle paralysis. Hepatotoxicity and epistaxis.	Toxoplasma. Cat: 25–50 mg/kg divided TID. Dog: 10–40 mg/kg divided TID. Do not use with erythromycin, chloramphenicol.
Clindamycin (Cleocin) (Antirobe)	Subconj. inj.	30 mg	Gram-positive organisms: Staphylococcus, anaerobes, causing keratitis.	Minor GI side effects in cats. Dose-dependent neuromuscular blockage causing skeletal muscle paralysis. Hepatotoxicity and epistaxis.	Do not use with erythromycin, chloramphenicol.
Clodronate	PO		Hypocalcemia agent. Preparation for parathyroidectomy.		
Cloxacillin	PO	10 mg/kg QID for 4–6 wk	Discospondylitis due to Staphylococcus intermedius.		Beta-lactamase resistant.
Codeine	PO	1–2 mg/kg q12 hr	Postoperative pain.	Constipation.	Least affected of the opioids by hepatic metabolism.
Colchicine (Colchicine)	PO	0.03 mg/kg/day SID–TID	Chronic hepatic fibrosis.		

798

Drug (Trade name)	Route	Dosage	Indications	Toxicity	Comments
Colistin (Polymixin E) (Colymycin S)	Subconj. inj.	15–30 mg	Endophthalmitis. Bactericidal for gram-negatives, including Enterobacter, Escherichia coli, Klebsiella, Salmonella, Pasteurella, and Pseudomonas spp. Bone grafting.	Hepatotoxic parenterally.	
Cyclophosphamide (Cytoxan)	PO, IV	50 mg/m² PO 4 days/wk, or 200 mg/m² IV	Lymphoreticular neoplasms; mammary, lung, ovarian neoplasms; miscellaneous carcinomas; arthritis; immune-mediated diseases.	Leukopenia, anemia, thrombocytopenia, nausea, vomiting, sterile hemorrhagic cystitis, constipation, alopecia.	Wear gloves.
Cyclosporine (Sandimmune)	Eye drop	1% in olive oil SID–BID	Keratoconjunctivitis sicca. Chronic immune-mediated keratoconjunctivitis syndrome in dogs. T-lymphocyte inhibitor.		Prepare in pharmaceutical-grade olive oil. Not reliable as sole treatment for canine xerosis.
Cyclosporine (Sandimmune)	PO	Various	Prevention of renal allograft rejection.		Dosage titrated to maintain a blood level of 500 ng/ml. Used synergistically with prednisolone.
Cyproheptadine (Periactin)	PO	2 mg BID–TID (cat)	Appetite stimulant.	Sedation and drowsiness.	
Cytosine arabinoside (Cytosar)		20 mg/m² intrathecal	Lymphoma, myeloproliferative disorders.		
Cytosine arabinoside (Cytosar-U)	SC, IV	100 mg/m²/wk (BID for 2–4 wk)	Combination agent. Lymphosarcoma, myeloproliferative disorders.	Leukopenia, thrombocytopenia, anemia, nausea, vomiting, diarrhea, anorexia, constipation.	Alternative doses: 100 mg/m²/day SC for 4 days every 3 wk; continuous 4-day infusion at 100 mg/m²/day IV in saline.

800

Drug (Trade Name)	Route	Dose	Effects and Medications	Side Effects	Comments
Cytosine arabinoside (*Cytosar*)	IV	150–200 mg/m² (BID for 2–4 wk topical)	Lymphoma. Antineoplastic agent in combination.	Leukopenia, thrombocytopenia, anemia, nausea, vomiting, anorexia.	
D-Penicillamine (*Cuprimine*)	PO	10–15 mg/kg BID	Chelating agent for lead, copper, mercury. Prevents cysteine urolithiasis.	Vomiting.	Administer on empty stomach.
Dacarbazine (*DTIC*)	IV	200 mg/m² for 5 days every 3 wk	Malignant melanoma, sarcomas.	Leukopenia, thrombocytopenia, anemia, nausea, vomiting, diarrhea (often decreases with later dosage cycles).	
Dactinomycin—see actinomycin D (*Cosmegen*)					
Dantrolene sodium (*Dantrium*)	PO, IV	2–4 mg/kg IV; 3–15 mg/kg PO in divided doses	Malignant hyperthermia (>41°C, 106°F); somatic functional urethral obstruction.	Generalized muscle weakness, hepatotoxicity with long-term use.	Maximum dose 10 mg/kg.
Dehydrocholic acid (*Decholin*)	PO	10–15 mg/kg TID for 7–10 days	Stimulates bile flow.	Do not use in biliary obstruction.	
Demerol—see meperidine (pethidine)					

Drug	Route	Dose	Indication	Precautions	Comments
Desmopressin acetate (DDAVP)	IM, IV, SC	1 μg/kg	Vasopressin analog. To prevent prolonged bleeding due to altered platelet function caused by azotemia, or von Willebrand's disease in Dobermans.	Hypersensitivity reactions.	Also used intranasally or by conjunctival instillation for central diabetes inspidus.
Desoxycorticosterone acetate (Percorten)	IM	1 ml/12 kg q25days. Titrate to effect	Hypoadrenocorticism.		Each 25 mg releases 1 mg DOCA/day for 1 mo.
Dexamethasone (Maxidex)	Eye drop	0.1%	Local immunosuppressant. Inhibition of pigmentation, vascularization.	Potentiation of proteases.	Use with extreme caution in brachycephalic dog. Stimulates herpesvirus felis in cats.
Dexamethasone (Azium)	Retro-orbital inj.	10–15 mg	Reduction of orbital swelling after replacement of a prolapsed globe.	See above.	See above.
Dexamethasone (Azium)	IV	2 mg/kg	Reduction of edema around CNS tumors.	May decrease concentration of chemotherapeutic agents in tumors.	Do not exceed two doses. See above for precautions.
Dexamethasone (Azium) (Decadron)	IV	0.1–0.2 mg/kg	Potent glucocorticoid. At induction of anesthesia, then immediately after adrenalectomy.	See above.	0.25 mg/kg q8h; may be used the day before adrenalectomy as well.
Dexamethasone (Azium)	IV	0.1 mg/kg	Before tracheostomy.	See above.	See above for precautions.
Dexamethasone (Azium)	IV	0.2–1.0 mg/kg	Reduction of laryngeal edema after surgery and after trauma.	See above.	Continue orally for 3–5 days.

Drug (Trade Name)	Route	Dose	Effects and Medications	Side Effects	Comments
Dexamethasone (*Azium*)	IM, IV	0.2–1.1 mg/kg for 2 days	Cerebral edema and increased intracranial pressure.	See above.	See above for precautions.
Dexamethasone (*Azium*)	PO	0.2 mg/kg for 3 days	Intervertebral disc disease with strict cage rest.	See above.	See above for precautions.
Dexamethasone (*Azium*)	PO, IV	2–4 mg/kg	Hypovolemic shock, preoperative preparation in gastric dilation–volvulus.	See above.	See above for precautions.
Dexamethasone (*Azium*)	IM	0.2–1.1 mg/kg	Medical treatment of atlantoaxial instability.	Polyuria, polydipsia, adrenal suppression, colonic perforation in neurosurgical patients.	Possible fetal death and resorption; avoid elective use in pregnant bitches. After neurosurgery, 1–2 mg/kg IV, IM, then 0.5 mg/kg every 6 hr with dose halved daily and stopped by the 5th day.
Dexamethasone	IV	6–8 mg/kg	Soluble corticosteroid. Acute therapy in septic and hypovolemic shock, hypoadrenocorticism.	See above—multiorgan side effects.	Low-dose dexamethasone suppression test: 0.01 mg/kg IV. High-dose dexamethasone suppression test: 0.1 mg/kg IV.
Dextran	IV	20 ml/kg/day	Colloidal plasma substitute for hypovolemia/acute blood loss. To prevent edema in hypoproteinemic patients.	Andidextran antibodies; hemorrhagic diathesis if given too rapidly due to antithrombotic effect.	Low MW (40,000; dextran 40)—half-life 2 hr. HMW (70,000; dextran 70)—half-life 6 hr. Infuse at 40–50 ml/kg/hr until blood pressure is 90% of baseline; then reduce rate.

Drug	Route	Dose	Indications	Side Effects	Comments
Dextrose	IV	5% 5 ml/kg during anesthesia.	For hypoglycemia in pancreatic beta cell carcinoma/hypoadrenocorticism. During anesthesia in diabetics, fluid replacement. To prevent seizures after metrizamide contrast imaging.		To prevent metrizamide seizures—1–1.5 g/kg (20–30 ml 5% solution).
Diazepam (*Valium*)	IM	0.2–0.4 mg/kg; 2–10 mg TID PO	Muscle and skeletal muscle relaxant, anticonvulsant. Functional urethral obstruction.	Sedation.	Benzodiazepine derivative.
Diazepam/morphine	IM	0.2 mg/kg; 0.2 mg/kg (dog)	Sedative, analgesic, neuroleptanalgesic.		
Diazepam/oxymorphone	IM	0.2 mg/kg; 0.1 mg/kg (dog)	Sedative, analgesic, neuroleptanalgesic.		
Diazoxide (*Proglycem*)	PO	5–30 mg/kg BID	Oral hyperglycemic for use in insulinoma.	Anorexia, vomiting, diarrhea.	May be synergistic with hydrothiazide (2–4 mg/kg BID PO).
Dichlorphenamide (*Daranide*)	PO	2–4 mg/kg BID–TID	Carbonic anhydrase inhibitor. Used in acute glaucoma.	Panting, disorientation, anorexia, diuresis.	
Diethylstilbestrol (*Stilbestrol*)	IM	1.1 mg/m² once IM, then 1 mg q72h PO	Perianal adenomas, adjunct for prostatic neoplasms; estrogen-responsive urinary incontinence, benign prostatic hyperplasia.	Bone marrow toxicity, feminization.	0.1–1.0 mg/day for 3–5 days PO, followed by 1.0 mg/kg/wk for maintenance for incontinence.
Dihydrotachysterol (DHT) (*Hytakerol*)	PO	0.02 mg/kg/day in three divided doses	Vitamin D analog. To prevent hypocalcemia after parathyroidectomy.		Onset of action 3–5 days.

803

Drug (Trade Name)	Route	Dose	Effects and Medications	Side Effects	Comments
Dimethylsulfoxide	IV	1 g/kg of <10% solution over 2 hr	Reduction of cerebral edema after cardiac resuscitation. Feline urological syndrome (FUS).		For FUS 10 ml 10% instilled into bladder for 10 min and then removed.
Diphenhydramine (Benadryl)	PO, IV, IM	2–4 mg/kg BID-TID PO; 1–2 mg/kg BID IV, IM	H₁ receptor antihistamine, antiemetic. Gastric ulceration with mastocytomas. Prevents transfusion reactions.	Sedation, anticholinergic.	Do not use IV in cats.
Dipyramidole (Persantine)	PO	2 mg/kg BID	Prevents platelet aggregation. Used 3–4 days before vascular surgery to prevent thrombosis of grafts.		
dl-Methionine (Methigel)	PO	0.2–1 g/kg TID (dog); 0.1–1 g SID (cat)	Urinary acidifier.	GI side effects. In high doses can cause hemolytic anemia, hemoglobinemia, and Heinz body formation.	
Dobutamine (Dobutrex)	IV	2–8 μg/kg/min in lactated Ringer's	Alpha, beta-1, and dopaminergic agent for heart failure, renal vasodilation, hypotension, septic shock, prostatic abscess.	Tachycardia, vasoconstriction.	ICU monitoring required.
Docusate sodium (Colace) (Doxinate)	PO	To effect	Fecal softener for use in perineal hernia.	Nausea.	Latent period to effect is 1–3 days. Also available as enema.

Drug	Dose	Route	Indications/Comments	Side Effects/Notes
Dopamine HCl (Inotropin)	2–30 µg/kg/min	IV	Inotrope for heart failure, e.g., in septic shock, renal vasodilator for renal failure, pressor agent in hypotension, alpha, beta-1, and dopaminergic agent. Operative support of blood pressure in bradycardia. Presurgically in hepatic portosystemic shunt repair.	Tachycardia, vasoconstriction, arrhythmias.
Doxapram (Dopram)	5–10 mg/kg IV once	IV	Respiratory stimulant, xylazine antagonist. Recovery from anesthesia or after caesarean section. Hepatic congestion after portosystemic shunt correction.	Blood pressure support. Requires ICU monitoring. Also used in gastric dilation volvulus, diaphragmatic hernia repair, prostatic abscess, and renal support after trauma.
Doxorubicin (Adriamycin)	30 mg/m^2 every 3 wk	IV	Lymphosarcoma, osteogenic sarcoma, various carcinomas, sarcomas.	Few drops beneath the tongue to effect in puppies/kittens, or via umbilical vein. Less effective than yohimbine or tolazoline as a xylazine antagonist.
Doxycycline (Vibramycin)	10 mg/kg SID	PO	Arthritis due to ehrlichiosis, borreliosis. Also for chlamydia, rickettsia, hemobartonella.	Leukopenia, anaphylaxis, bone marrow suppression, thrombocytopenia, nausea, vomiting, cardiac toxicity, reactions during administration.
Droperidol (Innovar-Vet) (Innovar)	Combined with fentanyl	IM	Antiemetic, sedative. Anesthesia induction in pheochromocytoma; for aggressive dogs.	Anorexia, depression.

Used while awaiting serology, in differential diagnosis of immune mediated polyarthritis. Do not use in puppies, kittens, or pregnant patients.

Can be given orally in aggressive dogs (by syringe).

Drug (Trade Name)	Route	Dose	Effects and Medications	Side Effects	Comments
Edrophonium (Tensilon)	IV	0.11–0.22 mg/kg (dog); 0.25–1 mg/kg (cat); 1–1.2 mg/kg as NNBD	Diagnosis of myasthenia gravis, antagonist for nondepolarizing neuromuscular blocking agent (NNBD).		
EDTA-Ca	Eye drop	1%	Protease inhibitor useful in severe ulcerations, removal of calcium deposits after parotid duct transposition.		Adjust pH to 7.4.
EDTA-Ca (Versenate)	SC	100 mg/kg/day for 5 days; give in four divided doses	Lead poisoning.	Painful, nephrotoxicity.	Dilute in 5% dextrose solution.
Emepronium bromide	PO	10 mg/kg/day in divided doses BID–TID	Urinary urge incontinence in bitches.		
Enalapril (Vasotec)	PO	0.25–0.5 mg/kg SID–BID	Vasodilator, hypertension, congestive heart failure.	Hypotension, weakness, anorexia.	Avoid in renal failure.
Enrofloxacin (Baytril)	PO, IV	2.5–10 mg/kg BID	Broad-spectrum bactericidal fluoroquinolone. Prostatic abscess, urinary infections.	Articular cartilage erosion in immature animals, anorexia, vomiting, confusion, dizziness.	Do not use in puppies or kittens. Norfloxacin and ciprofloxacin are approved for use in man. Norfloxacin is concentrated in urine.

Drug	Route	Dose	Indications	Side Effects/Comments
Ephedrine (*Ephedrine sulfate*)	IV	0.05–0.2 mg/kg; 20–50 mg BID (dog); 2–50 mg BID–TID PO (dog)	Bronchodilator. Urethral incompetence due to postprostatic or posturethral disease, ectopic ureter syndrome.	
Epinephrine (*Adrenaline*)	Intraocular inj.	1:100,000	Hemostatic, mydriatic in intraocular surgery. Included in infusion fluids.	
Epinephrine (*Adrenaline*)	IV	0.02–0.2 mg/kg, 0.05–0.3 μg/kg/min	Alpha- and beta-adrenergic agent for cardiac support, bronchodilation, anaphylaxis.	Vasoconstriction, tachycardia, ventricular fibrillation if sensitized by halothane. Arrhythmias. Give early and in high doses (1 mg/10 kg) for cardiac resuscitation. *The most important drug to administer during CPR!*
Epoetin (*Epogen*)	SC	100 units/kg three times/wk	Anemia of chronic renal failure and chemotherapy. Recombinant human erythropoetin. Used before elective surgery.	Use until RBC levels increase, then once a wk.
Erythromycin (*Erythrocin*)	Subconj. inj.	50–100 mg	Bactericidal/bacteriostatic depending on the dose and organism. Used especially for *Staphylococcus* spp., *Chlamydia*, *Campylobacter*, *Mycoplasma*, *Rickettsia*.	Pain, swelling at injection site.
Erythromycin (*Ilotycin*) (*Erythrocin*)	PO, IV, IM	10 mg/kg TID	See above.	GI dose-related side effects. Pain and swelling if given by injection.

807

Drug (Trade Name)	Route	Dose	Effects and Medications	Side Effects	Comments
Estradiol cypionate (ECP)	IM, SC	0.1–1 mg weekly or monthly	Estrogen-responsive incontinence in spayed bitches. Termination of pregnancy.	Bone marrow toxicity.	Termination: dog—20–40 µg IM up to 5 days after breeding. Do not exceed 1 mg. Cat—250 µg IM 40 hr after mating.
Ethanol	Inhalation	25–50% inhalation; 5.5 ml/kg IV q4h for 5 doses, then q6h for 4 doses	Lowers surface tension and breaks down frothy pulmonary edema; ethylene glycol toxicosis (IV).	CNS depression.	
Etomidate (Amidate)	IV	0.5–1.5 mg/kg	Hypnotic for induction of anesthesia. Negative inotropic effect, lack of cardiac and respiratory depression.		Can be used in sight hounds; also propofol.
Fentanyl/droperidol (Innovar-Vet)	IM	1 ml/10–25 kg	Sedative, analgesic, neuroleptanalgesic. Fentanyl used in geriatric patients, trauma, liver disease, pheochromocytoma, orthopedic surgery, control of aggression.		
Flavoxate (Urispas)	PO	100 mg TID–QID	Urge urinary incontinence.		
Flucytosine (Ancobon) (Ancotil)	PO	100 mg/kg BID	Used in Aspergillus, Cryptococcus.	Renal, bone marrow, and hepatotoxicity. Do not use during pregnancy.	

Drug	Route	Dosage	Indication/Action	Side Effects/Comments
Fludrocortisone (*Florinef*)	PO	0.1 mg/kg BID	Replacement mineralocorticoid. Hypoadrenocorticism.	Hypertension.
Flumazenil	IV		Antagonist for diazepam, midazolam, tiletamine-zolazepam (Telazol).	
Flumethasone (*Flucort*)	PO, SC, IM, IV	0.06–0.25 mg SID (dog); 0.03–0.125 mg SID (cat)	Anti-inflammatory, corticosteroid.	Cortisone-related side effects.
Flunixin meglumine (*Banamine*)	IV	0.5–1 mg/kg; maximum 3 days dosage	Nonsteroidal anti-inflammatory agent, analgesic. Inhibits prostaglandin synthetase, decreases aqueous protein concentration.	Gastric ulceration when given with corticosteroids. Platelet coagulopathy.
Fluorescein	IV	15 mg/kg	Assessment of viability of GI vasculature.	
Fluorouracil (5-FU) (*Fluorouracil*) (*Efudex Cream*)	IV	150–200 mg/m²/wk; 2–5 mg/kg/wk	Antimetabolite. Various carcinomas and sarcomas, cutaneous tumors.	Leukopenia, thrombocytopenia, anemia, anorexia, vomiting, nausea, diarrhea, stomatitis. Do not use in cats.
Flurbiprofen (*Ocufen*)	Eye drop		Reduction of formation of plasmoid aqueous before intraocular surgery.	Not for continuous use in uveitis. Not approved for use in dogs by U.S. Food and Drug Administration, but wide extralabel use worldwide. Do not use in cats.

Drug (Trade Name)	Route	Dose	Effects and Medications	Side Effects	Comments
Furosemide (*Lasix*)	PO, SC, IM, IV	2–4 mg/kg BID–TID (dog); 0.5–2 mg/kg BID–TID (cat)	Increases renal blood flow and water and solute excretion after trauma. Postoperative increased intracranial pressure, acute renal failure in septic shock, hypercalcemia, congestive heart failure, hypertension, ascites, fluid retention.	Hyponatremia, hypokalemia, and hypochloremia acidosis. Dehydration.	5 mg/kg, then 5 mg/kg/hr to enhance calciuresis in severe hypercalcemia. Prednisolone 2 mg/kg may be added. Use for cerebral edema and to restore consciousness after CPR with mannitol, corticosteroids.
Gemfibrozil (*Lopid*)	PO	150 mg 10 kg BID (dog)	Antihyperlipidemic.	Nausea, GI upset.	Dosages empirical.
Gentamicin	Subconj. inj.	10–20 mg	Broad-spectrum bactericidal antibiotic, aminoglycoside. Intraocular penetration.	Toxic to retina when injected intraocularly. See below.	Serious infections only. Ineffective orally.
Gentamicin	IM, IV, SC	2 mg/kg TID, 10–20 mg subconj. inj.	Broad-spectrum bactericidal antibiotic, aminoglycoside. Intraocular penetration. Peritonitis, endophthalmitis, keratitis, urinary infections, pancreatitis, presurgical prophylaxis.	Toxic to retina when injected intraocularly. May cause neuromuscular block, especially administered intraperitoneally or intrathoracically. Nephrotoxicity, ototoxicity.	
Glucose	Eye drop	40%	Reduces corneal edema.	Irritation on instillation.	
Glycerol 50%	Eye drop		Reduces corneal edema.	Irritation on instillation.	
Glycerol 50–75%	PO	1–2 g/kg	Reduces intraocular pressure.	Vomiting.	Give chilled to avoid vomiting.

Drug	Route	Dose	Indications	Comments
Glycopyrrolate (*Robinul V*)	IM, IV, SC	0.005–0.01 mg/kg	Anticholinergic. Prevents salivation, bradycardia.	Mydriasis, ileus.
Gonadotrophin-releasing factor	IV	50 µg once	Vaginal edema in bitches.	Possible development of ovarian cysts if given in early pro-oestrus or with immature ovarian follicles.
Heparin	Intraocular inj.	2 units/ml	Reduction of formation of plasmoid aqueous.	
Heparin	IV	200–400 units/kg (2–4 mg/kg)	Anticoagulant before cardiac bypass or vascular surgery. Neutralized by an equal amount of protamine sulfate.	Prolonged prothrombin times.
Heparin	IV, SC	5–10 IU/kg/hr IV; TID-QID SC	Treatment of disseminated intravascular coagulation.	Neutralized with protamine sulfate. Monitor prothrombin times to prevent spontaneous hemorrhage. Heparin dose adjusted to keep activated partial thromboplastin time 1.5–2 times normal.
Hetastarch (hydroxyethyl)	IV	100 ml/kg	Replacement for hypovolemia; volume-expanding effect lasts 24–36 hr.	Similar hemodynamic effects to albumin.
Hydralazine (*Apresoline*)	IM, IV, SC	0.2–0.5 mg/kg	Vasodilator, arteriolar smooth muscle relaxant. Duration of action 2–8 hr. Use for operative hypertension.	With prolonged use: systemic lupus erythematosus, neuritis, blood dyscrasias.
Hydrochlorothiazide (*Aldoril*) (*Hydrodiuril*)	PO	2–4 mg/kg BID, then SID or decrease 50%	Diuretic. Synergistic hyperglycemic effect with diazoxide in insulinoma.	Hypokalemia, dehydration, exacerbates digitalis toxicity.

Drug (Trade Name)	Route	Dose	Effects and Medications	Side Effects	Comments
Hydroxyurea	IV	15 mg/kg	Suppresses erythropoiesis in feline polycythemia rubra vera.	Extreme myelosuppression.	Monitoring of hemogram necessary.
Hydroxyzine (Atarax)	PO	1–2 mg/kg BID–TID (dog); 0.5–1 mg/kg BID–TID (cat)	H₁ receptor antihistamine. Allergic skin disorders.	Sedation.	
Imipramine pamoate (Tofranil)	PO	0.5–1 mg/kg TID	Urge urinary incontinence, decreased bladder contractions, increased urethral resistance.	Depression, myocardial depression, GI side effects.	
Indomethacin	Eye drop	1%	Inhibits prostaglandin synthetase, decreases aqueous protein concentration.		Useful for acute uveitis; before cataract extraction.
Indomethacin (Indocin)	PO	1–1.25 mg/kg	Nonsteroidal anti-inflammatory agent for degenerative joint disease.	Gastric ulceration and side effects.	
Isoetharine (Bronkosol)	Inhalation	0.5–1 ml 1% solution diluted in three parts saline TID	Beta-2 adrenergic agonist for bronchodilation.		
Kanamycin	Subconj. inj.	10–20 mg	Intraocular penetration.		
Ketamine (Ketaset)	IV	5 mg/kg IV sedation, minor procedures (dog); 11 mg/kg IM restraint (cat)	Dissociative anesthetic.	Muscular tremors, salivation, respiratory depression, laryngospasm.	4–10 mg/kg IM in kittens. Not used in renal disease. Also used 1:1 or 2:1 with diazepam.

Drug	Route	Dose	Indication	Side Effects	Comments
Levobunolol (*Betagan*)	Eye drop		Beta-adrenergic blocking agent. Glaucoma.		Efficacy poor. Not suitable alone.
Lidocaine (*Xylocaine*)	IV	0.5–4.0 mg/kg bolus (dog); 0.25–1.0 mg/kg slowly (cat)	Reduction of cardiac arrhythmias. Gastric dilation volvulus.		Continuous infusion of 40–80 µg/kg/min for control of refractory arrhythmias. Maximum total dose 8 mg/kg.
Lincomycin (*Lincocin*)	Subconj. inj.	50–150 mg	Intraocular penetration.		
	PO	10–20 mg/kg BID	Staphylococcal and anaerobic infections, *Mycoplasma*.	Minor GI side effects in cats. Dose-dependent neuromuscular blockade causing skeletal muscle paralysis. Vomiting, hepatotoxicity.	Do not use with erythromycin, chloramphenicol.
Lomustine (*CEENU*)	IV	50–80 mg/m²/6–8 wk	Confirmed glial tumors.	Bone marrow suppression, nausea, vomiting, CNS toxicity, and others reported in man.	Reported with chlorambucil in canine ovarian tumors.
Mafenide acetate (*Sulfamylon*)	Topical	BID	Broad spectrum, sulfonamide. Prevention of bacterial infection in burns. Rapid penetration of burn eschar.	Pain on application, metabolic acidosis.	Secondary agent after silver sulfadiazine.
Mannitol	IV	1–2 g/kg; 0.5 g/kg bolus for renal function	Presurgical reduction of vitreous volume, reduced intraocular pressure, reduction of CNS tumor–associated edema, maintenance of renal function after trauma and during anesthesia, restoration of consciousness after CPR.	Diuresis, dehydration.	

Drug (Trade Name)	Route	Dose	Effects and Medications	Side Effects	Comments
Medetomidine	IM	0.01–0.02 mg/kg	Sedative, muscle relaxant, analgesic.		Reversal agent: yohimbine.
Medroxyprogesterone (*Depo-provera*)	IM, SC	10–20 mg/kg (cat)	Urine spraying in cats.	Local alopecia and change in hair color at injection site.	Inject SC in inguinal region for cosmetic reasons.
Megestrol acetate (*Ovaban*)	PO	2 mg/kg/day for 7 days	Appetite stimulant. Given in early pro-oestrus to prevent vaginal edema in predisposed bitches. Urine spraying in cats.	Prevents ovulation.	Second choice to medroxyprogesterone for urine spraying. Regimen: 5 mg/kg/day reduced to 5 mg/wk at intervals of 2 wk. Terminate treatment in 2–6 wk.
Melphalan (*Alkeran*)	PO	1.5 mg/m² for 7–10 days	Alkylating agent. Multiple myeloma, monoclonal gammopathies, lymphoreticular neoplasms.	Leukopenia, thrombocytopenia, anemia, anorexia, nausea, vomiting.	Repeat dosage cycles used.
Meperidine (pethidine) (*Demerol*)	IM, SC	5–10 mg/kg (dog), 2–4 mg/kg (cat)	Analgesic, sedative. Duration 1–2 hr.	Sedation, depression, seizures, hypotension with overdosage.	Opioid agonist. Short duration (2–4 hr).
Mephentermine (*Wyamine*)	IV	0.1–0.75 mg/kg	Sympathomimetic. Increases myocardial chromotropy, inotropy. Operative heart failure and bradycardia.		

Drug	Route	Dose	Description	Adverse Effects	Comments
Mercaptopurine (6-mercaptopurine) (*Purinethol*)	PO	50 mg/m^2; 0.5–0.8 mg/kg IV	Antimetabolite. Canine nonerosive immune-mediated arthritis, lymphosarcoma, acute lymphocytic leukemia, granulocytic leukemia.	Leukopenia, nausea, vomiting, hepatopathy.	
Metaraminol (*Aramine*)	IV	0.05–0.2 mg/kg	Sympathomimetic. Increases peripheral vasomotor tone. Operative bradycardia and heart failure.		
Methadone (*Dolophine hydrochloride*)	PO, SC, IM	0.1–0.2 mg/kg (dog)	Analgesic. Duration 4 hr.		
Methazolamide (*Neptazane*)	PO	2–4 mg/kg BID–TID	Carbonic anhydrase inhibitor. Reduced intraocular pressure, diuresis.	Vomiting, panting, acidosis, disorientation.	
Methenamine mandelate (*Mandelamine*)	PO	25 mg/kg BID	Forms ammonia and formaldehyde at pH 5–6 in urine.	Do not use in cats if preparation contains methylene blue.	No bacterial resistance demonstrated. Adjust urine pH with ammonium chloride or sodium acid phosphate.
Methicillin	Subconj. inj.	100–200 mg	Intraocular penetration.		
Methimazole (*Tapazole*)	PO	5 mg SID–TID (cat)	Feline hyperthyroidism. Inhibit formation of T4.	Anorexia, vomiting, reversible leukopenia and thrombocytopenia.	Monitor CBC until euthyroid. Preferable to propylthiouracil.
Methocarbamol (*Robaxin*)	PO	20–45 mg/kg	Muscle relaxant. Intervertebral disc protrusion.	Ataxia, ptyalism, emesis, sedation.	Cage rest important to prevent further protrusion when pain is relieved.

Drug (Trade Name)	Route	Dose	Effects and Medications	Side Effects	Comments
Methohexital (*Brevital sodium*)	IV	5–10 mg/kg	Ultra-short-acting barbiturate, general anesthetic.	As for barbiturates.	Alternative to thiobarbiturates in sight hounds.
Methotrexate	PO	2.5 mg/m²/day PO, 0.5–0.8 mg/kg IV	Antimetabolite. Lymphoreticular neoplasms, myeloproliferative disorders, various sarcomas and carcinomas.	Leukopenia, thrombocytopenia, anemia, stomatitis, diarrhea, hepatopathy, renal tubular necrosis.	
Methotrexate (amethopterin) (*Folex*)	PO, IV, IM	0.06 mg/kg SID PO; 0.5–0.8 mg/kg/wk IV; 2.5 mg/m² SID PO, IV, IM	Antimetabolite. Inhibits folic acid reductase. Chemotherapy and immunosuppression.	Leukopenia, hepatotoxicity, GI hemorrhage.	
Methoxamine (*Vasoxyl*)	IV	0.05–0.2 mg/kg	Sympathomimetic alpha-1 adrenergic agonist. Increases peripheral vasomotor tone. No myocardial inotropy or chromotropy.		
Methylcellulose	Intraocular inj.	1–2%	Intraocular viscoelastic.		
Methylcellulose	Eye drop	1–2%	Tear replacement.		
Methylprednisolone (*DepoMedrol*)	Intralesional		Repository corticosteroid. After laser laryngeal surgery (10–15 mg). Antiendotoxin in prostatic abscess (30 mg/kg IV), spinal cord protection during decompression (30 mg/kg IV). Feline asthma (10–20 mg IM).	Contraindications and effects of cortisone.	

Drug	Route	Indications	Comments
Metoclopramide (Reglan)	PO, SC, IM, IV	0.2–0.4 mg/kg BID–QID	Antiemetic. Enhances GI motility, stimulates gastric contractions and emptying, stimulates small intestinal smooth muscle, reduces postoperative nausea and vomiting after abdominal procedures. Prostatic abscess and reflux esophagitis.	Can be added to IV fluid at 1–2 mg/kg/hr. Contraindicated with phenothiazines, narcotic analgesics. Blocked by atropine.
Metronidazole (Flagyl)	PO	15–30 mg/kg BID (dog), 5–15 mg/kg BID (cat)	Septic peritonitis, surgical wound infections, anaerobic infections of mouth, liver, pulmonary, and GI tract; also Giardia, Entamoeba, Balantidium, Pentatrichomonas, Trypanosoma spp.	May increase seizure activity.
Midazolam/butorphanol (Versed/Torbutrol)	IM	0.2 mg/kg; 0.2 mg/kg	Sedative, analgesic, neuroleptanalgesic, pediatric anesthetic, preanesthetic for geriatric/trauma patients.	Dose-dependent CNS signs: anorexia, vomiting progressing to ataxia and nystagmus. Hepatotoxicity.
Misonidazole	PO	10.5–15 g/m² (total dose)	Radiosensitizer.	Midazolam used alone and in combination with butorphanol, ketamine, and oxymorphone.
Misoprostol (Cytotec)	PO	6 mg/kg q12h	Antisecretory prostaglandin E₁. Cytoprotective effects against gastric/duodenal ulceration from nonsteroidal anti-inflammatory drugs and hemorrhagic gastroduodenitis secondary to mastocytoma.	Nausea, vomiting, neurotoxicity.

Drug (Trade Name)	Route	Dose	Effects and Medications	Side Effects	Comments
Morphine	IM, SC	0.5–1 mg/kg (dog), 0.05–0.1 mg/kg q4–6h	Preanesthetic, emetic, postoperative analgesic, sedative, vasodilator. Duration 3–4 hr.	Vomiting, CNS and respiratory depression. Histamine-mediated hypotension. Hyperexcitability in cats.	Opioid agonist.
Morphine	IV	0.5 mg/kg + 0.1–0.2 mg/kg/hr (dog)	Analgesic, vasodilator. Duration is as long as the infusion.	CNS and respiratory depression. Histamine-mediated hypotension, nausea, vomiting.	After thoracotomy: 0.2 mg/kg IV with further increments of 0.1 mg/kg to effect.
Morphine	Epidural	0.1 mg/kg preservative free (dog)	Analgesic, vasodilator. Duration 12–24 hr.	CNS and respiratory depression. Histamine-mediated hypotension, nausea, vomiting.	
Morphine	IM, SC	0.05–0.1 mg/kg (cat)	Analgesic, vasodilator. Duration 3–4 hr.	CNS and respiratory depression, excitement.	
Morphine	IM	0.2–0.4 mg/kg (dog)	To induce preoperative vomiting.	CNS and respiratory depression. Histamine-mediated hypotension, nausea, vomiting.	
N-(2-Mercapto-propionyl)-glycine (MPG)	PO	15 mg/kg (dog)	Increases solubility of cystine urinary calculi.		
Nalbuphine (Nubain)	IM, IV, SC	0.03–0.2 mg/kg	Analgesic, sedative, antagonist of opioid agonists, preanesthetic. Does not totally remove opioid analgesia as does naloxone. Duration 2–4 hr. Opioid-induced respiratory depression.		Opioid agonist/antagonist. In opioid-induced respiratory depression, some analgesia remains after reversal with this agent.

Drug	Route	Dose	Indications	Side Effects/Comments
Naloxone (Narcan)	IM	0.005–0.04 mg/kg	Antagonizes opioid agonists, including removal of analgesia. Opioid-induced respiratory depression; removes analgesia.	Few drops beneath the tongue for puppies and kittens to effect. Narcotic effect may last longer than naloxone.
Nandrolone acetate (Deca-Durabolin)	IM	5 mg/kg, 200 mg/wk IM (dog), 1 mg/kg/wk (dog)	Anabolic steroid, appetite and bone marrow stimulant.	
Neomycin	Subconj. inj.	100–500 mg	Intraocular penetration.	
	PO	20 mg/kg QID	Broad-spectrum aminoglycoside antibiotic. GI bacterial overgrowth and hepatoencephalopathy. Also used in combination with bacitracin and polymixin in eye drops.	Not absorbed orally. Allergic reactions, especially periocular, recorded occasionally.
Neostigmine (Stiglin) (Prostigmin)	IV	0.02–0.04 mg/kg	Nondepolarizing neuromuscular blocking antagonist.	Not useful for anaerobic infections.
Nitrofurantoin (Macrodantin) (Dantefur)	Topical	4 mg/kg q8h PO	Surface infections, urinary bacterial infections. Bactericidal. Many urinary pathogens resistant.	Useful topical agent. Vomiting after oral use.
Nitrogen mustard (Mustargen)	IV	5 mg/m²	Alkylating agent. Lymphoreticular neoplasms.	Leukopenia, thrombocytopenia, nausea, vomiting, anorexia, contact dermatitis.
Nitroglycerin (Nitro ointment)	Topical	0.5–4.0 cm/day (dog), 0.25–0.5 cm/day (cat)	Transdermal venodilator for use in congestive heart failure.	Hypotension. Cautious topical application (10 mg/50 cm² water). Apply with gloved finger to pinna or inguinal area.

Drug (Trade Name)	Route	Dose	Effects and Medications	Side Effects	Comments
Nitroprusside (Nipride)	Slow IV drip	0.5–10 μg/kg/min	Vasodilator, direct arteriolar and venular smooth muscle relaxant. Operative hypertension, induction of hypotension in neurosurgery.	Avoid in hepatic or renal failure. Total dose less than 1.5 mg/kg/2 hr. Large doses cause cyanide toxicity. Treat with sodium nitrite 0.5–0.75 mg/kg slow IV, then 5–15 μg/kg/min.	Continuous blood pressure monitoring during administration.
Norepinephrine (Levophed bitartrate)	IV	0.02–0.2 mg/kg, 1–10 μg/kg/min	Sympathomimetic. Increases peripheral vasomotor tone. Variable myocardial inotropy and chromotropy.		
Norethandrolone (Nilevar)	PO	0.25–3 mg/kg/day	Androgenic steroid.	As for nandrolone.	
Norfloxacin (Chibroxin)	PO	22 mg/kg	Broad-spectrum bactericidal fluoroquinolone, concentrated in urine. Urinary infections.		
Noscapine (Coscopin) (Vetinol)	PO	0.5–1 mg TID–QID (dog)	Antitussive.	Nausea, drowsiness.	
o,p'-DDD (Lysodren)	PO	50 mg/m²/day to effect, then every 7–14 days	Adrenocortical tumors, hyperadrenocorticism.	Adrenocortical insufficiency.	
Oxazepam (Serax)	PO	2.5 mg SID–BID (cat), 0.2–1 mg/kg SID–BID (dog)	Appetite stimulant.	Sedation, and incoordination.	Benzodiazepine derivative.

Drug	Route	Dosage	Indication	Side Effects	Notes
Oxtriphylline (*Choledyl*)	PO	4–10 mg/kg	Bronchodilator.	Vomiting, diarrhea, hyperexcitability.	
Oxybutynin (*Ditropan*)	PO	5 mg BID-TID	Urge urinary incontinence; direct antispasmodic effect on smooth muscle increases bladder capacity.	Urine retention.	
Oxymorphone (*Numorphan*)	PO, SC, IM, IV	0.05–0.1 mg/kg (dog), 0.03–0.05 mg/kg (cat)	Analgesic, sedative, preanesthetic and postoperative analgesic. Useful for depressed trauma patients in small increments. Duration 3–4 hr.		Opioid agonist.
Oxytetracycline—see tetracyclines (*Terramycin*)					
Oxytocin (*Pitocin*)	IM, SC	5–25 units q30min (dog), 2 units/kg q30 min (cat), milk production 2–10 units, IM	Ecbolic, vasopressive, antidiuretic. Stimulates uterine contraction and involution and reduces uterine hemorrhage and fetal membrane retention. Stimulates milk flow.		Dose conservatively initially due to fetal hypoxia at higher doses. Warm syringe before injection.
Pancuronium	IV	15–20 µg/kg	Nondepolarizing neuromuscular blocker. Duration 10–90 min.		Reversal agents: neostigmine, pyridostigmine, edrophonium.
Penicillin G	Subconj. inj.	300,000–1 million units	Intraocular penetration.	Hypersensitivity reactions: cutaneous eruptions, fever, angioedema, anaphylaxis, anorexia, vomiting, minor GI side effects.	

821

Drug (Trade Name)	Route	Dose	Effects and Medications	Side Effects	Comments
Penicillin G	PO, SC, IM, IV	40 mg/kg QID for 4–6 wk	Discospondylitis due to beta-hemolytic *Streptococcus*. Effective for anaerobic infections except *Fusobacterium* and some *Bacteroides* and *Clostridium* spp.	Hypersensitivity reactions: cutaneous eruptions, fever, angioedema, anaphylaxis, anorexia, vomiting, minor GI side effects.	Crystalline penicillin for wound irrigation 20,000–40,000 units/kg parenterally q6–8h. Less effective orally.
Pentazocine (*Talwin V*)	PO, SC, IM, IV	1–4 mg/kg (dog), 2–6 mg/kg PO	Analgesic, sedative, antagonist of opioid agonists. Duration 2–4 hr.	Salivation, sedation.	Opioid agonist/antagonist. Reverse with naloxone.
Pentobarbital	IV	20–30 mg/kg (cat)	Barbiturate, general anesthetic.		
Pentobarbital (*Nembutal*)	IV	10–30 mg/kg anesthesia, 2–8 mg/kg seizures	Anesthetic. Status epilepticus, strychnine toxicity.	Respiratory depression, hypotension.	Do not use in sight hounds or with diazepam.
Pethidine—see meperidine (*Demerol*)					
Phenobarbital	PO	1–2 mg/kg BID–TID, 10–15 mg/kg IV	Sedative. Long-acting barbiturate for seizures.	Ataxia, sedation, polyuria, polydipsia.	Hepatotoxicity with long-term use.
Phenoxybenzamine (*Dibenzyline*)	PO	0.2–0.4 mg/kg BID (dog), 2.5 mg SID–BID (cat)	Alpha-adrenergic blocker, sympatholytic, alpha-receptor blocker. Decreases hypertension. Functional urethral obstruction. Decreases urethral resistance. Pretreatment before removal of pheochromocytoma.	Postural hypotension, tachycardia, vomiting, miosis.	See Chapter 171 for further details.

Drug	Route	Dose	Indication	Toxicity/Side Effects	Comments
Phentolamine mesylate (*Regitine*)	IV	0.02–1.0 mg/kg by bolus	Reduction of hypertension during manipulation of pheochromocytoma.		See Chapter 171.
Phenylbutazone (*Butazolidin*)	PO	10–22 mg/kg q8h (dog)	Nonsteroidal anti-inflammatory. Symptomatic treatment of degenerative joint disease.	Bone marrow depression, depression, anorexia, vomiting, fever, petechiation.	Toxicity more common at doses of 200–600 mg/day in divided doses, for prolonged periods of 1–4 mo.
Phenylephrine (*Neosynephrine*)	IV	0.05–0.2 mg/kg	Sympathomimetic. Increases peripheral vasomotor tone.		
Phenylpropanolamine (*Dexatrim*) (*Ornade*)	PO	12.5–50 mg BID (dog)	Urethral incompetence due to postprostatic or posturethral disease, ectopic ureter syndrome, hormone-responsive incontinence.	Restlessness, anxiety, dizziness, hypertension, urinary retention.	Titrate dose to effect. If over-the-counter, use with caffeine.
Phenytoin (*Dilantin*)	PO	10–40 mg/kg TID (dog)	Anticonvulsant.	Ataxia, vomiting.	Rapidly metabolized. Monitor liver function. Agent of second choice.
Pilocarpine	Eye drop	2% eye drops q15min for 1 hr, then q3h	Acute glaucoma.	Pain on instillation.	Not useful for chronic glaucoma.
Potassium bromide	PO	65 mg/kg SID	Anticonvulsant. Used with phenobarbital.	May potentiate sedation, incoordination with phenobarbital.	

Drug (Trade Name)	Route	Dose	Effects and Medications	Side Effects	Comments
Potassium chloride	IV	1 mEq/kg/day, 0.125–0.25 mEq/kg/hr	Treatment of hypokalemia (<3.5 mEq/dl), hypodynamic septic shock in peritonitis to increase cardiac output.	Do not exceed 0.5 mEq/kg/hr.	Administration in glucose or maintenance fluids preferable. Do not exceed 0.25–0.5 mEq/kg/hr. Monitor serum potassium regularly and infuse slowly. Given with 25% glucose lactated Ringer's with 1 unit regular insulin/g of glucose.
Potassium citrate (Urocit-K)	PO	1 mEq/kg/day divided BID-TID	Dissolution of oxalate calculi.		Efficacy unproven, dose approximate.
Pralidoxime chloride (Protopam chloride) (2-PAM)	IM, IV, SC	40–50 mg/kg over 2 min, then q12h SQ (dog), 20 mg/kg (cat)	Reactivates cholinesterase inactivated by organophosphates.		
Prazosin hydrochloride (Minipress)		1–5 mg once daily or in divided doses	Sympatholytic, alpha-receptor blocker. Functional urethral obstruction. Decreases urethral resistance.	Postural hypotension, tachycardia.	
Prednisolone	PO	1–2 mg/kg for 3 days	Reduces formation of plasmoid aqueous before intraocular surgery.		
Prednisolone	PO	Various. 60 mg/m² daily to 20 mg/m² q48h	Lymphoreticular neoplasms, CNS tumors.	Hyperadrenocorticism, secondary adrenocortical insufficiency.	

824

Drug	Route	Dose	Indication	Comments
Prednisolone	PO	40 mg/m²/day for 7 days, then 20 mg/m² q48h	Mastocytoma.	See above.
Prednisolone	PO	1–4 mg/kg/day	Stimulates gluconeogenesis in preoperative therapy of insulinoma, reduction of laryngeal edema after surgery and after trauma.	See above. Continue 3–5 days.
Prednisolone	PO	2.2–4.4 mg/kg/day divided BID for 7 days	Immune-mediated thrombocytopenia.	
Prednisolone	IV	1–2 mg/kg IV, 0.5–1 mg/kg PO maintenance	Degenerative joint disease. Establish the lowest possible maintenance dose, e.g., 0.5–1 mg/kg every 2nd or 3rd day.	Polyuria, polydipsia, hunger.
Prednisolone or prednisone	PO	0.2 mg/kg/day	Replacement after hypophysectomy.	
Prednisolone sodium succinate (Solu-Delta-Cortef)	IV	15–30 mg/kg	Reduction of CNS tumor–associated edema. During manipulation of the liver if congestion occurs in treatment of portosystemic shunts.	
Procainamide (Pronestyl)	PO, IV, IM	6–8 mg/kg IV slowly, 6–20 mg/kg q4h IM, 6–20 mg/kg q6h PO	Controls premature ventricular contractions in dogs, gastric dilation volvulus, surgery and after surgery.	Hypotension, tachycardia. 6–15 mg/kg IM q4–6h for infrequent arrhythmias; 0.5–1 mg/kg IV for refractory arrhythmias. Not recommended in cats.

Drug (Trade Name)	Route	Dose	Effects and Medications	Side Effects	Comments
Prochlorperazine (Compazine)	IM, SC	0.1–0.4 mg/kg	Antiemetic.	Sedation, hypotension.	Do not use in epileptics.
Propantheline (Pro-Banthine)	PO	0.2 mg/kg BID–TID (dog), 1/4–1 tab SID–BID (cat)	Anticholinergic. Diarrhea, bradycardia, urge urinary incontinence, detrussor hyperreflexia.	Decreased uninhibited bladder contractions, urine retention.	
Proparacaine	Eye drop	0.5%	Topical anesthetic.	Toxic to epithelium.	For diagnostic purposes only, extreme oral toxicity.
Propofol (Diprivan)	IV	4–8 mg/kg	General anesthetic. Rapid onset, short duration. Cesarean section, geriatric patients.		
Propranolol (Inderal)	IV	2.5–5 mg q8h before surgery. 0.02–0.06 mg/kg IV to effect	Beta-adrenergic blocker. To decrease resting heart in hyperthyroid cats to <240 beats per minute. Reduces cardiac contractility and heart rate, prolongs atrioventricular conduction and decreases blood pressure. Supraventricular arrhythmias, feline hypertrophic cardiomyopathy.	Anorexia, depression, ataxia, bradycardia.	Not given to patients with congestive heart failure. During anesthesia 0.1 mg only if needed. Potentiates atrioventricular nodal depression with digoxin and calcium channel blockers.
Propylthiouracil (PTU)	PO	10 mg/kg BID–TID	Feline hypothyroidism. Prevents formation of T4.	Anorexia, vomiting, lethargy, immune-mediated hemolytic anemia.	Methimazole is the drug of first choice due to less frequent side effects.

Drug	Route	Dosage	Indications	Comments
Prostaglandin F$_{2alpha}$ (*Lutalyse*)	SC	0.25 mg/kg SID 3–7 days	Open cervix pyometra. Abortifacient at 31–35 days.	Panting, salivation, vomiting, diarrhea, tachycardia for 30 min.
Protamine sulfate	IV	1 mg/100 units heparin	Reversal of hemorrhage after heparin.	Hypotension. Give slowly over 10 min. Reduce dose to 50% if heparin given 1 hr previously and to 25% for 2 hr previously.
Pyridostigmine bromide (*Mestinon*)	IV	0.1–0.2 mg/kg IV, 0.2–2.0 mg/kg BID–TID PO (dog)	Nondepolarizing neuromuscular blocking antagonist. Used PO to treat myasthenia gravis.	Vomiting, diarrhea, salivation.
Quinidine sulfate	IM, PO	6–20 mg/kg q4–6h	Ventricular dysrhythmias in gastric dilation volvulus.	For refractory arrhythmias 0.04–0.08 mg/min IV. Not recommended in cats.
Ranitidine (*Zantac*)	PO	2.2–4.4 mg/kg BID	H$_2$ histamine receptor antagonist. Reduction of gastric ulceration from histamine release in treatment of mastocytoma. Zollinger-Ellison syndrome from gastrinoma, GI failure in sepsis.	See also cimetidine. Not recommended in cats.
Rifampin	PO	10 mg/kg	Bactericidal antibiotic. Gram-positive and many gram-negatives including *Mycobacterium*. Synergistic with streptomycin and isoniazid against *M. tuberculosis*.	Anorexia, vomiting, mild pruritus. Turns tears, saliva, urine, and feces red. Induces hepatic microsomal enzyme production.
Silver nitrate	Topical	0.5% aqueous solution	Broad-spectrum antibacterial for burn wounds.	Brown staining of tissues. Leaches sodium and potassium from the wound, may cause hyponatremia. Bulky wet dressings required.

Drug (Trade Name)	Route	Dose	Effects and Medications	Side Effects	Comments
Silver sulfadiazine (*Silvadene*)	Topical	1% water soluble cream SID–BID	Topical antimicrobial for burn wounds. Gram-positive and negative bacteria, *Candida* spp.		Pseudoeschar is removed before application. Gram-negative bacteria become resistant with protracted use.
Sodium bicarbonate	IV	1 mEq/kg	Reduction of acidosis during resuscitation, hyperkalemia, hypovolemic shock, metabolic acidosis, regulation of acid-base imbalance.		
Sodium bicarbonate	Inhalation	1–2% solution	Reduction of viscosity of respiratory mucus.		
Sodium chloride	Eye drop	5%	Reduces corneal edema.	Irritation on instillation.	
Sodium hyaluronate (*Hyaluron*)	Intraocular inj.		Intraocular viscoelastic agent. Used to reconstitute anterior chamber and protect corneal endothelial cells.		Removed before closure.
Sodium nitrite	IV	0.5–0.75 mg/kg slowly	Used to treat cyanide toxicity from nitroprusside therapy.		Follow with sodium thiosulfate IV 200 mg slowly.
Sodium thiomalate (*Myochrysine*)	IM	1 mg/kg/wk	Rheumatoid arthritis.		

828

Drug	Route	Dose	Indication	Comments
Somatostatin (SM 201-995)	IM	10–30 μg BID–TID	Somatostatin analog inhibits growth hormone, insulin, glucagon, and gastrin. Used in treatment of insulinoma, gastrinoma.	
Spironolactone (Aldactone)	PO	1–2 mg/kg BID (dog)	Potassium-sparing diuretic.	Monitor potassium. Used with other diuretics (with hydrochlorothiazide [Aldactazide]).
Stanozolol (Winstrol)	PO	1–2 mg BID (cat)	Appetite stimulant for anorexia, debilitation, anemia.	Contraindicated in pregnancy.
Streptomycin	Subconj. inj.	50–100 mg	Intraocular penetration.	Alternate dose: 25–50 mg IM.
Streptomycin	IM	20 mg/kg BID for 5 days	Discospondylitis due to Brucella canis.	
Streptozotocin (Zanosar)	IV		Antineoplastic activity against pancreatic islet cells in insulinoma.	Highly nephrotoxic in dogs. Not recommended for clinical use.
Sucralfate (Carafate)	PO	500 mg TID (<18 kg), 1 g TID (>18 kg)	Gastrointestinal protectant to prevent ulceration, e.g., septic shock, mastocytoma, Zollinger-Ellison syndrome.	Interferes with absorption of cimetidine. Constipation, interferes with drug absorption from GI tract. Give cimetidine 45 min before or 2 hr after sucralfate.
Sulfadiazine (Suladyne) (Tribrissen)	PO	90–120 mg/kg BID	Bacteriostatic agent for toxoplasmosis, nocardiosis.	Keratoconjunctivitis sicca. Idiosyncratic reactions of sulfonamides. Trimethoprim added for broader spectrum and bactericidal activity. Other agents preferable for surgical infections.

Drug (Trade Name)	Route	Dose	Effects and Medications	Side Effects	Comments
Sulfadimethoxine (Albon) (Bactrovet)	PO	50 mg/kg, then 25 mg/kg/day after 1st day	Bacteriostatic agent for toxoplasmosis, nocardiosis, coccidiosis, discospondylitis.	Keratoconjunctivitis sicca, nephrotoxicity, hypersensitivity, idiosyncratic reactions of sulfonamides.	Rapid renal elimination.
Sulfamethizole (Proklar) (Thiosulfil)	PO	50 mg/kg QID	Bacteriostatic agent for urinary tract infections.	Idiosyncratic reactions of sulfonamides.	
Sulfasalazine (Azulfidine)	PO	22–55 mg/kg TID (dog), 10–20 mg/kg BID 3–5 days	Anti-inflammatory effect on colon. Ulcerative and idiopathic colitis.	Keratoconjunctivitis sicca. Do not use for more than 3–4 consecutive days. Blood dyscrasias, vomiting.	
Sulfisoxazole (Gantrisin)	PO	50 mg/kg QID	Bacteriostatic agent for urinary tract infections.	Idiosyncratic reactions of sulfonamides.	Rapid absorption and renal excretion.
Sutilains ointment (Travase)	Topical	Apply QID	Chemical burn débridement.		Use early while eschar is moist and pliable. Inactivated by antiseptics.
Tamoxifen citrate (Nolvadex)	PO	10–20 mg BID	Antiestrogen. Mammary adenocarcinomas with estrogen receptors.		
Taurine	PO	125–300 mg SID (cat)	Feline degenerative cardiomyopathy, central retinal degeneration.		

Drug	Route	Dose	Indication/Use	Notes
Testosterone cypionate (*Depo-testosterone*)	IM	200 mg/mo	Testosterone-responsive urinary incontinence.	None in dogs.
Tetracyclines	PO	25 mg/wk (small dog)	Eliminates color from tear staining.	Substitutes for pigment porphyrins.
Tetracyclines	PO	20 mg/kg TID for 3 wk	Discospondylitis due to *Brucella canis*.	Streptomycin used for the first 5 days with this treatment at 20 mg/kg BID IM. Tetracycline is used for 3 wk, then streptomycin is repeated for 5 days.
Tetracyclines	PO	10–22 mg/kg TID for 3 wk	Broad-spectrum bacteriostatic antibiotic. Useful for *Brucella, Chlamydia, Mycoplasma, Rickettsia*. Also for pleurodesis, urinary tract infections, tooth root surface decalcification.	Mild GI disturbances in cats, discoloration of erupting teeth, nephrotoxicity. Pleurodesis: 20 mg/kg in 4 ml saline/kg. Do not administer in last third of pregnancy or with antacids, dairy products, or intestinal adsorbents.
Theophylline	PO	6–11 mg/kg TID	Bronchodilator.	
Thiamylal sodium (*Surital*) (*Biotal*)	IV	4–8 mg/kg	Ultra-short-acting barbiturate, general anesthetic.	Restlessness, vomiting.
Thiopental (*Pentothal*)	IV	5–10 mg/kg	Ultra-short-acting barbiturate, general anesthetic.	
Thyroxine (levothyroxine) (*Soloxine*)	PO	0.02–0.04 mg/kg/day	Replacement after hypophysectomy. Treatment of hypothyroidism.	

831

Drug (Trade Name)	Route	Dose	Effects and Medications	Side Effects	Comments
Thyroxine (levothyroxine) (Soloxine) (Synthroid)	PO	0.1 mg/5 kg BID (dog), 0.05–0.1 mg SID (cat)	von Willebrand's disease. Increases platelet adhesiveness. von Willebrand's factor: Ag concentration. Corrects bleeding times.	Thyrotoxicosis.	
Tiletamine/zolazepam (Telazol)	IV	0.5–3 mg/kg	Dissociative anesthetic.		Zolazepam can be reversed with flumazenil
Timolol (Timoptic) (Apotimolol)	Eye drop	0.5% BID	Beta blocking agent for glaucoma.		Small-pressure reductions only. Will not control glaucoma alone.
Tobramycin (Nebcin)	Subconj. inj.	20–40 mg	Intraocular penetration, endophthalmitis, ulcerative keratitis. Broad spectrum.		
Tobramycin	IM, IV, SC	2 mg/kg TID	Broad-spectrum aminoglycoside antibiotic.	May cause respiratory arrest. Nephrotoxicity, predisposed by fever and dehydration. Synergistic nephrotoxicity with furosemide and flunixin. Vestibular ototoxicity in cats.	Not useful for anaerobic infections.
Tolazoline (Priscoline)	IM	3–5 mg/kg	Antagonizes alpha-2 agonists: xylazine, medetomidine.	Hypotension, tachycardia, abdominal pain, nausea.	

Drug	Route	Dose	Indications / Description	Side Effects / Comments
Tranexamic acid (*Vasolamin*)	PO, IV	25 mg/kg, 10 mg q6h maintenance	Hematuria after nephrotomy. Inhibits urokinase, which activates plasminogen and fibrinolysin (plasmin).	Less toxic than aminocaproic acid.
Triamcinolone (*Kenalog*) (*Vetalog*)	Retro-orbital inj.	10–20 mg	Reduction of orbital inflammation, swelling.	Corticosteroid effects.
Triamcinolone (*Kenalog*) (*Vetalog*)	PO, SC, IM	0.1–0.22 mg/kg, 1 mg/cm² of tumor q14days	Intermediate-acting corticosteroid. Tracheal stenosis. Mastocytoma.	Hyperadrenocorticism, polyuria, polydipsia, adrenal suppression.
Triiodothyronine (*Cytobin*)	PO	406 µg/kg TID	For hypothyroidism when unable to convert T4 to T3.	Thyrotoxicosis, polyuria, polydipsia, nervousness, panting, tachycardia.
Trimethaphan (*Arfonad*)	IV	0.4–4.0 µg/kg/min	Vasodilator, direct arteriolar smooth muscle relaxant, postsynaptic ganglion blocking agent.	Parasympatholytic effects, releases histamine.
Trimethoprim/sulfadiazine (*Tribrissen*) (*Ditrim*)	PO, SC, IM	15 mg/kg BID	Broad-spectrum bactericidal agent, plus *Toxoplasma*, *Nocardia*, and *Pneumocystis* spp.	Idiosyncratic reactions: fever, lymphadenopathy, cutaneous eruptions, hepatitis, focal retinitis, anemia, leukopenia, thrombocytopenia, glomerulonephritis.

Drug (Trade Name)	Route	Dose	Effects and Medications	Side Effects	Comments
Trimethoprim/ sulfamethoxazole (Bactrim) (Septra)	PO, SC, IM	15 mg/kg BID	Broad-spectrum bactericidal agent, plus Toxoplasma, Nocardia, and Pneumocystis spp.	Idiosyncratic reactions; fever, lymphadenopathy, cutaneous eruptions, hepatitis, focal retinitis, anemia, leukopenia, thrombocytopenia, glomerulonephritis.	
Trypsin		0.5–1.5 ml per sinus	To dissolve mucus in the nasal sinuses, after surgery to assist drainage.		Dissolve 1 part trypsin powder in 2 parts sterile water.
Tylosin (Tylan)	PO, IV	5–10 mg/kg BID	Macrolide antibiotic used for colitis.	GI dose-related disorders. Pain and swelling at injection site.	
Valproic acid (Depakene)	PO	60–220 mg/kg TID (dog)	Control of seizures.	GI side effects. Hepatotoxicity with chronic use.	Not agent of first choice.
Vancomycin (Vancocin)	IV	15 mg/kg BID	Antibiotic, gram-positive bacteria, especially Staphylococcus. Synergistic with gentamicin and tobramycin.	Deafness, skin reactions, fever, anaphylaxis, thrombophlebitis at injection site.	
Vasopressin (Pitressin)	IM	0.2 IU/kg	Used for replacement after hypophysectomy for 1–2 wk. Diagnosis of central or neurogenic diabetes insipidus.	Pain at injection site.	Do not inject oil suspension IV.

Drug	Route	Dose	Use	Comments
Vecuronium	IV	10–20 µg/kg (dog), 20–40 µg/kg (cat)	Nondepolarizing neuromuscular block. Duration: 20–40 min (dog), 10–15 min (cat).	Reversal agents: neostigmine, pyridostigmine edrophonium.
Verapamil (*Calan*) (*Isoptin*)	PO	1.0–4.4 mg/kg BID-TID	Calcium channel blocker for supraventricular tachyarrhythmias. Also used to reverse multidrug resistance in chemotherapy.	Not used with beta blockers.
Vinblastine (*Velban*)	IV	2 mg/m²/wk	Plant alkaloid. Lymphosarcoma, various carcinomas.	Leukopenia, nausea, vomiting.
Vincristine (*Oncovin*)	IV	0.5 mg/m²/wk	Plant alkaloid. Transmissible venereal tumor, lymphosarcoma, immune-mediated thrombocytopenia.	Peripheral neuropathy, paresthesia, constipation.
Vitamin D	PO	10–20 IU/kg/day, 500 IU/kg food/day	Used in rickets in immature animals and osteomalacia in adults, after parathyroidectomy.	Hypervitaminosis D with elevated calcium, phosphate levels.
Vitamin K_1 (*Aquamephyton*) (*Mephyton*)	PO, SC	Load 2.5–3.3 mg/kg multiple sites SC, 1.1–3.3 mg/kg BID PO	Warfarin, pindone, and indandione toxicity. Used to control prothrombin time to three times normal after warfarin use in vascular surgery.	Hematomas by IM, anaphylaxis by IV injection. Do not give IV.
Warfarin (*Coumadin*) (*Panwarfin*)	PO	1–2 mg/kg in two divided doses daily	Anticoagulant after vascular surgery.	Prolonged prothrombin time and clotting abnormalities. Monitor prothrombin time; control with vitamin K, to less than three times normal.

Drug (Trade Name)	Route	Dose	Effects and Medications	Side Effects	Comments
Xylazine (*Rompun*)	IM	0.5–1.1 mg/kg	Sedative, muscle relaxant, analgesic, alpha-2 agonist. Emetic in cats (IM). Postoperative hyperthermia.	Cardiac arrhythmias, hypotension, sensitization to halothane.	Note: reversal agent is yohimbine.
Xylazine/oxymorphone	IM	0.5 mg/kg, 0.05–0.1 mg/kg	Sedative, analgesic, neuroleptanalgesic.		
Yohimbine (*Yobine*)	IV	0.2 mg/kg	Antagonizes alpha-2 agonists such as xylazine.	Excitement.	

CNS, central nervous system; GI, gastrointestinal; CBC, complete blood count; CPR, cardiopulmonary resuscitation; HMW, high-molecular weight; ICU, intensive care unit.

Cross Index by Trade Name of Drugs Listed in Appendix I

Trade Name	Generic Name
2-PAM	Pralidoxime chloride
Acepromazine	Acepromazine
Adrenaline	Epinephrine
Adriamycin	Doxorubicin
Albon	Sulfadimethoxine
Aldactone	Spironolactone
Aldoril	Hydrochlorothiazide
Alkeran	Melphalan
Amethopterin	Methotrexate
Amicar	Aminocaproic acid
Amidate	Etomidate
Amiglyde-V	Amikacin
Amikin	Amikacin
Amoxi-drops	Amoxicillin
Amoxi-tabs	Amoxicillin
Amoxil	Amoxicillin
Ancobon	Flucytosine
Ancotil	Flucytosine
Antirobe	Clindamycin
Apotimolol	Timolol
Apresoline	Hydralazine
Aquamephyton	Vitamin K_1
Aramine	Metaraminol
Arfonad	Trimethaphan
Ascriptin	Acetylsalicylic acid
Aspirin	Acetylsalicylic acid
Atarax	Hydroxyzine
Augmentin	Amoxicillin clavulanic acid
Azium	Dexamethasone
Azulfidine	Sulfasalazine
Bactrim	Trimethoprim/sulfamethoxazole
Bactrovet	Sulfadimethoxine
Banamine	Flunixin meglumine
Baytril	Enrofloxacin
Benadryl	Diphenhydramine
Betagan	Levobunolol

Trade Name	Generic Name
Betasone	Betamethasone
Betoptic	Betaxolol
BICNU	Carmustine
Biotal	Thiamylal sodium
Blenoxane	Bleomycin
Bretylol	Bretylium tosylate
Brevital sodium	Methohexital
Bronkosol	Isoetharine
Buprenex	Buprenorphine
Butazolidin	Phenylbutazone
Calan	Verapamil
Calcet	Calcium gluconate 10%
Capoten	Captopril
Carafate	Sucralfate
CEENU	Lomustine
Centrine	Aminopentamide
Chibroxin	Norfloxacin
Chloromycetin	Chloramphenicol
Chlor-Trimeton	Chlorpheniramine
Choledyl	Oxtriphylline
Cipro	Ciprofloxacin
Clavamox	Amoxicillin/clavulanic acid
Cleocin	Clindamycin
Colace	Docusate sodium
Colchicine	Colchicine
Colymycin S	Colistin (polymixin E)
Compazine	Prochlorperazine
Coscopin	Noscapine
Cosmegen	Actinomycin D
Cosmegen	Dactinomycin—see actinomycin D
Coumadin	Warfarin
Cuprimine	*d*-Penicillamine
Cytobin	Triiodothyronine
Cytosar	Cytosine arabinoside, cytarabine
Cytosar	Cytosine arabinoside
Cytosar-U	Cytosine arabinoside, cytarabine
Cytotec	Misoprostol
Cytoxan	Cyclophosphamide
Dantefur	Nitrofurantoin
Dantrium	Dantrolene sodium
Daranide	Dichlorphenamide
DDAVP	Desmopressin acetate
Decadron	Dexamethasone

Trade Name	Generic Name
Deca-Durabolin	Nandrolone acetate
Decholin	Dehydrocholic acid
Demerol	Meperidine (pethidine)
Depakene	Valproic acid
DepoMedrol	Methylprednisolone
Depo-provera	Medroxyprogesterone
Depo-testosterone	Testosterone cypionate
Dexatrim	Phenylpropanolamine
DHT	Dihydrotachysterol
Diamox	Acetazolamide
Dibenzyline	Phenoxybenzamine
Dilantin	Phenytoin
Diprivan	Propofol
Ditrim	Trimethoprim/sulfadiazine
Ditropan	Oxybutynin
Diuril	Chlorothiazide
Dobutrex	Dobutamine
Dolophine hydrochloride	Methadone
Dopram	Doxopram
Doxinate	Docusate sodium
DTIC	Dacarbazine
ECP	Estradiol cypionate
Efudex Cream	Fluorouracil (5-FU)
Elspar	Asparaginase
Ephedrine sulfate	Ephedrine
Epogen	Epoetin
Erythrocin	Erythromycin
Flagyl	Metronidazole
Florinef	Fludrocortisone
Flucort	Flumethasone
Fluorouracil	Fluorouracil (5-FU)
Folex	Methotrexate
Fungizone	Amphotericin B
Gantrisin	Sulfisoxazole
Geopen	Carbenicillin
Hyaluron	Sodium hyaluronate
Hydrodiuril	Hydrochlorothiazide
Hytakerol	Dihydrotachysterol
Ilotycin	Erythromycin
Imuran	Azathioprine

Trade Name	Generic Name
Inderal	Propranolol
Indocin	Indomethacin
Innovar	Droperidol
Innovar Vet	Fentanyl/droperidol
Innovar-Vet	Droperidol
Inocor	Amrinone
Inotropin	Dopamine HCl
Isoptin	Verapamil
Jenotone	Aminopropazine
Kenalog	Triamcinolone
Ketaset	Ketamine
Lasix	Furosemide
Leukeran	Chlorambucil
Levophed bitartrate	Norepinephrine
Lincocin	Lincomycin
Lopid	Gemfibrozil
Lutalyse	Prostaglandin F_{2alpha}
Lysodren	o,p'-DDD
Macrodantin	Nitrofurantoin
Mandelamine	Methenamine mandelate
Marcaine	Bupivicaine
Maxidex	Dexamethasone
Mephyton	Vitamin K_1
Mestinon	Pyridostigmine bromide
Methigel	*dl*-Methionine
Mexate	Methotrexate
Minipress	Prazosin hydrochloride
MPG	*N*-(2-Mercaptopropionyl)-glycine
Mucomyst	Acetylcysteine
Mustargen	Nitrogen mustard
Myochrysine	Sodium thiomalate
Narcan	Naloxone
Nebcin	Tobramycin
Nembutal	Pentobarbital
Neosynephrine	Phenylephrine
Neptazane	Methazolamide
Nilevar	Norethandrolone
Nipride	Nitroprusside
Nitro ointment	Nitroglycerin

Trade Name	Generic Name
Nolvadex	Tamoxifen citrate
Noroxin	Norfloxacin
Nubain	Nalbuphine
Numorphan	Oxymorphone
Ocufen	Flurbiprofen
Oncovin	Vincristine
Ornade	Phenylpropanolamine
Ovaban	Megestrol acetate
Panwarfin	Warfarin
Pentothal	Thiopental
Percorten	Desoxycorticosterone acetate
Periactin	Cyproheptadine
Persantine	Dipyramidole
Pitocin	Oxytocin
Pitressin	Vasopressin
Platinol	Cisplatin
Priscoline	Tolazoline
Pro-Banthine	Propantheline
Proglycem	Diazoxide
Proklar	Sulfamethizole
Pronestyl	Procainamide
Propagest	Phenylpropanolamine
Prostigmin	Neostigmine
Protopam chloride	Pralidoxime chloride
PTU	Propylthiouracil
Purinethol	Mercaptopurine (6-mercaptopurine)
Regitine	Phentolamine mesylate
Reglan	Metoclopramide
Ridaura	Auranofin
Robamox-V	Amoxicillin
Robaxin	Methocarbamol
Robinul V	Glycopyrrolate
Rompun	Xylazine
Sandimmune	Cyclosporine
Septra	Trimethoprim/sulfamethoxazole
Serax	Oxazepam
Silvadene	Silver sulfadiazine
SM 201-995	Somatostatin (analogue SM 201-995)
Solganal	Auriothioglucose
Soloxine	Thyroxine (levothyroxine)
Solu-Delta-Cortef	Prednisolone sodium succinate

Trade Name	Generic Name
Stiglin	Neostigmine
Stilbestrol	Diethylstilbestrol
Suladyne	Sulfadiazine
Sulfamylon	Mafenide acetate
Surfak	Docusate sodium
Surital	Thiamylal sodium
Synthroid	Thyroxine (levothyroxine)
Tagamet	Cimetidine
Talwin V	Pentazocine
Tapazole	Methimazole
Telazol	Tiletamine/zolazepam
Tenormin	Atenolol
Tensilon	Edrophonium
Terramycin	Oxytetracycline—see tetracyclines
Thiosulfil	Sulfamethizole
Thorazine	Chlorpromazine
Timoptic	Timolol
Tofranil	Imipramine pamoate
Torbugesic	Butorphanol
Torbutrol	Butorphanol
Tracrium	Atracurium
Travase	Sutilains ointment
Tribrissen	Trimethoprim/sulfadiazine
Tribissen	Sulfadiazine
Tylan	Tylosin
Tylenol	Acetaminophen
Urecholine	Bethanecol
Urispas	Flavoxate
Urocit-K	Potassium citrate
Valium	Diazepam
Vancocin	Vancomycin
Vasolamin	Tranexamic acid
Vasotec	Enalapril
Vasoxyl	Methoxamine
Velban	Vinblastine
Velosef	Cephradine—see cephalosporins
Versed/Torbutrol	Midazolam/butorphanol
Versenate	EDTA-Ca
Veta K_1	Vitamin K_1
Vetalog	Triamcinolone

Trade Name	Generic Name
Vetamox	Acetazolamide
Vetinol	Noscapine
Vibramycin	Doxycycline
Winstrol	Stanozolol
Wyamine	Mephentermine
Xylocaine	Lidocaine
Yobine	Yohimbine
Zanosar	Streptozotocin
Zantac	Ranitidine
Zyloprim	Allopurinol

INDEX

Note: Page numbers in *italics* indicate illustrations; those followed by t refer to tables.

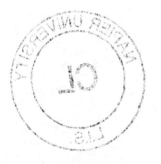

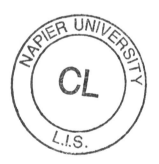